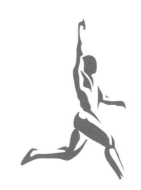

GAME

THE ART OF SPORTS SCIENCE

CHANGER

DR. FERGUS CONNOLLY
with PHIL WHITE

foreword by Jim Harbaugh

First Published in 2017 by Victory Belt Publishing Inc.

ISBN-13: 978-1-628601-18-3

The information included in this book is for educational purposes only. It is not intended or implied to be a substitute for professional medical advice. The reader should always consult his or her health-care provider to determine the appropriateness of the information for his or her own situation or if he or she has any questions regarding a medical condition or treatment plan. Reading the information in this book does not create a physician-patient relationship.

Cover design by Brett Chalmers
Book design by Justin-Aaron Velasco
Illustrations by Charisse Reyes & Justin-Aaron Velasco

Printed in Canada
TC 0117

CONTENTS

FOREWORD

I love the game of football.

Each morning I bound out of bed with excitement to get to work. The start of the season is like Christmas morning. This is a wonderful sport. It has everything: stamina, speed, skill, strain, and excitement.

To me, playing this game is the finest measure of a man. He is tested and tried in competition. The only thing that comes close to the ups and downs, the struggles and the triumphs of playing, is coaching.

There are few things as wonderful as coaching football. Each day we mold young men through physical and mental challenges. We pit player against player, forge iron with iron, steel with steel and toughen ourselves in the white heat of play. We suffer and strive to produce moments of magic that keep hundreds of thousands in awe each weekend.

Who's got it better than us?

I'm honored to write this foreword for Fergus. Anything that helps us as coaches helps the young people of this country, and this book can do just that. We have a privileged role and position and need to always be open to learning from experts, professionals and pioneers from all walks of life—whether that's sports, the military, business, technology, science, or any other discipline—who can help us reach our common goal: to win. To be part of a team that's striving to achieve a shared goal is the ultimate challenge, and one that Fergus and I have devoted our careers and lives to.

"The Team. The Team. The Team." As long as I can remember, those words have been ringing in my ears, whether on the practice field or at the breakfast table. Growing up as the son of a coach, I shared in all his experiences and listened to all his stories about coaching with and for greats of the game. When I was around the age of seven, my father took a job at the University of Michigan under the legendary Bo Schembechler, and that exposed me to a whole new world of excitement and learning. And that's how my childhood was, in a family where the currency was love and competition, most of it shared through the game of football.

From an early age, I knew I wanted to be a coach. This wasn't just a matter of wanting to continue my father's legacy or because my brother, John, followed him into the profession. It was also due to the profound influence of the coaches who've inspired me throughout my life. Growing up, the local Washtenaw County sheriff, Tom Minick, was another example of a man who taught us life lessons through football. Since then I've learned from many other great coaches and people, like my brother-in-law Tom Crean, Al Davis, Bo Schembechler, and, of course, my father, Jack Harbaugh. Coaches, like teachers and preachers, have the rare and special opportunity to positively impact youth in ways that go beyond the confines of the sports field.

While I love football first and foremost, all team sports can play a powerful role in forging young people. I continue to learn from sports like baseball, soccer, basketball, and many others. To me there is no finer measure of a man or woman than what they go through on the practice field and how they put what they've learned into action in the arena on game day. It's the embodiment of total commitment to a single goal.

People often ask me how coaching has changed. Our understanding of football has certainly progressed over the past few years, and we know more now about performance, training, nutrition, and so many other areas. After reading this book, you will too. But the goals of coaching and the nature of the people who play the game remain the same. So we need to keep learning, improving, and striving.

As a coach, my commitment goes beyond what happens on the field. I have a duty to each and every player as a person whose growth and development have been entrusted to me and my staff. That's one of the reasons that Fergus's model is so important: it puts the health of the player at the core of everything we do. The athlete is a person first and a player second. Another thing that's different about this book is its holistic look at the qualities that manifest themselves in practice and game play. All too often we only focus on strength, speed, power, and other physical factors. While these are obviously important, we must also give greater consideration to the technical, tactical, and psychological elements of the game, which you're going to learn more about in the following pages.

My father's phrase "Attack this day with an enthusiasm unknown to mankind" has been used often, though few know the second part of it: "and don't take any wooden nickels." This means that you shouldn't take any nonsense, listen to any foolishness, or let anyone take advantage of you. I implore you to approach this book with the same mindset, in the knowledge that there's a wealth of quality information here that will enrich you, challenge what you think you know, and, ultimately, make you a better, more engaged coach, player, or fan.

It's an incredible honor to coach this game, to work with dedicated professionals like Fergus and our coaching staff, and to see the growth of young people on and off the field every day. I hope you enjoy your journey to becoming a Game Changer and that once you've finished this book, you're better equipped to win, no matter what your game is.

JIM HARBAUGH

INTRODUCTION

Is anything as culturally pervasive as team sports?

In the United States, the NFL effectively owns Sunday—not to mention Monday night and now Thursday night, too.

During college football season, several million people spend their Saturdays in packed stadiums across the country, and in certain states, entire communities turn out under the Friday night lights to cheer on their high school football teams.

Meanwhile, college basketball dominates the entire month of March as Americans wager, watch, and, dare I say, stop working as favorites are upset, underdogs triumph, and a new national champion is crowned.

And just when it seemed that the NBA would never reclaim the glory days of Michael, Magic, and Larry, along came a new breed of superstars like LeBron James, Steph Curry, and Kevin Durant to bring pro basketball to an even greater domestic and international audience.

Across the Atlantic, people are just as fanatical about team sports, if not more so. The 2015 Rugby World Cup brought 460,000 fans from around the globe to Britain and saw a global audience of 120 million tune in for the final. In countries like Australia, South Africa, and New Zealand, the sport is even more popular, with every kid dreaming of one day pulling on a Wallabies, Springboks, or All Blacks jersey. And the Australian Football League has an equally fanatical following Down Under.

Then there is the globe's biggest game: soccer. More than a billion people watched the 2014 World Cup final, while there are 245 million registered participants in the game worldwide. The British often joke that their countrymen talk about only three things: the weather, politics, and the Premier League—and there's a lot of truth to this cliché. If American football owns Sunday in the U.S., then the "other kind of football" dominates Saturday in Britain, across Europe, and far beyond. When you look at countries like Brazil and Argentina, the sport is practically a religion.

Even in the U.S., which for so long was wary of this low-scoring, free-flowing game, soccer is booming, with more than three million kids turning out to play each week, a women's national team that has won two World Cups, and an increasingly competitive major league.

Such popularity means that team sports are big business. Very big.

ESPN paid $5.6 billion to broadcast the college football playoffs for twelve years, with Turner Sports/CBS shelling out $10.4 billion to show the national basketball tournament through 2024. The pros haven't exactly fallen on hard times, either. The most recent NBA TV deal came in at a cool $26.4 billion, while the NFL TV deal is worth $3.1 billion a year. And this is just TV revenue—there's also merchandise, ticket sales, and other commercial interests to consider.

As a result of this cash influx, spending has increased dramatically at the organizational level. Sixteen college athletics programs racked up more than $100 million in annual expenses in 2015. But that's child's play compared to the outgoings at the world's most valuable soccer team, Manchester United, which spent more than $500 million that same year.

The trouble is that all this spending often fails to yield better results. Teams in all sports have tried just about every gimmick to hack their way to better performance. But as they've gotten stuck in stats, mired in backroom politics, and diverted by the facilities arms race, many have lost sight of what should've been their primary focus all along: the game itself. Through my experiences with teams all around the world—in the NFL, college football, English Premiership soccer, the NBA, international rugby, and Australian rules football—as well as with elite military units, I've discovered that while there are obvious differences between these disciplines, there are also many commonalities. By breaking down these universal principles to their basic, elemental components, this book shows you how to better analyze each moment of any game, whether you play, coach, or watch.

And when you can break a game down into its basic elements, you can create valuable learning experiences in training, better evaluate the quality of your team's performance, and home in on what's working and what isn't. This book is essentially about how teams win games.

Another area of team sports that this book transforms is athlete and team preparation. Until now, coaches largely have focused on developing players' physical qualities. I propose turning that model on its head and show how athletes can advance technically, tactically, and psychologically at the same time. My approach not only helps players to continually progress but also stops treating them like disposable commodities, instead prioritizing athlete health and tapping into the technical and tactical value they have accumulated.

In addition, the coming pages explain specifically how to prepare a team for its next win by working backward from the game and revolutionizing how successful coaches and sports organizations operate, with a focus on players' game performances.

Bringing together the latest evidence-based practices and lessons from business, psychology, biology, and many other fields, this book is the first of its kind, helping coaches, athletes, and fans:

- Better understand what is *really* happening in team-sports games

- Build an analysis system based on what really happens in games

- Create a cohesive game plan that improves performance through aligned objectives, strategy, and tactics

- Put statistical analysis and technology into context, so that teams can bypass the hype and get meaningful results

- Improve their evaluation of a team and its opponents

- Identify players' dominant qualities to maximize during training and limiting factors to improve

- Create realistic, immersive learning experiences for individual players and the entire team that deliver defined outcomes

- Structure player development with a new, holistic model that puts athlete health first, reduces the risk of injury, and keeps players in the game longer

- Balance training load so that all squad members are fresh and ready to play at their best in competition

- Identify the root of common problems with athletes and teams and implement strategies to solve them

- Rethink coaching and organizational leadership and apply effective principles to enhance communication, group dynamics, and player interaction

- Create a sustainable-winning culture using best practices from business, technology, and the military

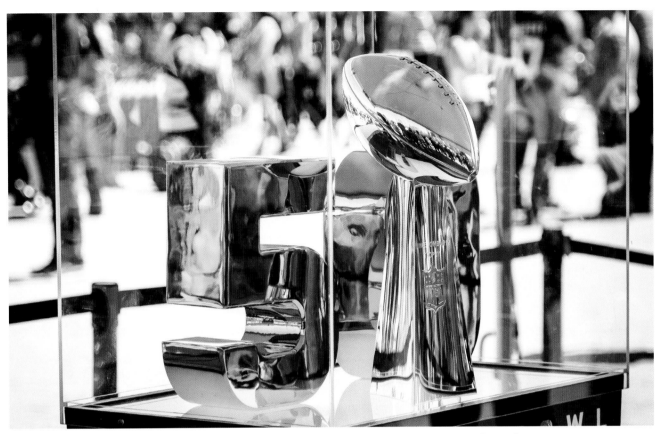

The Vince Lombardi Trophy, one of sport's most prestigious awards. Photo by Mobilus In Mobili (CC BY).

HOW TO USE THIS BOOK

Though this book is very detailed, it presents a simplified version of what goes on in team sports. It presents the *basis* of all team sports. As such, it's impossible to be completely accurate for every minor incident in a certain sport—but its principles are accurate. Think of an architect's rendering of a building: it represents what the building looks like, but it isn't the building itself. Even a three-dimensional model cannot show every detail.

It's the same with this book and the laws and principles it contains. What I do is provide a greater level of insight into the elements of team sports, but as this world and the athletes and coaches within it are infinite in their complexity, it's impossible to present them with 100 percent accuracy. Think of what you're holding in your hands as a guide, but not one that is free from error or foolproof.

I've arranged this book in a way that follows a logical progression. Because one of the central concepts is to work backward from the game itself, that section comes first. You need to understand what you're truly looking at when you watch a team play before you start thinking about how players can be better prepared to excel or how the way the coaching staff and organization as a whole function can be enhanced. So I'll introduce you to some fundamental principles of play that are common across all team sports and explain how each manifests itself during games. You might not expect to find chaos and systems theory in a book like this, but that's just what you'll encounter in "The Game," along with a new way to apply mathematical and scientific concepts like fractals, amplification, and turbulence to preparing for and playing team-sports games. Plus, I'll show you how we can break down every contest in macro and micro moments so that we can better identify what's working, what isn't, and what to focus on with individual players, units, and the entire team before the next time they take the field, pitch, or court. In addition,

I'll lead you through various conflict styles and show how these and concepts like *schwerpunkt*, surfaces and gaps, and the fog of war are just as applicable to sports teams as they are to the military.

After "The Game" comes "The Player." That's because the most valuable asset of any team (whether it's in sports, the military, or business) is its people. For too long, player health has been an afterthought, but as you'll soon see, it's the key to creating sustainable-winning organizations and people who have a good quality of life during and after their career. In this section, we'll also explore the impact of DNA, heredity, and epigenetics as part of a long-overdue reexamination of the nature-versus-nurture debate. You'll also find a different take on tribal and group behavior, a holistic view of how various bodily systems interact, and how best to manipulate players' dominant qualities and limiting factors to produce continual progression. I'll also reexamine the stats-obsessed narrative that has been framing team-sports analysis since the publication of Michael Lewis's *Moneyball* and explain why we must have a qualitative lens if quantitative assessments are to positively affect the scoreboard. After reading this section, you'll also see why we need to move past the present fixation on solving all performance issues by enhancing physical characteristics.

Next up is "The Preparation." On the wall where I work, in the building named after him, is a giant quote from legendary University of Michigan football coach Bo Schembechler that reads, "The team, the team, the team." While all players need to feel valued and should be developed to their fullest potential as athletes and people, and their overall well-being should be protected, they also must be willing to buy in totally to the higher ideals of the team and its objectives. In this section, we'll also look into how best to prepare a team to perform on game day, how to structure balanced training plans that avoid common pitfalls, and how to best harness the principles of stimulus and adaptation. I'll also slay some sacred cows, including the faulty implementation of periodization, trying to separate training and recovery, and attempting to reduce performance to isolated elements. Plus, you'll learn the importance of developing technical, tactical, physical, and psychological

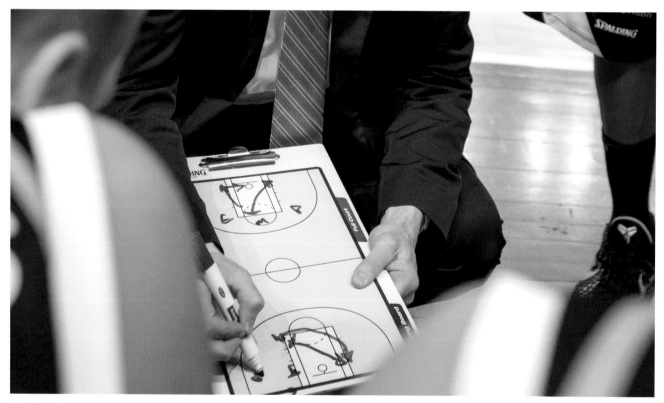

The planning is more important than the plan. Photo by Pavel Shchegolev / Shutterstock.com.

coactives concurrently in rich learning experiences that produce outcomes directly applicable to the next game.

The fourth and final section is "The Coach." In sports, business, and the military, we often overlook the significance of strong and capable leaders and the impact they have on their teams. It's often not until they leave that we truly appreciate great leadership—see Manchester United's poor results after iconic manager Sir Alex Ferguson retired, Apple's floundering after Steve Jobs left in the 1980s, and the U.S. Army's struggle to fill the void left after General Patton was relieved of his command. In this section we'll explore what makes a great head coach and how they can better manage their players in an age of 24/7 media scrutiny, unrealistic expectations, and superstar players. You'll learn how the best coaches build a culture on solid core values that lead to winning habits and behaviors, not just in the locker room or on the sideline but also in every position and at every level. On the flip side, we'll also dive into how to preempt the kind of issues that sink all too many teams when possible and handle problems when they do arise. I'll also share what I've learned about the importance of communication, functional ergonomics, and how to get the most out of a small back-office staff. In addition, we'll take a close look at innovation, see how data without context is meaningless, and cover how to use the latest technology to ask better questions, not as a be-all and end-all solution.

In an ideal world, you'd read this book from cover to cover. That said, I know what I usually do when I get a new book: I go straight to the section that will interest and benefit me the most. So if you're an athlete, you'll likely make a beeline for "The Player," and if you're a coach, "The Preparation" or "The Coach" might be your first destination.

There's nothing wrong with that. But if you do jump ahead, I implore you to go back and read the other sections closely later. Just as the systems in this training philosophy are interrelated (which you'll learn more about throughout the book), so too are the sections of this book and the principles you'll find in each section. If you read just a quarter of the text, you'll get only a small portion of the benefits to the holistic approach that I present.

PART ONE

THE GAME

The silence and loneliness of a Super Bowl quarterback is a beautiful paradox. It's the quiet at the eye of the greatest storm in the world.

One hundred sixty million eyes are watching him, but Tom Brady doesn't seem to notice. Or if he does, it certainly doesn't show. Thousands of flashing lights, screams, cheers, insults: it's just white noise.

This "white noise" is what the military refers to as the "fog of war." But for Brady, his depth of experience means that this fog isn't as thick as it was when he was a rookie. He is fully in "ignore the noise" mode, a favorite mantra of his head coach, Bill Belichick.[1]

He's been here many times. He's seen it all before.

Brady allows himself to fall into something of a natural trance. His nervous system relaxes to a state of calm alertness and begins to prioritize functions. This is his autopilot mode, which enables him to block out all distractions and focus on the most critical information.

Brady jogs onto the field, buckling his chinstrap, as he's done thousands of times before. He automatically shouts a word of encouragement to his left offensive tackle, who happens to be walking out on his right-hand side. On the last play, this teammate struggled a little to keep his feet steady. Brady knows that upon hearing his quarterback's support, his comrade will get a psychological lift.

Turning around, Brady slaps the running back on the backside as he jogs past and shouts more words of encouragement. During this short trot out to the huddle, he is thinking of his teammates and their energy. He knows, without consciously focus-

ing on it, that this is the time when his offensive unit reacts to—and feeds on—his energy and leadership.

He gives them a lift by calling out to them. What he says is largely irrelevant—it's his facial expressions, the positive sounds, and the contagious enthusiasm that will elevate their mood and performance levels.

The offensive linemen have been grinding hard for three quarters, protecting Brady and giving him the space he needs to pick off the opposition. They are carrying the piano; he's playing it. And today, the music has been beautiful. But Brady knows that winners drive home success. He's not letting anyone give anything less than 100 percent on his watch.

For a fraction of a second, as he approaches the huddle having cheered his teammates, he gets a sudden flashback of emotion. It's a reminder of how much he loves these moments. He tries to ignore its distraction but use the energy. His directions in the huddle are clear, concise, upbeat, and, most of all, businesslike. This team, his team, has a job to do.

The huddle breaks and Brady takes his position behind the center. Now that the offense has lined up, the opposing defense has reciprocated.

Brady looks up, glancing left and right. He doesn't see what you and I see—men, numbers, and personalities. He observes green turf, skills, and opportunities. He doesn't focus on one specific thing but rather scans, allowing his eyes to identify open spaces. He is looking with what some call his "quiet eye"— seeing the opposition's structure, the gaps created, and the personnel skillsets in front of him.

Brady recognizes but ignores a slight positional lineup error on his side: his receiver is a yard too wide. He chooses not to correct it. Instead, he's drawn to watching an unusual body lean by the outside linebacker. This veteran's experience and ability to close space quickly has been an issue for Brady and his team all game long, but he's making a mistake with this lean, which gives this most clinical of quarterbacks a hint as to his intentions.

Slowing his breathing, Brady does something simple. He looks up and motions for the tight end on his left to come inside a little more. It's an irrelevant move—complete misdirection on his part—but Brady wants to see if the deep safety is paying attention and reacts or moves, and if, as a result, the linebacker does. This reaction will give him enough information to know whom the defense is focusing on or prioritizing.

The safety doesn't move, but the linebacker takes a small step to his right. Few others notice, but Brady does. What he doesn't actually see but his brain subliminally perceives is that the safety glances sideways. Brady's brain is processing hundreds of minor movements and readjustments in milliseconds. Some he is conscious of, but many more he is not. His ability to stay on autopilot allows his brain to manage them.

The game restarts, and it's time for Brady to move—and move quickly. He barks out signals and the ball arrives from the center safely into his hands. Brady readjusts the ball's placement with ease, knowing where the stitching is as he steps back.

New England's five offensive linemen surround their star quarterback, each blocking a defender, forming a horseshoe shape and leaving Brady about a one-yard radius of turf in which to work. Brady is not going to flee the pocket, so edge rushers aren't a concern. He just needs enough time in the middle.

His feet send micropulses of neural feedback to his brain with each step backward. Some signals don't even make it all the way to his brain and instead go to the spinal cord as his feet readjust automatically. Other messages speed to the brain and tell his cerebellum, the part of the brain responsible for balance, how he's moving in three-dimensional space. Meanwhile, his eyes are still registering millions of pieces of information.

The linemen are by now struggling under the force of the pass rush. Pads crash and grind against pads, stitching tears, groans fill the air, and the smell of fresh sweat is everywhere. The powerful linemen are battering against the masses of strength and power trying to get to Brady.

But Brady doesn't see any of this. He's looking over them, although he knows they are there. While his eyes aren't focusing on them, his peripheral vision recognizes the space closing in on him fast. His football-specific spatial intelligence in the pocket is exemplary. The offensive line gives him the space to have time to look up in what seems like an explosion of colored jerseys.

As Brady expected, the opposing team's outside linebacker initiates a move to cover the tight end. Although he anticipated it, Brady is still a little surprised that the experienced Pro Bowler is falling for this deception so readily. So to gently encourage him to fully commit to his initial decision, Brady turns his shoulder to that side first, and the linebacker goes for the bait. The misdirection is complete.

The tight end was being covered already, but it doesn't matter. Brady knows that the only way to get the ball to any of his men is to create space, and the only way to do so is to move the defensive players toward each other.

There is a sliver of space in the center now. The safety is moving in that direction. The gap opening up in front of him perhaps panicked him a little. Brady knows the safety who's meant to be covering that gap is a rookie and thus is likely to take the bait faster and with less-subtle clues than an experienced veteran. He steps up so his offensive linemen can create more space.

At this stage, only Brady knows what he has planned. Even his coach can't anticipate what's going to happen. Brady is adjusting to a different move than the play initially called for. But he has a small problem: he needs time.

Brady hasn't shown his hand fully, but he's hoping that the receiver on his right—the one who was positioned slightly incorrectly on the line—will be the one to go deep and take the space the safety is exiting. It's a risky gamble, but if it works, it will pay off big-time.

The defensive back covering Brady's receiver is quick, but also slow. It seems paradoxical, but he's fast in short spaces and slower over longer distances. This is common in slightly older DBs. Brady and the receiver both know it. The man covering the run does, too, which is why he's getting ready to make up for his diminishing physical gifts with the technical and tactical know-how he has acquired over his career competing at football's highest level.

Since the defensive back can't watch Brady or the ball, he has to focus on the receiver. The roar of the crowd and the wide receiver's reaction usually tell him when the play is over. But on this down, there's been no such confirmation. This means the play is still on, and now he's having to run deep with the receiver. He realizes that he's in a pure and simple foot race against a very fast pass catcher.

Brady is still in the pocket, moving slightly, hips open, head on a swivel, feet registering millions of proprioceptive messages, big toe managing balance, brain processing millions of sounds, shadows, and shades that tell him exactly how much territory he has around him and how fast it's closing. It's a constantly changing movie of color and space. And space makes time. But the movement in front of him isn't constant; in fact, it's constantly changing speed, slow to fast and then back again. The movement of space is reactive. The defense watches the ball, basing all its movement on the orchestrator, Brady. All eyes are fixed on him.

Ball movement can be fast, such as in a quick handoff to a running back, or slow, as in this play. Brady is in the pocket, his brain processing more signals than we even know how to measure. The longer he can hold the ball, the more space the wide receivers, tight ends, and running backs crucial to the team's passing game can create and move into.

Meanwhile, the Patriots' TE is lined up to be hit by the linebacker in an expression of the incredible violence that NFL fans come to see every week. The safety also has taken the bait, moving to cover the space left by the linebacker. This cascade of movements has created space for Brady's receiver to cut into. The race with the cornerback is on.

But to all but the most experienced viewers who have played or coached football, it's still not clear what is happening. The world still doesn't see who Brady is going to target. Patriots fans are starting to feel fear because of this uncertainty. They also know that the longer Brady stands in the pocket with the ball, the greater the chance one of the opposing players can get to him.

Time in possession increases the probability of dispossession.

For all the pressure, however, Brady is the calmest man in the stadium. He's in that moment of peace, and the space is a sanctuary to him. He focuses on the receiver. His brain processes the speed of movement and the confidence of the run and the angle. He still isn't actually thinking but instead is focusing on where to put the ball so it's clearly in the path of the receiver. Brady's brain knows how fast he can throw, so the only complicating factor is the angle of the WR's run—slightly away from him this time, making it a little harder. A rookie quarterback might panic, but Brady has been here before. Many times. He judges the perspective and angle just right.

Brady steps back. This is purely for biomechanical leverage, as he's already in sufficient space. His brain has been processing foot placements since the snap, so the extra force he transmits to the ground registers as a placement to throw. His hips are open, his soleus and gastrocnemius pre-tension, and his Achilles tendons load for the final, decisive step. His left, gloved hand comes off the ball as he winds up, back arching and loading. His eyes and brain are focusing on the receiver's movement but still registering the closing space in the pocket. The left side of the line battle is closing in marginally faster than the right. But this doesn't matter, as Brady knows instinctively how much time he's got—not in milliseconds, but in emotion.

Now his brain switches completely over to processing throwing mechanics and action. Brady's windup is over, and he brings his arm, hand, and ball forward in one long, smooth arc. But it's not over; Brady is still capturing every movement of the receiver. He notices the DB closing in on his intended target, so even as the arc is in mid flow, he makes a tiny adjustment to push the ball more to the outside of the receiver. This minimal recalibration will amount to merely a two- or three-inch difference in the catching mechanics of Brady's target but will allow him to get his body in front of the defender.

Brady's final acts of microsecond brain processing involve a long, smooth follow-through that improves the accuracy of the flight and the application of optimal spin to offset the slight wind effect he perceives on the ball.

All this is done without a single sound. The ball leaves Brady's fingertips, spiraling its way toward either a reception, an incomplete pass, or an interception.

As the ball leaves Brady's fingers—some 2.3 seconds after the snap and just before the linebacker bursts through the middle to smash into him—he switches focus and readies his body for impact. Speed and changes in shade and shadow tell him that the left side of the O-line has collapsed. He knows he won't be able to get out of the way, so he relaxes a little to absorb the hit rather than try to match the 290 pounds of fire-breathing defensive end driving at him.

Meanwhile, thirty-two yards downfield, the Patriots' receiver has run smoothly into the path of the ball. Its flight was at an angle to allow him to see it, follow its path clearly, and reach out to gather it in safely just before he is pulled to the ground in the end zone.

Tom Brady doesn't see the catch, nor does he need to. The instant the ball left his fingertips, he knew it would be perfect. He's seen it many times before. Brady is on his back on the ground underneath a big, heaving, sweating mass of an opponent whose sole motivation was to bring him down as hard as possible. Brady hears the crowd reaction, and the cheering confirms what he already thought: his gamble worked, and his team has pulled ahead with minutes left on the clock. He mentally checks his body for any sign of pain or injury and, as the lineman begrudgingly rolls off him, he switches out of autopilot for the first time.

Brady's 2.3 seconds of chaos are over.

He smiles.

Unfortunately, much of the practice and training we see in team sports is based on misplaced understandings. The reality is perhaps not surprising: essentially, there is a universally poor (or, at best, misplaced) understanding of "the game" and what really happens in it.

Most training and practice tasks are performed simply because they have always been done that way, or because there is a misplaced belief that the only way to improve something is through repetition and more repetition. Yet to train players and teams to win more often, we must first know the game.

This section looks at the game from a new perspective and offers a completely new approach to assessing teams, players, and games. This approach then forms the basis for training players and teams in an entirely unique and effective way, as we'll explore in later sections.

The models, principles, and laws outlined in this section will allow you to apply methods developed over many years to improve athletes and teams in every major field and court sport.

ONE

WHAT'S REALLY HAPPENING

Before we look at how to prepare to win games, I want to introduce you to a language and system of understanding team-sports games. I've developed and adapted such a methodology in my game model, which provides a way to understand the dynamic systems on which all team-sports games are based.

CHAOS

1.1

Watch any team sport—whether it's Premier League soccer, the NFL, college football, or the NBA—and at first there appears to be no pattern to the plays. It all seems chaotic. Look longer and more thoughtfully, however, and you may think that you see patterns or repeated interactions of some sort…but you can't be sure. The aim of this section is to provide a method for really understanding the patterns of a game so that we can prepare and practice for it more effectively.

> *Possibly the model of the world as a great organization can help to reinforce the sense of reverence for the living which we have almost lost.*
>
> —Ludwig von Bertalanffy

We live in a chaotic world. Chaos appears in heart failure; in the rise, spread, and adaptation of viruses; in weather; in the stock market; in prey-predator relationships; and in the human immune system. No book has done more to explore and expose this reality than James Gleick's *Chaos: Making a New Science.* In this seminal work, Gleick noted the paradigmatic character of this new scientific development:

> Now that science is looking, chaos seems to be everywhere, chaos appears in the behavior of the weather, the behavior of an airplane in flight, the behavior of cars on an expressway, the behavior of oil flowing in underground pipes. No matter what the medium, the behavior obeys the same newly discovered laws. That realization has begun to change the way business executives make decisions about insurance, the way astronomers look at the solar system, the way political theorists talk about the stresses leading to armed conflict.[2]

Since sport is a subset of life, it too is chaotic. A game of football—or any other team sport, for that matter—is a confrontation between chaotic deterministic systems and fractal organization—in other words, between an unpredictable system and the way parts of it form patterns. The outcome of any game is determined by the nature of the confrontation between two complex systems (two teams) and is characterized by the alternation of successive states of order and disorder, stability and instability, uniformity and variety.[3]

A game of football—or any other team sport, for that matter—is a confrontation between chaotic deterministic systems and fractal organization.

Chaos theory is a way to look at and make sense of the nonlinear, unexpected, and unpredictable. While we're conditioned to believe that we live in a somewhat predictable world, this isn't true. Yes, phenomena like gravity, time, and electrical energy are, if complex, certainly regular and constant, and we're taught that such things can be understood and planned for. But anyone who has played, coached, or even closely watched team sports knows that such logic doesn't extend into this domain. So for some level of understanding of what happens when two teams play each other, we can turn to chaos theory.

At its heart, chaos theory models nonlinear phenomena. These are things that we cannot understand fully, that are composed of events that don't happen in a repeatable sequence, and that are impossible to control or predict. In many cases, nonlinear phenomena are things we have collected incredible volumes of data about. Examples include environmental phenomena, like the weather, and man-made phenomena, such as the stock market—and, of course, team-sports games.

CHAOS, FRACTALS, SYSTEMS THEORY, AND PRINCIPLES

1.2

Just like nature and weather, sport is a highly complex and chaotic environment, yet in a game, some actions appear to occur multiple times despite being unplanned. This complexity is often described and explained using a science referred to as "fractal mathematics." A fractal is a figure in which a close-up detail resembles the figure as a whole. For instance,

if you look closely at a tree branch, you'll see that it resembles almost exactly the tree itself. In many chaotic systems, there is a fractal aspect of complex, repeatable, chaotic behavior—it can be seen, for example, in snow, clouds, and streams. Fractal mathematics are highly applicable to sports, too.

Our social, biological, and economic systems are interconnected in a way that impacts what we see manifested as physical performance in sport. While it is impossible to accurately predict or control complex, intertwined chaotic ecosystems such as team-sports games, by applying chaos theory, we can at least begin to understand and evaluate them.

Chaos theory and fractals help us recognize how certain patterns and events in games are interconnected and appear to replicate themselves over and over again. They also help us understand the context of events and elements in the chaos of a game.

The greatest irony of chaos theory is that chaos may not exist, because it's a human construct! It is a concept we have created to help us explain random complexity that we cannot understand or control. There may be no real disorder or randomness in the universe—we simply observe it as such through our structured perspective. In reality, there's likely incredible order and patterning in the universe and games alike; we just don't have the capacity to fathom or substantiate it.

Chaos represents the uncontrolled and unexplainable. For now, anyway.

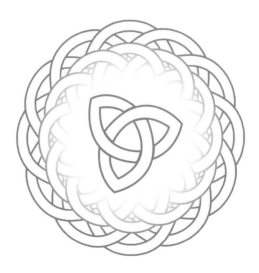

The concept of fractals is fundamental to all team sports.

THE MICRO PRINCIPLE OF DYNAMIC FEEDBACK   1.2.1

Games are inherently complex and can become incredibly chaotic in the presence of feedback, such as goals, tackles, passes, and other events. The moment a game kicks off between the team at the top of the league and the team at the bottom of the league, there begins a dynamic chaotic system. Should the bottom-ranked team score, the resulting feedback affects the context of the dynamic system. The same happens if the top team scores, but the feedback is different and changes the game in a different way. Heisenberg's uncertainty principle says, essentially, that there is a fundamental limit to how well you can simultaneously know the position and momentum of a particle. As you measure something, it is moving, so as you watch a game, the projected result is continually changing. Similar to Heisenberg's uncertainty principle, there's a fundamental limit to how well you can understand and play the game at the same time.

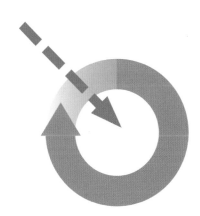

The game is constnatly subject to dynamic feedback.

We see this in events outside of sports, too, such as in the stock market. As the value of a certain stock rises or falls and the resulting feedback concerning the company's altered valuation goes into the system, the subsequent actions and reactions of people and algorithms influence buying and selling. This in turn affects the price of that stock and others in the market, creating a new context for more feedback and interactions and perpetually encouraging the chaos.

Even without observers, the action of the game itself supplies a dynamic feedback that affects the game. The best example of this is in how teams change their playing style when they take the lead in a game. Even though the players may not have changed and the situations are exactly the same— for instance, third down and goal in football—the players' mindsets are altered. The scoreboard affects how coaches and players make decisions, and it is constantly changing. Such dynamic feedback affects attitudes and decisions even though the key elements haven't changed.

Take a free kick in soccer, a conversion in rugby, or a free throw in basketball. This isolated action is essentially the same whether it occurs at the start of a game or at the end, but the scoreboard and game clock create the perception that it's completely different and has greater or less significance.

> **"**
>
> *Nothing in Nature is random....A thing appears random only through the incompleteness of our knowledge.*
>
> —Baruch Spinoza **"**

THE MICRO PRINCIPLE OF NONLINEAR AMPLIFICATION   1.2.2

Just as a major team-sports event like a goal can affect the outcome and contextual feedback, very small events can, in the end, lead to major consequences. For example, the child of a pro team's strength coach may pick up an illness at school and transmit the virus to the coach, who goes to work anyway—the end result is that a large portion of a team falls ill.

There is an amplification of consequence based on the environment in which the event occurs. This "butterfly effect" describes phenomena such as how a hurricane in China could be attributed to a butterfly flapping its wings in New Mexico. In stock market terms, a misunderstood comment in a crowd about exploratory mining in Africa might cause a sudden surge on Wall Street. The same effect is clearly seen in nuclear physics and many other fields. These amplified consequences may take a long time to develop, but the effect is real. There is always a consequence to any action and its reaction.

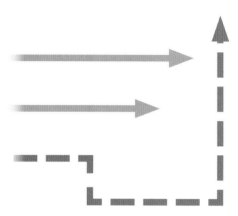

The context, timing, and event dictate the ultimate outcome of the game.

The butterfly metaphor is used to illustrate the importance of context and timing. *Context* means the initial conditions of the event, while *timing* underlines the importance of an event occurring at a particular spot in space-time. It also shows how any effect can amplify itself far beyond the initial force or action. In other words, the quantity of the initial action is inconsequential—the wind generated by the butterfly's flapping its wings is almost negligible, yet it can end up causing a hurricane.

So when we try to rate football or soccer players by the number of tackles or passes they've made, we're focusing on the wrong thing: we must consider the context, timing, and amplification of each tackle or pass. These have effects far beyond the actual tackle or pass itself.

THE MICRO PRINCIPLE OF TURBULENCE   1.2.3

In games, as in life, various interconnected and dependent chaotic systems affect each other: unpredictable times unpredictable. This means that two similar elements, hypothetically affected by the same conditions and occurring at the same moment in time and space, will have completely different paths and terminations due to the turbulence of the other. The second law of thermodynamics tells us that entropy always increases—and it does so in a way that is nonlinear.

Let's consider a football game in which one team loses a key linebacker to injury in the first play of the game. As a result, the team concedes a touchdown soon afterward. Either event, alone, can be overcome easily enough. But losing the fulcrum of the defense *and*, moments later, allowing a touchdown affects the game and the mindset of the team and its opponent in a completely different way.

Or consider a Tier 1 Special Operations assault team raiding a house or compound. Not being able to breach a main entrance, not being fast enough, an alarm being raised before they reach the main entrance, and losing a key member early in the conflict to injury (or worse) are all major events—but the team has been trained to overcome these. However, if multiple events occur on top of or after one another, it can change the control of the engagement multiple times.

THE MICRO PRINCIPLE OF DYNAMIC STABILITY   1.2.4

According to experts in chaos theory, there are apparent states of order and disorder in chaos. I'm not going to tell some of the most brilliant people in the world that they're flat-out wrong, but in team sports at least, the theory that any point in a game is either stable or unstable is debatable. In my experience working with elite teams worldwide, there are only transitions between states of low disorder and high disorder. In other words, there is instability even in states of apparently great stability, even if it's minor.

Think of any game in which one team is attacking at breakaway speed. This may seem highly organized and stable, but in reality it is an unstable state where one error could leave the team unbalanced defensively and exposed to the opponent's counterattack. There is never total stability, only a perception of it.

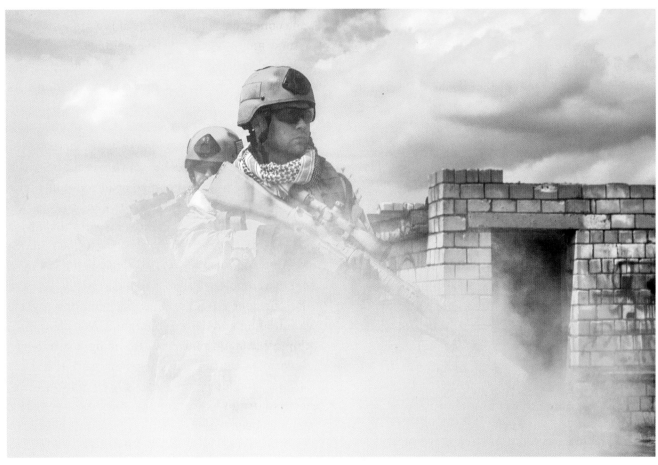

In sport and conflict, thriving in chaos is critical.

THE MACRO PRINCIPLE OF UNPREDICTABILITY   1.2.5

When we combine the principle of dynamic feedback and the principle of nonlinear amplification, we get the macro principle of unpredictability. This simply means that because we expect to (possibly) know only the initial conditions, we cannot predict outcomes. I say "possibly" because in many cases, we don't have all the information about even the initial conditions (despite what the prophets of the Big Data movement might try to tell you). We know from the principle of nonlinear amplification that any small inaccuracy, error, or missed detail can have a major effect or consequence. Despite what sports commentators might say, we cannot hope to accurately predict the ultimate fate of a complex system, as anything can happen at any moment in a game.

THE PRECISION PARADOX   1.2.6

Do not confuse this incredible complexity with inaccuracy or lack of precision in sports. Chaos is a paradoxically precise chaotic behavior. The fact that a model of a chaotic system does not predict every event or outcome exactly does not mean that it is wildly inaccurate. The effect of chaotic systems cannot be predicted with certainty due to unstable coefficients, feedback, and phase changes, but a model can predict the probability of overall patterns.

THE CHAOS OF SPORT   1.2.7

These principles outline a number of important conclusions. First, they frame how complicated and nuanced a team-sport game truly is. For generations, smarter coaches have attempted to look for patterns

The statistical probability that organic structures and the most precisely harmonized reactions that typify living organisms would be generated by accident is zero.

—Ilya Prigogine

and broad generalizations and have advanced their aims with strategies and general tactics. In recent times, though, many others have tried to break down the game into microscopic elements and enhance and control each one. The principles of turbulence and nonlinear amplification reveal the foolishness of this reductive approach. Second, these principles lead to a macroscopic, big-picture approach that acknowledges that everything is interconnected. Each event in a game matters and affects the outcome.

Chaos theory describes the specific range of irregular behaviors in a system that moves or changes. The thrust of this theory is that small inputs in a closed system may produce large, unpredictable consequences, and that these systems may jump from ordered states to chaotic states and back again, based on those small inputs. Chaos operates in a closed system, so it does not, as is commonly believed, describe a nondeterministic phenomenon. So we should stop trying to quantify and measure every aspect of sports in the hope that it will allow us to better manage the outcome. It won't, because there are too many variables interacting with each other, and these variables change from game to game.

The critical point to understand is that these are the principles that will affect your team and your next opponent equally. Recognizing this impacts the approach we use in the run-up to each contest.

CATCHING LIGHTNING   1.2.8

The whole point of chaos theory is that the fate of the system is determined by small factors that become magnified over time. These factors are too numerous to pin down and too small to fully comprehend, meaning that the system we see in sports is unpredictable.[4] This is why we see a non-league team upset a Premier League high-flyer in the Football Association Challenge (FA) Cup, a small-college team defeat a Division I powerhouse in the NCAA basketball tournament, and an underdog team like Japan upend mighty South Africa in the Rugby World Cup.

If the outcomes of sports games could be preordained, what would be the point of watching, playing, or coaching them?

The importance of understanding the basic principles of fractals, chaos, and chaos theory is that although sport is chaotic and appears random, it is possible—using certain approaches—to create a model to understand and manage it.

CARTESIAN REDUCTIONISM   1.2.9

Western science was guided and built up on the contributions of classic rationalism, inherited from Aristotle and developed by, among others, Descartes. The science was developed on the following fundamental principles:

1. Divide each problem or difficulty into the largest possible number of sections to be better able to resolve them.

2. Neatly guide the issues, beginning with the simplest objects and easiest to understand, to show how, little by little, by successive degrees, they become complex.

3. Always complete the questioning and assessments as generally as possible to ensure that nothing is omitted.

In preparing athletes, the traditional, simple specificity model is inadequate because the game itself is so complex and there are so many intertwined variables. Instead, you need a specific, tactics-driven game model—a system of play based on a full understanding of the sport.

One issue we face when addressing individual or team performance problems is that the analytical model we're used to gives way to structural-

> *We must rethink our way of organizing knowledge. This means breaking down the traditional barriers between disciplines and conceiving new ways to reconnect that which has been torn apart. We have to redesign our educational policies and programs. And as we put these reforms into effect we have to keep our sights on the long term and honor our tremendous responsibility for future generations.*

—Edgar Morin

ism and develops from reductionism, the fragmentation of the whole (that is, the "whole is equal to the sum of its parts" objective thinking, as advocated by Descartes), to the supremacy of the whole over the parts (that is, the Aristotelian dictum "the whole is more than the sum of its parts"). In sports, we've struggled to understand both the collective as well as the nature of the organization as a system.

The study of cybernetics, a transdisciplinary approach for exploring regulatory systems and their structures, constraints, and possibilities, has been used to help understand chaos in sport. Norbert Wiener defined cybernetics as "the science of control and communication in both the animal and the machine." Developed from the concepts of general systems theory, this area of knowledge transcended the Cartesian division of mind and body, conceiving the mind as the very process of life and not as a distinct entity.

NEWTON'S ERROR
1.3

We have been taught to think of the world in a structured way, with a deterministic, mechanistic, reductionist Newtonian view. Because they're so complex, however, it has become apparent that this notion is inadequate for understanding conflict and team-sports games. The writings of Einstein, Heisenberg, Gödel, Morin, Bertalanffy, and Prigogine all describe in detail concepts that provide an alternative, more holistic way to look at the world and, more importantly, to systematically address challenges.

The method in this section builds on such a systemic, model-based view to refine the understanding of dynamic systems for the sporting context. It encour-

TRADITIONAL THINKING VS EMERGING THINKING	
REDUCTIONISM	HOLISM
LINEAR CAUSALITY	MUTUAL CAUSALITY
OBJECTIVE REALITY	PERSPECTIVE REALITY
DETERMINISM	INDETERMINISM
SURVIVAL OF THE FITTEST	ADAPTIVE SELF-ORGANIZATION
FOCUS ON DISCRETE ENTITIES	FOCUS ON RELATIONSHIPS BETWEEN ENTITIES
LINEAR RELATIONSHIPS	NONLINEAR RELATIONSHIPS
NEWTONIAN PHYSICS PERSPECTIVES	QUANTUM PHYSICS PERSPECTIVES
WORLD IS PREDICTABLE	WORLD IS NOVEL AND PROBABILISTIC
MODERN	POSTMODERN
FOCUS ON HIERARCHY	FOCUS ON HETERARCHY (WITHIN LEVELS)
PREDICTION	UNDERSTANDING
BASED ON 19TH-CENTURY PHYSICS	BASED ON BIOLOGY
EQUILIBRIUM / STABILITY / DETERMINISTIC DYNAMICS	STRUCTURE / PATTERN / SELF-ORGANIZATION / LIFE CYCLES
FOCUS ON AVERAGES	FOCUS ON VARIATION

ages us to approach challenges very differently and makes it easier to interpret what happens in every team-sports contest than if we just try to break down performance into dozens of separate elements, as has been the trend for the past few years.[5]

THE PRINCIPLE OF EMERGENCE AND SELF-ORGANIZATION   1.3.1

Order Out of Chaos by Ilya Prigogine was one of the first books to present the concept of self-organization as an important part of chaos theory. Prigogine believed that although certain systems—like a sports game—are inherently chaotic, order will emerge out of this chaos because the elements (for our purposes, athletes) self-organize in response to their environment.[6] As a result, certain patterns emerge during the game that can tell us how individuals, units, and the team as a whole tend to react in certain moments and situations.[7]

The principle of emergence and self-organization also applies to the opposing team. Though we can't say, "The defense always does this when . . ." or "The midfield is bound to do this . . ." we can at least identify tendencies that can be used to evaluate performance outside of either the box score or the mind-numbing range of statistics that many teams have defaulted to as they seek to isolate certain elements of the game.

CHAOPLEXITY   1.3.2

The term *chaoplexity* brings together the theory of complexity and chaos theory. In addition to describing systems that are both chaotic and complex, a key principle of chaoplexity is that dynamic patterns that at first glance seem complex are, in fact, underpinned by an unexpected simplicity. As James Gleick discusses in *Chaos: Making a New Science* and Mitchell Waldrop explores in *Complexity: The Emerging Science at the Edge of Order and Chaos*, the complexity of the game exists in a world founded on chaos.[8] Combine this with social laws, the rules of competition, and training or practice schedules, and we see that players are experiencing what can only be described as chaoplexity.

The complexity of the game exists in a world founded on chaos.

FRACTALS AND GAME PRINCIPLES   1.3.3

Think for a moment about what you see when you go to a window to watch snow fall. At first, you're aware of the big picture—the prevailing whiteness, the sense of beauty, the hush as the flakes gently land. It all seems ordered, cohesive, and logical, but you know it's actually chaotic and random.

Each flake is unique. It forms and crystallizes in the atmosphere as it falls. In addition, every flake has a slightly different shape and takes a different course from the air to the ground. Yet each one is a fractal, or a representative part of the bigger picture.[9]

The paradox here is that a series of random, uniquely constructed flakes combine to create a uniform effect. Similarly, in a game of football, basketball, soccer, or rugby, everything appears to work smoothly in an orderly, cohesive manner at first glance; the fact that there are two teams with equal numbers of players competing in the same conditions furthers this impression.

The game experience is not simply about one team or the other, either. It's about two teams moving and interacting in space and time to create a game.

Each tackle, interception, and turnover is its own unique, chaotic, seemingly unrelated event. But these events interrelate to form a dynamic and apparently stable system. Within any team-sport game, there is chaos but also equilibrium due to the constraints of a fixed-size field, pitch, or court and the influence of the sport's rules.[10]

This apparent dichotomy is precisely the reason that we need a model to help us understand what the game really is, the moments it is composed of, and how its disparate, seemingly conflicting parts combine to create a relatively harmonious contest between two teams. As Aristotle famously said, the whole is greater than the sum of its parts. Another way to explain this is through the words of the Sufi teacher Jalaluddin Rumi, who said, "You think because you understand one you must understand

MODELS OF FOOTBALL TRAINING			
Dimensions of Analysis	Analytical model	**Structural model**		Systemic model
		Traditional perspective	Functional perspective	
Thought	Dualism	Holism		Holism (complex)
Object	The parties	The whole and the parts	The whole and its context	The whole, the parties & their context
Objectives	Isolated	Each task has goals for each of the players	Each task has goals for each of the player groups	Based on the principles of team play model
Theoretical Foundation	Behaviorism (mind) and mechanism (body)	Cognitivism (information processing)	Cognitivism (constructivism)	Ecological theory and dynamical systems
Process Central Mechanism	Execution	Decision (static)	Decision (dynamic)	Perception
Learning Conception	By association (associative behavioral)	By association (cognitive associations)	By restructuring (comprehension)	By restructuring (adaptation)
Teaching	Fragmented	Global: interaction of the parts/structures to target one	Global: interaction of the parts/structures to focus the cognitive	Global: Interaction of the parties to focus the whole and the parts
Orientation of the Teaching	It is part of the sport to reach the player	Be part of the players and their structures to make the team		It is part of the team (game model) to reach the player
Teaching Techniques Tend to	Direct instruction	Teaching by searching (discovery followed predominates)		Teaching by searching (predominantly problem-solving)

two, because one and one makes two. But you must also understand *and*."[11]

The whole is greater than the sum of its parts.

THE ART OF WINNING   1.3.4

"Decision making is an art, which requires the decision maker to combine experience and education to act."[12] So states the U.S. Marine Corps' instruction manual on making choices on the battlefield. This statement also is highly applicable to team sports. We must remember that a sports team is a fluid and functioning system, not a robot-operated assembly line that gives consistent output that can be easily measured and quantified. Sports are, or should be, a people business, and so the methods used to manage sports are an art. Sun Tzu's most famous text refers to this in its very title: *The Art of War*. It's not the *science* of war. That's why you should consider this book to be about the *art* of winning, not the science of winning.

The truth is that understanding the game is the fundamental starting point for all winning teams. If the game as a whole is not understood, you're just operating in isolation, and the progress of individual players as well as the team will be limited. After gaining a deeper and broader insight into the nature of the game itself, we can begin to look at how to

All religions, arts and sciences are branches of the same tree. All these aspirations are directed toward ennobling man's life, lifting it from the sphere of mere physical existence and leading the individual towards freedom.

—Albert Einstein

train for the situations that athletes encounter in a team-sports contest. The biggest mistake fitness and strength and conditioning coaches make is to assume that this is not important and that the physical ability of a player is all that matters.

THE CHAOS TO WIN   1.3.5

The philosophical thrust of chaos theory is that uncertainty can be caused by small changes that, even if anticipated, result in an unpredictable system. This doesn't mean that the behavior of the system is totally unpredictable. Long-term trends can be distilled with a certain level of probability, and we can estimate the range of change, at least to some extent.

Any game appears chaotic when watched from afar or with an untrained eye. But in reality, a game is a series of simple actions that create interactions that appear complex. What we see is chaos, but it can appear as a dynamic and somewhat poetic interaction. Watching Pep Guardiola's Barcelona and Bayern Munich sides, Bill Belichick's Patriots, or Phil Jackson's Bulls at their peak showed us teams that appeared to work in unison. What we really saw, though, was the emergence of order within a complex, adaptive system. Over the course of a game, unique events involving two or more players (such as a tackle or shot on goal) combine to create global properties that can differ greatly from the behavior of the individuals involved.

The more we can model, the less is left to chance.

This is an important point for the design of game models. It may seem like an unusual statement, but good coaches do not know how exactly their teams will win. They simply know that the win will occur through the evolution of the complex, adaptive system.

The more we can model, the less is left to chance. Jim Schwartz once said of the Patriots and Bill Belichick: "Probably the biggest thing I learned from Bill is that there isn't anything that is not important. Anything that touches the team is important. That philosophy of 'Don't sweat the small stuff'? Yeah, that was never his philosophy."[13]

THE POWER OF COMPLEXITY   1.3.6

A game is a never-ending series of chaotic feedback loops. The seemingly small interactions between teammates and their opponents create larger effects, which in turn influence what chaos theorists call "agents." In team sports, these agents are the players, coaches, staff members, and anyone else involved with the organization.

One key ramification of emergence is that reductionism cannot be successfully applied to complex systems. Since emergent behaviors do not predictably arise from a simple linear combination of inputs and outputs, reductionism is ill suited to analyzing the behaviors of complex systems. This means that on the sports field, we can't simply look at a statistic or the action of one individual and expect to draw meaningful conclusions.

Already, you can start to see why sports *science* has failed for so many teams.

Another fundamental behavior of complex systems is adaptive self-organization. Massively disordered systems can spontaneously "crystallize" a high degree of order. Good coaches trust that the system or group will evolve and develop over time. Self-organization of the team and game model will arise as the system reacts and adapts to its externally imposed environment. So if the team is trained in the manner that prepares it best to adapt, that preparedness will reveal itself on game day—what Bill Walsh called "letting the score take care of itself" because he'd prepared his players so well.

A third important behavior of complex systems is evolution at the edge of chaos. Games are never stable or in equilibrium but are always unfolding, always in transition. There is no end to team evolution—it's a constantly determining and adapting network. The team can itself evolve to address the future challenges it perceives and anticipates in the moment.

It's critical to recognize the edge of chaos so that as you start to use a game model, you begin to see the game itself as the embodiment of an evolving approach that is addressing a complex challenge. It's also important to recognize that coaches and players are solving a problem together and preparing an eventual answer that you can't yet know; you have to trust that the team's play will evolve to provide a long-term solution.

> **Evolution is chaos with feedback.**
>
> —Joseph Ford

> **We grow in direct proportion to the amount of chaos we can sustain and dissipate.**
>
> —Ilya Prigogine

To do this properly, the best teams implement the game model and principles that are derived from the theory of military conflict, chaos theory, and many other contributing concepts from mathematics, biology, warfare, and more. The next section explores how these principles can be applied to any team-sports game to improve our understanding and evaluation while informing team preparation that leads to improved performance.

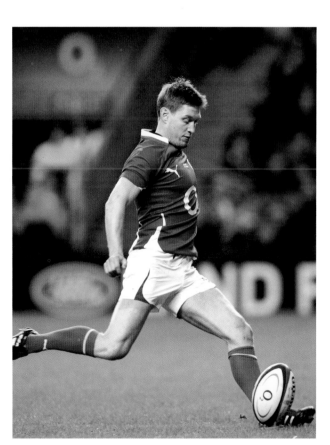

Ronan O'Gara, Munster Rugby legend, the epitome of calmness in chaos. Photo by Mitch Gunn / Shutterstock.com.

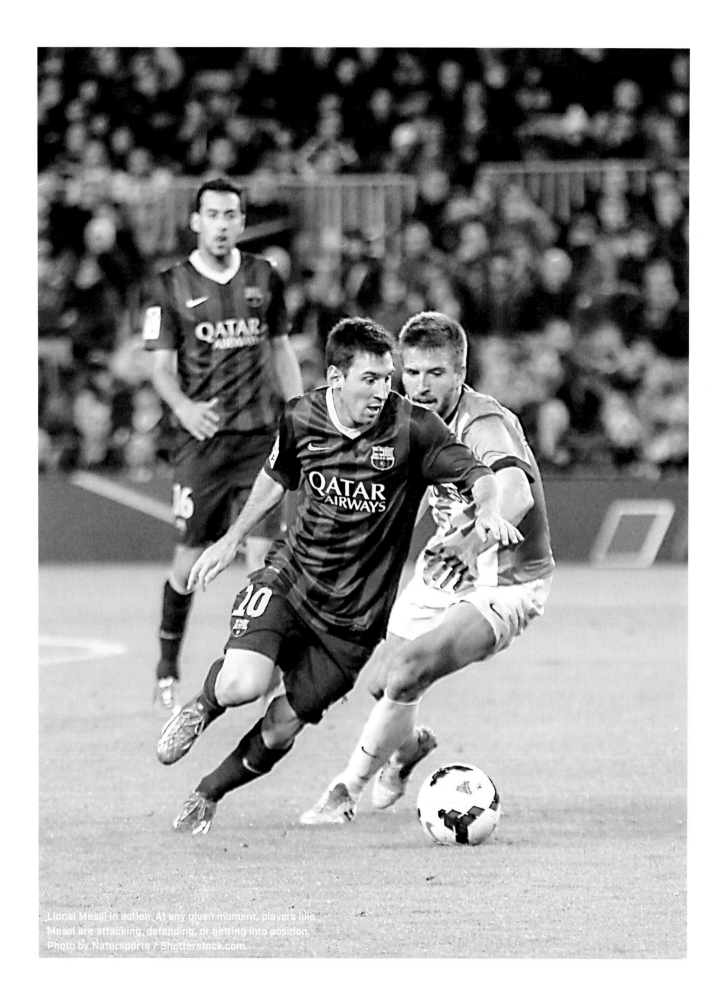

Lionel Messi in action. At any given moment, players like Messi are attacking, defending, or getting into position. Photo by Natursports / Shutterstock.com.

TWO

PRINCIPLES OF THE GAME

Now that we recognize that sport is chaos personified, let's look at what that looks like in practice. The first thing to consider is that all team sports involve a formation or starting point for players, who have certain intentions. All team sports involve the movement of a ball or, in military terms, a target. The movement of the players is always relative to their goal, either offensively or defensively. Finally, the players' actions occur in a moment that has context. You're either attacking or defending. And if you're not attacking or defending, you're moving into position to either attack or defend.

PRINCIPLES OF TEAM SPORTS
2.1

Principles are the beginning, not the end; the point of departure, not of arrival. Take any small section of a game, period, or play—from whistle to whistle, if you will. What I will show you, and what most people don't realize, is that every sport at every level—from a playground pickup game to the NBA Finals—has the same four basic principles.

Ignore where, on the field, an event occurs; just focus on what *happens*. One player has the ball. Every other player takes up a position relative to the sidelines, the end zone or its equivalent, and each other—as well as to the ball (the principle of structure). Attackers typically spread out from their team-mates to create space (the principle of player circulation). Defenders will be much nearer to the other teammates in their defensive unit and will either stay very close to an opponent or fill a space that an attacker could move into.

The whistle blows, and now the dance begins. As the attacker with the ball moves, everyone else changes their position relative to the ball, with attackers moving away into space to accept the ball and defenders coming into space to intercept or pressure it. The attacking team also attempts to move the ball in an effort to create space and time (the principle of ball circulation). Defenders arguably have a little more work to do—just as in the observation that Ginger Rogers had to do everything Fred Astaire did, but backward and in heels. Defenders have to play their role by watching the ball and their man while anticipating upcoming actions. All these movements are interdependent and, if performed effectively, timed to perfection (the principle of relationship, or the interplay of sequencing and timing).

THE MACRO PRINCIPLE OF STRUCTURE (FORMATION)
2.1.1

All plays start with original positioning from kickoff/tip-off or a restart. So in rugby this could be a line-out, in football a kickoff, in basketball an inbounds play after a timeout, and in soccer a free kick or corner. To play the correct role in each structural situation, players need to be aware of where they are in relation to teammates, opponents, and the ball. They must also know where they are on the pitch, court, or field before the ball goes live. In an offensive situation, positional structures exist to create a scoring opportunity; in a defensive situation, to prevent one.

Just like our earlier snowflake analogy, all plays are essentially fractals, repeating with similar principles. But each play is individual and unique in some ways. For example, a football team could run the same play a hundred times. The main elements—whom the quarterback is targeting, the wide receivers' routes, the setup of the offensive line, and so on—would be the same. But the exact way the team executes the play is slightly different each time because of the varying ways that each player performs as well as changing conditions from play to play and game to game.

Effective offensive positioning aims to create space, while defensive positioning tries to condense it. But both are initially attempting to misdirect the team's true intentions. The best players adjust, assume good positions, and have heightened awareness of their location in space at every restart. Even in basic drills or small-sided games, smart players

know where they are in relation to the ball and the sideline plus how much operating space they have. This knowledge is essential, because once the ball starts to circulate, players need to have excellent spatial awareness.

THE MACRO PRINCIPLE OF BALL (TARGET) CIRCULATION 2.1.2

Watch any game and focus on the movement of the players and the movement of the ball. Ignore colors and teams and observe those two things: ball and player movement. Sometimes it helps to watch at double speed from a high-up view that shows the whole court or field. You will see that the movement of the ball influences the movement of both teams. This influence is greatest in games where there is no man-marking (think man-to-man defense in basketball). We sometimes think that players following the ball occurs only in youth sports, but watch carefully and you'll see that it's also true, to a different degree, at the elite level.

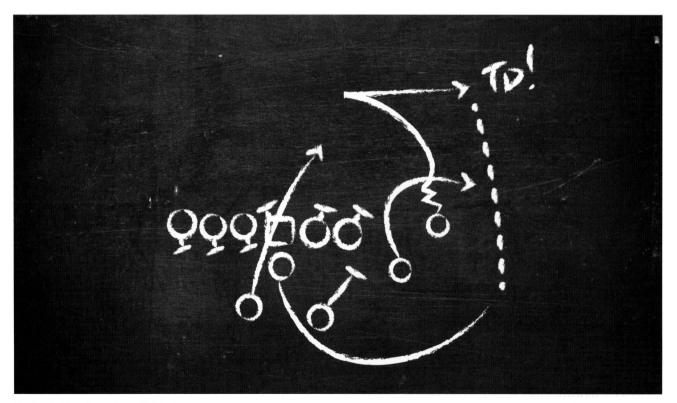

Sprint right option—"The Catch."

Smart players and teams know how to use the ball to move people and eventually create space. Players attacking and defending will both move to and follow the ball. Watching Barcelona, you see a team moving the ball around the pitch and constantly changing the angle of attack. As they advance, the ball is eventually worked into the space just outside the eighteen-yard box, and gaps develop as impetuous opposition defenders attempt to close down space.

THE MACRO PRINCIPLE OF PLAYER CIRCULATION (MOVEMENT)

2.1.3

The next thing you'll notice, especially if the ball slows or becomes stationary, is how the players move in relation to each other. Defenders will try to fill space or track a man, whereas attackers will move into space to accept the ball.

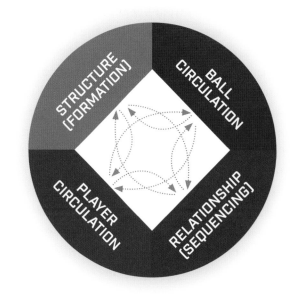

The four macro principles of all team sports.

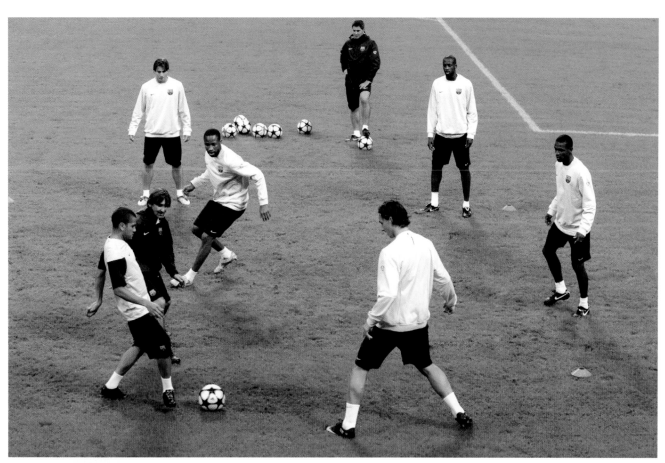

The rondo helps players develop tactical ball circulation, skills, and timing, all at a very high speed. Photo by Paolo Bona / Shutterstock.com.

By moving to a different point on the field, an offensive player not only puts pressure on the defender but also creates space for the other players on his or her team. Player circulation often includes elements of deception or misdirection to confuse the defense and obscure the true intention of the attacking move. It also creates too many possibilities for defenders to choose among, impairing their decision-making. For example, in basketball, the defending team often struggles to defend the pick-and-roll because either the player setting the screen or the teammate for whom the screen is set can become the shooter. Or the offensive team may mix it up further still by having the player setting the pick pop out to take a shot instead of cutting to the basket.

THE MACRO PRINCIPLE OF RELATIONSHIP (SEQUENCE AND TIMING)   2.1.4

The final element in every play is relationship. This is the sequence or order in which events happen and the timing with which they occur. Effective attacking or offensive play will demonstrate good initial positioning, smooth player circulation to accept the ball and move into space, and precise ball circulation to exploit it. The best teams and players do this with effortless timing and in an order that befuddles and breaks down even the most potent defenses. This seems almost preprogrammed and like a dance when observed from a distance, but as we will see, it is far more complex.

The players are not trying to do as much as possible but rather as much as is *necessary*—a highly efficient skill that makes the team appear to be playing effortlessly and with the precision of a Swiss watch. Look at the poetry in motion of the Dutch "Total Football" teams of the 1970s, the unstoppable offense of Bill Walsh's San Francisco 49ers, and the San Antonio Spurs dynasty under Gregg Popovich.

What you see on the field that seems to be chaos, then, is not a linear sequence of events but actually a series of principles at work that *tame* chaos with a game plan or intention that guides players' decisions and actions.

COHESION OF MACRO PRINCIPLES
2.2

When you see these four macro principles come together, you're witnessing almost telepathic nonverbal communication—just like in the Tom Brady example at the start of this chapter. At the highest level of any sport, basic skills are executed at incredibly high speed. The sequencing of players' actions appears to create and close space almost at will. The positioning, timing, and constant movement are on par with those of any world-class orchestra.

These four basic principles are essential to understanding effective movement and game play in all sports. They allow us to analyze stages of any game and identify issues with poor play and how to correct them or exploit them in an opponent. The principles are also a critical teaching resource for coaches. By using these four macro principles, coaches can help players begin to see where they need to improve. Careful application of this part of the game model allows coaches to use training and practice more purposefully to build expertise in the players and team.

THE COMPLEXITY OF THE SIMPLE RONDO   2.2.1

One impressive demonstration of these macro principles in game preparation is seen in the warm-ups of teams like Barcelona FC or Real Madrid when they use rondos. At first glance, this drill appears to involve seven or eight players simply kicking a ball to one another as one or two others chase and try to intercept it. In reality, though, you're looking at a fundamental development of all games with ball circulation, whether played by schoolchildren or by elite pros. The stress and decision-making of positioning and player movement are removed so that tactical ball circulation, contextual skill execution, and timing can be emphasized and practiced—all at very high speed. This directly relates to how quickly a team is able to move the ball around come game time. The simplest version keeps players stationary,

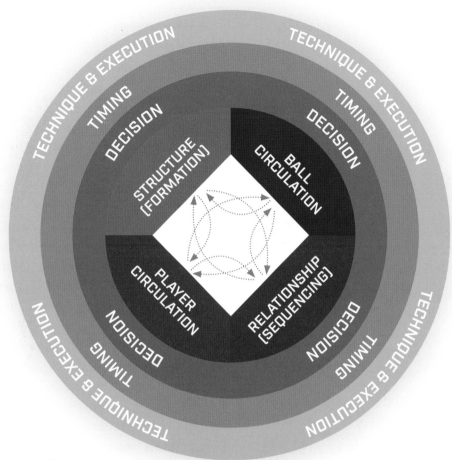

The macro principles in practice.

moving the ball, circulating it among themselves, and using the ball to move the defenders with precise timing. The next progression is the movement of the outside players, then on from there with an objective like scoring a goal.

THE FUNDAMENTALS   2.2.2

These four macro principles form the basis of every moment in a team-sports game. The purpose of viewing the game in this manner is to allow players and coaches to problem-solve and develop athletes' skills continuously. As we saw in the Brady example at the beginning of this chapter, every player's first and primary action is to see where they are and what's happening around them. What is their position relative to the field as well as scoring and defensive areas? Before you can do anything in a game, you need to know your overall position. As the athletes move, they begin to process their exact location relative to that knowledge.

When coaches review film or players look back on their performance, the first thing they should observe is positioning. In the team setup, this is relative to the planned structure or lineup. One of the first things we should teach in youth sports to help kids better understand the game is to assess where they are at any given moment. For example, are they close enough to the sideline or far enough from an opponent to execute a skill, and do they feel they can close or exploit the space that's available to them?

All this is related to spatial intelligence and the ability to process the moving space. Good vision is important; however, effective spatial awareness is also predicated on the athletes' ability to process what they see. We know from experience that nonspecific vision training improves the player's ability in nonspecific testing but not in game-specific demands. For this reason, we need to train vision, perception, and game-specific spatial intelligence all at once, by playing the game.

EXAMPLES OF MACRO PRINCIPLES

To better understand the four macro principles of team sports, let's look at real-life examples of each.

POSITIONING/FORMATION

An unusual structural decision by the attacking team often confuses the defense (even if it's well organized), leading to a better scoring opportunity. For instance, Eric Cantona's setting himself up at the edge of the penalty area for a corner kick in the final minutes of the 1996 FA Cup final enabled him to receive the ball when it was punched clear by the goalkeeper. This allowed him to take the Liverpool defense by surprise with his remarkable volleyed goal. The defense simply stood still because they weren't expecting danger to come from such an unusual spot on the pitch.

Another example is in close-quarter conflict (or battle). Correct positioning is critical before engagement, not just to avoid friendly fire, but also so soldiers are aware of each other's roles, arcs of fire, and areas of responsibility when clearing rooms and buildings or engaging with enemy combatants. Correct positioning and formation is the fundamental basis for the speed of attack and application of overwhelming force. Going back to sports, take the Boston Celtics' seemingly endless list of set plays that coach Brad Stevens chooses from to confuse the opponent coming out of a timeout. While an assistant and then head men's basketball coach at Butler University, Stevens always kept paper and a pen beside his TV so that he could sketch out plays in the pro and college games that he watched obsessively. Now he's using this cribbed playbook to create open looks after the game restarts, enabling his Celtics to shake free of defenders and get high-quality scoring opportunities when the pressure is on and mere seconds remain on the game clock.

One reason these plays are effective is that instead of automatically going to the team's best player, Stevens has run sets for just about everyone on the roster to get a shot. This is another example of misdirection and using the element of surprise. Such crafty positioning earned Stevens high praise from six-time NBA championship coach Gregg Popovich: "Brad is one of the top coaches in the league. He's a clinician, he's a technician, he's detailed."[14]

Purposeful player movement is also essential if the offense is to create scoring opportunities. Bill Shankly's philosophy at Liverpool FC was not just "pass" but "pass and move." In soccer, rugby, and Australian rules football, player movement is more spontaneous and requires endless invention on the part of the players. In more-structured team sports such as basketball—and even more so in American football—players must grasp how to move within the context of the playbook, knowing that positioning is more influential.

This is not to say that there's no creativity or that there's no place for audibles or read-based decision-making. But synchronized player movement has to occur on a group level if a team is to implement its plays within the game plan. As 49ers coach Bill Walsh once said about player movement done right, "The variation of movement of 11 players and the orchestration of that facet of football is beautiful to me."[15] In the case of the 49ers, the results weren't just aesthetically pleasing but also effective, as Walsh's tutelage began a run of five San Francisco Super Bowl wins between 1981 and 1994, including rare back-to-back victories in 1989 and 1990.

BALL CIRCULATION

There are two ways to create space when attacking in team sports. The first is what legendary Dutch soccer coach and father of "Total Football" Rinus Michels called "ball circulation."[16] Simply put, this is the movement of the ball between players on the same team. If you look at clubs whose style of play involves retaining a high percentage of possession, such as Barcelona FC in soccer, you can watch several minutes of the game and the only thing that seems to move when they have possession is the ball (aka the tiki-taka style of play). Only when they see an opening in the defense does a player burst into space. And because they have proven goal scorers like Lionel Messi, Luis Suarez, and Neymar, such penetration often leads to a high-quality scoring opportunity.

For the team trying to defend a ball circulation–heavy side, the effect of the ball constantly moving is that players are pulled out of position all over the pitch, court, or field. Indeed, if you took a bird's-eye view of your favorite team sport, you'd see that, for the most part, players follow the ball. I'll cover defensive aims a bit later, but suffice it to say for now that effective ball circulation frustrates defenders' attempts to achieve compactness and cohesion and to apply man-to-man pressure.

Regardless of whether a team favors a fast or slow attack (lots more on that in a little while), ball movement is a foundational pillar for any offense. As Tex Winter, the man who architected Phil Jackson's famous "triangle offense," puts it in his famed book *The Triple-Post Offense*, "Pass the ball. Do not massage the basketball. A good basketball player can receive a pass from a teammate and make his play within three seconds of receiving the ball."[17]

A different way to view ball movement is through the eyes of Liverpool's Shankly: "Our approach was to use the ball like a baton in a relay race. You pass it to me, I pass it to him, he passes it on. It's the ball that is covering most of the ground—not the players."[18]

Another reason to move the ball a lot is to wear down elite offensive players so that they're less able to exert themselves in the attacking game as the contest wears on. When talking about how his San Antonio Spurs grind down the opposition, Popovich explained to ESPN the impact of his team's exemplary ball movement: "Let's say you have a great offensive player like Steph Curry. You want to make him work on defense, but to do that you need a great one-on-one player to give the ball to. We don't have a Kevin Durant, a LeBron [James], a James Harden, so we have to do it with pieces. And the only way to do that is to move the basketball and make the people guarding you move with it."[19]

Such emphasis on ball circulation certainly had the desired effect in the 2014 NBA Finals, as Miami's James Jones confirmed after his Miami Heat fell to the Spurs. "It was exhausting," Jones said after the series ended. "I don't think we'd ever seen them move the ball that much, that well."[20]

PLAYER CIRCULATION   2.2.3.3

The other way to create space in any team sport is for players to move. By relocating to a different point on the field, a player not only puts pressure on the defender but also creates space for the other players on his or her team. Player circulation often includes an element of deception or misdirection to confuse the defense and obscure the true intention of the attacking move. We use the word *circulation* to underscore that players are in continuous motion, not executing one simple movement that starts and stops. It also underlines the fact that players circulate through space, often taking the place of others in a play.

Circulation also creates too many options for defenders, impairing their decision-making. For example, in basketball the defending team often struggles to defend out-of-bounds plays after a time-out as there is so much misdirection and the attacking team's best shooters may end up being decoys rather than the intended target.

In highly structured sports with even more players, such as American football, player circulation often is even more important to creating penetration and scoring opportunities than in free-flowing team sports such as rugby and soccer. There are so many possible variations for player circulation that even the best defenses struggle to identify the quarterback's intended target, let alone stop him from reaching his desired position unchallenged.

RELATIONSHIP (SEQUENCE AND TIMING)   2.2.3.4

Some teams appear to play effortlessly, with the precision of a carefully orchestrated Broadway or West End play. Well-sequenced teams in any sport are characterized by a fluid combination of ball and player movement that pulls opponents' defenses apart possession after possession, game after game, year after year. In addition, each player is positioned exactly where she needs to be to take advantage of the two types of circulation, player and ball.

The best teams sequence and time positioning, ball circulation, and player circulation very quickly and to devastating effect, achieving a seemingly effortless synchronicity. Think about George North streaking away to score a forty-yard try in a Six Nations game after a perfect pass to the flank from a Welsh center. The intricate passing move before this final decisive pass has lured the defense away from the wing, giving North space to operate out wide untouched.

If the ball is passed to North when he's already running and has nothing but grass ahead of him, taking the ball home becomes a simple enough task. But if his teammates have not set up the move well and instead get North the ball when he's in traffic with two defenders clogging the wing, his chances of scoring on that try are greatly reduced.

It's the same in all team sports: sequencing, timing, and synchronicity are everything when it comes to execution.

THE MOMENT

2.3

The four macro principles exist in every sport regardless of field position or time in the game. In practice, while the time, location on the field, and score make no difference to the actual action, the context in which actions happen is important to understand.

So while a particular pass between two players in the first minute of a soccer game with no score may occur in the same situation during the final minute of the game, the context is different. Perhaps one team is in the lead and the other is pressing hard to even the score with seconds remaining until the final whistle. So they are identical actions, but not the same. Once the context changes, it's a different event, and it should be assessed as such.

This is another area in which statistics fall short of their promise to improve our understanding of the game.

CONTEXT

2.3.1

The real point of this section is that players never perform the same action twice: it's always slightly different. Some people may try to tell you that a shot is always "textbook" from a certain player. This could be true if you exclude the psychological aspect of the action, but I work in the real world, and the real world doesn't function like that. The psychological and the physical aspects of skill execution are indivisible.

THE DRUNK, THE POLICEMAN, AND THE PRIEST

2.3.2

Vítor Frade, professor at the Sports University of Porto, told me the following parable: A fan travels to a foreign city he's never been to for an away game his team is playing in. When he gets off the bus, he needs directions.

The first person he meets on the street is a drunk. Needing to find the stadium, the fan asks him the best direction to start walking. The drunk tells him to continue down the street, turn left at the first liquor store, keep going until he comes to a big new bar, and at the bar turn right and go on for three hundred yards. The drunk says that the stadium will then be right in front of him.

So the fan sets off. On the way, he passes a police officer. Questioning the drunk's inebriated directions, he asks the cop how to get to the stadium. "Go down to the courthouse, turn right, keep going until you reach the main police station, and then turn left just after it," the policeman says. "Go on for another hundred yards and you'll find one of my colleagues standing on the corner. He'll get you rest of the way."

So once again, off the fan goes. On his way, he meets a priest. "It won't hurt to make sure I'm going the right way," the tourist thinks. He asks the priest for directions and is told to walk back to the old basilica on the hill, go around it, keep going until he comes to a synagogue, then turn left fifty yards after it and continue on to the stadium.

Any of these sets of directions would've gotten the fan to the stadium. The three people he spoke with all knew where the stadium was located; they just had different perspectives on how he should get there. Each spoke based on his own experience and perspective. The drunk tied his instructions to alcohol, the cop used legal-system landmarks, and the priest focused on places of worship.

The lesson here is that context is one of the most important things in sports. Ask a strength coach, a data analyst, and a defensive or offensive coach the same question, and you'll get different answers based on those individuals' experiences, education, and lingo.

CONTEXT IS PERSPECTIVE   2.3.3

At any point in a game, a team is in one of four moments. It is either attacking, moving from attacking to begin to defend, defending, or moving from defending into attacking. Each is what we call a moment—or context. By breaking up our game analysis into these four moments, we can provide context for the actions and decisions we're making and better evaluate how well the game plan objectives are being executed.

MACRO PRINCIPLES OF MACRO MOMENTS   2.3.4

We now can start to frame the four macro principles with one of four game moments. This gives us context for the analysis of the actions and a goal for the four macro principles. (And yes, I know that's a lot of fours—and a lot of principles!)

In an attacking moment, for example, the goal is to score. So positioning, ball circulation, player move-

ment, and sequencing combined are intended to lead to a scoring opportunity. In transitioning from defense to attack, the aim is to move the ball into an attacking area—all four macro principles should be aimed at this. This gives us a focus and direction for action.

At any level—be it high school, college, or professional—a game involves all four moments. There are obviously offense and defense, but if the ball is turned over, the game switches into one of the two transitional moments, either into or out of possession. First there's a moment as you move to execute an attack with possession, and then there's another moment as you try to regain possession.

Even in small games, like five-a-side soccer, or in military engagements, these four moments exist in the same way. You are either attacking, defending, or moving from one to the other. The execution of the basic skills exists in this context. Special operators will tell you that they do three things very well: shoot, move, and communicate. Notwithstanding that all three are predicated on excellent planning and preparation, every single engagement often will be refined to these basic principles. These skills are performed in all four game moments, during which their execution and the implications of how effective the actions are vary.

We can use these moments to form a basis for infinitely better analysis of the data and, with that, grasp the opportunity to improve performance.

> *Invincibility lies in the defense, the possibility of victory in the attack. Invincibility depends on oneself, but the enemy's vulnerability on himself.*
>
> —Sun Tzu, *The Art of War*

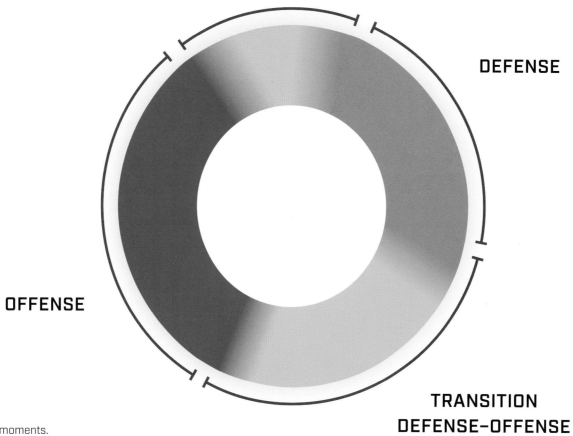

TRANSITION
OFFENSE–DEFENSE

DEFENSE

OFFENSE

TRANSITION
DEFENSE–OFFENSE

Game moments.

MACRO MOMENTS   2.3.5

Just like the macro principles, the four macro moments need to be clearly defined so that they can give us context for a complete understanding of situational decision-making.

While each moment is defined by the team's primary aim in that moment, they aren't about how the team should achieve that aim. These moments are simply states of the game and are not defined by space or positions on the court, pitch, field, or battlefield. The scoring-threat zone or moments can change or be determined by such things as scoring range and/or physical location of the play. The way athletes and teams go about executing in each of the four moments will depend on their structure, strategy, tactics, and personnel, as well as what the opponent is doing at any given time.

OFFENSIVE MOMENT   2.3.5.1

An offensive moment occurs when the team that has possession has moved the ball into an area from which it can score. The team is no longer trying to win the ball, pass it, or move the ball into a scoring zone but is actually in a position to try to put points on the scoreboard. In conflict, it is the moment when an operative's eyes are on a target that they can now "reach out and touch."[21]

During the offensive moment, the attacking team's primary intent is to score. To make this happen, they use various approaches. Some use short touches and lots of passing (the tiki-taka approach in soccer or the San Antonio Spurs' exemplary ball movement), and others try to make a single, decisive long pass (like the Dutch soccer team that beat favorite Spain

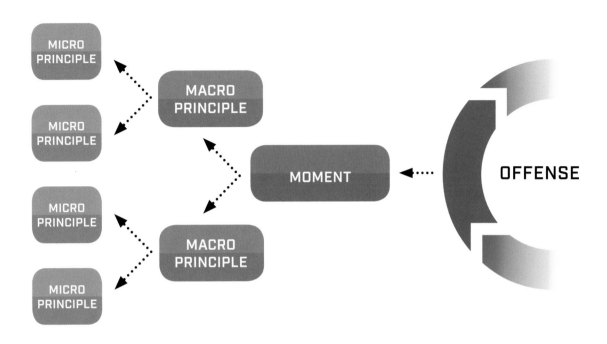

Moments and principles.

5–1 in the 2014 World Cup). The actual techniques or tactics do not affect the moment, which is the final phase of execution. The construction of these moments will be explained later, but they often involve creating space, moving the ball fast, aggressively compressing players, and creating chances.

DEFENSIVE MOMENT   2.3.5.2

This is essentially the same as an offensive moment but from the opposite perspective. While it may be considered the defensive moment, because the aim is primarily to stop the other team from scoring, I do not look at it like that. Instead, I consider it to be simply an offensive moment without possession. How this is done or executed is defined by each team's game model, but the basic action in the moment is always the same: to prevent scoring.

Defenses can reduce opportunities by closing space or preventing movement in areas where the attacking team can create scoring opportunities. The defense has to disrupt the attacking team so that it's prevented from implementing the objectives of its game plan. Being aggressive on the defensive end forces the attackers to reckon with pressure, which complicates and slows their decision-making.

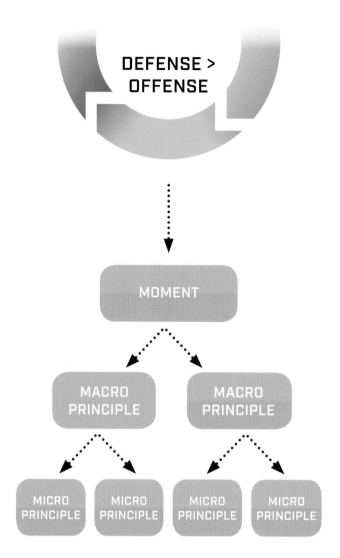

Transiitonal moments and principles.

TRANSITION-TO-OFFENSE MOMENT   2.3.5.3

When the ball is turned over, a transitional moment begins. This can occur after a score, a pick, a tackle, or a fumble, but regardless of how the changeover occurs, the transitional moment starts when possession switches from one team to the other. The defense-to-offense moment starts when you have been in a defensive moment, forced a turnover, and now are attacking to score. In a conflict context, this is the transition from a defense moment to locating or stalking.

For the team that is now on the offensive, the aim is to move the ball as quickly as possible. In most sports, ball movement is lateral or forward, but in the case of rugby, it is lateral or backward.

Depending on the game, the offensive moment can last from mere seconds (twenty-four in the NBA and thirty in college basketball) to many minutes. So there are, of course, differences in how quickly the offense must try to move into enemy territory and get into position to take a shot. But the essential elements of attacking are the same in any team sport.

Rapid ball movement creates space and allows the attacking team to take full advantage of the element of surprise. It also puts the attacking team in command and stymies the defense's ability to stop the offensive move and prevent a scoring opportunity. Advancing the ball quickly also presents defenders with too many options—particularly if they're outnumbered, such as when on the wrong end of a three-on-one fast break in basketball.

The result is that the defense's options are compromised on both the individual and the team level. This in turn slows down the very actions needed to arrest the breakaway momentum, making it almost impossible for the defense to deny the creation of a high-quality scoring opportunity. The faster the offensive team can move the ball forward and get players up in support, the more scoring choices they will have and the less likely the overwhelmed opponent will be to stop them.

TRANSITION-TO-DEFENSE MOMENT   2.3.5.4

The offense-to-defense moment begins when you have been in an offensive moment, were attacking and scored or turned the ball over, and now have to retreat to a defensive moment—or, rather, an offensive moment without the ball. This is where there is (or at least should be) a fluid movement to organize and attack without the ball.

There are two primary situations leading to the offense-to-defense moment. The first is when the attacking team scores and the game restarts. In some sports, such as American football, this moment is more drawn out and involves a break as different units take the field. But in others, like basketball, it's a lot shorter and the other team starts attacking immediately after conceding points, unless a time-out is called.

The second transition of this type follows a rapid change in ball possession, such as a fumble or interception in football, a steal or turnover in basketball, or a broken-down passing move in soccer or rugby. This kind of offense-to-defense moment is harder for the team that loses possession to defend than the offensive moment because of the speed at which it unfolds and the urgency of the situation.

Once your team loses control of the ball, the attacking team will try to gain ground rapidly and create a scoring opportunity while you're on the back foot. They will usually attempt to go through their offensive phases much more quickly than if they had started an attacking move from scratch, which in turn forces the defending team to make faster decisions and act without delay.

The most important thing for the team that's now defending is to slow the opponent's offense down. If the attackers are allowed to continue the helter-skelter pace that follows a change in possession for more than a few seconds, they're likely to create a high-percentage scoring chance.

So the first required step is to disrupt the movement of the attacking player who has the ball. If the defensive team can put the ball under enough pressure, it can buy time to get bodies back to support the defense, compress the playing field, and cut off space for the offense. As this happens, the moment of crisis can be averted and the defense can move from a state of chaos into one of readiness and organization, with players moving either to the attacker they're supposed to be guarding/marking in a man-to-man system or into their designated area in a zone scheme.

TRANSITIONS IN FOOTBALL

Some argue that there are no transitions in football, but they do exist. Any kickoff, turnover, or interception is a transition. Proactive teams attempt to not simply stop the ball but intercept the ball, turn it over, and exploit any disruption in the game and movement.

GAME DECISION-MAKING AND MACRO PRINCIPLES   2.3.5.5

An analytical decision-making process occasionally benefits a novice player because less real-world experience is required to make a decision and any complexity is systematically simplified during analysis. But in the fast-moving environment of elite sports or military conflict, we usually don't have this luxury, so the decision-making process relies on instinct. Decisions must be made with insufficient information when not enough data has been gathered. Instinctive decision-making relies on intuitive, emotional, and multisensory pattern recognition. In common parlance, it's called "gut instinct" or "intuition."

In sports, we want the decision-making process to occur so fast that it combines (1) the know-how to distinguish the key elements of a particular problem, (2) intuition, (3) experience, based on an aggregate of learned conditions and previous exposures, and (4) pattern recognition—we subconsciously recognize factors in the current situation that are similar to a previous one. The macro principles facilitate such decision-making, but in the context and with the direction of the overall game model.

MICRO MOMENTS   2.3.6

When you understand the rationale for identifying the game as four macro moments, you have the opportunity to further refine your understanding by separating each of these moments into three distinct micro moments. Doing so enables us not only to understand what is happening in the game more specifically but also to pinpoint limiting factors, which can then be minimized through training-based learning experiences between games.

Focusing on each micro moment in turn also makes it easier for players to see how effectively they're executing their game plan objectives and to understand how they can do better. Beyond pivotal events—say, a goal scored or missed or a red-card tackle—it's difficult for players to assess their performance across the whole game because of the fog of war and the need to focus intensely in the moment. Using a micro-moment-based approach breaks the game down into more-digestible chunks so that players and coaches can work together to build on positives and identify areas of potential improvement.

The four macro game moments are not always linear and can occur in any order, given the fluid nature of a game. So, for example, a basketball team may start with an offensive possession only to have a defender steal the ball, suddenly starting the offense-to-defense transition. The player who lost the ball recovers, blocking the shot and starting a defense-to-offense transition. This is only one of an almost limitless number of ways in which game moments can be sequenced in competitive play.

In contrast, the micro moments of a game moment are sequential and linear. Each one might last for a shorter or longer period than the others, but the micro moments occur in a certain order if the game moment is allowed to run to completion. So, for example, the attacking team always constructs before it penetrates and penetrates before it executes, even if one or more of these micro moments lasts for just a few seconds. A team may not have the opportunity to go through all the micro moments if the opposition disrupts it, so it could be dispossessed after the construction micro moment of the offensive moment before getting to penetration.[22]

OFFENSIVE MICRO MOMENTS   2.3.6.1

The nature of each team sport dictates how long each offensive micro moment lasts—whether the game is structured or free-flowing, and whether the offense is under time constraints, like a shot

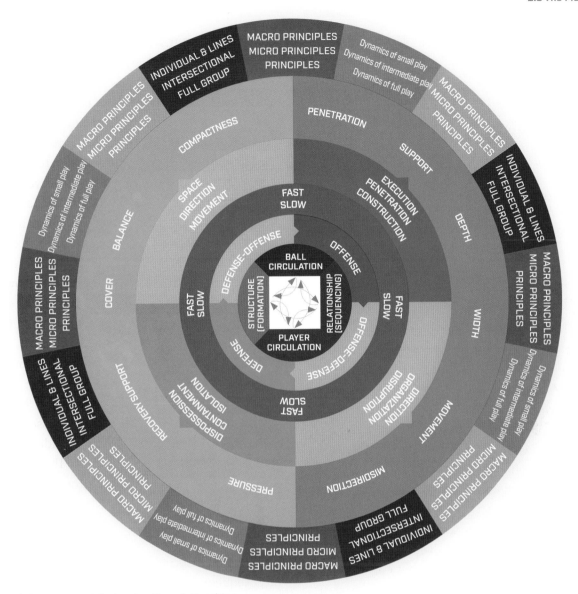

The complete game model, showing the relationships
among macro moments, micro moments, and principles.

clock. Yet regardless of how long the entire offensive moment and its constituent parts last, coaches need to know which micro moments to emphasize on the training ground in order to increase the chances of scoring on game day.

Construction Micro Moment   2.3.6.1.1

During the construction micro moment, the offense is trying to set up the conditions needed for scoring. Foremost among these is creating sufficient functional space—that is, space in which the ball, the players, or both can move. In certain schemes, construction can be a patient stage that sees the attacking team retain possession for long periods, string many passes together, and wait for the defense to leave a gap open or lose its shape. Alternatively, a coach's plan for the construction micro moment might be to strike quickly before the defense is set so that a scoring opportunity can be fashioned before the opponent has a chance to react.

Some teams use the quick-strike tactic only a few times during a game, while for others it is the de facto option. One of the most famous examples is coach Mike D'Antoni's "Seven Seconds or Less" approach with the Phoenix Suns, which saw Steve Nash pick apart defenses across the league on his way to back-to-back NBA MVP titles. More recently, D'Antoni used the evolution of this strategy to transform an underperforming Houston Rockets team into a championship contender.

Penetration Micro Moment   2.3.6.1.2

While the penetration micro moment (getting into scoring range) might involve getting as close to the opposition's goal, basket, or red zone as possible for a high-percentage scoring opportunity—like a two-yard run in football, a soccer tap-in, or a dunk in basketball—it can also be minimal. For example, a rugby team might want to get its best kicker within range for a drop goal, or a basketball team might go to a catch-and-shoot play for its best three-point shooter.

The extent of penetration depends not only on the offense's game objectives but also on how it reacts to what the defense will allow. So if a soccer team starts trying to play long balls into the penalty area but is consistently thwarted by the aerial superiority of two towering center backs, it will have to adapt and try to create greater penetration on the ground.

Execution Micro Moment   2.3.6.1.3

The execution micro moment is about creating the best possible scoring opportunity for the final player to receive the ball at the culmination of an attacking move. In sports such as basketball, in which both teams have many possessions during the game, the results of occasionally failed execution are somewhat less severe. But in sports in which offensive and defensive moments last longer and scoring opportunities are few and far between, execution is far more important—not to mention in the military, where this final offensive micro moment is often quite literally a matter of life and death.

> *The more you prepare beforehand, the more relaxed, creative, and effective you'll be when it counts.*
>
> —Bill Parcells

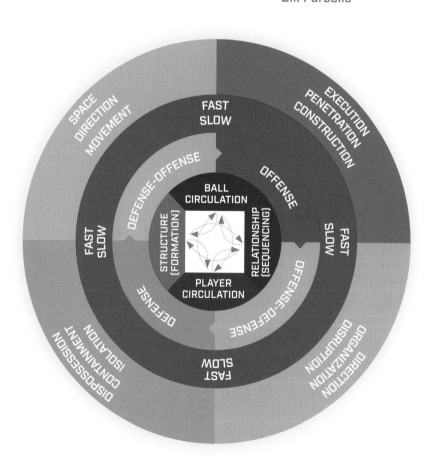

Moments, micro moments, and the influence of ball speed on the phase of play.

AN EMOTIONAL INSTINCT FOR SCORING

When working on offense during practice sessions, the coaching staff should focus most of their time and effort on improving the construction and penetration micro moments and largely let execution become a learning experience. To put it simply, talented attackers in any sport must develop an emotional instinct for scoring.

Those who score are at their most effective when they're focused but at ease and when their instincts can take over to convert scoring opportunities. The coaches can help them by not pressuring them or focusing too much on the final offensive micro moment of execution. If the coaching staff overemphasizes execution, the player taking the shot will feel stressed and anxious, which will only slow decision-making and negatively impact his or her actions.

We see this in penalty shootouts and game-ending free throws, conversions, and field goals. Players choke because the moment and their own expectations are placing too much emphasis on execution.

During all of the offensive micro moments, the more space the attacking team can create, the more time it will have. The more time is available to make decisions, the more relaxed and therefore accurate the player who is trying to score will be.

Slow is smooth and smooth is fast.

—Sniper saying

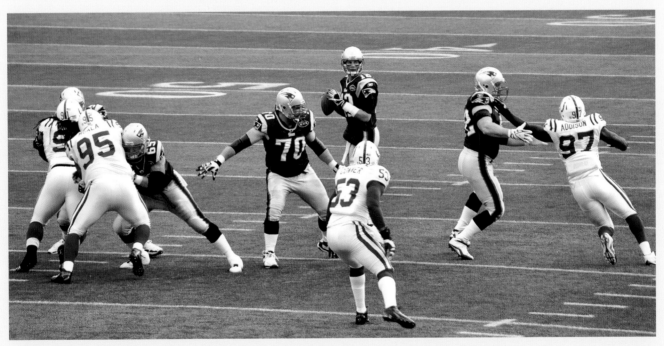

A relaxed but focused Brady looks for an open receiver as his offensive line creates space around him.
Photo by Jack Newton (CC BY-SA).

The more space attacking players have during the execution micro moment, the more time they have and the more likely they are to succeed. The more time players have and the less pressure they are under when taking a shot, the more accurate they typically are. If you give Tom Brady acres of space in the pocket, he's going to pick his spot and find that wide-open receiver with little trouble. This is just as true for military personnel. If a sniper is in the correct position to take a shot and has time to compose himself, he's going to hit the designated target more often than not.

There are, of course, instances in which a player has *too much* time—think of a soccer striker putting her head in her hands after missing an open goal or a basketball guard clanging a wide-open three-pointer off the front of the rim. This is more of an issue for inexperienced players, who can start thinking too much before taking action. But as a rule, teams convert more uncontested scoring opportunities than contested ones, showing the need to create space during the construction micro moment and time the final pass just right.

TRANSITION-TO-DEFENSE MICRO MOMENTS   2.3.6.2

Within the defensive macro moments, there are now smaller micro moments that help us describe the activities that occur within certain phases of the larger moment.

Disruption Micro Moment   2.3.6.2.1

The goal of the transition-to-defense moment is to slow the other team down in order to dispossess them. The first step is disruption: to have at least one player put pressure on the ball and try to stop the player with the ball from proceeding in a straight line to where he or she wants to go. If the momentum of the ball can be halted, it will prevent the offense from creating space and give other defenders the time they need to get back into solid defensive positions. In basketball, we've all seen lazy transitions to defense lead to a breakaway in which the ball handler streaks all the way down the court for an uncontested dunk. What you want is the opposite—rapid ball pressure, everyone sprinting back in transition, and a concerted effort to disrupt what the attacking team wants to do.

Organization Micro Moment   2.3.6.2.2

After the ball changes hands (or feet), the attacking team will try to create chaos and confusion to prevent the defense from settling into its planned defensive setup. To counter this aim, defenders must organize themselves as quickly as possible. This involves players talking to each other, managing the direction of the ball, and then getting into their designated areas in a zone defense or picking up their marking assignments in a man-to-man defense. If it is to prevent the attackers from quickly transitioning through their offensive micro moments and getting a scoring chance, the defensive unit must try to become compact and cohesive immediately.

Direction Micro Moment   2.3.6.2.3

The attacking team will want to get into its opponent's danger zone as quickly as possible so that it gets a high-quality chance to put points on the scoreboard. To prevent this, the defense must force the attackers to change the direction of both player and ball movement. The aim is most often to use the placement of your players and the sideline to force the attackers into confined places—making the field as small as possible for them. This allows progression to the final defensive micro moment, dispossession (see page 48).

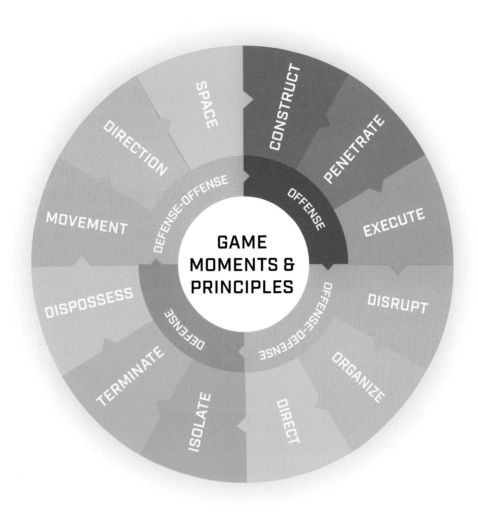

Micro moments and their principles.

TRANSITION-TO-OFFENSE MICRO MOMENTS   2.3.6.3

During the transitional moment from defense, the following micro moments outline the phases that the team goes through to move into offense.

Movement Micro Moment   2.3.6.3.1

When a team captures the ball, it has the advantage, as the opposition will be in disarray and struggling to get back into their defensive scheme. To make the most of this advantage, you have to move quickly to create space and give the defense too many options to consider. This will allow you to move quickly through the offensive micro moments while defend-

ers are still stuck trying to observe what's going on around them and organize themselves. This delays their ability to decide and act, enabling the offense to penetrate and create a scoring chance.

Direction Micro Moment   2.3.6.3.2

The next step in befuddling the defense, once your offense has started moving and advancing the ball, is to create motion in different directions. Using width and depth (i.e., lateral and forward motion) will help create multiple attacking options for players to move the ball into and will confuse and frustrate the defense as it tries to create cohesion and compactness. The concept of direction is used by coaches in all sports during offensive drills, such as three- and five-man weaves in basketball. The more variety there is in direction, the less likely backpedaling defenders are to make the right predictions about where the ball is going to go next.

Space Micro Moment   2.3.6.3.3

Once the offense has initiated movement and used direction to create width and depth, it needs to get players and the ball into space as quickly as possible. The faster space is created and exploited and the larger the functional area that can be used, the more effective the counterattack will be and the more likely it is that a scoring opportunity will be set up and executed successfully.

DEFENSIVE MICRO MOMENTS   2.3.6.4

During the three defensive micro moments explained below, the team without the ball must try to minimize the functional area in which the offense can operate by compressing space. The defense must also aim to restrict ball and player movement and disrupt the offense's game plan as much as possible. Defenders should also aim to be offensively minded, forcing attackers to become reactive rather than proactive and interfering with their decision-making to force errors.

Isolation Micro Moment   2.3.6.4.1

For an offense to get into its rhythm and control the tempo of the game, it must enable multiple players to connect with each other and the ball in sequence. The aim of the defense's isolation micro moment is to prevent this by blocking as many potential pathways for the ball as possible. The defense also needs to cut off offensive players from their teammates and do what it can to disrupt communication among players in the attacking unit. Isolation forces offensive players to switch their focus from achieving their game plan aims to reacting to the actions of the defense.

It is possible for a defensive unit to isolate its foes in a normal defensive scheme, but a temporary, more intense type of defense can also be employed to apply greater pressure. Common examples include a full-court press in basketball, a blanket defense in soccer, and a blitz in American football. Such tactics are often unsustainable for an entire game but, when used correctly, may enable a team to transition through the three defensive micro moments more quickly and effectively.

Termination Micro Moment   2.3.6.4.2

If the defense is able to apply constant pressure to each attacker and limit passing options, it will terminate offensive players' role in the game. This makes it difficult, if not impossible, for the offense to control the tempo of the game. Termination has the side effect of producing frustration and forcing the attacking side to exert more energy to maintain possession. If the defense can keep up its pressure for the duration, it can start to take a toll on the offense in the waning minutes of the game, leading to critical errors that present chances for late winners.

Dispossession Micro Moment   2.3.6.4.3

Once players have been isolated and have no available support from teammates, it is easier to dispossess the attacking team and take control of the ball through a tackle, steal, interception, or turnover. This is where the tactical and technical transition takes place.

THE FOUNDATION: MACRO MOMENTS, MICRO MOMENTS, AND MACRO PRINCIPLES

2.4

As we can see, all games have the same principles of positioning, ball movement, and player movement acting in a complex relationship and sequence. Every team-sports contest transitions between four universal moments, each composed of a series of micro moments. These are generic models that are applicable to all situations, but none dictates a certain method or system of play. Instead, they give us a basis or structure from which we can develop everything else.

The role of micro moments is to allow further analysis of the game in context. Understanding micro moments facilitates the construction of training scenarios and experiences in the exact game manner that allows us to improve them. This is the foundation for everything—team training, nutrition strategy, analysis, statistics, and so on. The next stage is the development of your game model.

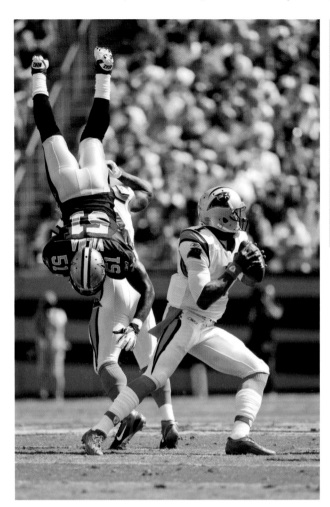

Saints linebacker Jonathan Vilma is flipped while Panthers quarterback Cam Newton sets up to pass.
Photo by Action Sports Photography / Shutterstock.com

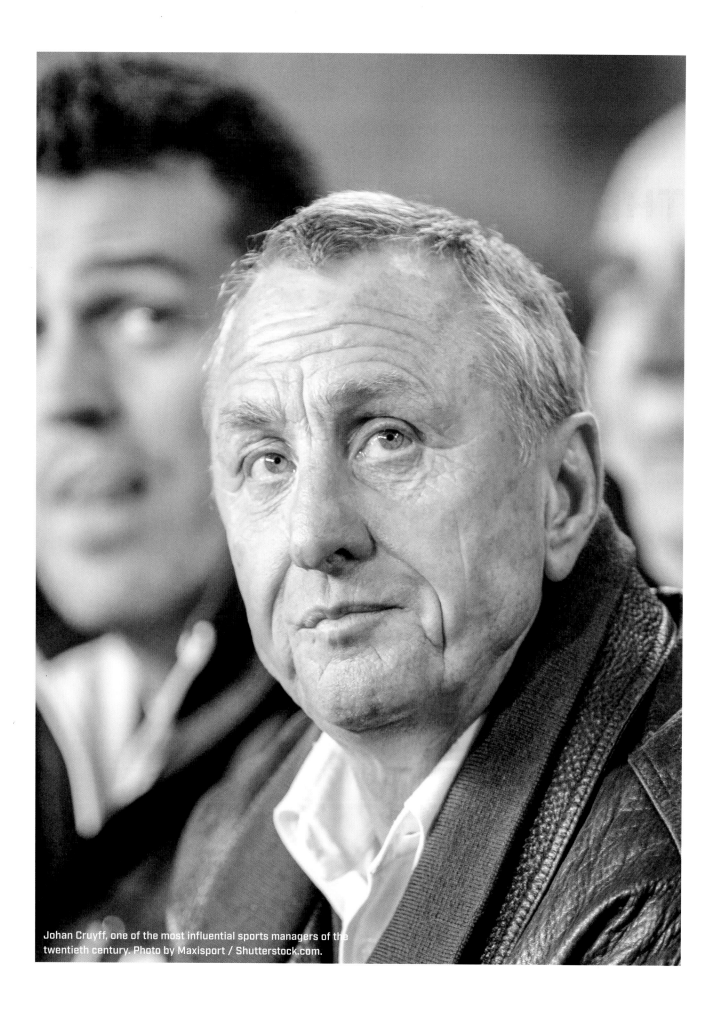
Johan Cruyff, one of the most influential sports managers of the twentieth century. Photo by Maxisport / Shutterstock.com.

THREE

THE MODEL

Now that we understand how the game is seen and have a system with which to analyze it, we can start to plan how to win. To do so, we're going to construct and apply a game model. All teams have one, whether they know it or not. It's a system of play that is derived from a model of how they see their sport and game played.

While it's impossible here to design an individualized game model for every team or sport, I'll explain the optimal approach to winning that's most universally applicable. Don't take my word as gospel, though—challenge, refine, and develop the model to find the best version for your team. Although we keep striving to improve, a perfect model is unattainable because it is constantly being refined. The model guides the process for playing through concrete principles of a collective and an individual nature. These principles develop the collective organization while individual players express them in a pattern of behavior, decided on by the coach with a team objective in mind, using principles of play during various moments of the game.

> *To me, the most important aspect in my teams is to have a defined game model, a set of principles that provides organization.*
>
> —José Mourinho

> *All models are wrong, some are useful. The problem is to determine how wrong the model is before it is no longer useful.*
>
> —George Box

Here are some of the characteristics of the game model:

- It's a dynamic, living, and evolving idea.
- It's the way the team philosophy emerges on the field of play.
- It's something observable that identifies and distinguishes itself.
- It's always open-ended.

DEVELOPMENT OF A GAME MODEL

3.1

As we develop a game model, it's important to recognize that this model encompasses all areas of performance, from tactics to physical training. As we develop it, we will see how it respects the theories of chaos and complexity.

Development of a game model is something of a study in ethnomethodology, which can be defined as the study of the everyday methods people use to help explain their worldview and the social order. The approach was originally developed by Harold Garfinkel, who attributed its origin to his work investigating the conduct of jury members in 1954. In a sporting context, it's a process that teams use to explain the game and game model.

The idea of a game model was best expressed by José Guilherme Oliveira, the Portuguese professor whose tactical periodization approach profoundly influenced José Mourinho, Jorge Jesus, Aitor Karanka, and other coaches in this golden age of Portuguese soccer management. Oliveira wrote:

> The model of play is an idea, a conjecture of the game consisting of principles, sub-principles, sub-sub-principles...representing the different stages and phases of the game, which hang together, manifesting on its own a functional organization, or an identity. This model, as a true model, is always assumed as a conjecture and is permanently open to individual and collective additions, so it is in permanent construction. It is never, nor will it be, a given object. The final model is always unattainable, because it is always under evolving reconstruction.[23]

What is the game? How is it played? How should it be assessed? These are three fundamental questions that this section seeks to answer. They may seem like basic questions with simple answers, and yet, even at the highest echelon of sports, many people fail to ask them. And it is only by evaluating the principles, moments, and micro moments of any game that we can better understand how to achieve the primary aim of all teams: winning.

THE EMPEROR HAS NO CLOTHES   3.1.1

One of the central contentions of this book is that sports science, analytics, and technology have not delivered on their overinflated promises. A fundamental reason why they're not being applied correctly is that very few people truly understand the

The less versatile you are, the better you have to be at what you do well.

—Bill Belichick

theater in which team sports are played out—namely, the game itself. If coaches, players, and staff can't comprehend what we're seeing when we look at and try to evaluate the game, how on earth are we going to apply the lessons and methodology of sports science to it effectively?

The simple answer, of course, is that we're not. Or we're going to utilize them in the wrong way. We will also be unable to adequately prepare athletes and teams or structure team-sports organizations appropriately if we fail to comprehend the game at its most elemental level. This is why there is a need for a game model.

For all the statistics and tracking that are now prevalent in team sports, particularly at the elite level, there is widespread failure to diagnose problems and then find and apply the correct solutions. In our fervor to gather more and more data, we're focusing too much on the *quantity* of outcomes at the expense of assessing the *quality* of what occurs during the game. Simply looking at metrics is useless if they're not evaluated in context and if we forget to match them up with subjective and qualitative interpretations. We're in danger of losing our way in pages of numbers that, when taken at face value, have little bearing on how games are contested, won, and lost. This book represents an attempt to remedy the situation.

By seeing what is truly happening on the playing field, court, or pitch through a game model, my hope is that you'll be able to create a more effective game plan, see which aspects of it work and which don't, and make the necessary corrections before the next contest. This will lead to continual improvement of individual athletes and the team through more effective, game-focused preparation, which in turn will positively influence game-day results.

THE CHAOS OF TEAM-SPORTS SCIENCE 3.1.2

When looking at team sports through the construct of the game model, I freely admit that there are elements that contribute to winning and losing that we simply cannot understand—this is why such a model is critical. Every game also unfolds at a speed that makes it impossible to process what's going on in its entirety. There are so many interactions—at the team level, between teammates, and in individual matchups with opponents—that they'll render us helpless if we try to examine them in totality.

That's why we need to establish a framework and principles by which we can better evaluate the elements that compose any sporting contest. Even though we can't hope to fully quantify or measure every single facet of the game—particularly those intangibles involving players' emotions and motivations and the complex interactions among biological and neurological processes—we can at least implement a blueprint that acknowledges each of them.

The perfect game model isn't obtainable, because if it were, there'd be no more quibbling over coaching methods, preparation and recovery, or strategy and tactics. But you can construct the right game model for your team. This allows you not only to better understand and evaluate the game but also to reduce the negative effects that arise from the frictions of the game—the things we cannot plan for once two opposing sides clash (see page 61).

We cannot hope to re-create reality or the perfect game in training because what happens during a game is in many ways random, just as life is random. Plus, there are an almost infinite number of possible scenarios. But if we can learn to understand the game on a deeper level, we can accurately evaluate each team's and athlete's performance within its construct. Then we'll be able to help players prepare more appropriately by creating realistic learning experiences that directly apply to game-day scenarios.

Despite the limitations of any plan, we can still use a game model to assess performance in a more holistic and sophisticated way than in the past, and use this all-encompassing analysis to inform real-world practice. The better each team and its players are prepared, the more able they are to focus on the unexpected events that occur in every game, and the less overwhelmed they will be in the thick of the action. This is just as applicable to warrior-athletes, although their learning experiences—such as mock hostage situations—are preparing them for contests with much higher stakes.

For the individual, richer preparation for either game day or combat allows more of the functional reserve to be left intact for adapting to new situations and for easier orientation during individual moments in the game (more on this when we start discussing John Boyd's OODA Loop / the observation-action cycle on page 126). When extrapolated to the team level, this means better decision-making and more successful outcomes, no matter the sport. But before we get to this point, we need to back up and identify what the game truly is and what it is not. Only then can we work backward to the athletes, team, and organization.

TEAM IDENTITY 3.2

We must remember that from the environment, the team's identity emerges. Former Porto and Chelsea players have said that while José Mourinho's principles didn't change for specific matches, his game model was adaptable, so he would present them with dossiers on their opponents. "One of the most important aspects about José, which I support, is that the other team has to be the one making the changes, you have to keep your own identity," said former Porto defender Francisco Costinha. "Of course, he would give us detailed information about the team we were facing next at the start of the training week and more precisely about the player that would be closest to our area of play. 'What was the player like? Did he have a tendency to get many cards? What kind of movements did he make?' It was new for many of us back then, but it was very helpful and meant we were much better prepared for each match."[24] While Mourinho altered his tactics depending on the habits and preferences of each opponent, his team's identity remained constant.

CULTURE AND ENVIRONMENT 3.2.1

Most people ignore the reality that the actual environment and location of a team is the origin of all game models. The model for every team must be born from the people to whom it is most exposed.

> *The best way to find yourself is to lose yourself in the service of others.*

—Mahatma Gandhi

Do not confuse this with the team players, who are secondary to the environment.

A manager who arrives at a new team and attempts to impose a game model must first understand the nature of the majority of the people in the building, to whom the players will be exposed on a daily basis. The local culture will be a constant presence for the team—for example, if the team is located in a working-class area, the values and culture of the area will affect the players. This does not mean the coach must resort to a working-class style, but he or she must respect its constant influence and develop a game model that respects it and emerges in the societal context.

Here's a real-world example: Basketball "purists" in the Midwest are used to a slower, more player-dominated offense and often sniff at the run-and-gun playground style of inner cities, which is less structured and played at a much faster pace. Or look at Brazil's fast, highly skilled soccer players, who grew up playing either in small urban spaces or on the beach. They also played a lot of five-a-side futsal, which emphasizes rapid ball movement. So the tempo at which they play is a lot different from that of English or German players who grew up playing on full-sized pitches and in wide-open parks.

COHERENCE 3.2.2

The most critical aspect of a game model is coherence. This means that all principles and, in turn, methods must be coherent with each other and not conflict. These all evolve from the environment and culture of the people who make up the team. In the game model, it means that all principles must complement, not oppose, one another.

The most successful teams I've worked with have had a clear identity and clear coherence of game principles. This is observed as the team's playing identity, which has evolved from its history.

It may be useful to think of the team as a family. A family has some of the characteristics of and is influenced by its predecessors, but each generation has its own distinct identity. Now I want to underline that culture and identity can also impact formation of the game model.

Once this model has been created, there must be a single coherent message throughout the entire organization and even in the game plan, strategy, and tactics. This need for coherence begins at the game model.

MACRO AND MICRO PRINCIPLE COHERENCE 3.2.2.1

Game principles, macro principles, and micro principles must be cohesive, complementary, and not contradictory. This facilitates clear teaching of the game model and allows players to own it and then in time develop the model for themselves. Players selected, recruited, or drafted must have the personality to execute the game model. Think of players who didn't fit in on certain teams. Often this isn't because of their skillsets but because of their attitudes, emotions, and psychologies. The game model doesn't exist in isolation as a tactical model. As we will see later, it is an entity that uses and exploits emotional and personal attributes.

Think of a traditionally skillful team, or one whose identity is rooted in its physicality. It encourages that image, and players aspire to uphold it. So rugby players on a physical team will want to tackle hard and intimidate their opponents. Players on a skillful soccer team like Brazil will try to run rings around the opposition with tricks and fancy footwork. The game model tends to reflect this, and players who best match this model will play best for it.

When players understand the game objectives and try to advance the principles, sub-principles, and sub-sub-principles outlined, they start to understand and eventually expect each other's actions. This eventually leads to the emergence of a coherent level of play.

For a defensive or offensive unit to achieve its aims within the game plan, it must function as one. We often hear commentators deriding a shooting guard who fires at will, taking wild shots over multiple defenders at the expense of passing to open teammates. Such criticism is leveled because this player isn't playing within the team's cohesive plan of attack—or maybe the plan was inadequate to begin with.

THE COHESION CODE   3.2.3

Cohesion is also an essential part of a team's game plan to thwart its opponent. Pioneering military strategist John Boyd said that if the game plan is set and acted upon, it's easier to "generate uncertainty, confusion, disorder, panic, chaos…to shatter cohesion, produce paralysis and bring about collapse" in your opponent.[25]

Shattering a foe's cohesion on the playing field or battlefield isolates them and takes them out of the team concept completely. Pressuring a player and cutting her off from her teammates clouds her judgment, slows her decision-making, and prevents her from executing her objectives. Preventing cohesion forces the opponent to decrease its chances of success and increase the number and severity of errors it makes. In this way, disrupting the opponent's cohesion is every bit as important as creating and maintaining it within your own team and unit.

GAME MODEL AND LANGUAGE   3.2.4

In order for the game model to be used effectively, those involved in its creation, implementation, and assessment must be aware of certain core concepts that impact how the game is played. It's imperative that we establish common terms that can be used across the organization. This is significant when considering all the different roles and expertise of front-office and back-office personnel.

Many times, terminology is wielded in different and contradictory ways. Take the term *speed*. An American football fan might think of speed in terms of a player's forty-yard dash time at the NFL Combine, or the top speed reached in some in-game stat. A strength and conditioning coach will be thinking of explosive power, while the wide receivers coach might be planning how to get his unit to complete their routes faster. The team physio is considering how a player's old ACL injury might be limiting his speed and what techniques she can deploy to return the player to his old self. The head coach could well have yet another interpretation.

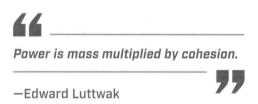

Power is mass multiplied by cohesion.

—Edward Luttwak

While we can't (and shouldn't) completely change specialists' mindsets about the connotation of certain terms, we can at least establish some elemental language that all areas of the organization can use to assess player and team performance on game day and then to work backward to enhance the team's preparation so that they keep improving. In order for communication to be effortless among the various roles and levels of the organization, we must define the right lexicon to describe the game itself.

ORGANIZATION AND COMMUNICATION COHERENCE

3.2.5

Communication is a vital component of cohesion and coherence. For a team to deploy its game plan effectively, a cohesive, clear, and consistent message must flow among all levels of the organization in an unconscious, subliminal manner. Such a message can be conveyed effectively only if the lexicon is understood in all disciplines and units. Using precise, clear, and universally agreed-upon language to discuss the game, how to prepare for it, how to evaluate it, and which adjustments to make afterward is of even greater significance in the multicultural and multilingual locker rooms that exist in all team sports today, from college to the pros.

When special operatives are engaged in combat, there's no time to say something twice or have hesitation or ambiguity. Clarity of language has also become more necessary than ever in professional sports like soccer, where there are often several nationalities represented on each team and the "same" word in multiple languages can not only mean different things but also imply different levels of emphasis.

GAME PRINCIPLES

3.3

As we've seen, every game has a series of moments. Within each macro moment, a team and its players have a goal they achieve through the use of the macro principles. These are key tenets underlying and anchoring something that appears random—in this case, a team's collective performance. A principle isn't a lengthy treatise but rather a clear, concise definition of an action or series of actions with a goal.

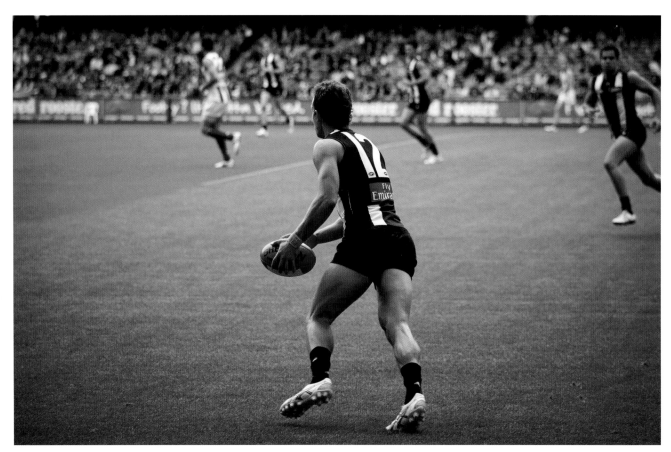

Luke Ball, capturing the cohesion of principles and moments. Photo by Neale Cousland / Shutterstock.com.

The objectives for any team in every sport are:

Objective 1: When in possession, score.

Objective 2: When not in possession, get possession. Then see objective 1.

Go to any playground or watch any NBA or NFL game and that's the summary. The game model is a model for how these objectives are met. But as we break the game down into macro moments, we can be more specific about the principles in each moment.

BASIS FOR THE MACRO PRINCIPLE SYSTEM   3.3.1

By establishing principles for each macro moment, we clearly outline what the tasks are for the team as a whole. This has the added benefit of making goals and principles team focused. Note that I haven't mentioned anything about a specific sport or team

Obey the principles without being bound by them.

—Bruce Lee

yet in discussing the game model. Why? Because it doesn't matter. The job of every coach and player is to win, so the sport and team are irrelevant. Sure, we'd prefer if players in certain roles performed exactly as planned, but things can and will go wrong during the game, and so we have to compromise. The concept of using principles like this comes from *schwerpunkt*, a German term meaning "organizational focus." *Schwerpunkt*, John Boyd wrote, "represents a unifying medium that provides a directed way to tie initiative of many subordinate actions with superior intent as a basis to diminish friction and compress time."[26]

WHAT IS A WIN?

A primary goal of any coach, player, and team is obviously to win as many games as possible. But coming out ahead on the scoreboard is only one validation of the game model and its execution. A world-class team playing against one from a lower division in a cup competition can play poorly and win on the scoreboard but not class the result as a win. The execution of the game plan may have been sloppy and inefficient, and so the coach and team might be disappointed in their performance. On the other hand, a lesser-quality team might have executed the game plan, strategy, and tactics to the best of their potential and consider the game a win despite scoring fewer points.

We shouldn't discount the significance of winning, but neither should it be the only thing that matters. If a team plays better than it did the game before, then that's a small victory, even if it loses. Similarly, if the players implement the game plan, execute well, and still lose, they've done all they can. How the coach chooses to frame such advances can help determine whether the team will keep progressing. (More on this to come in "The Coach," starting on page 347.)

SCHWERPUNKT   3.3.2

The origin of the game model system and its facilitation have been heavily influenced by conflict approaches. The reason is that no other domains face challenges as serious and complex as military forces. *Schwerpunkt* was originally a German military idea that essentially helped direct military strategy toward singular aims without preventing ground troops from taking the initiative.

In effective teams, *schwerpunkt* connects players and groups of players who are working concurrently and at several levels. The players close to the action operate in tactical situations, and teammates operate in bigger supporting roles. These groupings of players act in sequence and harmony with each other. When everything is on a similar level, feedback from tactical actions guide decisions at every level, and vice versa. Ultimately, *schwerpunkt* results in a focused achievement, such as when a rugby team breaks through a gap that opens for just a second to score a try despite the defense focusing intently on trying to stop them.

The important point of *schwerpunkt* is that the micro principles of the offensive moment—such as misdirection, movement, or support, which we'll explore later on—must all be focused and aligned to achieve a singular objective. It's key for coaches to develop principles in a way that is both cohesive and complementary. Games, like war, are interactive. An advance leads to a retreat. Taking fire leads to returning fire. For every action there is an equal and opposite reaction, the response to which must be managed. By establishing the aims as team aims, we set the goal as a team target. Later we can establish the individual roles and responsibilities needed to achieve this, but these are not the starting point.

COMMANDER'S INTENT   3.3.3

The game plan is the collection of objectives and aims that a team and its individual players have for each contest. But the overarching aim of any athlete or warrior-athlete engagement couldn't be simpler or more obvious: to win. We call this the Commander's Intent. All other aims are secondary to this—and they must be cohesive with it.

It's a surprising truth that in team sports, the Commander's Intent sometimes becomes obscured. When we fail to create a plan in which all roads lead to this big-picture imperative, players, coaches, and staff can start chasing aims that subvert or even sabotage such an intention and the sub-goals below it. Take, for example, the selfish striker whose hunger for goals means that she virtually ignores her fellow attackers, choosing to pepper the opponent's goal with hopeless shots from impossible angles instead of setting up teammates who are in much better scoring positions.

It's not just players themselves who can short-circuit the Commander's Intent. Occasionally position coaches confuse the directives from the head coach and cause confusion among his or her team unit (such as the defensive line in football or the backs in rugby). The overreliance on statistics in recent years has led many teams down rabbit holes that they believe will lead to better game-day performance but instead merely divert attention from things that have a real impact on the scoreboard.

For example, soccer teams remain far too fixated on the number of meters each player covers in the game, a metric that has leaked into on-screen statistics and colored fans' views of player effort. Such a number fails to take into account that in some ways, team sports are like a boxing match, in which the fighters move back and forth across the ring together. If a right back is marking a winger for ninety minutes in a soccer match and the attacking player makes repeated long forays into her opponent's half, then the defender has little choice but to follow. Similarly, if the right back then pushes up to support her team when they're on the attack, her "meters run" number will continue to climb until the final whistle (more on this kind of misleading metric later in this section).

The next game may see the same right back playing against a team that lacks an active attacker on the right side, preferring instead to penetrate down the middle. Or maybe the opposition's tactics won't allow this player to move forward on counterattacks anymore. Suddenly, her end-of-game total is down by a couple of thousand meters.

The coaching staff (not to mention the team's supporters) now assume that the right back didn't put in as much effort or that she lacks stamina. So now the team dials up her endurance training, leading to overexertion and a season-ending hamstring injury. A false, statistics-driven impression led to a decision that runs afoul of the law of unintended consequences, and suddenly the team is less likely to achieve the Commander's Intent of winning its last three games of the year.

COHERENCE BEATS CONFUSION

3.3.4

Frequently coaches give players too many aims within the game plan. Of course, a lot of concepts can be covered during practices in the days leading up to the next fixture, as the coaching staff creates learning experiences applicable to attacking, defending, and transitioning. But on game day itself, even the most intelligent, cerebral players do not have the capacity to focus on a long list of objectives once the ball is in play. This is also true of soldiers going into combat—perhaps more so, given the life-or-death pressure exerted upon them.

Giving athletes too much information stagnates their decision-making and spreads their physical and mental efforts too thin. It also increases the chances of mistakes and causes fatigue—a problem in sports and a potentially fatal issue for military personnel. That's why the most effective coaches and military commanders never give their players or soldiers more than three aims for competition or battle. These should be so clear and simple that the player can easily repeat them back if asked by a coach, "What are you going to achieve in today's game?"

The first should be the Commander's Intent: "win the game." The second could be focusing on an attacking target for the player's unit, such as when a basketball team's front line is told to secure more offensive rebounds than the opposition. The third could be limiting a tendency or strength of the other team, such as when a rugby team is told, "Don't let player X break away." In an effective game plan, all smaller objectives are stark in their simplicity and descend from the Commander's Intent.

Each game moment will have an objective (micro principle) that is subservient to the team's overarching aim for the game. If achieved, it will increase the chances of achieving the main objective. So, for example, a soccer team might state that in the defensive moment, the micro principle is "prevent possession in the penalty area." Or a basketball team may outline "get to the rim" as its main priority for the offense-to-defense transition moment.

When it comes to outlining objectives for the team, its units (e.g., the receivers in football, the forwards in rugby, the guards in basketball, and the midfielders in soccer), and its individual players, function should trump form. Often, a team will try to copy the style of a successful opponent. This is a mistake on several levels. First, it doesn't have the same personnel. And second, the championship-winning squad it's trying to emulate isn't necessarily winning consistently because of its style. Rather, its way of playing is a by-product of the game plan objectives being executed correctly.

YOU DON'T KNOW WHAT YOU DON'T KNOW

3.3.4.1

The starting point for all performance is function and the achievement of goals, not technique or style. The best example was Michael Johnson's running form. People became obsessed with his unusually upright posture and short, super-efficient stride pattern, but they were missing the point. His focus was not on running in an upright position with a quick stride—that is, form—but instead on going faster—function. He found that he could beat all comers with a certain form, so he adopted it to fit his functional goals. The results are indisputable—breaking Pietro Mennea's sixteen-year-old two-hundred-meter world record by a remarkable four-tenths of a second and capturing the four-hundred-meter world record and four Olympic gold medals.

Or look at high jump pioneer Dick Fosbury. Until he came along, every athlete was using either the scissors or straddle method in the event. But Fosbury couldn't get as high as he wanted with either, so he broke the mold by going over the bar backward.

This led to his claiming the American and Olympic records in winning gold at the 1968 Olympics and, more importantly, completely revolutionized the high jump. Fosbury's goal was not to do something new but rather to jump as high as possible. Again, he adapted his form to meet his functional objective.

Going back to team sports, it's the responsibility of the coaching staff to similarly put function above form. The coaches should give their players functional goals within the game plan and then empower them to use whatever form is needed—concocted from their skills, experience, and creativity—to achieve them. The use of specificity has no place within game plan objectives. Coaches can tell players what their goals are but should not tell them exactly how to achieve them. This is for the athlete to determine during the game itself, and how each aim is achieved should not be a cause of concern to the coaching staff as long as goals are met and the player's technique is not harming them.

Instead of issuing direct "thou shalt do it this way" orders, a coach should try to help his or her players form positive habits by creating realistic experiences during individual and team training. By preparing players in such situations, the coach will help them reinforce motor patterns that are accessed automatically and unconsciously on game day. Athletes should be told as little as possible about the drills they participate in and should instead be allowed to learn through discovery.

The accumulation of this training-ground experience leads to faster and more informed decision-making, which not only increases the likelihood of achieving game plan aims but also reduces the mental and physical strain accumulated throughout the course of the game. If players know what to do and have done it many times before, they will be less anxious and stressed, so their body systems will be better able to focus on execution instead of managing negative emotions.

With the correct game plan and the use of my game model to assess the concepts in this section and the four game moments, the common mistakes of overplanning, setting contradictory goals, and undermining the Commander's Intent can be avoided. By keeping the ultimate aim in mind, assigning a small number of goals to each player and team unit, and making sure these sub-objectives contribute to the imperative of winning, teams will be able to outline, communicate, and execute their objectives more effectively.

THE BAUHAUS RULE

The Bauhaus was an art school in Germany that combined crafts and fine arts and was famous for the approach to design articulated by its founder, Walter Gropius. Its motto was quite clear and pragmatic: Form follows function. The belief was that if an item was created first to be functional and effective, its style or form would naturally evolve. There is a perception that in sports, style is important or a predesigned act. The reality is that it develops out of function. Never be confused; in sports, as at the Bauhaus school, form follows function.

THE FOG OF THE GAME   3.3.5

In the heat of battle or a sporting contest, there is so much going on and so much information to process at high speed that athletes have to maintain laserlike focus on the moment just to compete or, in the military context, to survive. This is why it's so difficult for warrior-athletes to recall precisely what happened afterward and why their accounts often differ.

The dissonance is enhanced by the extreme mental, physical, and emotional toll that a military operation or, to a lesser degree, sports game takes on the participants. The fog of war (or fog of the game) is one of the reasons coaches rely so much on film to analyze what happened, find limiting factors, and create training scenarios to reduce their impact on the next game.

THE FRICTIONS OF THE GAME

3.3.6

Even the most disciplined team going into a game in a high state of readiness and preparedness cannot control the unpredictable elements that inevitably manifest themselves from the first second the ball goes into play. Events resulting from the random, chaotic nature of team sports and military conflict are often referred to as *frictions*.

The best way to prepare a team to handle these frictions is to prepare thoroughly during training so that, as a coach, you're in command of the things that you can control and influence on game day.

War is the realm of uncertainty; three quarters of the factors on which action in war is based are wrapped in a fog of greater or lesser uncertainty.

—Carl von Clausewitz

Sometimes, a lot of factors in team sports appear to be random and thus uncontrollable. But if coaches and their scouts can look a little closer at team performance, they'll notice more factors that at first appeared to be variable and yet have patterns.

The same impacts of frictions are found in ordinary life. Suppose a particular route is the fastest way to work each morning. The annoying thing is that several times a week, it becomes traffic-jammed and you have to choose an alternative. The jams happen at different times of day, so they appear to be random. But one day, you start to write down the times that you are able to get to work fast or are stuck in traffic. You soon realize that on certain days and times, due to circumstances that you don't completely understand, there is a pattern to the seemingly chaotic events. So now you see that the seemingly random problem—traffic jams—does in fact have a pattern and is therefore somewhat manageable.

The same is true on game day. If coaches and scouts break the analysis down into the four macro moments and individual events and ask players what was going on in certain situations, they'll likely discover that they are less subject to the frictions of the game than at first glance. This will then leave the team free to concentrate on those factors that are truly outside of their control.

Everything in war is very simple, but the simplest thing is difficult.

—Carl von Clausewitz

Walking and talking athletes through as many scenarios as possible and having them mentally rehearse strategies for adversity and surprise, as Bob Bowman did with Michael Phelps in preparing him to capture a record-setting Olympic medal haul, will help the team feel confident in any circumstance. Such preparation will also enable warrior-athletes to avoid wasting invaluable energy panicking when faced with the frictions of the game and will help them better manage their emotions.

INTENDED, ACTUAL, PERCEIVED, AND OBSERVED ACTIONS

3.3.7

Based on our understanding of chaos theory, we know that as you watch a game, you're seeing an outcome of complex interactions and intentions. You're seeing an evolution, not a planned event.

It's true that depending on your familiarity and experience with the sport (not least if you've played or coached), you might assume certain things about the reasons behind certain actions or about the style of play. You may watch an NFL game and see your favorite team run a lot of plays through the middle or down the wing. These are examples of observed actions. Of course, where and how you are viewing affects this. Watching a game on TV, you will be shown more action around the ball. But when you attend a game in person, you can see the whole playing area and contributing actions off the ball.

You may observe certain patterns—the quarterback being forced to throw sooner than appears normal or a team's midfielders making a lot of runs out wide—and form an assumption about what the coach and players intended. This illustrates some of the differences between intended, actual, perceived, and observed actions. For any action in a sporting contest, there's what the coach instructed, what the player understood, what the opposition allowed, and what you perceived—all of which can be very different. This underlines how complex and difficult it is to interpret a performance correctly.

It is no different from a recipe that is written by chef, interpreted by a home cook, and then tasted by a hungry son or daughter. The intended, perceived, and actual results don't always line up.

LAWS OF THE TEAM GAME
3.4

Over the years, I've come to recognize a number of basic laws as critical to winning in team sports. These fundamental laws of winning must be part of a coherent overall game model.

THE LAW OF EXPECTED EMERGENCE
3.4.1

There is one universal law in team sports: success is dependent on the ability to execute skills in a chaotic environment against an enemy who will expect them. This is in essence the summation or refinement of team sports. You know what your enemy will most likely do and what it will resort to, and you must stop it. The other key thing to remember is that because there is more and more visual information about every play you and your opponent have made, there are no longer any secrets. On the positive side, this makes it easier for your team to know what to expect

of its next opponent, but it also means the opposing team is more likely to know your team's tendencies, preferences, and habits. The law of expected emergence states that experts will execute in competition based on the instincts they've developed and what they anticipate is about to happen.

> "
> *Every art should become science, and every science should become art.*
>
> —Friedrich von Schlegel
> "

Your only task is to do what you've done repeatedly, faster and better than your opponent (who expects it) can stop you from doing it. The only differences as the season goes on are that the pressure—internal or external, perceived or real—increases, as does the chaos created by circumstance and the opponent.

If you are going to try to stop Steph Curry or Alex Morgan, you know what they are going to do—there is an expected emergence from the chaos and game. The challenge is actually stopping them from doing it.

THE LAW OF INDIVIDUAL INFLUENCE
3.4.2

The fact remains that not all players are equal. In team sports, there is a need to reduce the influence of the key players. Jiang Ziya (Lü Shang), a Chinese noble in the eleventh century BC, was the first strategist to explain the unequal importance of individuals in a group. In any team, not all players are equal. This holds true for all other areas, too. The law of individual influence states that because not all players are equal, select players can express unequal influence on a game. This ultimately dismisses the myth that we should or can treat all players equally in terms of performance (though of course we must still try to preserve the health and well-being of every member of the squad).

You definitely go through a stage, most coaches do, where you see a good player and you get enamored, you really like what the player does, but then when you put him into your system, it's not quite the same player that he was in another system. He has some strengths, but you can't utilize all those strengths. If you try to utilize all his strengths, you end up weakening a lot of other players who are already in your system.

—Bill Belichick

It's also a fact that not all injuries are the same. If the Cleveland Cavaliers lost any of their bench players for the year, they'd probably still be okay. But if LeBron James were to suffer a season-ending injury, the Cavs would have little to no chance of winning the NBA championship. The same applies even in sports that feature a greater number of players on the field. No Peyton Manning, far less hope of a Denver Broncos Super Bowl victory in 2016. Few teams have the resources and depth to persevere and survive without their star players. Some that do, like the All Blacks, have incredibly intense practices, but this is not the norm.

THE LAW OF SPACE AND TIME   3.4.3

Space creates time, but time cannot always create space. The most important law in all sports, regardless of moment, context, or micro moment, is the law of space and time. Often you hear people refer to an athlete who seems to have more time on the ball, or a player who creates time for others. In reality, what is being referred to here is the creation of space. Time and space are both created using the four macro principles of team sport. The law of space and time states that space can create time. This law is not reversible in sports—time does not necessarily create space.

To create space in one area, we compress players in another. We move the players through force, the ball, or misdirection. Phillip Meilinger suggested that this is "based on the premise that telescoping time—arriving at decisions or locations rapidly—is the decisive element in war because of the enormous psychological strain it places on an enemy."[27]

Olympic and NBA-championship-winning coach Chuck Daly summed up the vital importance of this when he said, "Offense is spacing and spacing is offense." When a quarterback drops back into the pocket, the more time he has to look downfield and evaluate his passing options, the more likely he is to convert the pass. In this scenario and others like it, space creates time rather than the other way around.

TECHNIQUE, SPACE, AND TIME   3.4.3.1

All great players appear to have more time than their peers. This generally comes down to the ability to create space. The greatest athletes—Michael Jordan, Mia Hamm, Zinedine Zidane, Richie McCaw, Joe Montana—could all create space through the execution of superior technique.

Better technique creates space (and therefore time) in two ways. First, it can make players more biomechanically efficient than their opponents. Simply put, they can move faster and with less effort. Second, the superior athlete enters and exploits the opponent's decision-making cycle. In simple terms, he or she makes the opponent think. Thinking causes a pause. Pause and you're dead.

Space and time aren't just created by physical attributes like speed. Technically, players can apply movement, balance, and misdirection on an individual basis. Or, tactically, they can use strategies to do the same in the team context, with the ultimate goal of creating space and, therefore, more time to act.

CONTROLLING SPACE: EFFECTIVE FIELD

3.4.3.2

The total size of the pitch, court, or field is virtually irrelevant. What is truly significant is how much *usable* area, or *effective field*, there is. A team that's on the attack can create a larger effective field through movement.

When in the offensive moment or defense-to-offense moment, effective field is often defined as the space that the person with the ball can pass or move into. This varies by player, position, and sport. From a defensive perspective, the goal is the opposite—to limit effective field by closing down space and restricting movement.

Effective field can be represented graphically with circles around attacking players. The edge of the circle represents the limit of each player's passing range or the area he or she can run into. The circles can be color-coded to show the fact that players are typically more accurate the closer they are to the intended recipient, although in the case of excellent long-ball players, like David Beckham, there are exceptions.

The future is uncertain...but this uncertainty is at the very heart of human creativity.

—Ilya Prigogine

Faster athletes and those with greater passing abilities will have bigger circles.

Some coaches have taken this approach to new heights. The prime example is "Clarko's Cluster" in Australian rules football. Hawthorn Hawks coach Alastair Clarkson, aka Clarko, recognized that a traditional fifteen-man zone wasn't helping his team win games, so he came up with a radical new concept: a grid formation that closes in like a vise around the player with the ball and prevents him from doing anything within his effective field area. If the opponent passes wide, then the Hawk's defense converges on this wing. The only way to counter this unusual tactic is to move the ball very quickly outside the perimeter of the cluster, something few

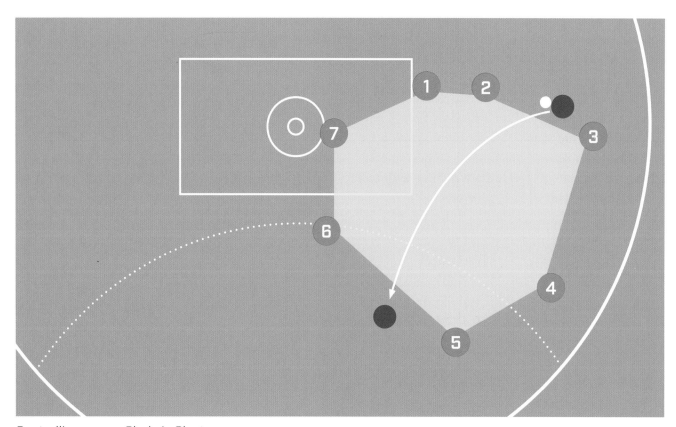

Controlling space: Clarko's Cluster.

teams have done successfully against Clarko and his now-famous tactic. As former AFL player-turned-commentator Gerard Healy has said, "Take on the grid in the corridor at your peril."[28]

THE LAW OF BALL SPEED   3.4.4

The concept of ball speed or target speed is a critical aspect of any game or sport, as it determines many subsequent actions and reactions. When it comes to analyzing game play and tactical play, we see what are referred to as *fast ball* and *slow ball*. In football, this is not the ball-throwing speed but the length of time between the snap and the handoff or pass. Certain elements, like whether the quarterback executes a five- or seven-step drop-back, impact this ball speed.

The law of ball speed states that the complexity and rate of all decision-making are determined by ball speed, not player speed. In rugby this can be the speed with which the backline moves and passes the ball, while in soccer it can be a combination of passing and dribbling speeds. Every sport has its own ball speed. But remember, this is not solely the actual speed of a single pass or player running; it's also the combination of pass and transport, carry, and dribble.

Why? The ball is the key target in the action play, and it determines the tempo of both actions and decision-making. Ball speed naturally affects the length of each game moment and the micro moments within it, effectively setting a rhythm of play. The choice of either fast ball or slow ball also influences how quickly the defensive team must act.

FAST BALL   3.4.4.1

Teams like Real Madrid, Fiji, and South Africa's rugby sevens team and the Golden State Warriors are effective in large part because they play fast. This enables them to make rapid, instinctive, subconscious decisions when there is no time to think. Fast ball is not more physically or mentally demanding if the game model is clear. Yet fast ball can wear down the opposition, leaving them too tired physically and mentally to implement their game plan.

SLOW BALL   3.4.4.2

Slow ball can be a very effective method, too. It can promote frustration among opponents, and with ill-disciplined teams the tendency to commit errors increases when frustration arises. Because slow ball means longer time in possession, the technical ability of all players must be far superior. They must also be very patient and be able to identify moments when a gap opens so that they can then speed up the game to create scoring opportunities.

FAST OR SLOW BALL?   3.4.4.3

Naturally, the question will be asked, "Which is better, playing fast or slow?" The answer is that teams with robust systems can deploy both methods very effectively. The most synchronous teams have something else, too: tempo. In this context, *tempo* means the ability to change pace from slow to fast and back again. (We'll dive more into tempo on page 100.)

While some of the best teams have mastered the art of fast ball, the tactic is arguably even more useful for inexperienced clubs with less talent. A great team might prefer to play fast, but when push comes

EXPLOITATION OF BALL SPEED

Barcelona is a great example of a team that chooses ball speed carefully. It turns down quick counterattacking opportunities from within its own half if support and balance are not available. It is rarely seen moving completely from box to box, counterattacking. However, when possession is regained inside the opposition half, Barcelona is more likely to exploit the space and counterattack in the shorter spaces because there is more confusion to exploit and a greater chance of regaining defensive shape should it lose possession.

to shove, it can also be effective at a slower speed if forced by an opponent's defensive scheme.

For a rebuilding team full of younger players or a newly promoted squad with fewer stars, slow ball is usually a bad decision because it gives the players too much time to think and too many options. This can slow, delay, or even paralyze decision-making, increasing the frequency of errors and empowering a more-experienced opposition to take command. Of course, fast decision-making can sometimes be poor, but it is frequently superior when it comes to a young team that lacks the real-world knowledge to slow down and use proven movement patterns and actions within the pressure of the game.

THE LAW OF SPACE   3.4.5

Since all team sports have fixed physical boundaries, the creation and compression of space is the most critical aspect. As we will see later on when we explore the origins of this idea, maneuver war-

> ## SCORE FIRST, THEN WE'LL DISCUSS THE BEST OPTION

A perfect example of less-skilled teams using fast ball effectively was clear in the 2015–16 Premier League season, in which a low-budget Leicester City team given odds of 5000–1 before the start of the campaign shocked the sports world by claiming the title. An article in *The Economist* explained, "Leicester were toothless when building slow attacks—but ruthless on swift counterattacks. Leicester's staff identified that players such as Jamie Vardy, Riyad Mahrez and Danny Drinkwater—all unremarkable in 2014–15—were suited to such guerrilla tactics."[29]

fare, like sports, revolves around the compression of space and exploiting the expansion of space. While directly related to the compression of players, it is not about just the movement of players. In offensive terms, compressing space is achieved through misdirection and the movement of attacking players. The law of space states that if space is unavailable in one location, it must exist elsewhere. This means that by compressing and occupying space in one area, a team can create it in another.

COMPRESSION AND EXPANSION   3.4.5.1

At its most basic level, we try to compress space with players and create space elsewhere. It doesn't matter if it's an A or B gap in a line of scrimmage or a cornerback out of position in football, a defensive line blitzing in rugby, or midfielders pressing in soccer.

In conflict situations the principles apply similarly, but with slight variations. In military operations with Tier 1 assault teams or raids, the vital factor is not control of space but movement through it, so compression of the enemy combatants is the concern. Another factor, of course, is that the fastest way to achieve compression is to reduce the number of targets to be compressed.

THE LAW OF EXPOSURE   3.4.6

The best players and teams are forged in the furnace of competition, which only heightens their ability to move quickly through their decision-making cycles and play fast. The law of exposure states that players and teams consistently exposed to the highest speeds of movement and complexity are those that can execute the best under pressure. One of the reasons Michael Jordan excelled to such a degree and for so long is that the players guarding him and the rest of the opposing team brought their best against him every single night—doing anything less would have resulted in a rout. So Jordan was forced to consistently raise his already-high level of play so that he could continue decimating defenses. This didn't apply just to the game but also to practices and his off-season preparation. He knew that every team in the league would be gunning for him and trying to dethrone his Bulls, so he had to put in the effort to prevent this from happening.

THE LAW OF OFFENSE   3.4.7

The law of offense states that in successful teams there exists only offense and a proactive mindset. There is no such thing as reaction or defense. I don't believe in either. You're either attacking with the ball or attacking the team in possession to get the ball back. So even though we do, technically, talk about "defense," in reality there should be no such thing as passive defense—at least not with winning teams. The defense must get into and stay in attack mode until it can take possession—in other words, play offense without the ball. This involves putting the opponent under sustained pressure, so that it becomes reactive rather than proactive. In doing so, the defensive team has the chance to steal not only the ball but also the momentum.

To see yourself as on "defense" means that you are psychologically accepting the status quo. Instead, the team without the ball must make a psychological statement that it is going to win the ball back. Do not think that this is purely semantic. Having this mindset means that every defensive moment or move is made with the intention to counter. It's never a static or resigned action; it's a process used to regain the momentum.

The clearest example was demonstrated by a young Mike Tyson. One of the best defensive actions Cus D'Amato taught Tyson was constant movement. This wasn't just for movement's sake but rather, as explained in the excellent book *Confusing the Enemy* by Scott Weiss and Paige Stover, to help Tyson avoid contact while generating great power to counter-attack—in other words, employing an offensive defense. Later I'll show you how great teams like Barcelona and others do this in team sports through their principles of play.

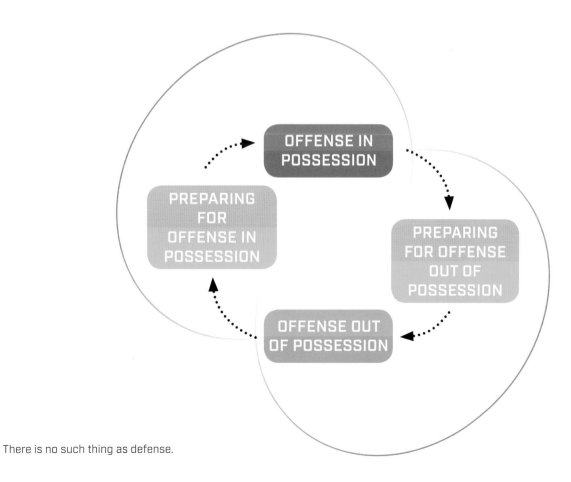

There is no such thing as defense.

PARADOXES OF THE GAME

3.5

There are an increasing number of assumptions in team sports today that have no basis in fact or human performance. These assumptions, such as "The fittest team always wins," have become accepted by many coaches without any critical analysis. In this section, you'll see how many of these are completely false.

THE PARADOX OF POSSESSION

3.5.1

A cliché you hear a lot within team-sports organizations is "Possession is nine-tenths of the law." This belief is pervasive among sports media outlets and broadcasters, too, particularly in rugby and soccer. Almost every write-up of a game in these sports includes a mention of which team had more possession, and often a breakdown of the areas of the field where each squad held onto the ball most.

The implication is that whoever had the most possession dominated the game, created more chances, and "deserved" to win. This is one of the fallacies of our outcome-obsessed sports culture and the flawed way in which stats-fixated analysis creates false impressions on fans, players, coaches, and staff.

As José Mourinho put it, "Sometimes I ask myself about the future, and maybe the future of football is a beautiful, green grass carpet without goals, where the team with more ball possession wins the game."[30] Of course, the Portuguese soccer manager was being sarcastic, but given the continued media and statistician obsession with possession, his scorn is justifiable.

Now, for some teams, gaining and holding possession may be an important and valid part of their game plan and an objective of the coaches and players. It doesn't exist in isolation, though. This aim will be connected to the team's other objectives and may even be necessary to achieve them. Simply put, some teams need a lot of possession to score enough to win.

And yet there are many elite teams in all sports that do not require a lot of possession to create scoring opportunities or put points on the board. Instead, they exploit gaps in their opponents' defense with aplomb, take advantage of moments of relative superiority, and punish mistakes and errors, even if these moments are few and far between. Frequently, such teams end games with less possession time than their opponents, often quite dramatically so. But despite this supposed imbalance or deficiency, they end the season with a winning record.

This is often the case for teams and offensive units that have a lot of experience playing together, are highly skilled, and are battle tested at the highest level. It also applies to elite military units, who need only one chance to meet their mission objectives and have been drilled in doing so over and over again, so that success is almost automatic.

On the flip side, a poor team may have a lot of possession but be unable to make the most of it. It might fail to create penetration, to use ball and player circulation purposefully, or to take advantage of defensive mistakes. Just because the media or fan comments assert that the team with the greatest possession time was "robbed" because it didn't win doesn't make this impression true.

In masterminding Leicester City's unlikely Premier League title, manager Claudio Ranieri did the exact opposite of just about every other manager. Most soccer coaches don't want their team's opponents to get within striking distance of the goal, as they fear this will lead to more scoring chances. So they play a high defensive line. In complete contrast, Ranieri wanted the other team to get deep into Leicester's half and soak up the pressure. When it did so, his defenders and midfielders would force mistakes, get possession, and then initiate a rapid counterattack that enabled Riyad Mahrez, Jamie Vardy, and Leicester's other attacking players to rapidly create scoring opportunities before the defense could react.

So Ranieri instructed his defenders to sit deep, cede possession, and then pounce when the attacking team turned the ball over. Only two teams saw less of the ball in the season. The results were evident, as Leicester beat its big-money rivals and topped the table.[31]

POSSESSION EXCEPTIONS   3.5.1.1

Of course, some teams can win with very high levels of possession, but this is not the reason for their success. The level of technical and physical ability must support the style of play. Barcelona under Guardiola managed more than 50 percent possession in each of his 183 games in charge up to 2011. You have to go all the way back to May 2008 to find a game where Barcelona was outpassed (a 1–4 loss to Real Madrid). Yet teams without a Messi, Neymar, or Suarez who've tried to copy the Guardiola approach (which is, in some ways, an evolution of Dutch Total Football—see Jonathan Wilson's work for more on this) haven't been able to replicate it, or they just try to pass more because it's what Barca and Bayern did to win. The key to winning is matching your tactics to the strengths of your squad and the overall objectives for each of the four game moments.[32]

THE PARADOX OF OPPORTUNITY   3.5.2

Similar misconceptions come into play when evaluating the number of opportunities a team creates in a game. In one Premier League fixture in the 2015–16 season, Liverpool had fourteen shots on goal and Manchester United just one. If I asked you to guess who won the game, you'd probably say Liverpool, yes? And yet it was England's record goal scorer Wayne Rooney who proved decisive in this game between bitter rivals, converting United's only scoring chance while Liverpool squandered all fourteen of its opportunities.

This example shows just how overrated the number of opportunities can be, even when analysts take it up a notch to look at not just "shots" but "shots on goal," "shots in the penalty box," and all manner of other numbers ("shots dominance" and "total shots ratio," to name two more). Just like possession statistics, such metrics can be highly misleading if they're not looked at in the proper context and through the macroscopic lens of the game model. One of the things I like to do to evaluate the effectiveness of a team's analytics approach is to take the stats report after the game and go through each objective key performance indicator. Then I look at the final score. If the indicators fail to tell the story of the game and let me accurately predict which side won (or at least get close), then these stats are largely irrelevant, and the team should consider excluding them, or at least not letting them influence its game plan or strategy.

The opportunities stat often falls into this dubious category. As Chris Anderson and David Sally put it in *The Numbers Game*: "That is the thing with soccer: it does not always reward those who take more shots or complete more passes. It only rewards those who score more goals."[33] The same is true of any sport. In basketball, a team's taking twenty-three three-point attempts doesn't tell you anything. If the team doesn't have good long-range shooters, or if those players were having an off-night, perhaps it missed twenty of these shots, gaining only nine points.

In contrast, a team with one or more excellent three-point shooters perhaps took only eleven three-pointers in the same game. But because it had someone like Kyle Korver on the team, it made eight of them and put twenty-four points on the board. Again, the total number of three-point opportunities meant little in the end.

This is not to say categorically that every team should avoid including the creation of a high number of opportunities in its game plan. If there are a dearth of quality attacking players, such an objective may well be a necessity, as the coaching staff knows that unless their athletes create a lot of scoring chances, they're unlikely to convert enough to prevail. Or perhaps the quality of the defense they will be facing is a factor. If a team's scouting report shows that its adversary has an elite defensive unit or perhaps a dominant player—such as a miserly goalkeeper in soccer or an intimidating, shot-blocking machine of a center in basketball—then they may decide that creating a lot of scoring opportunities is a valid aim for that particular game.

If a team with that objective did create many more chances than its opposition, as was intended, it isn't enough to say that it fulfilled this component of the game plan. The question remains: what impact did this have on the most important stat of all—the final score? Say Team A fashioned twenty-five shots on goal, scored on three of them, and won 3–0. Then it executed well offensively and defended adequately. Two thumbs up!

But say, in contrast, that Team A created twenty-five chances but lost 0–3. The coaching staff should then deduce that yes, their players fulfilled the goal of getting a lot of shots on goal, but they failed to execute well and also defended poorly. Having identified limiting factors that are hampering performance, they can now use this insight to inform the training sessions before the next game: the coaches can create learning scenarios that encourage their strikers and attacking midfielders to be more accurate and decisive in front of the goal.

THE PARADOX OF CONTROL
3.5.3

So much statistical and subjective analysis focuses on what players do when they have the ball that their actions without it are often overlooked or ignored completely. On the defensive end, how players move without the ball is essential to creating pressure and disrupting the attacker's game plan. Positioning is a key component, as defensively astute players will know exactly where they need to be to prevent the opponent from carving out and capitalizing on space. The defender should always try to disrupt attackers' decision-making cycles by making them reactive instead of proactive and constantly forcing them to make adjustments.

In the offensive and offense-to-defense moments, playing without the ball is also important. Moving into space not only provides more attacking options but also helps spread the defensive players apart, which is essential if facing a compact, well-drilled defensive side. Misdirection is another way to fool the defense and obscure the offensive unit's true intentions. If a team moves well without the ball, it can dominate and win games without relying on a possession advantage.

THE PARADOX OF FITNESS
3.5.4

Oh, distance covered, what an overused stat you are! For many years, statisticians have tracked how far individual players move during team sports, with the results showing up in postgame reports and in-game displays alike. Distance covered has also found its way into mainstream "health" culture, first with pedometers and now with fitness trackers and GPS-enabled smartphone and smartwatch apps. We've been conditioned (pun intended) to think that distance is the be-all and end-all when it comes to measuring physical output.

Bill Walsh believed that we've got it all wrong when it comes to a quantity-over-quality approach to conditioning. "Physical strength and speed are important advantages, but even more advantageous is having the training that permits you to respond intelligently to whatever confronts you," Walsh told the *Harvard Business Review*. "That means more precision, better execution and quicker responses than your opponents. Under the extreme stress of game conditions, a player must condense his intellect and focus it on thinking more quickly and clearly than the opposition."[34] Coaches like Jill Ellis, Bo Schembechler, Eddie Jones, Alex Ferguson, and Jack, John, and Jim Harbaugh all subscribe to this approach.

So in terms of increasing game-day performance, distance run in training—or, for that matter, in the actual game itself—is largely irrelevant. If you ran around and around in a circle like a headless chicken for the duration of a sporting contest, you'd certainly cover a lot of ground. But it would be purposeless.

Beyond this, those responsible for measuring such key performance indicators rarely look at the percentage breakdowns for different paces within the distance within each moment. It may look impressive to see that a soccer player ran seven or eight miles during a game, but in reality this was mostly a combination of short sprints and walking. It's not as if the total distance covered was completed at a Mo Farah–paced ten thousand meters.

Another issue with the distance-covered metric is that team sports are in some ways similar to two partners dancing together. Just as one partner leads and the other follows on the dance floor, so it goes in the sporting arena. When a basketball player attacks, the player guarding him or her responds by moving. If WNBA star Skylar Diggins runs a long route across the baseline and back to the top of the key, her opposite number will chase after her. Played out over the course of a full game, both Diggins and her marker will have totaled roughly the same total distance.

A similar pattern is repeated in most team sports. We look at cumulative metrics like distance covered to make blanket statements about an athlete's effort and even their character. How many times have you heard someone say that a certain player is "lazy" because they don't run a lot of yards or seem to be exerting that much effort? Sometimes players are very effective when it comes to executing their team objectives without racking up distance.

THE OBJECT OF THE GAME   3.5.4.1

To paraphrase General George Patton, the object of the game is not to run the most but to make the other guy run the most and still win. Zlatan Ibrahimovic, Thierry Henry, Eric Cantona, and Dimitar Berbatov are perfect examples in soccer. All four have been derided for their supposed "laziness," yet their languid approach to the game is belied by their fantastic goal-scoring records. These players would be near the bottom of the rankings in terms of distance run per game, but this says literally nothing about their effectiveness in achieving their primary objective: putting the ball in the back of the net.

This is not to take anything away from players who run a lot and are effective, as there are plenty who check both boxes. Rather, I'm trying to make the point that many people within the team-sports establishment put way too much stock in distance covered. Identifying the "top fifteen hardest-working players" just by the amount of meters or yards they've run, as *Talk Sport* did, is faulty logic.[35]

It's often thought that Barcelona works harder than the average team, but their distance-covered figures from the 2016 UEFA Champions League are quite revealing. On average they covered 110.465 km per game, compared to 110.644 km run by second-place Manchester United. Both figures are less than the 112.040 km average of all teams in the competition. Barcelona's season-high distance covered was 116.624 km, which was dwarfed by the overall competition high of 124.503 km. Clearly, the long periods spent playing a relatively low-intensity passing game help to balance out high-intensity pressing.[36]

THE PARADOX OF SPEED   3.5.5

We all love speed, don't we? The one-hundred-meter finals are always a top draw at the Olympics because we want to see who the fastest men and women are. NASCAR and Formula 1 are wildly popular because of how fast the cars go. This speed fascination carries over to team sports, too. After every one of Usain Bolt's Olympic triumphs, sports columnists busied themselves pondering how fast he could complete football's standard measure of top-end speed, the forty-yard dash.

In football itself, the quest for a fast forty has become an obsession for players and fans alike. Stopping the clock at the NFL Combine doesn't just win you bragging rights, a higher draft position, and popularity among fantasy league players—it has also become lucrative.[37] Adidas paid Trae Waynes, Phillip Dorsett, and Kevin White $100,000 each for being the three fastest athletes signed to the company at the 2015 NFL Combine.[38] Nice work if you can get it!

Top-end speed is measured not just during player evaluations but also in games themselves. "Five wide receivers came in with top speeds of over 21 mph during Week 13," announced an article from December 2015.[39] "Is Panthers WR Ted Ginn Jr. the fastest player in the NFL?" wondered another sportswriter during the same month.[40]

It certainly doesn't hurt to have rocket boosters for legs, like Ginn Jr., NBA speedster John Wall, or late rugby great Jonah Lomu (who boasted a 10.7-second hundred-meter time at 260+ pounds).[41] But team-sports games are not a hundred-meter final nor a forty-yard straight-line dash. They are contests of applying speed while avoiding obstacles—often obstacles moving toward each other at a great rate.

Frank Gore was arguably one of the toughest players I've ever had the pleasure to coach, but his greatest skill was not his top speed but the speed of his decision-making and his ability to run at *optimal* speed—the best speed for the situation in front of him. Frank's brain works faster at processing information than all other backs.

Yes, it certainly is exciting to watch a basketball player race to the rim on a fast break, a rugby winger break away for a you-can't-catch-me try, or a special teams speed freak run the ball back eighty yards for a touchdown. Measuring top speed in a game is somewhat more beneficial than clocking forty-yard dashes because it is a more realistic scenario. But we have to also consider how effectively this speed can be applied, what the end result is, and what the cost is.

So if a player puts points on the board with a burst of quickness, that's terrific. If they did it at a pivotal moment, such as when the score is tied with seconds remaining on the clock, all the better. But lamentably, this is often not the case. Think about the basketball player who streaks downcourt, throws down a dunk, and blows out her knee on landing. Or the football player who is so taxed by his unlikely interception and touchdown run that he needs oxygen on the sideline and is below par for the rest of the game. Or the rugby player who makes it half the length of the field, only to get poleaxed into touch and ruled out for the remainder of the contest.

In these scenarios, reaching top speed is not only unhelpful but also harmful to the player and the team. These may be extreme examples, but the point stands: top speed is no guarantee of game-time success and is most often a useless measurement unless its impact on the scoreboard and achieving game plan objectives can be shown. Speed is also one example of how physical attributes are lauded while technical and tactical astuteness are undervalued. There are many players who have been dismissed as physically slow who compensate for their lack of raw athleticism with lightning-fast reflexes and decision-making—Larry Bird, Peyton Manning, and Teddy Sheringham, to name just three.

In close-quarters battle or close-quarters combat, speed—along with extreme violence and force—is the decisive factor, but even then it must be contextual and controlled. Later we will see that tempo is the critical overriding factor with speed control.

Despite the fact that a great many Hall of Famers compensate for lack of physicality with superior technical-tactical and psychological acuity, developing speed remains a priority in team sports. Over the past few years, we've seen more and more speed coaches employed by pro clubs and rich college programs. Similarly, if you asked a strength and conditioning coach what they hoped their athletes will achieve, they'd likely include "get faster" or "get more

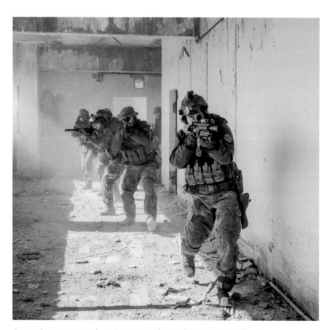

As snipers say, slow is smooth and smooth is fast.

explosive" in their answer. This shows the impact of speed and other such metrics at the organizational level, which we'll explore in more detail later on.

THE PARADOX OF INTENSITY   3.5.6

Intensity is a difficult thing to define, and it is also a very difficult part of team sports to measure. Sometimes people will look at a game and say a team failed because they weren't fit enough, but this is often a mistake. Players or teams can appear on the surface to be moving slowly and with a lack of intensity, when in reality they're being just fast and intense enough to get their job done well. What we usually don't see when watching a game is the effort players make to get into position to receive the ball and what they do after they've passed it to a teammate. There's a lot of hidden exertion in each contest, much of it in off-the-ball movement.

We also overlook the fact that each player has a different functional reserve, which as the game goes on is drained on by physical, mental, and emotional factors. Cognitive decline is just as big a challenge at the end of the game as physical fatigue, if not more so. It's the job of each player (and the coach, with regard to substitution patterns) to manage his or her intensity and effort level throughout the game with the big picture in mind. Burn yourself out in the first few minutes and you'll be as unsuccessful as the inexperienced five-thousand-meter runner in the Olympics, who mistakenly sets out fast only to fall victim to the old issue of "fly and die" and fade with two laps still to go.

COMPARING PLAYERS AND WORK RATE   3.5.6.1

Soccer writer Isaiah Cambron wrote an entry for *Barcelona Football Blog* in which he compared the distance covered by certain players over several games. He found that Lionel Messi covered 44,027 meters in 482 minutes, scoring five goals and racking up three assists. His teammate Xavi covered 56,552 meters in 441 minutes. So if someone were going to identify the "hardest-working" player by dis-

tance covered, they wouldn't pick the record-setting Argentinian forward. And yet he had the most goals and assists of any of his teammates in the games surveyed—the output was there to help win Barcelona those matches. Now let's put the stats into context. If we take his goals and assists into account and their impact on the outcome of each game, Messi has the lowest distance divided by the highest number of goals plus assists. Therefore, you could say that he was the most efficient (not to mention effective) player on his team. So even though he ran less than Xavi or any other Barcelona player, this had no bearing on how well he accomplished his objectives or positively impacted the game. This example shows how careful we have to be in using individual statistics to make claims about "working hard" or being "lazy." Often, the numbers *do* lie, when they're not examined with the big picture of the game in mind.[42]

THE PARADOX OF TACKLING   3.5.7

The number of tackles frequently appears on statistics websites, during draft discussions and combines, in game reports, and even during TV broadcasts of football, soccer, and rugby. It even makes it into transfer/trade news. For example, when Manchester United acquired Morgan Schneiderlin in the summer of 2015, newspapers were quick to evaluate the deal based on the number of tackles he had made. "According to Squawker, the Frenchman won the most tackles in the English top flight since winning promotion with previous club Southampton in 2012," *Metro* announced.[43]

Not to take anything away from the unquestionably talented Schneiderlin, but this statistic is largely meaningless. While the above-mentioned *Metro* article asserted that he was the "best ball winner" in the Premier League and that this could be proven or disproven with a detailed assessment, just having the highest number of tackles means little to nothing. A player could attempt twenty-five tackles in a game and yet fail to win possession in twenty-three of them. On the other hand, a teammate might try tackling twelve times and come out with the ball ten times. The latter would clearly be the more effective tackler in this particular game.

Tackles in football and steals in basketball are similarly overrated. Players in the top five for steals in college are often thought of as having "NBA-ready defense," and if they can repeat the feat in the pros, they'll likely be included in Defensive Player of the Year conversations. The trouble is that the steals stat doesn't show how many attempted steals it took to get the desired results, or what the impact of failed attempts was.

The same goes for tackles and sacks in the NFL. Unquestionably, bringing down a quarterback with regularity can earn a defensive end or defensive tackle (note the inclusion of the term *tackle* in the position name) a big contract and can strike fear into any QB. But again, obsessing over tackles and sacks in isolation, without the framing context of the game model, is a risky proposition for statisticians and the coaches to whom they supply numbers.

Plus, there are cases in which a football team gets a low number of sacks and yet has a dominant defense—see the 2015–16 Jets, who ranked number one in both scoring and total defense, yet were twenty-eighth in sacks.[44] This is because their positional defense was excellent, and team coverage minimized the need for league-leading tackling and sacking numbers.

The ultimate example of a great soccer player avoiding the tackle-happy approach is AC Milan and Italy legend Paolo Maldini. His positional defense was so advanced that while anchoring one of the best back lines in history, he averaged just one tackle every 1.8 games.[45] That's because his vast experience—he made 904 appearances for AC Milan in a twenty-four-year career—allowed Maldini to close down space and take away what attackers wanted to do without sliding in to dispossess them. As Maldini famously put it, "If I have to make a tackle then I have already made a mistake."[46]

Not every player can be a Maldini-like model of restraint when it comes to tackles and steals. But it's not just the frequency of attempts to reclaim possession that we should examine. The context and timing of attempted tackles or steals is also a factor that is usually overlooked. Were they early in the game while the player was fresh, or late in the game when he or she was fatigued? Which game moments did the tackles or steals occur in, and what was the impact if successful? (In the defensive moment, did they claim possession? In the offense-to-defense transition, did they stop the other team on a dangerous counterattack?)

If the tackle failed, what were the consequences? Did the other team get or convert a scoring chance? Did the player attempting the tackle leave a gaping hole that the opposition exploited? Did the player cause or sustain an injury? Maybe he or she drew a penalty in football or rugby or a yellow card in soccer. Or did a failed steal attempt leave the player a basketball guard is supposed to be defending wide-open to knock down a shot? Such examples show that looking at statistical outcomes like tackles and steals without taking into account their context and timing in the game is of questionable value.

THE PARADOX OF VICTORY   3.5.8

Part of the problem in analyzing sports is the phenomenon of victor's bias. This impacts the team that won, the team that lost, and those watching the game, and colors our subjective analysis of each team's performance and how it jibed with the objectives for each game moment.

Let's look at a common example. If a rugby game was tied until the sixty-five-minute mark and then Team A ran in three tries in the final fifteen minutes, commentators would often assert that Team B's legs failed them and that Team A's superior fitness levels proved to be the difference. The dejected personnel in Team B's locker room might come to the same conclusion, as might the victors. Now, this deduction could be correct, and Team A's late-game success could be rooted in superior off-season conditioning. In which case, well and good.

But this conclusion could just as easily be the faulty outcome of victor's bias. There are many possible reasons why Team A pulled away at the end of the game. Fitness could be one element, but then so could better decision-making, learning experiences on the training ground, and execution.

Victor's bias poses two major challenges. First, managing expectations and having humility are essential to proper continuous improvement—and ignoring the score is the only way to achieve these. Second, in assessment of the enemy or opposition, failure to remove the score and emotion from the critical analysis will lead to failure to see the improvement in the opponent and, more importantly, failure to see what kind of opposition you will face in future engagements.

Technical skill and tactics play underrated roles in late-game wins. If two boxers fight over fifteen rounds, the one with better tactics and superior technical skills often prevails over the more powerful puncher. Many times, we see the freak athlete come out with a flurry of blows, attempting to pull off a first-round knockout. This can work, but if his opponent can absorb the barrage in the early rounds, his conservation of energy will pay off as the fight wears on. He can then use his skill to pick off the big puncher, who has now exhausted much of his functional reserve (see the earlier example about Mike Tyson's fight strategy, or George Foreman punching himself out against Muhammad Ali in the Rumble in the Jungle).

This is not a hard-and-fast rule, but it does illustrate the crucial role of skill and tactics. The current team-sports system is geared toward creating über-athletes, yet teams without a whole roster of such specimens frequently prevail through superior technical skill and wiser tactics. And yet when it comes to subjectively analyzing the game, all too often we fall into the trap of assuming that the winning team triumphed because of superior athleticism, endurance, or some other physical attribute.

This then leads the coaches of the losing squad to continue the arms race of physicality when they should be focusing on developing leadership, decision-making, and skills through realistic learning experiences. So the team may get fitter, but it will continue to lose because the objective is false. There can also be other unintended negative consequences from pushing players who are already adequately fit too hard, not least of which is increasing injury rates. So we see that sometimes a team's faulty analysis of why it won or lost leads it to pursue an objective that contradicts or undermines the Commander's Intent.

The fallacy of victor's bias is another reason the game model is necessary, so that both winning and losing teams can overcome such flawed thinking and get to the root of why they really won or lost. They can then make more-informed decisions about what to focus on in individual and team preparation so that errors are corrected and the impact of weaknesses is mitigated in forthcoming fixtures, while overall aims remain intact.

THE PARADOX OF INJURY   3.5.9

A myth that is often promoted is that team injury rates are related to success. But as we saw earlier with the law of individual influence, not all players are equal. Therefore, not all injuries are equal.

This also means that the rates and degrees of injury are irrelevant as a general observation. The Patriots have had one of the highest injury rates over the past few seasons, but this statistic is misleading. Tom Brady is significantly more important to the Patriots than any other player, and he has missed very few games. An injury to Brady would be a bigger problem for Bill Belichick than if another Patriots player got hurt. This is not to say that we shouldn't do our utmost to keep every player injury-free.

MACRO PRINCIPLES OF TEAM SPORTS   3.6

Having outlined the concept of game moments, cohesion of tasks, focus of *schwerpunkt*, and the Commander's Intent, we now move on to outlining the series and sequence of macro and micro principles behind successful play. Each game moment has a series of principles that must be respected to achieve optimal performance.

OFFENSIVE MACRO PRINCIPLE: BALL SPACE   3.6.1

In the offensive moment, the primary factor is the creation of space. Once space is created, teammates can move into it and time runs, movements, and actions to exploit it. The overall aim of all attacking approaches is to create space; the aim of defenses is to deny it. Some teams want to talk about making time for shooting or about how some players make time for themselves, but this isn't correct. They create space. Space makes time.

TRANSITION-TO-OFFENSE MACRO PRINCIPLE: BALL SPEED   3.6.2

The phrase "speed kills" is overused in elite sports, but as an overall principle of attack it is critical. Nonetheless, it is not to be misinterpreted. The speed of the ball forces very fast decision-making. It's not the speed that kills; it's the failure to think fast. Ball speed is one of a series of methods used to force the opponent to think faster. At the highest level, the key is for the player with the ball to make decisions faster than the person trying to prevent skill execution can react. Skill and tactics are used to achieve this aim. As soon as a team has possession, it must try to move the ball quickly and cause maximum disruption. Constant movement causes constant decision-making and creates in the defense a reactionary mindset.

BLITZKRIEG AND TRANSITION TO OFFENSE   3.6.2.1

English military theorist B. H. Liddell Hart is considered by some to be the conceptual father of the modern blitzkrieg concept. Several high-ranking German tank commanders, such as Guderian, von Manstein, Balck, and Rommel, spoke in depth about how it

works in practice on the battlefield. Deploying the "lightning war" method in World War II led Germany to, as John Boyd put it, "conquer an entire region in the quickest possible time by gaining initial surprise and exploiting the fast tempo/fluidity of action...as basis to repeatedly penetrate, splinter, envelop, and roll-up/wipe-out disconnected remnants of [the] adversary organism."[47] This should also be the aim of good teams. If you can set up and execute scoring opportunities before the opponent can react, then your game plan is highly efficient and difficult to stop, even when the opponent knows what you're going to do. The blitzkrieg principle can also be used in the other game moments. A primary example of its application in the defensive moment is the blitz in football.

TRANSITION-TO-DEFENSE MACRO PRINCIPLE: BALL PRESSURE   3.6.3

Once a team has lost possession, the most important thing is to pressure the ball (to put pressure on the player in possession). This slows the counterattack enough to allow reorganization and a return to the defensive game plan. Initiative is regained and, if done properly, the moment is reversed. The overall aim is to get possession back, of course, but in the moment, pressure is the immediate goal.

DEFENSIVE MACRO PRINCIPLE: MAN PRESSURE   3.6.4

In this moment, the team must try to take back the initiative and win possession by recapturing the ball or forcing an error on the ball or man. By pressuring every opposing player within the effective playing area (the area the ball can be moved into by passing or player movement), it increases the chance of forcing an error and regaining possession.

MICRO PRINCIPLES OF TEAM SPORTS

3.7

Our ultimate aim is to build a group of players who constantly adapt and learn—even during a game. In *Team of Teams*, retired army general Stanley McChrystal outlined an excellent interpretation of adaptive organizational principles, showing how the best teams decentralize decision-making during training and learn to apply this on the playing field or battlefield. Former All Blacks coach Graham Henry said that he knew his team was learning when they could make adjustments and overcome adversity in the middle of games without his intervening. By using a methodology based on principles, we achieve two things: we avoid micromanaging events that we cannot prepare for, and we enable our players to make decisions based on the best available intelligence at that time.

MICRO PRINCIPLES AND RESILIENCE

3.7.1

In their article "Organizational Extinction and Complex Systems," Russ Marion and Josh Bacon write that robust systems are characterized by "rich patterns of tight, moderate and loosely coupled linkages; chains of interdependency branch in complicated patterns across nearly every actor in a broad network of interaction. Such complex patterns of interaction protect the organization against environmental shock by providing multiple paths for action. If one pattern of interdependency in a network is disrupted, the dynamic performed by that subsystem can usually be rerouted to other areas of the network. Such robustness makes it difficult to damage or destroy the complex system, for complex interaction lends it amazing resilience."[48]

To build a robust and resilient organization, we need to develop it thoughtfully and purposefully from the very beginning. Because the entire system is developed from its smaller parts (what Marion and Bacon call "micro structures"), the principles of conflict or play must reflect this.

THE CELLULAR APPROACH

3.7.2

The optimal way for a group to adapt in turbulent environments such as sports games or military conflicts is to act in a "cellular" manner as part of a bigger network. This is an idea included in John Boyd's views on command and control. Cells operating within networks allow teams to be self-organizing and self-controlling. Special operations teams and elite business groups already facilitate this. We will look at this idea from the organizational perspective later.

Sub-groups of players, whether organized by position or task, are small interactive teams operating relatively autonomously, pursuing and exploiting opportunities as they present themselves—with respect to the principles outlined. Just like the small, nimble groups of special operatives McChrystal describes in *Team of Teams*, units like the backs and forwards in rugby need to be able to have some degree of autonomy and must be trusted to apply their expertise to achieve the objectives of the game plan during competition.

DECENTRALIZED DECISION-MAKING

3.7.3

In rapidly changing sports games or military engagements, the decisions cannot all be made on the sidelines. Events may outpace communications, and lower levels must understand the overall intent and make decisions independently. In war, this is referred to as "decentralized command." This concept scares many coaches, but in reality it's the most important aspect of sustainably successful teams.

This is most common in modern irregular conflict (asymmetrical warfare). The greatest challenge to winning such an encounter is to adapt, and the faster adaptation occurs, the sooner success is reached. But responding to changing conditions demands the development of a complex adaptive conflict unit.

The critical word: *adaptive*. To sustain success, each unit—and I include coaches in this as well—needs to be able and allowed to adapt.

The key aspect of sustainably successful teams is that the members share know-how among themselves. Freedom of activity and self-learning is the key to enabling self-organizing behavior: as the environment changes, cells develop, new reactions occur, and old methods can be disbanded as necessary—but always with respect to the underlying principles.[49] So as long as a group of players keeps the Commander's Intent and its sub-objectives in mind, how they achieve these is irrelevant. They must be the ones who decide how to execute in the heat of the action.

GENERAL MICRO PRINCIPLES OF OFFENSIVE PLAY   3.7.4

Now we're going to take a look at some elemental concepts that are universal across all team sports, at every level, and should be used when analyzing each game-day performance and planning training.

But before we continue, let's review where we are. We now appreciate that a team game is composed of fractals of interactions. These are based around four macro principles, which occur in moments in time, and each moment has a context. In these moments there are natural micro moments that occur in sequence if the moment is allowed to run its course. You may have noticed that we haven't really looked

TRADITIONAL	EMERGING
LINEAR	NONLINEAR
STATIC, CAUSE-EFFECT VIEW OF INDIVIDUAL FACTORS	DYNAMIC, CONSTANTLY CHANGING FIELD OF INTERACTIONS
MICROSCOPIC, LOCAL	WIDE-ANGLE, GLOBAL
SEPARATENESS	RELATEDNESS
MARKETPLACE	ENVIRONMENT
REDUCTIONIST	NONREDUCTIONIST
COMPONENT THINKING	SEEING AND THINKING IN WHOLES
TIME CARDS, TASK ANALYSIS	COMPLEX ADAPTIVE SYSTEMS
PROBLEM-SOLVING	BUTTERFLY EFFECT, SYSTEM FEEDBACK
BRAINSTORMING	ENVIRONMENTAL SCANNING PLUS MAPPING
POLARIZATION	UNDERLYING PROCESS AND INTERACTIONS OF A SYSTEM'S VARIABLES CREATE SELF-ORGANIZING PATTERNS, SHAPES, AND STRUCTURES
PAYS ATTENTION TO POLICIES AND PROCEDURES THAT ARE USUALLY FIXED AND INFLEXIBLE	PAYS ATTENTION TO INITIAL CONDITIONS, INFORMATION, EMERGING EVENTS, AND STRANGE ATTRACTORS
STANDING COMMITTEES	AD HOC WORKING GROUPS, NETWORKS
POLITICS	LEARNING
PLANNING AS DISCRETE EVENT	PLANNING AS CONTINUOUS PROCESS
PLANNING BY ELITE SPECIALIST GROUP	PLANNING REQUIRES WHOLE SYSTEM INPUT
IMPLEMENTATION OF PLAN	IMPLEMENTATION FLEXIBLE AND CONSTANTLY EVOLVING IN RESPONSE TO EMERGING CONDITIONS
FORECASTING THROUGH DATA ANALYSIS	FORESIGHT THROUGH SYNTHESIS
QUANTITATIVE	QUALITATIVE
CONTROLLING, STABILIZING, OR MANAGING CHANGE	RESPONDING TO AND INFLUENCING CHANGE AS IT EMERGES
DINOSAUR BEHAVIOR	ENTREPRENEURIAL BEHAVIOR
CHANGE IS THREAT	CHANGE IS OPPORTUNITY
LEADS TO STAGNATION AND EXTINCTION	LEADS TO RENEWAL AND GROWTH

at technique or method but simply principles. In summary, we want to create space, which will in turn give us time to invade, move, and execute. The creation of space in a field can come only through the compression and dispersal of players and by using width and depth with the ball to pull the defense apart.

THE MICRO PRINCIPLE OF OFFENSIVE SUPPORT   3.7.4.1

The idea of support applies to both offense and defense (we'll look specifically at defensive support on page 82) and is a vital component of achieving the game objectives on both sides of the ball. Providing support in attack offers several benefits. First, it gives the player who has possession options for creating and exploiting space using ball movement. Second, it can help create a distraction and confuse defenders by presenting them with too many options. For example, if a rugby player has adequate support on both flanks, the defense is faced with at least three possibilities: the player with the ball goes right down the middle; the player moves to the left; or the player moves to the right. The more options the defensive players have, the slower their decision-making and actions will be. The principles of offensive support can be reinforced in practice during small-sided games.

Massed or Focused Support   3.7.4.1.1

Support can be focused (one or more persons supporting in one singular area/direction) or massed (many options in multiple directions). As a general rule, less-talented teams should employ multiple massed support structures. For the defense, having multiple options to defend against is both physically demanding and demoralizing.

The contrast between massed and focused support is best illustrated in conflict in the difference between German and Soviet military approaches in World War II. The more technically gifted Germany preferred the philosophy of a focused approach like *schwerpunkt*, or "organizational focus," which aims

for a few specific objectives and is more efficient. On the other hand, the Soviet philosophy of *glubokaya operatsiya*, or "deep operations," focused on multiple attacks that better utilized its less-prepared troops and took advantage of greater resources to break its enemies' spirit.

In the NFL, a great example of the massed approach is the Seattle Seahawks, who have multiple attacking options masterminded by head coach Pete Carroll. They have a powerful offensive line and a formidable running game, which complement the deep threat of their mobile quarterback, Russell Wilson.

THE MICRO PRINCIPLES OF WIDTH AND DEPTH   3.7.4.2

A primary aim of attacking play is to make the field as big as possible—to maximize functional space. The way to do this is by creating space through width and depth. The use of both varies from sport to sport and in the contextual moments of each game. For example, a quarterback whose team is pinned back in its own half wants to create as much depth as possible to gain maximum yardage—getting his offensive unit closer to its scoring objective and reducing the chance of his team's defense having to take over in a precarious position.

In contrast, if a central midfielder in a soccer match gets the ball in the middle of the field, she will first look to spread the ball wide to create space and construct a dangerous attacking move. Moving the ball to the wings stretches out the defense, preventing the opponent from maintaining compactness.

Sometimes, a certain scenario will prevent the use of depth or width. For example, a football team that has pushed all the way to the five-yard line no longer has the option of depth, so it must use player movement out wide to create a touchdown opportunity. In the opposite situation, if a basketball team's wing players are locked down by excellent defenders, the point guard will be forced to create penetration using depth down the middle, either by driving to the basket or by pounding the ball inside to the center or power forward.

In any game situation, neither depth nor width can exist in isolation. One merely precedes the other. An effective attacking team or unit must balance both to generate space for the ball to move into and to penetrate the defense. Player positioning becomes crucial in not allowing the defense to take away width or depth. By always having at least one player in a deep position, even a lone striker, the offense forces the defense to address the threat of depth. Similarly, by ensuring that wing players don't constantly drift into the middle of the field, a team makes the defense contend with width, even when the ball isn't played out wide.

As a general rule, in offense you want to achieve width first and then depth. While this may vary by sport, it's usually more difficult to create a truly threatening offensive depth before pulling defenders out wide. The risk-reward equation is much more complex. Of course it's also about perception, but the threat must be real.

SEQUENCING MICRO PRINCIPLES OF WIDTH AND DEPTH

When you attend a sporting event, sitting to one side is better than having a seat aligned with the middle of the playing surface if you're looking to assess width and depth. Though you'll see your team attacking from this perspective for only one half, the off-center position will still provide a more beneficial view for that time than if you spent the entire game on the halfway line.

THE MICRO PRINCIPLE OF BALANCE IN OFFENSE   3.7.4.3

A balanced or symmetrical attack provides multiple options for creating width and depth and for quickly taking advantage of a defensive lapse anywhere on the playing surface. If a team is balanced going forward, there are more opportunities to construct an effective play with ball and player circulation and less risk of the defense forcing dispossession.

THE MICRO PRINCIPLE OF PENETRATION   3.7.4.4

Once your offense has used width and depth to create space and enlarge the functional playing surface, it's time to exploit this and create a scoring opportunity. The method for doing this in any team sport is penetration. While goals or points can be scored from deep—whether it's a long drop goal or field goal, a freaky forty-yard strike, or a three-pointer from five feet behind the line (or, in Steph Curry's case, fifteen feet)—most teams create the bulk of their scoring opportunities by invading the opponent's danger area (aka the "red zone" in American football).

You can create penetration by using either man or ball movement. In soccer, a long ball over the top of the defense can be exploited by a speedy striker, or this forward could use fancy footwork to take the ball around her marker and into the penalty area. Penetration could also come from width, such as a corner or free kick out wide.

On the defensive side of the ball, a team can prevent or limit penetration by making the playing surface smaller. This is achieved by taking away the option of depth, width, or both. So a rugby team can pack the middle to prevent a charge up the middle or tightly cover the opposing wingers to prevent a breakaway out wide. It's a cliché to say that the best defender in any sport is the sideline, but it's true. If you can force attackers to this boundary and prevent them from advancing straight down the court or cutting inside, they're done for, as they can't go around the sideline and it never shifts.

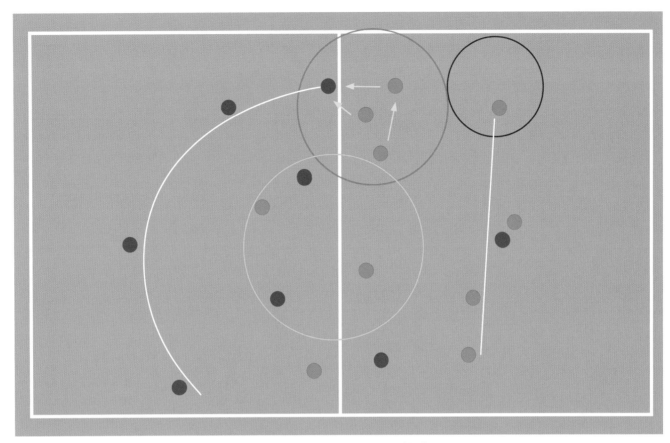

The micro principles of width and depth are essential to the macro principle of ball space.

THE MICRO PRINCIPLE OF MOVEMENT   3.7.4.5

There is a high physical cost to restarting momentum that has been halted. That's why it's essential that an offensive unit keeps its players and the ball moving as much as possible. Think about a basketball team that struggles to score. If you watch them closely on offense, you'll see that both player and ball movement become stagnant and they typically get bogged down in one-on-one isolation. Contrast this to high-scoring ball clubs who swing the ball around before taking a shot, who have a high assist percentage, and whose players are seemingly in constant motion.

Movement has to happen at the team level to prevent the defense from asserting itself and applying more pressure than the offense can handle. If just one player is moving, the defense has fewer options to consider and more time to react. Constantly moving players and the ball enables the offense to con-

sistently create space through width and depth and provides more opportunities to execute the game plan objectives. The more players who are open, the more chances there are to penetrate and score. (See pages 30 and 31 for more on ball and player circulation.)

THE MICRO PRINCIPLE OF MISDIRECTION   3.7.4.6

Sometimes the aim of player movement is to get into position to receive the ball. But the movement of players and/or the ball can also be used as a decoy to trick the defense and obscure the attacking team's true purpose. Misdirection can be applied to width or depth and can be utilized by an individual player—micro-level misdirection—or in the team context—macro-level misdirection. By sending one player or an entire team the wrong way, the attacking team buys time for the ball handler, which lends itself to creating and exploiting space.

In basketball, a player can drive to the basket without any intention of dunking or making a layup. This aggressive move forces the defense to collapse, lose its width, and give up cohesion and compactness. As a result, the ball handler has created space on the perimeter and kicks the ball back out to a wide-open teammate, who calmly nails a three-pointer. The crossover is another example of misdirection on the hardwood.

In soccer, misdirection is frequently employed on the wings. So the left winger makes a dummy run up her flank, drawing two defenders with her. But instead of passing to her, the central midfielder swings the ball to the right wing, who is now more open as the entire defensive line has been stretched out to the left. In play-dominated offenses in more-structured sports, like football, coaches and players elevate misdirection to an art form, and there can be multiple examples of it within a single play to create space amid the befuddled defense for the intended ball target. In football, there could be a fake handoff at the same time two receivers are running dummy routes to further confuse and frustrate the opponent.

These are all examples of active misdirection, but passive misdirection can be equally effective at tricking the defense. This is achieved by setting up your personnel in a certain structured way. For example, in soccer, a team might want its opponent to think that it's targeting the back post with a corner, when its real intention is to play it short. So it will send a couple of tall players to the back post to deceive the defense. Or a rugby team might position one of its highest leapers at a certain spot in the lineout to trick the defense into thinking he's the target, when in fact another player rises to receive the ball.

Variety is essential with misdirection. If a basketball player overuses a ball fake or crosses over defenders only from left to right, opponents will get wise and stop biting. Or if a team has only one or two out-of-bounds set plays, it won't take a scouting genius to figure out what they're really up to. John Boyd believed that variety was essential if you were to short-circuit your opponent's decision-making. Surprise leads to shock, which then gives you an opportunity for exploitation.[50]

GENERAL MICRO PRINCIPLES OF DEFENSIVE PLAY   3.7.5

As with offensive play, the aim of defensive micro principles is to align defending players' actions in a sequenced and synchronized pattern that forces the offense to be reactive. The micro principles of defensive play outlined remove offensive options from the opponent, allow the defense to seize the initiative, and help it to take possession back as quickly and efficiently as possible.

THE MICRO PRINCIPLE OF DEFENSIVE SUPPORT   3.7.5.1

When your teammate goes to dispossess an opponent or apply extra pressure, she needs support to be effective. If she is successful in taking the ball away, having teammates close by enables a faster and more effective transition to offense. They might also force a mistake that allows someone else to gain control of the ball.

Similarly, if the teammate fails to capture the ball, supporting teammates help mitigate the negative impact. For example, if a soccer player misses a tackle and she's the last defender, the attacker can have a clear run to the goal. But if she misses a tackle and has adequate support, there will be another line of defense that prevents a one-on-one with the goalkeeper and reduces the chances of the opponent scoring. Defensive support enables your team to maintain cohesion.

THE MICRO PRINCIPLE OF PRESSURE   3.7.5.2

The goal of defensive pressure is to force the attacker to contend with the defender and to focus on their actions rather than implementing the game plan. Pressure can be applied effectively in either man-to-man or zone defensive schemes. The U.S. Marine Corps and other military units have applied John Boyd's theories about the impact of pressure on decision-making to prepare their troops for combat. Former air marshal Curtis Sprague explained to an interviewer how rushing a gunman is unexpectedly effective in halting a shooting incident: "By closing the gap, you're resetting your adversary's Loop because now they have to re-orient themselves to an unexpected change in the environment."[51]

While it would be folly to equate what happens in a sports game to the scenario Sprague is referencing, the principle is still applicable. By applying consistent pressure, defenders can force their opponents to look for other options, which forces them to decide and act slower. It also increases the chances of the defense achieving its game objectives—limiting red zone penetration, for example—while reducing the effectiveness of the offense's own plan. As legendary UCLA basketball coach John Wooden put it, "My philosophy of defense is to keep the pressure on the opponent until you get to his emotions."

Pressure is not just a factor in the defensive moment but in the offensive and transitional moments, too. Employing constant ball and player motion when attacking will wear down even the best-conditioned defense eventually. As NCAA championship–winning basketball coach Rick Pitino has said, "The basic premise of my system is to fatigue your opponents with constant pressure defensively and constant movement offensively."

THE MICRO PRINCIPLE OF RECOVERY 3.7.5.3

When the ball is turned over, the players who now find themselves out of possession have to react quickly. Fast recovery will slow down the opponent's transition from defense to offense and limit their chances of creating a high-percentage scoring opportunity. The aim in such a situation is to close off space quickly. This gives teammates the chance to reclaim cohesion from chaos and set up their structure to prevent penetration. If a player takes a few moments to get back into the action after losing possession, that's okay, but she must put maximum effort into recovering.

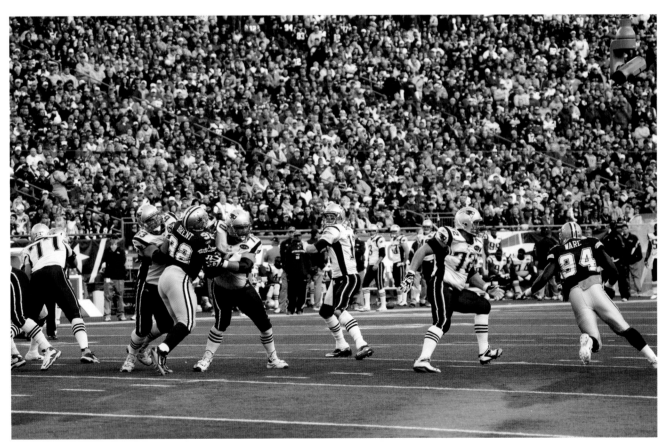

Tom Brady throws a pass from within the space provided by his offensive line, which gives him time to pick his receiver. Space creates time. Time does not create space. Photo by Joseph Sohm / Shutterstock.com.

Think about LeBron James having the ball stolen. The man who was guarding him streaks up the court, and if James just stands in place and throws his hands to the sky, the other team scores easily. But we've all seen him do just the opposite—sprint back on defense and swat his opponent's layup attempt out of bounds. Indeed, his block of Andre Iguodala's layup attempt was the pivotal moment in game seven of the 2016 NBA Finals.

THE MICRO PRINCIPLE OF COVER   3.7.5.4

Cover and support are closely related concepts. When the offense breaks down and possession is lost, there needs to be backup in place for the team that is now playing defense. Often, this means that teammates must stay close enough together to prevent their opponents from exploiting space if the ball changes hands.

Failure to provide such cover will result in the opposition quickly adjusting to having possession and creating penetration through width and depth quickly and look to rapidly fashion a scoring opportunity. While cover can come into play defensively through movement in that moment—such as when a basketball player switches onto another man on a pick-and-roll—cover is often more effective when it's part of the offensive plan.

So in soccer, for example, if a left back goes on a roving run up the wing, one of the central defenders moves to the left a little to cover the vacated area of the pitch. Similarly, the midfield could also realign itself to provide extra cover in case the left back loses the ball and the offense exploits this by attacking up that side of the pitch.

THE MICRO PRINCIPLE OF BALANCE   3.7.5.5

Balance is as essential in defense as in offense. The offensive side's misdirection, use of width and depth, and ball penetration can cause the defense to become imbalanced, which gives the attacking side space and time to execute a scoring opportunity. If a defense can stay organized and retain balance, it's less likely to leave gaps and is better able to close these gaps before the offense can take advantage of them.

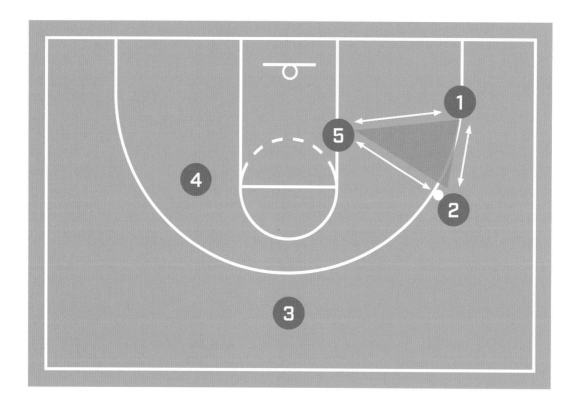

The triangle offense, popularized by Tex Winter.

THE MICRO PRINCIPLE
OF COMPACTNESS   3.7.5.6

When in the defensive moment of the game, the more compact your team is, the easier it is to provide cover and support for your teammates. Remaining compact also enables the defensive unit to close down attackers' space and to apply pressure to each offensive player and the ball. By setting up a compact defense, a team can prevent the opposition from accelerating and achieving penetration, two of the conditions necessary to create a threat to the goal, scoring zone, or basket.

Obtaining defensive compactness means that each defensive player covers less space, helping them to conserve energy throughout the game. Relatively even spacing also makes it more difficult for the offensive team to take advantage of certain defensive players' shortcomings. Furthermore, if a defense can remain compact, then connection to and communication among teammates will be improved.[52]

Cohesion is essential if compactness is to be maintained, as it is a team concept. If defensive play-ers aren't communicating, they will have trouble remaining compact and will struggle to exert control over the space that the attacking team wishes to exploit. The defensive unit needs to understand which areas of the playing surface are important to control and which are superfluous, so they can focus their attention on the danger areas and exert greater spatial control over them through compactness, support, and cover.

Offenses can disassemble compactness by using misdirection, depth and width, and continuous ball and player movement to pull the defenders out of position and create gaps in the areas vacated by the now-stretched back line. If a team knows that certain defenders have certain weaknesses, such as a lack of pace or poor stamina, players can try to make them cover more space with player and ball movement that isn't necessarily aimed at creating penetration or scoring chances. Forcing the defense to reposition itself with player movement is usually easier when facing a man-to-man scheme.

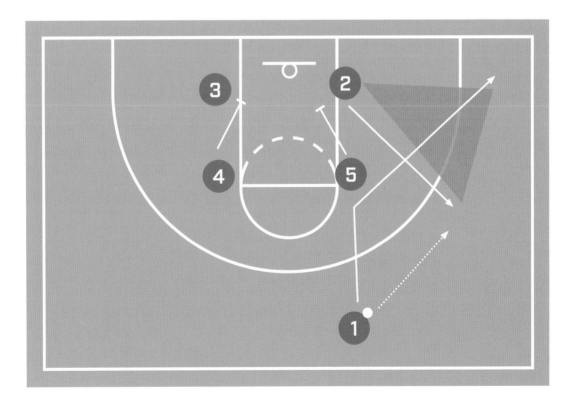

In the triangle offense, structure and movement are used to compress and create space.

THE GAME PLAN
3.8

I've established a system for game analysis and modeling. Next is the development of the game plan, which determines how a team will play. A game plan consists of structure, strategy, and tactics. *Structure* refers to the physical starting point of the players at each restart. The macro principle to which this relates is positioning (page 29). Structure does not refer to specific people in specific locations but rather to general positions on the field or court that should be established. Obviously, there are preferred players with ideal skillsets who can make the most of these positions, but this is secondary to structure.

> *The characteristic of the organism is first that it is more than the sum of its parts and second that the single processes are ordered for the maintenance of the whole.*

—Ludwig von Bertalanffy

Strategy concerns the specific adaptations of the game model to address each opponent. It's a style or method to defeat the opposition. Such adaptation should not change a principle or affect the cohesion of the overall model; it must respect its overarching principles. It's important to understand that the richer the game model, the more options the team will have to call on. *Tactics* refers to the detail of how exactly the strategy is executed.

STRUCTURE AND FORMATIONS
3.8.1

Structure is the formation that a team adopts at every restart. The coaching staff will change this structure as the game progresses and the scenario shifts. But for every single play, whether the formation is static, like in football, or dynamic, like in AFL, basketball, or soccer, the original positioning of each player is referred to as the team structure. As we saw above, this is all subject to such principles as misdirection and balance.

As the game is invariably mutable, structure must adapt to meet the evolving strategy and the tactics that comprise it. Structure can be used to promote certain elements of the game plan within each of the four moments. So if you're a soccer coach and one of your team's objectives is for the midfielders to "get the ball wide," you might line up with two defined wingers in a midfield structured within a 4-4-2 formation. If the defense shuts down one or both of the wingers early in the first half, perhaps you'll have them occupy a position closer to the central midfielders or further up the field.

When planning the team's structure for the next game, the head coach (and, in some sports, the various unit coordinators and assistants) must consider how to align the players to achieve the Commander's Intent and its sub-objectives, in keeping with the game model and macro and micro principles. Strategy is the positioning of the team to impact the other team's game model, its aims, preferences, and habits in each of the four game moments.

> *You can play hard. You can play aggressive. You can give 120%. But if one guy is out of position, then someone is running through the line of scrimmage and he is going to gain a bunch of yards.*

—Bill Belichick

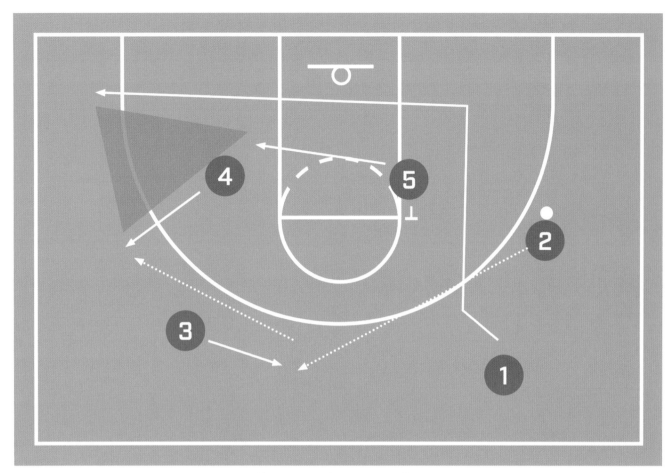

Speed and sequence are used to maximize the effectiveness of the triangle offense.

The same goes for how structure operates within set plays, when the ball comes back into play (such as a throw-in, lineout, or inbounds pass), and before and after game restarts (such as after time-outs or quarter and halftime breaks). While some games flow more than others, all have an inherent structure to some degree.

It's often said in team-sports circles that there is nothing new when it comes to tactics. While it's true that, assuming there is some level of scouting, the opposing team will have seen most of what you want to do, this doesn't rule out the potentially game-changing impact of springing surprises. In the documentary *A Football Life*, Bill Belichick revealed that unorthodox movement on the offensive line was key in fooling the opponent's defense and enabling his teams to win division titles and Super Bowls. Such unexpected tactics increase the degree to which the other team has to deal with a friction of the game: uncertainty.

The same is true of imaginative out-of-bounds plays drawn up by basketball coaches late in the game. If the other team knows that a predictable play will be used, it can set up accordingly to stifle it. But a creative coach will use decoys, screens, and player movement in innovative ways to create space and a potentially game-winning last-second shot.

What is strategy? A mental tapestry of changing intentions for harmonizing and focusing our efforts as a basis for realizing some aim or purpose in an unfolding and often unforeseen world of many bewildering events and many contending interests.

—John Boyd

STRATEGY   3.8.2

Strategy has several meanings in various contexts. The term has its origin in the Greek word *strategos*, which is normally translated as "general" or "art of the general." Colin Gray wrote, "Strategy is the bridge that relates military power to political purpose. It tells one how to conduct a war, or how to achieve political objectives, using the military instrument."[53]

In its simplest terms, strategy is an action plan that's focused on achieving a defined purpose. In the case of sport and conflict, this is the Commander's Intent and its sub-objectives. A coach's strategy is the series of decisions he or she makes as the game unfolds and the combination of tactics employed. Once the opposition starts reacting to and trying to thwart the game plan, the coach must make adaptations and corrections that improve the team's ability to reach its objectives and win the game in the conditions in which it finds itself. Tactical decisions are of increasingly vital importance the longer the game goes, particularly if the team is losing. Substitution patterns, tweaks to formation, and drawing up new plays are all ways that the coach can help the team prevail through strategy.

All men can see these tactics whereby I conquer, but what none can see is the strategy out of which victory is evolved.

—Sun Tzu

Although a head coach and his or her assistants must be adaptable and able to mold strategy as the game progresses based on the opposition's style and own adaptations, they have to stick to the team's core principles. A true principle cannot be malleable and change from game to game; otherwise it's not a principle at all but just hot air. The Patriots in their most successful years have used thirteen different starting lineups on their offensive line, the most of any NFL team over more than twenty years, and they have tried multiple combinations in a single season. Such squad rotation is successful because no matter which players take the field, they remain true to the team's core principles.

Strategies can also be used to overcome shortcomings in the squad. We've already seen how Ranieri used the counterattack so much because of Leicester's limitations in patient build-up play. Similarly, Bill Walsh created what became known as the West Coast offense because his quarterback at the Cincinnati Bengals, Virgil Carter, was not adept at completing long passes.[54] Once he had a better QB in Joe Montana at the 49ers (not to mention the perfect target for shorter passes in wide receiver Jerry Rice), Walsh's strategy became even more effective.

TACTICS   3.8.3

Tactics are the actions a team takes to execute its game plan and the aims within it. Tactics are a key part of strategy, and while a certain degree of adaptive pragmatism is needed, the tactics must fit within the boundaries of the game plan's goals for each moment. The execution of tactics depends on the athletes' ability to apply what they have learned in

> *I see tactics as an emergence which orders in a particular way each of the other dimensions. The process of tactical emergence has to do with what the cooks do, that is, the handling of spices for cooking a dish, and afterwards, a flavor emerges.*
>
> —Vítor Frade

training and games (i.e., their game-based education) and their technique.

Every team-sports athlete must have a baseline level of both. If they have technique but lack education, they will understand the skill that is needed, such as setting a pick in a basketball pick-and-roll, but will lack the correct judgment of when to use it. The result is failed execution. Similarly, if a player has had the in-game and training education to know when to do something, such as using a handoff in rugby right before being tackled by a defender, but lacks the technique to pull it off, the player won't be effective.

When it comes to tactics, too many coaches want to show how advanced their thinking is, so they overcomplicate matters when adopting Georgetown basketball coach John Thompson's mindset would be better: "Keep it simple. I'm not interested in trying to prove to my players that I'm a genius."[55]

The most important aspects of tactics are the macro principles: structure, ball circulation, player circulation, and the relationship (sequence and timing) among these (see pages 29 to 32). Rather than giving the team a complex list of what to do before a game—that is, specific ways of doing things in each game moment—it's better to provide them with a few very simple and obtainable objectives and let them use their experience to react as needed during the contest. Control should be relinquished in favor of guidance—coaches are not playing a video game! One of the issues with rigid tacticians' coaching is that it's impossible to plan for every eventuality in a game. Denying athletes permission to improvise compromises their ability to execute and meet pregame expectations.

If players are restricted by a defined tactic, they're going to feel too much pressure to do their job in a certain way, whereas if they're given freedom of decision-making, the outcomes are likely to be more positive, as the players will feel more relaxed and like they have the trust of the coaching staff to make the right call.

"We want to keep a certain level of randomness because we want our guys to use their talent, their reads, their ability, their understanding of the game—nothing's better than when five guys on the court figure it out," Boston Celtics head coach Brad Stevens said in an interview. "I don't want these guys to feel like they're robots and I don't want to coach them like they're robots, because ultimately you're going to have to use all that you know to win the game. We want our guys to feel like they're given the freedom to play."[56]

There are few game models, but there are infinite variations of tactics. There is also an unlimited variance in defensive schemes, but they are all based on three fundamental types of defense that are universal across different team sports: man-to-man defense, zone defense, and a hybrid of these two.

No matter which defensive scheme a team uses, it is essential that the defensive unit maintains organization, focus, and discipline until the final whistle or buzzer sounds if it is to limit the frequency, duration, and effectiveness of the opposition's offensive moments. As the defensive moment extends itself, the tendency is to lose concentration, make mistakes, and expose gaps that will quickly be exploited, particularly by an experienced, creative, and ruthless offense.

STRENGTHS AND WEAKNESSES

Rick Venturi, who was a Cleveland Browns assistant scout from 1991 to 1995, said of Bill Belichick, "Everybody in football wants to take away what you do best. The difference is Bill would go to an extreme to make you play left-handed. That's Belichick's absolute genius: pragmatism. When other coaches say it's important that we take away an opponent's best receiver, only Bill would commit four defenders on a receiver and play the rest of his defense with the other seven."[57]

The key takeaway from this example is that you have to be able to identify the weaknesses of the opposition so you can exploit them by removing their strengths.

THE MAN-TO-MAN DEFENSIVE TACTIC   3.8.3.1

Man-to-man defense is likely the oldest tactic ever invented. It is predicated on a defender applying constant pressure to a certain attacker. The objectives of a man-to-man scheme are easier to understand than those of a zone or hybrid approach, and there can be no confusion over dividing up territory. This makes it useful for young or inexperienced teams. It is often used based on the misplaced belief that it is more easily analyzed and hence quantified.

Man-to-man defense tends to encourage coaching personnel to attack physical advantages that the opposing offense possesses, the aim being to remove certain threats. It's very much a Newtonian approach to a problem, but it can be effective in some instances. For example, if a center is tall and explosive, a coach can nullify these attributes by guarding him with a similarly rangy and athletic player. Man-to-man defense can also enable a team to save the energy of its best player by assigning them to cover a lesser offensive threat.

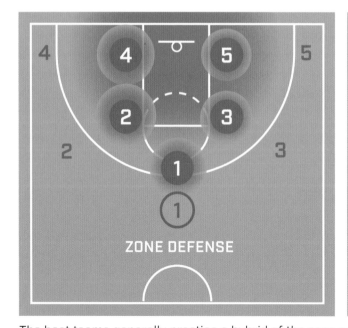

ZONE DEFENSE

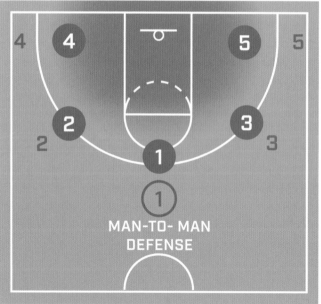

MAN-TO-MAN DEFENSE

The best teams generally practice a hybrid of the zone and man-to-man defenses.

THE ZONE DEFENSIVE TACTIC   3.8.3.2

There is a lot of confusion about what a zone defense is. At its most elemental level, a zone system involves each player defending a designated area of the field, pitch, or court, rather than another player. The keys to making a zone defense work include every player knowing their assigned area and getting to it quickly during offense-to-defense transitions. This requires discipline and intelligence.

In an effective zone defense, the defender must be proactive. The player must attack the ball the moment it comes into his or her area. The player can't be too late and has to be fully committed. This concept is often misunderstood, with players applying pressure when a *player* comes into their individual zone instead of the *ball*. This fails to slow the movement of the ball and allows the attacking team to quickly create a scoring opportunity.

THE HYBRID DEFENSIVE TACTIC   3.8.3.3

A hybrid defense combines the principles of zone and man-to-man defense. This strategy is often used when the opposing team has an extremely talented offensive weapon that the rest of the defensive scheme would struggle to contain. Most of the defenders play in a zone, but the best defender focuses on the threat posed by that particular player—like a box-and-one in basketball.

EXPECTATIONS AND ANTICIPATION   3.8.4

During a game, a player can expect a certain pattern to develop based on his or her prior experiences and knowledge of the opposing team's tendencies and preferences. This creates a certain level of anticipa-tion and causes the athlete to subconsciously prime mind and body to move in a certain way. However, nothing in sport can be predicted with anywhere close to 100 percent accuracy, so each player must be ready to adjust to the reality of what's happening, even when it contradicts their expectations and anticipation. As Vítor Frade said, "Reality pre-exists in our conception of things. The question is whether the idea adjusts to it."[58]

PATTERNS AND CONDITIONED RESPONSE   3.8.5

When Pavlov conducted his famous experiment with dogs, training them to salivate at the sound of a bell because it rang every time dinner was served, he showed the power of a conditioned response. Now, athletes obviously have a higher level of cognitive function than dogs, but the lesson is still valid in team sports. To reduce the amount of energy it consumes, the brain is constantly surveying the outside world to try to find patterns. When it does so, it prefers to output conditioned responses, as these are more efficient than having to do something new every time a scenario arises. So it is in a sports game, too. Athletes may not know it, but when they engage in competition, they are subject to the same kind of operant conditioning as Pavlov's dogs. The key is to make sure that the patterns they identify and the conditioned responses that these patterns elicit are appropriate for the situation and will further the achievement of the game plan objectives.

SCENARIOS   3.8.6

In a game, millions of possible situations can arise at any moment, against any opponent. It's impossible to plan for each and every one. However, head coaches can prepare their athletes to make better decisions and create learning experiences that help players apply the game plan to virtually any scenario.

Porto goalkeeper Vítor Baía discussed the extent of José Mourinho's meticulous preparation in this area in an article in *The Blizzard*:

> Sometimes it was as though he could see the future. I remember a specific incident against Benfica, when throughout the week he prepared us for what we should do after we scored a goal….He told us that [the Benfica coach José Antonio] Camacho would make a specific substitution and change his tactics, which was what happened. So we already knew what to do when he did it; we were completely prepared for it. For the same match, we also prepared to play with ten players, because José knew the referee would not be able to take the pressure and would show a red card along the way. That also happened, but we had already seen that movie during the week, so we knew what to do and got a narrow win.[59]

PATTERN RECOGNITION AND NONVERBAL COMMUNICATION   3.8.7

Arizona Cardinals football coach Bruce Arians was once asked how long it took legendary receiver Larry Fitzgerald and his quarterback to develop an understanding and feel comfortable in the offense. "Two solid years to learn all the things that are there for him," Arians said. "He had always been the X receiver. When you get in the middle of that hashmark area, there's so much more to learn and more balls to catch."

It wasn't just Fitzgerald who took time to build a rapport with his quarterback and fully comprehend the game plan. Arians revealed that it also took "over a year…for Carson to trust him to make the decisions the same way. If [Fitzgerald] had two-way goes or three-way goes, which one was he going to take? That's the hardest part for the quarterback and receiver, when I give you three-way options, up, out, in or out. At first, it was like, 'Where's he going?' Now, it's like 'Pop, there he is, he's going this way.' Carson sees his body language, and they see it the same way."[60]

This example shows that athletes need to play together consistently over an extended period to truly feel comfortable with one another. Once they reach a certain point, teammates can begin to read nonverbal cues and recognize patterns to predict what's coming next. This is one of the reasons excellent teams play together so smoothly.

THE SECRET IS IN PATTERNS AND CUES   3.8.7.1

In the course of a long season, it can be tempting for a head coach to tinker with the lineup to find the best combination of players. This is perfectly fine to a point, but if the coach messes around with the starters and the bench too much (not to mention calling up players from the reserves), the result will be instability in the organization and a lack of continuity on the field. If athletes are to get used to playing together to the point that they can use patterns and cues to be one step ahead, there must be some degree of squad stability.

When Leicester won the Premier League title, only eighteen players started a game (the lowest total in the league), and eight were called on by Ranieri to make at least thirty starts—the most in the league. So another factor of the Foxes' success—in addition to Ranieri's unorthodox counterattacking style and the outstanding play of Kante, Vardy, Drinkwater, and Mahrez—was consistency.[61]

PATTERNS AND DECISIONS 3.8.7.2

Decisions are not usually the result of conscious thought processes (except during the initial phases of learning—the verbal cognitive phase) but rather come from the subconscious.

So the goal of decision-making training should be to make athletes more attuned to specific environmental cues by manipulating constraints of the game. Coaches should allow athletes to discover solutions and guide them to these during learning experiences that allow experimentation, rather than simply tell them what to do.

Attuning players to specific cues in a game, teaching them tactical principles, and allowing them to make decisions on their own are key parts of team preparation. Instead of only running set plays, a coach should evaluate the strengths and weaknesses of the team and the opposition and then tailor tactics and strategy accordingly within the framework of the game plan.

SKILL AND THE GAME MODEL 3.8.8

So often we prioritize physical attributes in team sports and neglect the positive and negative impacts that skill and technique (or the lack thereof) can have on winning and losing. If players have insufficient skills, their decision-making cycles are going to be too slow in situations that demand the use of these skills. This means that unless they're able to apply superior physicality to a more skilled but athletically weaker opponent, they will come out second-best.

Technically proficient players often execute more often and more decisively because applying deeply grooved motor patterns requires less mental effort and so is less of a drain on their functional reserve. This gives them more energy to use on the action itself and reduces late-game fatigue. Effective players have cultivated the ability not only to master individual skills but also to select appropriate techniques and motor patterns unconsciously very quickly.

CHANCE AND GAME THEORY 3.8.9

It's possible to prepare almost perfectly for a game and still fall victim to the first friction of the game: chance. Perhaps the teams are tied going into the last minute and a deflected shot leaves the goalkeeper stranded and ends up in the back of your net. Or perhaps a key player is lost to injury, giving the other team a moment of relative superiority that they can exploit decisively. Maybe a referee makes a series of bad calls that tip the balance. All of these factors are outside any team's control.

That being said, the coaching staff can ensure that they have walked their players through adverse situations like these so that they have a compensatory routine to automatically adopt when facing a negative event that can be chalked up to chance. A great example from individual sports came when Michael Phelps was partway through the final of the two-hundred-meter butterfly at the 2008 Beijing Olympics. One of the eyecups on his goggles started leaking and then the other, until both were filled with water. This is the kind of situation that most athletes would use as an excuse for failing to win or medal.

Not Phelps. His preparation by coach Bob Bowman was so thorough and so meticulous that the Baltimore Bullet had mentally rehearsed entire races swum in difficult conditions. So when his goggles threatened to sabotage his bid for yet another gold medal, Phelps didn't do what most of us would have done: panic. Instead, he estimated the number of strokes remaining, timed his trademark burst of closing speed to perfection, and reached for the wall at exactly the right moment. The result? Not just a gold medal but also the unlikeliest of his many world records. "If I didn't prepare for everything that happens, when my goggles started filling up I'd have probably flipped out. That's why I swim in the dark," Phelps told *The Telegraph*. "We want to be ready for literally anything that comes our way. I never want to leave that comfort zone."[62]

Team-sports coaches can help mentally prepare their athletes in a similar manner. While there will always be unusual, chance-based events that nobody would think of, players and coaches can still explore various problem situations and develop coping/adaptation strategies that are applicable to a wide range of scenarios. This way, the athlete will feel ready, come what may, and will not waste valuable energy freaking out when fortune throws a curveball.

THE CERTAINTY OF UNCERTAINTY   3.8.10

While you can scout and assess each opponent's team game plan for every offensive moment, analyze their habits and patterns to predict what they're going to do, and adjust your strategy and tactics accordingly, there will still be events in each game that are unpredictable. The very nature of team sports means that there are myriad possibilities in every second of every game, and not all games follow the script that the athletes or their coaches have rehearsed. The other team also can do things that are unexpected, which are outside the scope of even the best and most comprehensive scouting report.

However surprising occurrences can be in a game, they need not be difference-makers when it comes to the final score. The better athletes and teams are prepared for what is likely, the more they are in command of what they can control within the game, and the more they buy into the coach's game plan and its principles, the better able they will be to deal with uncertainty and the game-time aspects over which they have little or no control.

THE GAME PLAN AND MITIGATED RISK   3.8.11

To reduce the impact of the opposing team's doing something unexpected during the game, a team must prepare diligently for each upcoming fixture and run through as many potential situations as time allows. This requires the head coach to show up at practice with every minute planned out so that the session remains high-quality while enabling the coaching staff to cover a lot of ground.

Bill Walsh explained how such meticulous legwork paid off when it came time to implement the game plan while mitigating risk during competition: "Calculated risks are part of what you do, but… I preferred the position of being able to take lower-risk actions with higher reward potential. That sounds like a situation that rarely exists—low risk, high reward—but it's exactly what my pass-oriented, ball-control system offered on the majority of our plays. In order to make it work, I applied great energy and expertise to a methodical process of anticipating, planning and practicing for every conceivable situation."[63]

QUALITATIVE ASSESSMENT
3.9

As I explained previously, a game evolves and presents itself to the coach and players. It cannot be scripted or predetermined. That being said, a series of characteristics can be observed in all games. It's important to understand that this is an assessment of the quality of game plan principle execution. The majority of coaches focus explicitly on winning. This is fine, but it does not lead to the kind of sustainable success that can come only from an assessment of how the team executes its principles within each context. John Wooden famously never focused on winning itself but on improving performance each time his team took the court. The result was a record eighty-eight-game winning streak.

There is a misconception that great teams compete against themselves. In reality, they reach a stage where they define themselves only against their best possible performance. Ideally, all teams should do this from the beginning, but very few do. A proper game model, developed and consistently expressed with respect to the game principles, will lead to this natural conclusion: the qualitative assessment of the performance.

Remember that a game is not simply an assessment of the players' or team's ability. It is a measure of the coaching process and the player experience. It's an assessment of the quality of training and teaching and then the players' execution. It's also an evaluation of the game model itself.

ANALYSIS OF THE EXPERIENCE
3.9.1

Three major factors contribute to proper analysis of any team sport. They are: looking at performance quality, not just statistics; examining the cohesiveness of the game model; and focusing on solutions, not problems.

QUALITATIVE BEFORE QUANTITATIVE
3.9.1.1

After a game ends, attempting to quantify the performance has become the go-to assessment method. It is true that this is measured to some extent by the scoreboard, but to assess in a manner that facilitates improvement, it's critical to evaluate how the team played with a combined quantitative *and* qualitative manner. One reason for focusing on qualitative as opposed to quantified analysis is that the players know that they have license to make the best decisions for the situation they face, not chase fixed statistics. Therefore, any quantitative analysis can be based only on principles. This means actions are already measured in context.

GAME MODEL COHESION
3.9.1.2

The analysis process is a reflection of the overall player experience. The constant reinforcement of the principles of the game, especially during evaluation, ensures a cohesive game model. It's important that all analysis is done with the cohesion of this model in view.

OUTCOME AND EFFECT
3.9.1.3

The primary focus of analysis is not simply to find mistakes or errors. Any analysis should be conducted with the aim of correcting or developing a habit. So the question among the coaching staff should always be how best to solve a certain problem. If it can be addressed by making a change without providing an explanation to the players, this is fine.

Development of Habit
3.9.1.3.1

As players enter formation, they look at how an individual or the opposing team is positioning itself, predict what the opposition is going to do next based on their experience and what's happening in the game, and act appropriately to thwart the opposition. In certain sports, the term *reads* is used, such as in American football, in which quarterbacks look at—*read*—how the defense is lined up and adjust their next play accordingly. Reads are also sometimes referred to as *keys*.

In *The Power of Habit*, Charles Duhigg recounts how Tony Dungy helped the Tampa Bay Buccaneers improve their performance by rewiring their on-field habit loops. When working with his squad on the under defense, Dungy noticed that outside linebacker Derrick Brooks occasionally hesitated at the start of a play and realized that he was trying to gather too much information from his read of the running back, quarterback, and guard.

Dungy didn't want Brooks to discard the cues he was accustomed to interpreting but rather to sequence them so that he focused on one at a time. "First, focus only on the running back," Dungy advised Brooks. "That's it. Do it without thinking. Once you're in position, *then* start looking for the QB." The result, Duhigg states, was that "it removed the need for decision-making. It allowed Brooks to move faster because everything was a reaction—and eventually a habit—rather than a choice."[64]

Even in team sports that don't typically use the word *reads*, players are still constantly looking at what's going on in the game, assessing it, and making split-second choices. Players' preparation (including learning the opponent's patterns and habits), on-field experience, and ability to process information will determine how quickly they can go through their decision-making cycle and how effective the outcome of their chosen action will be.

Typically, coaches should follow Tony Dungy's example and advise their players to look for three things, one at a time. So if Cristiano Ronaldo is lining up a free kick, he might look first at the far upper corner for a direct shot on goal, then the near top corner (taking into account the goalkeeper's positioning, the distance, and all the usual factors, which he can evaluate based on experience), and finally the third option of curling the ball over the wall and onto a teammate's head.

QUALITATIVE OBSERVATIONS

3.10

Not all observations are necessarily quantifiable, nor do they need to be. But the quality of the play still must be observed. Here are factors to consider.

EFFICIENCY AND EFFECTIVENESS

3.10.1

Being efficient during a game means executing with the least amount of effort possible. Teams that are more efficient need fewer possessions and scoring opportunities to put points on the board and win games. Efficiency is a primary measure of quality. Using the game moments construct, it's possible to assess how efficient a team was during offense, defense, offense-to-defense, and defense-to-offense. In doing so, coaches can identify roadblocks that led to inefficiency, which in turn wasted opportunities and energy and compromised the game plan.

EFFICIENCY

3.10.1.1

Players tend to be more efficient when they have a greater number of passing opportunities and more available space. Efficiency is the economy of motion and effort, and having more options typically improves efficiency. For example, if a football team's wide receivers time their routes optimally and more than one receiver gets open, the quarterback will have a much greater chance of completing a pass to one of them, and his efficiency rating will go up.

The overarching goal of any team should be to become as efficient as it's able in all stages of the game and to force the opposition to become highly inefficient by being active and disruptive on the defensive end. The result of this imbalance is often the difference between winning and losing.

EFFECTIVENESS

3.10.1.2

The other side of the efficiency coin is effectiveness, which concerns how well a team is executing to reach the Commander's Intent and satisfy the secondary aims of the game plan. A team can be very efficient in the construction and penetration micro moments of the offensive moment and yet fail to score because of poor execution. You can have the most efficient squad in the world, but if you're ineffective, it will not help you to win. The coaching staff's job is to find room for improvement in both efficiency and effectiveness using the game model and then to work on improving both during all four game moments on the training ground.

PATTERNS OF TEAM PLAY

3.10.2

Sometimes the myriad events that take place in the course of every game can seem random and disconnected, with player actions dependent on the demands of each unique situation in which they find themselves. These situations are complicated, but by using the system of moments and principles, we can better understand how the game can be described in a completely different light.

Since all games are in essence embodiments of human expression within these contexts, a team will demonstrate distinct tendencies. Every team and its athletes have certain propensities, preconditioned movement patterns, and predisposed reactions to stimuli that they default to automatically again and again, especially in certain scenarios.

It is possible to study how a team as a whole or its individual parts tend to react in offensive, defensive, and transitional (defense-to-offense and vice versa) moments. By doing so, an opponent can start to identify patterns that make strengths and weaknesses apparent within the context of the game.

SURFACES AND GAPS   3.10.3

A team's success or failure on game day is just as dependent on its knowledge of the opponent as it is on its understanding of itself. Of course, you cannot predict every possible situation, but this is not an excuse for being underprepared. As Sun Tzu puts it in *The Art of War*, "If you know the enemy and know yourself, you need not fear the result of a hundred battles. If you know yourself but not the enemy, for every victory gained you will also suffer a defeat. If you know neither the enemy nor yourself, you will succumb in every battle."[65]

The concept of surfaces and gaps is another takeaway from military strategy and, specifically, the teachings of William Lind, who built on John Boyd's work and contributed much to the theories of maneuver warfare. The teachings of Robert Leonhard are also highly relevant. Whether on the battlefield or the team-sports game field, surfaces and gaps relate to the creation, closing down, and exploitation of space. Compression can be thought of as a surface, while dispersal is a gap.

Gaps are created through player and particularly ball circulation. Moving opposing defensive players out of position makes more usable space available and creates gaps. Attacking players try to accelerate their decision-making cycles so that they're faster than those of the defense and they can take advantage of the gap. Consider a running back or rugby prop punching through a hole that appears in the defense for only a moment.

Another way to look at gaps is as enemy soft spots. Conversely, then, surfaces can be regarded as enemy strengths, which are to be avoided or negated as much as possible. What constitutes a surface and what is a gap is not static but instead varies situationally. As the U.S. Marine Corps publication *Warfighting* suggests, "What is a surface in one case may be a gap in another."[66]

When applied to team-sports games, this could mean that a particular defender is very strong when a ball handler attacks her on the left side. Knowing this from the scouting report, the point guard would instead try to dribble right against this player.

GAME STYLE   3.10.4

In his writings about warfare, John Boyd identified three different types of conflict that can also be applied to team-sports games: attrition, maneuver, and moral. With regard to their own teams, coaches must assess the type of players they have and decide which of these three approaches will be most effective. Though a good team might switch effectively between these styles and adapt their application based on each opponent's strengths and weaknesses, the coaching staff's job is not to make their team proficient in all three. Rather, they must prepare their athletes to counter and disrupt other teams' use of each conflict type to defeat them.

Now let's take a look at each style and its key characteristics.

If equally matched, we can offer battle; if slightly inferior in numbers, we can avoid the enemy; if quite unequal in every way, we can flee from him.

—Sun Tzu

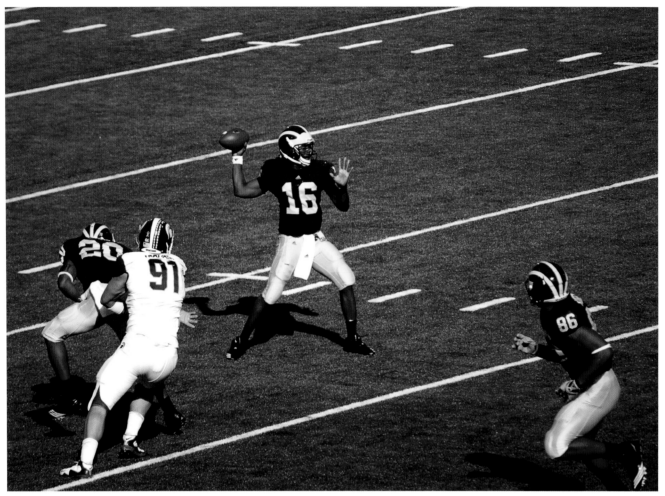

Denard Robinson prepares to throw a pass from within the pocket. Space creates time, and great players with time are very difficult to defend against. Photo by Susan Montgomery / Shutterstock.com.

ATTRITION STYLE   3.10.4.1

This style involves one side trying to grind its opponent down through persistence. It was used by both sides in World War I, by Pompey and Caesar's armies in ancient Rome, and by Napoleon. Boyd used this maxim to define attrition warfare: "Firepower is king of the battlefield."[67]

In team sports, we see attrition warfare in action when teams employ bigger, more powerful offensive and defensive lines in American football (the Steelers of the late 1970s), strong forward packs in rugby (England's 2003 World Cup–winning side), and "Twin Towers" (Tim Duncan and David Robinson on the Spurs' 1999 and 2003 championship-winning teams) on the front line in basketball. In summary, attrition warfare is most effective for teams that are bigger and stronger than their opponents. These advantages may not be telling early in the game, but as it progresses they take their toll on the other team, forcing it to fall apart late in the contest. Proponents of attrition typically have greater wealth in terms of personnel and can keep hammering their opponents all game long until they collapse.

In the 2015 AFC Championship, the Denver Broncos' offensive line used the attrition warfare approach to wear down the smaller, less powerful defensive line of the New England Patriots. This resulted in New England quarterback Tom Brady having less time than he needed in the pocket, which prevented him from putting in the kind of performance required to lead his team to a seventh Super Bowl appearance.

MANEUVER STYLE   3.10.4.2

Like attrition style, maneuver style was originally defined in the context of warfare. In both conflict and sport, the maneuver style revolves around creating space to invade. This can only come about through compression and expansion. Compression can be best achieved with the least physical cost through misdirection. Such misdirection can only be executed by exploiting speed and movement. By moving either players or the ball, we can create space or compress the opponents' defenders at varying speeds.

The one important difference between conflict and sport, of course, is that, in game theory parlance, team sports are something of a zero-sum game: there is fixed space to compress and expand into. This means that you can't compress without expanding somewhere else. This is why, in order to exploit space, synchronicity is vital.

When applied to team sports, maneuver warfare is characterized by the use of speed and counterattacking to create scoring opportunities through chaos and confusion. Bill Walsh adopted this approach with Stanford and Eddie DeBartolo's San Francisco 49ers. The greatest threat to the success of maneuver warfare is when the opposition slows or halts movement, allowing itself to exert strength and power.

Although General Rommel gets a lot of credit in terms of maneuver warfare results on the battlefield, Heinz Wilhelm Guderian probably formalized it best as a doctrine. Rommel stated, "In Germany the elements of modern armored warfare had already crystallized into a doctrine before [World War II]...and had found practical expression in the organization and training of armored formations."[68]

From a team-sports perspective, there are four very important lessons to be learned from Guderian's maneuver warfare work. One is the idea of misdirecting the opponent, which Rommel did to devastating effect in Africa before the main Allied landing in late 1942. The second is the importance of rapid attack and the impact of concentrated force at speed to occupy ground. Although *blitzkrieg* is an overused term, it is the most obvious example of maneuver warfare.

Third is the idea of communication in combined attack. Maneuver is not possible without the use of good communication. General Hermann Balck said, "The decisive breakthrough into modern military thinking came with Guderian, and it came not only in armor, but in communication."[69] This was not simply on a macro scale. Guderian also saw the value in a cellular approach by encouraging the use of autonomous five-man teams. Finally, and most significant, is the idea of combined attack. No one operates alone. Blitzkrieg succeeded with fast, mobile warfare, but the importance of efficient air support is often forgotten.

In sports, one team that has used maneuver warfare effectively is the Golden State Warriors, whose faster offense proved unstoppable during the 2014–15 and 2015–16 NBA seasons. The Cleveland Cavaliers tried to counter this in the 2015 NBA Finals with LeBron James leading a war of attrition with an old-school back-down post game reminiscent of Charles Barkley. The injury-ravaged Cavs couldn't overcome the Warriors in that series but did win a respectable two games. They went on to get revenge in the 2016 Finals.

The Smart Take from the Strong   3.10.4.2.1

One of the first innovators of the concept of small influential groups in conflict was Hamilcar Barca, a Carthaginian general who led a successful guerrilla war against the Romans in Sicily in the third century BC. His son Hannibal elaborated on this to provide some of the first examples of modern maneuver warfare, also against the Romans, at the Battle of Cannae in 216 BC. Napoleon adopted this approach successfully two thousand years later. Maneuver warfare was also employed to devastating effect by Ulysses S. Grant and Stonewall Jackson in the American Civil War and later by George Patton and Douglas MacArthur in World War II. And of course, German forces in World War II used it extremely effectively.

People like John Boyd saw maneuver warfare as a better way ahead for the U.S. military, rather than continuing to rely on the greater resources and firepower that had made attrition warfare the favored style. Today, small, elite, and nimble military units, like the British SAS and SBS and the Navy SEALs and Delta Force in the U.S., are leading proponents of maneuver warfare.

MORAL STYLE   3.10.4.3

Another term for this pattern is *guerilla* or *insurgency*. This style of conflict is chosen when a group recognizes that it has inferior firepower and may lack the mobility needed to successfully implement maneuver warfare. Famous wartime practitioners include Sun Tzu, the Mongols, and the Vietcong during the Vietnam War.

On the sporting field, we see teams use the moral style—so called because it's sometimes used in cause-based conflict—for similar reasons. Teams use skillful players to negate the brute power of an attrition approach and to define when, where, and how they engage their opponent. The moral style is closely related to the concept of relative superiority (which we will explain and explore later) in that teams who use it must exploit chances when they come along. This may not happen very often against a physically superior team with a well-drilled defense, against whom execution of scoring opportunities is vital. Teams sometimes combine or alternate between attrition and maneuver approaches, but the moral style is used exclusively by teams with limited resources.

The biggest upset of the 2015 Rugby World Cup was engineered through the use of the moral style. Japan's head coach, Eddie Jones, recognized that his players would be outmatched if they tried to go toe-to-toe with the behemoths on South Africa's front line. So instead, he took this size and power advantage away from the Springboks by employing a highly technical approach that created scoring chances by sowing seeds of uncertainty. Then they had the presence of mind and willpower to execute these chances and came away with the biggest victory in the history of Japanese rugby.

GAME AND TEAM TEMPO   3.10.5

At its most basic level, tempo in a team-sports context is the ability to change pace and alter the speed of ball and player movement. This depends on how well players work together and know each other's tendencies, and on how well the team can force the opponent into making poor decisions and then capitalize on them. Tempo is not speed itself but rather the gearing that enables a team to choose and move between different speeds. Just like on a racing bicycle, every gear has a different purpose—in the Tour de France, the yellow jersey holder will want to select one gear for flat sprints and another for long, arduous climbs.

To put it another way, it's not speed that kills but the *change* of speed. Muhammad Ali's most famous quote—"Float like a butterfly and sting like a bee"—perfectly illustrates the ability of the most effective athletes and teams to change speed on a dime and do so efficiently and gracefully. As explained earlier, the transition from fast to slow ball is the embodiment of tempo, but it also involves the movement of players and teammates. The difference between a very good team and an elite one is not speed itself but change in speed. This is not confined to sports but exists in close-quarter combat, too.

Tempo also varies between levels in team sports. At the elite end, there are certainly physiological differences. Players are bigger, faster, and stronger. But if you go to enough games at each level of team sport, what starts to become apparent is just how quickly the game moves in the NBA, NFL, Premier League, and national-level rugby. Players are not only more technically and tactically advanced, they're also making decisions at a much faster rate. Therefore, they're moving more quickly and changing pace—or shifting gears—more rapidly than at the lower levels of the sport.

In an article about World Cup– and UEFA Champions League–winning midfielder Xabi Alonso for *Sports Illustrated*, Grant Wahl wrote, "Because Alonso touches the ball so often in any given possession, he can influence the tempo of his team's passes, adjusting the metronome to a higher frequency to put pressure on the opposition, or to a lower frequency to settle the game down."[70] A transformative talent like Alonso can, then, influence the pace at which the entire team plays for portions of the game. The same could be said of the great basketball point guard Magic Johnson, whose command of the ball was so impactful that he could shift the gears of his "Showtime" Lakers from methodical, play-oriented attack on one possession to a freewheeling, run-and-gun fast break the next, keeping the defense in a constant state of uncertainty.

Tempo is also essential in the military. Special forces operatives move slowly and cautiously to get into position without detection and then act with incredible speed to storm a building and extract hostages within a couple of minutes. While moving and shooting are essential skills in such a situation, communication is also key, as is going through learning experiences so many times during training that responses are conditioned.

EMOTION, SPEED, AND THE GAME PATTERN
3.10.6

As speed and intensity vary throughout each game, the emotional state of each individual player and the team as a whole is highly contextual and ebbs and flows, too. Though we break the game down into moments, micro moments, and stages to better analyze it, it's impossible to make blanket statements or assumptions about a player's emotions at any point because there are endless variables.

Every dance has a particular rhythm. An elegant foxtrot requires smooth, controlled movements and restraint on the part of each partner. The tango, on the other hand, requires aggression and passion. The same is true of team-sports games and the athletes who play them. Every speed has a particular motivation and an accompanying set of emotions.

A team that is scared and intimidated by its opponent—such as a second-division side facing Arsenal in the FA Cup or a mid-major school taking on Duke in the NCAA Tournament—often plays slowly and hesitantly. In contrast, a championship-winning side that is confident will often advance the ball rapidly and without hesitation, its belief that it will win most games reflected in the tempo it adopts.

How much time is left on the clock also impacts emotion and, therefore, the pace of the contest. At the start of a game, many teams try to set the ground rules for engagement. So a big center may take an early hard foul on the opponent's star guard in a basketball playoff game to set the defensive tone. Or a rugby team may try to gain ground quickly and put points on the board in the first few minutes to serve notice that it will be on the attack for the entire game. From a physiological standpoint, players' heart rates and activity cycles are highly elevated at the beginning of a game and drop off dramatically after the first seven to twelve minutes, as the game settles into a certain tempo.

The end of a game also presents its own emotional and physical challenges that are situational. For example, being up 1–0 in a soccer game against a poor side with limited attacking options after eighty-five minutes will likely produce a very different emotional state in a team than having the same one-goal advantage over an opponent that has an embarrassment of offensive riches and could quickly level the score, like Real Madrid. In the first situation, players will likely feel comfortable and relaxed, while in the second, they're probably tense, anxious, and stressed. The coaching staff must be ready to make tactical adjustments and substitutions based on their assessment of the players' ever-changing emotional states.

Introducing a fast player can have devastating effects on a tired adversary, as seen in Manchester United's unlikely comeback win over Bayern Munich in the 1999 European Cup Final. Sir Alex Ferguson's introduction of speedy Ole Gunnar Solskjaer produced the stoppage time winner, as the Norwegian found space behind the Munich defense with seconds remaining in the contest. If speed kills, then late-game speed can prove particularly deadly.

> **"**
> *I don't want to be interesting. I want to be good.*
>
> —Ludwig Mies van der Rohe **"**

THE GAME LIFE CYCLE   3.10.7

All games have a natural life cycle. Of course, the principles of chaos affect the game and how it evolves. Strong starts are important for newer teams to reestablish and reinforce the belief in the game model and game plan, which are newer for them. Older teams can overcome relatively slower starts because established faith in the game plan will sustain players during periods of stress earlier on. We will look at team constructions and profiles later, but the profile of the team will dictate its resilience and ability to buy into the head coach's philosophy.

THE FITTEST TEAM NEVER WINS   3.10.7.1

One of the most used phrases immediately postgame is, "The fitter team won." This is a complete falsehood. The fittest team never wins—the best team does. Fitness alone has nothing to do with the outcome. Have you ever seen a winning team leave the field to comments of "They were not fit enough"? The aim of good teams is to make the opposition work harder. If a team is better technically and tactically, it is more efficient, and eventually its opponent becomes more fatigued. As we will explore more in a moment, this fatigue will accumulate and have a greater effect during the final plays and last quarter of the game. How this manifests itself depends on the limiting factors of the team, unit, and individual players. Occasionally, fatigue shows up in emotional issues, such as lack of self-discipline in committing a foul, or cognitive issues, in forgetting a play or position. But the perceived outcome is physical—seen as a separation, slowness, delayed reaction, or slow movement.

ACCUMULATED FATIGUE   3.10.7.2

Fatigue is not a one-off thing in team sports but rather an accumulation. As the game wears on, the physical, cognitive, and emotional load of different events and situations builds up on each player. The impact of fatigue depends on the individual profile of that player and how much functional reserve they have going into the contest. Often, when accumulated fatigue presents itself, it creates a tipping point that turns the match in favor of one team or the other.

So while the failure point may appear as a tactical or technical error, the actual fatigue may have been caused by something completely different, such as psychological fatigue. This is why efficiency is such a critical, and sadly underestimated, aspect of team performance: it delays the accumulation of fatigue in games.

THE FLOW OF ELITE TEAMS   3.10.8

Flow, as it relates to elite teams, occurs within a game when ball and player movement occur with as little wasted energy as possible. When a team is flowing offensively, its timing and sequencing are dialed in and the team as a whole is operating efficiently. Returning to the macro principles, this is when movement of ball and player are sequenced to match perfectly. Anticipation is a key aspect, but so is recognizing teammates' patterns, movements, and precursors to these movements.

But anyone who has experienced flow knows that the deep enjoyment it provides requires an equal degree of disciplined concentration.

—Mihaly Csikszentmihalyi

Conversely, the defense must aim to disrupt the other team's attacking flow and in its place sow the seeds of dissonance. Applying ball and player pressure prevents the establishment of a certain tempo and restricts the offense's ability to control the pace of the game. This is why in basketball, for example, if a coach knows that the team is facing a high-tempo, fast-ball offense, one of the primary defensive goals will be to "slow the ball down." The coach hopes that if the offense's aim to "push the ball" is derailed, it will be thrown out of its rhythm. If this happens, the offense will be unable to execute its game plan objectives for the attacking moment.

Obtaining defensive flow requires players to apply pressure together, cover for and support each other, and communicate well. We see a lack of defensive flow when players don't do these things and are disorganized, allowing the offense to do exactly what it intends.

RHYTHM 3.10.8.1

Rhythm is a series of repeated flows between game moments that make up the game as a whole. A team can get into a rhythm only if every player is executing connected actions with a shared goal in mind and at a similar speed. Sports commentators often say things like "The team is really struggling to find their rhythm today" when teammates are struggling to move themselves or the ball at a unified pace.

The teams that find their ideal rhythm early in the game and maintain it are often those that have been playing together for a long time. Familiarity among teammates on the training ground and in games enables athletes to understand how their comrades prefer to act in certain situations, to learn what their abilities and limitations are, and to identify their habits in each game moment and micro moment. So players are effectively creating a mini scouting report in their heads about their teammates, and the more time they spend with each other, the richer these reports become.

Such knowledge makes it easier for each member of the team to predict what the others will do in any game-time situation. This speeds up the decision-making process, which in turn leads to faster, more decisive actions. The quality of the decisions will also be better, increasing the chance of a successful outcome.

In the noise of a competitive game, verbal communication can become largely irrelevant; this is why the ability to recognize nonverbal cues is essential. There may be universal examples, such as a basketball player pointing to the sky when they want the point guard to throw an alley-oop pass toward the rim. But players also try to give each other many subtler indicators—gestures, eye movements, and so on.

A team's ability to establish flow and rhythm, particularly when attacking, largely depends on its ability to recognize and interpret such cues and incorporate them into the decision-making cycle. The goal for each player should be to instinctively know how teammates will act in a game scenario—such as how they will try to create or exploit space—so that each player can make the right decision. A series of correct autonomous choices helps create flow, which, when sustained, establishes rhythm.

FLUIDITY   3.10.8.2

A team that is having trouble getting into rhythm and flow will seem to be moving in fits and starts. This staccato rhythm is characterized by a profound lack of fluidity. Maybe it's a basketball team whose offense has broken down and is reverting to a series of one-on-ones to try to get points on the board, or a rugby team that frequently wins back possession only to throw the ball away again without getting close to scoring a try.

Then there are those times when a team is moving the ball quickly but without hurrying and is playing in sync like a well-conducted orchestra. The players' movements, both individually and collectively, are graceful and fluid and seem to be highly efficient. Every player seems to be trying to create opportunities for each other rather than just pursuing personal highlights. Take the Chicago Bulls team that won six championships, for example. When Tex Winter's triangle offense was flowing, Horace Grant said that the team was "a smooth operating machine. Baryshnikov in action! Picasso painting! A beautiful thing!"[71]

MOMENTUM   3.10.8.3

Creating momentum is the art of creating sustained effectiveness. Think about when a football team steadily marches up the field, gaining yardage and first downs as it progresses toward the end zone. Or when a basketball team goes on a run and turns a two-point deficit into a ten-point lead within a couple of minutes. Or when a rugby team scores two tries right after halftime to effectively end the game. Each of these scenarios involves a team creating and sustaining offensive momentum.

A defensive unit can also establish momentum by repeatedly shutting down and dispossessing the offensive group. In sports that require each player to both attack and defend, sustaining momentum on both ends can help a team fight back from a deficit. So if a basketball team applies sustained pressure and gets several stops defensively and then is able to convert on multiple successive possessions, two-way momentum can create a ten- or fifteen-point swing.

Each and every game is different because context is constantly changing. An intersquad scrimmage between a college basketball team's varsity and junior varsity squad is inherently different than a preseason exhibition, which is unlike a conference game, which has little in common with a tournament semifinal.

Comprehensive evaluation of team performance simply cannot exclude the context in which the game is played. Other factors to consider include recent run of form, prior history against the opponent, the number of injuries and how many games key players have missed, and the stakes of the game (from fairly meaningless preseason tune-up to national championship and everything in between). Also, is the game being played at home or away, and is it the only fixture that week or the second night of a back-to-back matchup? Only by establishing the setting and background of the game can we begin to frame certain deductions about it.

GAME EVENTS   3.10.9

We can use the following terms to identify the nature of events in a game or in conflict/combat events. It's important to be able to pinpoint each event and then determine which ones are key or pivotal. Doing this allows us both to understand the psychological resilience of the team and to find patterns in the play of both teams.

> *There is an old saying about the strength of the wolf is the pack, and I think there is a lot of truth to that. On a football team, it's not the strength of the individual players, but it is the strength of the unit and how they all function together.*

—Bill Belichick

KEY EVENTS   3.10.9.1

Key events involve two or more players. Just like regular events, they may not involve a majority of the team, but they can still be important. Examples include a double team trap and pick-and-roll in basketball, double coverage in football, a one-two in soccer, and a give-and-go in rugby. In the military, a key event could involve one operator providing covering fire while another advances.

PIVOTAL EVENTS   3.10.9.2

Pivotal events, unlike key events, have an effect on the entire team and the outcome of the game, even if the scenario didn't involve a direct contribution from each and every player. A pivotal event typically presents an opportunity to take advantage of relative superiority (which we'll discuss in more detail in a moment), such as a swift counterattack in soccer, an interception in rugby and football, and a three-on-one fast break in basketball. The timing of a pivotal event can have a great impact on the outcome of the game, particularly in low-scoring team sports like soccer. A team's ability to execute effectively is key to the success of pivotal events. Because, the law of individual influence tells us, some players are more influential—and skillful—than others, pivotal events often involve key players exhibiting moments of great skill.

RELATIVE SUPERIORITY AND ENGAGEMENT   3.10.10

In the seesaw of a game or military engagement, there are moments when each team gains the upper hand. A team's ability to take full advantage of these instances of relative superiority can determine the outcome.

The concept of relative superiority was first presented by Admiral William McRaven, former commander of Joint Special Operations Command (JSOC). The understanding of relative superiority in engagements is central to the understanding of how a diligent small force can overwhelm a larger force in conflict moments or game moments.

In basketball, a three-on-one fast break is an example of relative superiority in the defense-to-offense transition moment. An American football team running back an interception is another. In rugby, relative superiority can result as one team drives the other backward toward the goal line.

Relative superiority occurs in the two defensive moments, too. In basketball, the team that's defending achieves it when two players trap the ball handler. The same can happen in football when a defensive lineman punches through the offensive line and bears down on the quarterback. Defensive instances of relative superiority can prove just as pivotal as offensive ones if they're executed correctly.

While the motor patterns and habits that a player or multiple players deploy to take advantage of relative superiority are largely unconscious, concentration and focus can't just fall by the wayside. It's all too easy for a soccer player to take his eye off the ball and miss an open goal, a rugby player to pull a seemingly simple penalty wide of the posts, or a tight end to drop an easy catch.

The fewer scoring opportunities a team has in a game, the more important it is to take chances. We've all heard of players being described as "clinical" finishers or "clutch" performers, and that's exactly the kind of personnel who convert relative superiority into goals or points. The pressure of certain situations can make it more or less difficult to do so. Where some players flourish, others wilt.

> *There remains nothing, therefore, where an absolute superiority is not attainable, but to produce a relative one at the decisive point, by making skillful use of what we have.*
>
> —Carl von Clausewitz

The better prepared players are, the more good and bad situations the coaches have walked them through, and the more experience they have, the more likely they are to capitalize on relative superiority. Having familiar routines that precede the required action—like NBA superstar Kevin Durant's shoulder shimmy at the free-throw line or Welsh rugby fly half Dan Biggar's distinctive shuffle before attempting a penalty—also help reduce anxiety and increase the chances of success.

SYNCHRONICITY   3.10.11

The ultimate aim for all teams is a synchronicity that appears as a simultaneous sequencing of actions that are related and interact and appear almost causal. This comes about through the combination of things. First, timing and sequencing must be aligned. Second, the players must know each other's habits well enough to predict what's coming next and take instinctive, unconscious action. Third, the athletes involved must have both the experience and the technical proficiency to execute the required skills. Finally, they must act faster than the opposition can react.

THE MISINTERPRETATION OF WHITNEY AND FORD

3.11

At the end of the eighteenth century, American armed forces faced several big problems in preparing for a possible war with France and the specter of renewed hostilities with Britain, still smarting from its defeat in the Revolutionary War. One of these was a massive imbalance in armaments. The British Empire dominated more than a quarter of the nations on earth, and to maintain its dominance, its army had amassed an almost unlimited supply of firearms. The same went for France, a long-standing military power with a huge stock of rifles and muskets.

Recognizing that the U.S. Army would quickly be overcome if it faced France or Britain without addressing this imbalance, inventor Eli Whitney promised to manufacture ten thousand rifles within two years. Some scoffed at this lofty aim, as gun production was typically a slow process in which individual gunmakers painstakingly constructed each rifle from start to finish. Yet the army's top brass were convinced by Whitney's ambitious proposal and awarded him a contract in 1798.

Instead of having one craftsman assemble each gun from scratch with whatever components they saw fit, Whitney pioneered the interchangeable-parts approach. This meant assessing each kind of gun and breaking it down into a series of standardized components. A metalworker would then make a single part using one of Whitney's new milling machines. When put together, all of the individual parts formed a complete gun. Though his approach was initially slower than he'd anticipated and it took Whitney ten years rather than two to complete the order, he soon created new efficiencies that enabled him to fulfill the army's next order—this time for fifteen thousand rifles—in less than the two-year target.[72]

Fast-forward to the twentieth century, and Henry Ford utilized and improved upon Whitney's interchangeable-parts method to create his famed car assembly line. Ford not only assigned individual workers to specific parts but also knew exactly how many actions each task required and how long it would take to create and add each part.[73]

The legacy of this approach has influenced much of human productivity assessment ever since. In the past five years, we've seen misguided coaches and analysts try to apply a simplified interchangeable-part approach to the evaluation of team sports performance. The thinking goes that if you can measure each aspect of the game, break down each player's role, and then make each stop on the assembly line more efficient, you'll fix problems and win more games.

People are not machines, but in all situations where they are given the opportunity, they will act like machines.

—Ludwig von Bertalanffy

The trouble is that athletes are neither manufacturing components nor steelworkers performing standardized, routine tasks. They are, in contrast, complex organisms interacting with each other on multiple physical, emotional, and motivational levels. And unlike the predictable outcomes of the assembly line, there are an almost limitless number of possibilities in the course of each sporting contest. You can't find and fix inefficiencies in a team the same way you would on a factory floor, yet all too often, that's the way organizations have tried to improve, by channeling Henry Ford and trying to break down player performance to the minutest stats-monitored detail.

MEASURING HUMANS   3.11.1

There are numerous reasons why treating sports teams like an assembly line doesn't work. First, although coaches give players objectives as part of the game plan, these are subject to numerous internal and external factors that impact the athlete's ability to deliver on those objectives. A player's mental state, injuries and stiffness, illness, and the psychological specter of past failures all play a role in how effective the individual is in any particular game. Unless the game is played indoors, there are also environmental factors to consider, such as air temperature, humidity, and wind speed and direction. Even indoor games played in a dome or an enclosed arena will have different conditions.

Then factor in environmental elements like the crowd. As coaches and players know all too well, there's a huge difference between playing at home and playing on the road. At away games, you have to contend not only with the hostile reception from the other team's fans but also with the impact of being crammed into a plane or bus, changing time zones and elevation, and the effects of travel-related dehydration, jet lag, soft-tissue tightness, and so on. Then there are intangibles, such as the pressure of a cup final or playoff game, the nerves of rookie players, and the unspoken rivalries between squad members who don't get along. Plus, there are the worries of contract negotiations, upcoming trade windows, impending free agency, and so much more.

It's evident that neither interchangeable parts nor assembly-line thinking are useful when trying to assess the complex, dynamic system involving athletes, teams, and the games they play. We must stop applying reductionist approaches and instead view the game in a more comprehensive manner. Having said that, however, we cannot hope to look at the entire game as a whole, as there is simply too much too digest—it would be like trying to eat the proverbial elephant in one gulp.

This is why it's so important to consider the game as macro moments and micro moments. This allows us to subjectively and objectively assess a set of actions within a particular context, with the goal of identifying what is working and what isn't.

QUANTITATIVE ANALYSIS OF QUALITATIVE ASSESSMENT

3.11.2

Celtics coach Red Auerbach sniffed at numerical analysis, saying, "I don't believe in statistics. There are too many factors that can't be measured. You can't measure a player's heart." Those who coach and prepare elite players know that you cannot truly measure everything. There are intangibles. Having worked with winners like Justin Smith, Steven Gerrard, Frank Gore, Paul O'Connell, and Martyn Williams, I've realized that you can measure the heart as a muscle (when it comes to biomarkers like heart rate variability), but you can't, as Auerbach said, measure heart in terms of the commitment, desire, and will to win that the best athletes have.

There are two main kinds of analysis when it comes to team sports: quantitative (that is, objective, based on quantifiable measurements) and qualitative (that is, subjective, based on quality). Practitioners of the latter, such as Phil Jackson, look at sport as an art form and are concerned with the quality of the team's performance. Yet it is the quantitative approach that has become dominant in this post-*Moneyball* generation of sports analytics.

Nowadays sports analysis is predominantly about measuring outcomes. Every NBA team now has STATS SportVU tracking in its arena, and 80 percent of teams have analytics staff on the payroll. In baseball, 97 percent of teams have at least one full-time number cruncher.[74] Soccer is also becoming increasingly quantitative. When I joined the Bolton Wanderers as the first full-time sports scientist in the game, they had the most advanced analysis department in England. Now, almost every Premier League club has a "data scientist" or "analytics manager" on staff.

GAME MODEL

GAME OBJECTIVE

WIN GAME
SCORES FOR VS AGAINST

Each event can be assigned to a particular player, or, if an area is breaking down, then ONLY that area is interrogated for analysis.

DEFENSE

PREVENT SCORING CHANCES
OF OPPOSITION SCORING CHANCES CONCEDED

ATTACK

CREATE SCORING CHANCES
OF SCORING CHANCES CREATED

ATTACK -> DEFENSE

TURNOVER OPPOSITION BALL

QUANTITATIVE/ QUALITATIVE KPI

Dictates how hard the forward unit is working; applies across most types of defensive systems

DEFENSE

PREVENT POSSESSION INSIDE OUR SCORING ZONE

QUANTITATIVE/ QUALITATIVE KPI

If the defense is tight, number of clean possessions & passing options will be low

DEFENSE -> ATTACK

MOVE BALL TO ATTACK AS FAST AS POSSIBLE

QUANTITATIVE/ QUALITATIVE KPI

Ball speed essential to opposition disorganization

ATTACK

WIN BALL WITHIN SCORING ZONE

QUANTITATIVE/ QUALITATIVE KPI

We need to win ball in a scoring arc, defined; this dictates scoring chances

A game model forms the basis for a game plan.

American football is also riding the stats band-wagon. The stats website Pro Football Focus has increased its staff to more than eighty to make sure that it's posting up-to-the-minute numbers and dives so deep that it displays ball hang time to two decimal points and grades players in every position based on 106 metrics.[75] Twenty teams consult with the organization to get the latest numbers-based insights into current personnel, trade targets, and potential draft picks.

Despite the increase in doing sports by the numbers, not everyone buys into the promise of statistics. Super Bowl–winning coach Brian Billick told ESPN's *Mike & Mike* cohosts, "One of the most common questions I get is, 'Can you do *Moneyball*, for lack of a better term, in the NFL?' And the answer is, 'No, you can't.' You can't quantify the game of football the way you do baseball. It's not a statistical game. The parameters of the game, the number of bodies, and what they're doing in conjunction with one another."[76]

THE PLAYSTATION DELUSION   3.11.2.1

I completely agree with Billick that football is "not a statistical game." I suggest that there are an almost infinite number of actions, reactions, and inter-actions during each football game and that just because something can be measured doesn't mean that it should be. While a Big Data mindset can provide valuable insight in some ways, there are many human factors in sports that cannot be quantified. How, for example, do you evaluate a player's motivation, drive, and heart with metrics?

To be truly effective, quantitative analysis must be combined with assessing the quality of what happens on game day. British scientist Lord Kelvin wrote, "When you cannot measure it, when you cannot express it in numbers, your knowledge is of a meagre and unsatisfactory kind"—more commonly paraphrased as, "If you can't measure it, you can't improve it."[77] But when applied to team sports, this premise takes you only so far. Otherwise, with the current investment in analytics, we'd already have solved every problem, prevented every injury, and created leagues full of inerrant superteams.

The objective game-day outcomes that teams measure must inform what goes on during practice and future fixtures only if they fit with the Commander's Intent and the sub-objectives and principles of a team's game plan. Otherwise, as management guru Peter Drucker put it, "reports and procedures, when misused, cease to be tools and become malignant masters."[78] Numerical key performance indicators must be aligned with the quality focus of the game model. Bombarding players with spreadsheets full of numbers isn't going to help them improve their performance and will likely have the opposite effect—truly paralysis by analysis.

Certain advocates of quantitative analysis would have us believe that the more numbers they crunch, the more accurate the picture of the game is that they're presenting. Unfortunately, this flies in the face of reason. Heisenberg's uncertainty principle states that you can never measure the exact position and velocity of a particle simultaneously. If this is the case in quantum mechanics, why would it be any different when we're trying to analyze a team sports game?

Heisenberg also noted that the very act of measuring something has the effect of altering the measurement itself. For example, if a nature documentary team films lions in the wild, they're not going to get a true representation of how lions act, as the animals sense their presence and adapt their behavior in response.

A similar phenomenon can occur in a sporting context. Trying to evaluate player performance through certain metrics will impact their actions on the field. If a player knows that his tackling is going to be scrutinized, he will invariably bring a different mindset to the act of tackling. So the very fact that a team or third party is gathering statistics can have a detrimental effect—the opposite of the stats department's intention.

In contrast, breaking a game down into distinct moments and micro moments and talking through what happened in each will enhance athletes' understanding of what they need to do better to help the team improve. When it comes to applying game-day insights to training, coaches would be well advised to tell players as little as possible about what they should be doing, particularly in light of data-based analysis. Instead, the coaching staff should use qualitative analysis from the four game moments and a small number of quantitative measurements to create realistic drills. These must be based on minimizing the detrimental effects of limiting factors during the offensive, defensive, and transitional micro moments.

Giving players a long list of orders and objectives is counterproductive to a cohesive approach because they will tune them out and fail to experience what the coaching staff is asking them to do (see 3.3.4 Coherence Beats Confusion). But if they're allowed to make discoveries through immersive learning experiences, they will absorb the head coach's lessons on a profound level. It's like the difference between drilling one student on French verb conjugations and sending another to live in Paris for a semester on an exchange program. The first student might well be able to pass French-language tests, but the second will have a much richer cultural knowledge and a better grasp of how the language works in the real world.

THE FUTURE OF QUANTITATIVE ANALYSIS   3.11.3

Instead of trying to numerically assess individual performance, teams would be better off applying quantitative analysis to tactical performance. This has several benefits, including focusing on the team as a whole rather than on single players and putting player actions into the context of the game plan objectives. Such analysis can provide new insight into how players coordinate with each other and

how well units (such as the defensive line in football or the midfield in soccer) collaborate. A quantitative evaluation should also take into account the use of space and time by gathering spatiotemporal information on every player—in other words, where they are when they take certain actions.[79] In terms of evaluating performance in a quantitative way to improve preparation, this type of tactical analysis holds far more promise than the current approach of gathering as many individual player stats as possible.

QUANTITATIVE VS. QUALITATIVE   3.11.3.1

Whereas quantitative analysis is structured and clearly defined, qualitative assessment is more subjective and open to interpretation. In a numbers-focused approach, the expertise and prior experiences of the statistician have little bearing on what they record during or after the game, whereas in a qualitative approach, these factors lead to varying interpretations on the part of the analyst.

One way to bring both schools of analysis together is to focus on capturing data relating to how ball and player movement impacts execution and the application of the head coach's game plan. Such analysis can focus either on pivotal events—like scoring or conceding a goal—or on the occurrences within each of the four game moments. Tracking movement of the ball and athletes can also show how well strategy and tactics were implemented and how well the team adapted to adversity and the frictions of the game as the game unfolded.[80]

THE DANGER OF THE HAWTHORNE EFFECT   3.11.4

Henry A. Landsberger conducted productivity experiments between 1924 and 1932 at the Hawthorne Works, a Western Electric plant in Illinois. The company wanted to see if its employees would be more productive when working in abundant light or could maintain their output with less light. The workers' productivity seemed to increase at the time of the lighting changes, but then declined after the study was done. Later analysis concluded that there was an initial uptick in productivity because factory workers were told about the experiment and were motivated to work faster.[81] The same can be true in sports when quantitative analysis becomes the be-all and end-all of player assessment. If players know that they're going to be evaluated on the number of tackles they make and that this could potentially affect their next contract, then what are they going to do? Attempt more tackles. Measuring anything has an effect on coach and player behavior.

In any game, there are potentially hundreds of actions and events involving individuals, combinations of players, and entire teams. Statisticians are getting ever more detailed in their measurement of each event and its outcome, but we cannot focus on statistics at the expense of evaluating the *quality* of the actions and how they impact the achievement of game plan aims.

Key performance indicators (KPIs) and key performance objectives (KPOs) sometimes help in evaluating a statistic, such as when the stat sheet shows pass completions as well as total passes, or tackles that regained possession as well as the total number of tackles. In addition to looking at whether a player or the team as a whole can execute a particular action well, we must also consider frequency—that is, whether they can do something well over and over again. Then we need to see whether they can execute effectively late in the game, while fatigued.

In training, coaches can stress different elements of frequency. For example, they could set certain players a target of completing one hundred passes in a ten-minute small-sided game, or fifty over a twenty-minute game, depending on the desired result. The same emphasis should be placed on quality regardless of frequency.

GAME PARTNER

3.12

A game is played by two teams, not just one. So the execution of the game is based on what you can impose on your opponent and vice versa. This is why playing without a ball is a real and significant concept. When evaluating a single game performance, the game model provides the opportunity to identify limiting factors regardless of the opponent. This in turn allows the head coach to minimize their negative impact through focused learning experiences in training.

> *We analyze our rivals and we try to imagine how they will play against us. Using these thoughts we position certain players in certain positions according to the opposition's strengths and weaknesses. But these are only positional details. They don't interfere with our principles, or even with our system.*
>
> —José Mourinho

MAINTAINING YOUR GAME PLAN AND PRINCIPLES

3.12.1

To be effective from game to game all season long, a team should always focus on playing to its strengths. Scouting for each contest will enable the team to take into account and be cognizant of its opponent's limiting factors, but good coaches will not alter a game model. Rather, they will retain the team's core principles and objectives and add in only slight variations in aims and goals for individual players and the units/groups they comprise. This is the difference between maintaining a game model and developing a game plan.

Maintaining consistent principles from game to game ensures that players always know what is expected of them and, in broad terms, what they need to do for the team as a whole to achieve the Commander's Intent. For coaches to prepare the squad effectively, game-by-game variation should be minimized and case-by-case adaptations to strategy and tactics must be clearly communicated so that they can be understood and implemented effectively. I've often told coaches that if you give your players a solid game plan and they execute it and lose consistently, you should quit!

Another factor to consider is that the opposing team will almost always know what you intend to do on game day, no matter how good or bad the scouting is. While you can obscure certain intentions with misdirection, variation, and inventive set-piece moves, your focus should be on executing your game plan so quickly and effectively that no team can stop it.

For a team to effectively play against any and every opponent, the same methodology must be applied to assessing and scouting the opposition. In doing so, a team can see how best to adjust its tactics and strategy to be successful game to game, while sticking to its core principles. It is also essential that scouting reports use the same language and terminology that the team uses to discuss its own performance. That way, the team can use comparative analysis to see how another team's strengths, weaknesses, and limiting factors line up against its own. Sticking to the same lexicon also helps provide clarity among scouts, coaches, and players, which furthers the goal of establishing cohesion and clear communication among every layer of the organization.

As with looking at your own team, scouting reports on opponents must combine quantitative and qualitative analysis to be effective. It's not enough to look at an opposing team's statistical performance in the past few games, or even to examine KPIs for its past encounters with your club. This will only provide information about outcomes rather than the conditions and factors that led to them.

Instead, scouts should combine empirical data with qualitative assessment. What the coaching staff really needs to know is the opponent's patterns and habits. By analyzing game performance in each of the four moments (offense, defense, and transitions to each), a scout can pinpoint tendencies in individual players, offensive and defensive units, and the team as a whole. Identifying precursors to actions makes it easier to predict what players will do in any given situation, and thus to disrupt them.

The leaders who work most effectively, it seems to me, never say 'I.' And that's not because they have trained themselves not to say 'I.' They don't think 'I.' They think 'we'; they think 'team.' … This is what creates trust, what enables you to get the task done.

—Peter Drucker

By discovering and highlighting patterns, the scouting department can show the coaching staff what a team's game plan aim is within each moment. Only by knowing this can a coach strategize how to thwart his opposite number's objectives. He or she can then create learning experiences for players in the training sessions leading up to the next game that encourage them to obstruct the other team's intended actions. This will have the effect not only of interfering with individual players' decision-making cycles but also of making the entire opposing team reactive.

KNOW THY ENEMY—A LITTLE   3.12.2

In what situations were the team's last few games played? Were they preseason friendlies/exhibitions, league play, or playoff encounters? What has their form been of late, and is it exceeding or falling short of expectations? Whom did they play against, and what was the record of these opposing teams before these games? Although it might have a solid game plan that the players stick to consistently, the opposing team can play very differently from week to week, depending on the situation.

Knowing the background of the upcoming game itself can help your team figure out which version of the opponent it will face—a lackadaisical team that cares little about the outcome or a scrappy, intense, highly motivated foe fighting to secure a playoff berth, avoid relegation, or anything in between. The key is always to be aware of your opponent's tendencies and preferences but to focus on maximizing your own strengths. If you only try to cancel out the opponent's dominant qualities, then you're not really trying to win—you're playing not to lose. That's a cynical and often destructive approach.

Of course, there are other ways to gain an advantage. After being signed by the New England Patriots in September 2014, Caylin Hauptmann didn't help his new team win the Super Bowl with his on-field efforts. Rather, the offensive tackle contributed invaluable practice field insights about his former Seattle teammates and the plays that had helped them lift the Vince Lombardi Trophy the year before. "I was able to give [the Patriots] a sense of what [Seattle's] zone blocking looked like," Hauptmann told *SI*. "I'd tell them stuff like, 'On this play, they like to cut [block].'"[82]

It was this detailed, play-by-play knowledge that enabled Patriots cornerback Malcolm Butler to quickly read how the Seahawks were set up on the line of scrimmage with twenty-six seconds remaining in the Super Bowl and know that Russell Wilson was the intended passing target. Butler beat Wilson to his spot and intercepted the ball with twenty-three seconds left, securing the Patriots' victory. That said, knowing is not sufficient. As outlined in the law of expected emergence (page 62), you still have to stop them.

> *We prepared for everything. [I'm] not saying we perfected it, but we prepared for everything. There's no second-guessing or hesitation when you play for Bill. When you have to think on the field, it slows you down. When you know exactly what you're doing and how to do it and why you're doing it, that allows you to play faster, and your talent flows freely. It's like being in class. They hand you a test, you open it up, look at the questions and go, 'Wow, I know all the answers already.'*

—Kevin Faulk

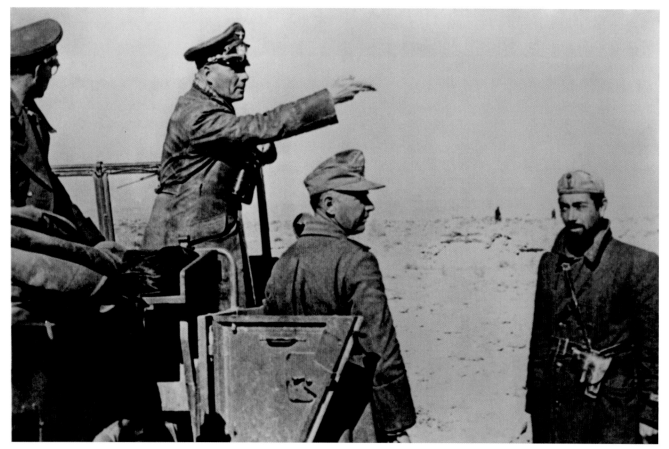

German general Erwin Rommel in North Africa in 1942. Rommel was influential in developing maneuver warfare (see page 99). Photo by Everett Historical / Shutterstock.com.

STRATEGY, TACTICS, AND STRUCTURE

3.12.3

How you assess the opponent is how you assess yourself. This is because you need a cohesive message all the way from scouting to practice to playing. The slight tactical adaptations to the game plan needed for each upcoming opponent will not affect the game model.

It's important to not only look at the capabilities of individual players but also evaluate what the opposition's tendencies are on the unit and team level within each of the game moments and its subcomponents. First, you want to know how certain players combine during offense, defense, and offensive and defensive transitions. What does the team prefer to do in each of these game moment scenarios?

Next, you want to find out what the team's structure looks like at each point of the game. This can include formation and go-to plays and also how the team employs player and ball movement to create space when attacking and to close it down when defending. How the team's tactics change throughout the course of the game is also influential, and how this varies if they're winning or losing.

Third, the scout should assess how the team likes to line up for restarts and dead-ball situations. Examples include jump balls and out-of-bounds plays in basketball; punts and kickoffs in football; corners, free kicks, and throw-ins in soccer; and line-outs and scrums in rugby. If the scout can identify patterns and preferences in each of these situations, the team will be better able to predict what's going to happen and stop it from occurring in the way their adversary wants it to.

By evaluating a team based on its style of play in each game moment, coaches can simplify their own pregame preparation and decide how to adjust strategy and tactics. So, for example, your scouts may find that in the defensive moment, five teams in your league play man-to-man defense, five favor a zone, and five employ a hybrid scheme. Now, instead of pulling your hair out preparing unique tactics to counter each opponent, you can prepare for the three styles of play by putting every team into one of those defensive moment categories. That way, each time you face that particular team, you're not starting from scratch. The same goes for analysis in the three other game moments. Remember, however, that the focus of a good team is not on the opponent but on how it will execute the game plan as per the game model with minimal change.

The job of the scouting and coaching staff is to assess the threats and strengths of the opponent in its totality, prioritize what's most important, and distill this down into small chunks that the players can easily digest. The key here is simplicity. Even if you have time until the next game, the key is to keep the teaching moments to a minimum and use the time to perfect them.

THE TYSON RULE   3.12.4

I always use the rule of three, or what I often refer to as the "Tyson rule," as a guideline for setting game plan objectives. Mike Tyson once said, "Everyone has a plan until they get punched in the face." I assume that every player will get punched, even if only metaphorically. If a player in the heat of battle is punched in the face, what three objectives will he or she recite back immediately afterward? Athletes can remember three things at most during a game because of all the other information they have to retain and process, so whatever you want them to recall going into a game had better be simple, clear, and easy to remember under extreme stress.

Coaches shouldn't just think about what they want each athlete to focus on when they're fresh at the start of the game but also what they want the players to recall when they're physically, emotionally, and mentally fatigued. Barry Trotz, head coach of the NHL's Washington Capitals, shared with *Sports Illustrated* that he tries to limit what he shares with his players about their next opponent: "You don't want them leaving the meeting going, 'I don't even know what to think about,'" Trotz said.[83]

Even the most intelligent, experienced, and cognitively advanced player has only a small amount of headspace to fill with goals and aims. If you try to get players to focus on too many things, they'll be overloaded and end up focusing on nothing. Plus, it makes them use up precious functional capacity that they need in order to apply their physiological gifts and skills during the game.

Instead, a coach should emphasize three very clear, simple goals, all of which the player should be able to explain before and after the game. The first should be a global, positional goal. So if you're a scrum half, your directive may be to spread the ball wide as much as possible. The second goal could be a group or unit goal. If you're a basketball forward, the coach might want your front line to secure more offensive rebounds than your opponent's forwards and center. The third and final goal can be specific to this particular game and opponent. For example, a cornerback may be told to smother a certain receiver and prevent him from catching deep passes.

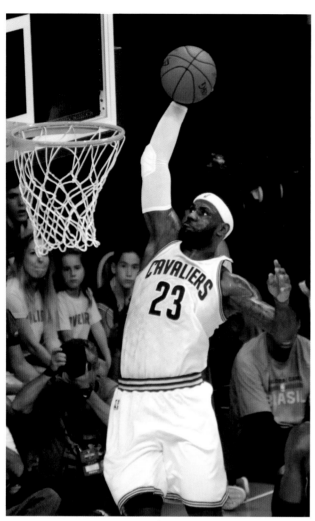

LeBron James. Photo by A.RICARDO / Shutterstock.com.

WORK BACKWARD FROM THE GAME

3.13

Outlining the game in terms of rules, laws, and paradoxes is critical to defining our fundamental problem in winning games. I always have believed in working backward from the game itself. Make no assumptions. It's a combination of a Machiavellian and a Bauhaus approach—define the problem exactly as it is.

In this section, I've demonstrated that the nature of sports is not what we've been led to believe. Our game is not one that is best described using structured, linear approaches. Instead, it's a chaotic environment with complex elements. In addition, I've highlighted the myths and paradoxes in the game and outlined the laws of play present in every sport. We can see now that quantitative approaches of analysis and assessment are incomplete unless combined with qualitative assessments.

> *It seems legitimate to ask for a theory... of universal principles applying to systems in general. In this way, we postulate a new discipline called 'General Systems Theory.' Its subject matter is the formulation and derivation of those principles which are valid for 'systems' in general.*
>
> —Ludwig von Bertalanffy

1 Mark Leibovich, "What Tom Brady Told Me During Deflategate, and What He Didn't," *New York Times*, May 8, 2015.

1 WHAT'S REALLY HAPPENING

2 James Gleick, *Chaos: Making a New Science* (New York: Viking, 1987), 5.

3 Julio Garganta, "Tactical Modeling in Soccer: A Critical View," *Proceedings of IV World Congress of Notational Analysis of Sport*.

4 Erich Jantsch, *The Self-Organizing Universe: Scientific and Human Implications of the Emerging Paradigm of Evolution* (Oxford, UK: Pergamon Press, 1980), 9.

5 Frans Osinga, *Science, Strategy and War: The Strategic Theory of John Boyd* (New York: Routledge, 2007).

6 Ilya Prigogine, *Order Out of Chaos: Man's New Dialogue with Nature* (New York: Bantam, 1984), 8.

7 Mick G. Mack et al., "Chaos Theory: A New Science for Sport Behavior?," *Athletic Insight* 2, no. 2 (May 2000), www.athleticinsight.com/Vol2Iss2/ChaosPDF.pdf.

8 Michael Lissack, "Complexity: The Science, Its Vocabulary, and Its Relation to Organizations," *Emergence* 1, no. 1 (1999): 110–126.

9 Benoit Mandelbrot, *The Fractal Geometry of Nature* (San Francisco: W. H. Freeman, 1982), 68–69.

10 Keith Davids, Duarte Araújo, and Rick Shuttleworth, "Applications of Dynamical Systems Theory to Football," in *Science and Football V: The Proceedings of the Fifth World Congress on Science and Football*, ed. Thomas Reilly, Jan Cabri, and Duarte Araújo (New York: Routledge, 2005), 537–550.

11 Quoted in Donella H. Meadows, *Thinking in Systems: A Primer*, ed. Diana Wright (White River Junction, VT: Chelsea Green Publishing Company, 2008), 12.

12 "Tactical Decision Making," Staff Noncommissioned Officers Career Distance Education Program, Marine Corps Institute, www.au.af.mil/au/awc/awcgate/usmc/tactical_decision_making.pdf.

13 David Fleming, "No More Questions," *ESPN The Magazine*, October 4, 2016, www.espn.com/espn/feature/story/_/id/17703210/new-england-patriots-coach-bill-belichick-greatest-enigma-sports.

2 THE PRINCIPLES OF THE GAME

14 Chris Forsberg, "The Scheme Dreamer: How Brad Stevens Draws Up Winning Plays," ESPN.com, March 9, 2016, www.espn.com/nba/story/_/id/14930372/boston-celtics-coach-brad-stevens-dreams-schemes.

15 Quoted in Richard Goldstein, "Bill Walsh, Former 49ers Coach, Dies at 75," *New York Times*, July 30, 2007, www.nytimes.com/2007/07/30/sports/football/31walsh.html.

16 Musa Okwonga, *Will You Manage? The Necessary Skills to Be a Great Gaffer* (London: Serpent's Tail, 2010), 108–109.

17 Fred "Tex" Winter, *The Triple-Post Offense* (Englewood Cliffs, NJ: Prentice-Hall, 1962; Lost Treasure Company, 2015), 10.

18 Paul Tomkins, "Paul Tomkins on Bill Shankly," Shankly.com, n.d., www.shankly.com/Article/2835/2.

19 Jackie MacMullan, "How Spurs' Majestic 2014 Finals Performance Changed the NBA," ESPN.com, June 9, 2015, www.espn.com/nba/playoffs/2015/story/_/page/PresentsSpursHeat/how-spurs-2014-finals-performance-changed-nba-forever.

20 Ibid.

21 Scott McEwen and Richard Miniter, *Eyes on Target: Inside Stories from the Brotherhood of the U.S. Navy SEALs* (New York: Center Street, 2014).

22 Luís Berkemeier Pimenta, "From Complexity Paradigm to Morphocycle: A Study-Map," 15, www.fotball.no/globalassets/trener/uefa-a-oppgaver/uefa-a-2014-oppgave-luis-pimenta.pdf.

3 THE MODEL

23 J. Guilherme Oliveira, "Organization of the Game of a Football Team: Methodological Aspects in the Approach of Its Structural and Functional Organization."

24 Jonathan Wilson, "The Devil and José Mourinho," *The Guardian*, December 22, 2015.

25 Osinga, *Science, Strategy and War*, 176.

26 Ibid., 157.

27 Phillip S. Meilinger, *Ten Propositions Regarding Air Power* (Washington, DC: Air Force History and Museums Program), 31–32.

28 Michelangelo Rucci, "How the Hawks' Squeeze Works," *The Advertiser* (Adelaide, Australia), May 15, 2008, www.adelaidenow.com.au/sport/afl/how-the-hawks-squeeze-works/news-story/cb35a35f9c687747e0f38527b6d91ca6.

29 "The Economist Explains: How Leicester City Staged the Greatest Upset in Sporting History," *The Economist*, May 2, 2016, www.economist.com/blogs/economist-explains/2016/05/economist-e.../tw/te/bl/ed/howleicestercitystagedthegreatestupsetinsportinghistory.

30 Dominic Fifield, "José Mourinho Strongly Defends Chelsea Style Against 'Boring' Criticism," *The Guardian*, April 27, 2015, www.theguardian.com/football/2015/apr/27/jose-mourinho-roman-abramovich-chelsea-style.

31 "The Economist Explains."

32 "What Makes Barcelona Such a Formidable Team?" (blog post), *The Backwards Gooner*, May 31, 2011, mr-renoog-videos.blogspot.com/2011/05/what-makes-barcelona-such-formidable.html.

33 Chris Anderson and David Sally, *The Numbers Game: Why Everything You Know About Soccer Is Wrong* (London: Viking, 2013), 8.

34 Richard Rapaport, "To Build a Winning Team: An Interview with Head Coach Bill Walsh," *Harvard Business Review*, January/February 1993, hbr.org/1993/01/to-build-a-winning-team-an-interview-with-head-coach-bill-walsh.

35 "The Premier League's 15 Hardest Working Players—Average Distance Covered Per Game in 2014/15," *Talk Sport*, March 6, 2015, talksport.com/football/premier-leagues-15-hardest-working-players-average-distance-covered-game-201415.

36 "What Makes Barcelona Such a Formidable Team?."

37 Michael Todisco, "NFL Scouting Combine Data Visualization," NYC Data Science Academy, February 1, 2016, blog.nycdatascience.com/student-works/nfl-scouting-combine-data-visualization/.

38 John Breech, "2015 NFL Combine: 3 Players Each Win $100K for Lightning Fast 40 Times," CBSSports.com, February 23, 2015, www.cbssports.com/nfl/news/2015-nfl-combine-3-players-each-win-100k-for-lightning-fast-40-times/.

39 "Next Gen Stats for Week 13," NFL.com, December 7, 2015, www.nfl.com/photoessays/0ap3000000596936.

40 David Newton, "Is Panthers WR Ted Ginn Jr. the Fastest Player in the NFL?," ESPN.com, December 15, 2015, www.espn.com/blog/carolina-panthers/post/_/id/17918/is-panthers-wr-ted-ginn-jr-the-fastest-player-in-the-nfl.

41 Owain Jones, "Who Is the Better All Black: Julian Savea or Jonah Lomu?," *Rugby World*, October 3, 2014, www.rugbyworld.com/countries/new-zealand-countries/better-black-julian-savea-v-jonah-lomu-39361.

42 Isaiah Cambron, "Of Messi and Distance: Limited Statistical Analysis of How Far Players Run and What It Means," *Barcelona Football Blog*, February 18, 2013, www.barcelonafootballblog.com/18698/messi-distance-limited-statistical-analysis-players-run-means/.

43 Mark Brus, "Manchester United Have Premier League's Best Ball-Winner in Morgan Schneiderlin, Stats Show," *Metro*, October 19, 2015, metro.co.uk/2015/10/19/manchester-united-have-premier-leagues-best-ball-winner-in-morgan-schneiderlin-stats-show-5448051/.

44 Pete Prisco, "After Further Review: Why Jets Have NFL's Top Defense Without Many Sacks," CBSSports.com, October 22, 2015, www.cbssports.com/nfl/news/after-further-review-why-jets-have-nfls-top-defense-without-many-sacks/.

45 Ed Smith, "Taxi for the Coach? Team Sports Could Do with More Mentors and Fewer Touchline Tyrants," *1843* magazine, January/February 2016, www.1843magazine.com/reading-the-game/what-sport-can-learn-from-classical-music.

46 Myles Palmer, "Gilberto, Maldini & Xabi Alonso Didn't Need to Tackle," *Arsenal News Review*, March 15, 2016, www.arsenalnewsreview.co.uk/gilberto-maldini-xabi-alonso-didnt-need-to-tackle/.

47 John Boyd, *Patterns of Conflict* (PowerPoint presentation), ed. Chet Richards and Chuck Spinney, January 2007, www.dnipogo.org/boyd/patterns_ppt.pdf.

48 Russ Marion and Josh Bacon, "Organizational Extinction and Complex Systems," *Emergence* 1, no. 4 (1999): 76.

49 Henry J. Coleman Jr., "What Enables Self-Organizing Behavior in Businesses," *Emergence* 1, no. 1 (1999): 33–48.

50 Brett McKay and Kate McKay, "The Tao of Boyd: How to Master the OODA Loop" (blog post), *The Art of Manliness*, September 15, 2014, www.artofmanliness.com/2014/09/15/ooda-loop/.

51 Ibid.

52 Tom Payne, "Tactical Theory: Compactness," *Spielverlagerung*, August 8, 2015, spielverlagerung.com/2015/05/08/tactical-theory-compactness/.

53 Colin Gray, *Defining and Achieving Decisive Victory*, Strategic Studies Institute, April 2002, ssi.armywarcollege.edu/pdffiles/pub272.pdf.

54 Bill Walsh with Steve Jamison and Craig Walsh, *The Score Takes Care of Itself: My Philosophy of Leadership* (New York: Portfolio, 2009), 211.

55 Coach Mac, "501 Awesome Basketball Quotes" (blog post), *Basketball for Coaches*, November 4, 2014, www.basketballforcoaches.com/basketball-quotes/.

56 "Brad Stevens: Give Kids the Freedom to Play," Positive Coaching Alliance, n.d., devzone.positivecoach.org/resource/video/brad-stevens-give-kids-freedom-play.

57 Fleming, "No More Questions."

58 Vítor Frade, in conversation with the author, August 2011.

59 Jonathan Wilson, "The Devil's Party (Part 1)," *The Blizzard*, December 17, 2016, www.theblizzard.co.uk/articles/the-devils-party/.

60 Jason Cole, "Bruce Arians Q&A: Cardinals HC on Teaching, Learning and Future After Football," *Bleacher Report*, June 3, 2016, bleacherreport.com/articles/2643499-bruce-arians-qa-cardinals-hc-on-teaching-learning-and-future-after-football.

61 "The Economist Explains."

62 Duncan White, "Michael Phelps Sets Mind's Eye on Triumphant Role in Final Part of Lord of the Rings Trilogy," *The Daily Telegraph*, July 15, 2012.

63 Walsh, *The Score Takes Care of Itself*, 211.

64 Charles Duhigg, *The Power of Habit: Why We Do What We Do in Life and Business* (New York: Random House, 2012), 79–80.

65 Sun Tzu, *The Art of War*, 46.

66 U.S. Marine Corps Staff, *Warfighting* (New York: Currency Doubleday, 1994), 94.

67 Jeffrey L. Cowan, *From Air Force Fighter Pilot to Marine Corps Warfighting: Colonel John Boyd, His Theories on War, and Their Unexpected Legacy*, master's thesis, Marine Corps University, 2000.

68 B. H Liddell-Hart, ed., *The Rommel Papers* (New York: Harcourt, Brace, 1953; Boston: Da Capo Press, 1982).

69 Ray Merriam, *General Hermann Balck: An Interview, January 1979* (Bennington, VT: Merriam Press, 1988).

70 Grant Wahl, "Bayern Munich's Mr. Cool," *Sports Illustrated,* June 29, 2016, www.si.com/planet-futbol/2016/06/29/xabi-alonso-bayern-munich-midfielder.

71 Nicholas Dawidoff, "The Obtuse Triangle," *New York Times,* June 23, 2015, www.nytimes.com/2015/06/28/sports/basketball/phil-jackson-knicks-triangle-offense-nba.html.

72 "Eli Whitney Biography," Biography.com, A&E Television Networks, April 28, 2017, www.biography.com/people/eli-whitney-9530201.

73 "Ford Installs First Moving Assembly Line, 1913," *A Science Odyssey,* WGBH, PBS, www.pbs.org/wgbh/aso/databank/entries/dt13as.html.

74 Trevir Nath, "How Big Data Has Changed Sports," *Investopedia,* April 27, 2015, www.investopedia.com/articles/investing/042715/how-big-data-has-changed-sports.asp.

75 Jenny Vrentas, "Football's Focus Group," The MMQB, *Sports Illustrated,* January 25, 2015, mmqb.si.com/2015/01/25/pro-football-focus-nfl-neil-hornsby-cris-collinsworth-analytics.

76 Doug Farrar, "Off the Grid: What the NFL's Moneyball Looks Like," SportsIllustrated.com, January 11, 2016, www.si.com/nfl/2016/01/13/off-the-grid-paul-depodesta-browns.

77 Joseph Loscalzo, "Can Scientific Quality Be Quantified?," *Circulation* 123, no. 9 (March 8, 2011): 947–950.

78 Peter F. Drucker, *The Practice of Management* (New York: HarperCollins, 2010), 115.

79 Daniel Memmert, Koen A. P. M. Lemmink and Jaime Sampaio, "Current Approaches to Tactical Performance Analyses in Soccer Using Position Data," *Sports Medicine* 47, no. 1 (June 2016): 1–10.

80 Ibid.

81 Henry A. Landsberger, *Hawthorne Revisited: Management and the Worker, Its Critics, and Developments in Human Relations in Industry* (Utica, NY: Cornell University Press, 1958).

82 Michael McKnight, "Best Practices," *Sports Illustrated,* February 1, 2016.

83 Alex Prewitt, "Restless Legs," *Sports Illustrated,* January 25, 2016.

PART TWO

THE PLAYER

The ball floats across the field to the left wing in a long, graceful but speeding arc. A cascade of flashes, lights, and screams explode just as the ball reaches the space in front of a diminutive soccer star. Lionel Andrés "Leo" Messi is one of the most masterful artists in the storied history of the world's most popular team sport. In a moment of skill defined by gentleness and deft, he lifts his foot and stops the ball dead in the air with such precision that he takes all kinetic energy from it and it falls to the ground, dead.

This brief moment of extreme skill is seen by millions but truly appreciated by only a few.

At that moment, Messi follows the flight of the ball as it makes its way across the field. He unconsciously knows exactly where he is in relation to the lines on the field. He is aware of his defender, only three yards in front of him, closing the space. He knows how far he is from the sideline on the left and from teammates and opponents on the other side. He can't see exactly who is to his right, but he instinctively knows, through perceiving the figure's shape, color, shadow, noise, and movement, that it is a teammate. This comes from a complex combination of knowledge and perception judged by experience—what we call intuition.

His brain is processing thousands, perhaps millions, of similar visual, auditory, and olfactory cues to give him a soccer-specific emotional awareness far superior to that of amateur players. His eyes follow the flight of the ball. Having recognized this pattern of spin, flight, angle, speed, and accuracy from a memory bank of thousands of similar previous experiences, he can afford to look away from the ball before the moment of impact to cast a glance at an advancing defender.

This opponent is approaching fast, closing down the space, hoping that he can reach Messi before the ball does. But the player slows now. He was hoping that Messi might focus on trapping the ball and be momentarily distracted. But no. Messi has done this so many times before that he multitasks his attention, flipping his concentration successively from ball to closing defender to surrounding teammates and prioritizing his attention.

The defender also was hoping that Messi would fail to control the ball and that it would spill so he could steal it. No such luck. Messi has watched the ball in flight, and his brain knows exactly how its speed and spin will affect the impact of his cleat upon it. He also knows from the glistening of the light on the ball how much water is on it and how wet and heavy it might be. All of these seemingly insignificant details are processed faster than a supercomputer could manage and result in Messi's left foot meeting the ball at the perfect height, with the right weight, control, and degree of force to absorb every possible joule of energy. The ball stops dead, and Messi and his would-be foil watch it fall to the ground, motionless.

Hardly anyone notices this, and not a single person in the crowd is focused on it.

They are already looking forward to Messi's next move, feeling the excitement of watching one of this generation's preeminent talents as he commands the attention of not only the defender in front of him, the other twenty players, and the 69,672 people in the stadium, but also the millions of viewers around the world. They anticipate Messi's next display of precision timing and control, synchronized with his teammates in a delicate tempo.

Messi seems to pause, the ball resting in front of him. For a moment he commands the anticipation of millions of people like a maestro conducting the London Philharmonic Orchestra.

He has space on three sides and is constrained only by the sideline to his left. He knows that the sideline is the best defender of all. It won't budge, and it can't be tempted or fooled. Messi is still waiting for the defender in front of him to make a move that he can avoid and counter. But he knows he can't wait long for that, either, as this player is trying to delay him long enough for his teammates to come over in support. This will close space even more and make things harder for Messi.

So Messi tempts him, leaving the ball momentarily out in front, hoping for an error, a movement, or anything that will give him the chance to blow by his opponent. He doesn't wait any longer than that moment, though. Instead, he nudges the ball forward gently with the outside of his left foot: once, then twice, brief touches that get progressively faster. Every nudge of the ball forces the defender to step backward to keep Messi in full view and, more important, to keep his peripheral vision as wide as possible for the support he hopes is coming from his fellow defenders.

Barcelona is an exquisite blend of some of the greatest footballers in the world, who define perfected team play. Not since the great Brazilian or Dutch teams of the 1970s have there been as many great footballers who play together so well on one single team. This Barcelona squad epitomizes efficiency and synchronicity. The players provide support and balance better as a team than any other club side before them.

This is what the defender is most concerned about. Yes, he is anxious at the prospect of facing possibly the greatest soccer player ever, but Messi's teammates pose a threat, too. This is what gives Messi the greatest advantage of all: fear. Rather than just trying to mark, tag, and tackle Messi, this defender has to consider Messi's teammates, the threat they pose, and the space they create, because simply closing Messi down creates opportunities for the other players.

And this is the essence of all attacking football—of attacks in any sport: the creation of space. Every team does it, but what Barcelona does better than most is create space in unison, cohesively and with flawless timing. And, most important of all, they do it faster than anyone else.

Again Messi nudges the ball forward, left foot always in front of the right. His arms move out from his sides a little now, like a bird about to take flight. His elbows start to come upward and outward, a little higher each time. He is creating balance and a wider base for his center of mass, which will allow him to move laterally if he has to. Not only this, but ever since he started to play as a child in Argentina, his elbows have been useful tools to protect him from larger defenders trying to impose themselves physically on him.

In comparison to his great nemesis of the modern era, Cristiano Ronaldo, Messi's posture is a little more conventional. Ronaldo stands very upright with the ball almost behind his hips and center of gravity as he readies his textbook physique to overwhelm a defender with pace and power. Messi is smaller, five foot seven to Ronaldo's six foot one, and uses his lack of stature to his advantage. Because he's lower to the ground, like that other Argentine wizard, Diego Maradona, he thrives on getting his body very close to the defender. Here, almost under the arm and chest of his opponent, he can keep himself between the ball and the man trying to take it away. This close, he also can spin tightly and change direction as quickly as an Allen Iverson crossover, delaying the reaction of his defender, sending him the wrong way, or causing him to stumble.

And this is exactly what Messi does next. He nudges the ball so far forward that the defender can almost touch it. Then he drives his right arm and shoulder forward and his left wrist back, and at the same time nudges the ball ever so slightly to the right. This is enough misdirection to convince the defender that Messi is going to try to sprint down the wing between him and the sideline. So he makes the mistake Messi expected and moves his right foot toward the sideline.

Messi knows from the defender's right step and the shape of his posture that he has transferred sufficient weight to the right foot to become unbalanced. The Argentine has the fraction of a second he needs. Before the defender has even placed all his weight on his right foot, Messi pulls the ball back to the center. His opponent notices this too late; he is already committed to the step, his center of gravity shifting. As with many who've tried and failed to stop Messi, it's too late.

Messi now pushes the ball fast to the defender's left. It's tantalizingly close, but momentum takes the slow-reacting opponent in the opposite direction, and all he can offer in protest is a flailing leg. Messi passes the defender as he loses his balance, falling backward. The five-time FIFA World Player of the Year glides past effortlessly. The ball appears stuck to his toe, as if on a string.

Now, another defender rushes forward.

Another vain attempt to stop the greatest soccer player ever to play the game.

As we have seen, the influences of tactical and cultural elements on team sports are far greater than many believe because each is quite complex. Nonetheless, the individual is a critical aspect of team-sport events. In this section, I present a model of the player as a person and as a multifaceted, complex performance system that we can now understand and improve in the context of the performance model.

My two main aims with elite athletes have always been to maintain and maximize basic functional health and to reduce factors limiting performance by identifying and improving them.

This section presents a holistic and complete model for the development of the player. Over the years, I've repeatedly found that on-field sustainable success is more often affected by inadequate basic health, lifestyle issues, poor diet, or dysfunctional relationships than by actual performance issues. So an athlete's inability to gain strength might be due to eating too much junk food, or insufficient recovery could be rooted in lack of sleep. A second and closely related issue is that the Kaizen approach of continuous advancement succeeds only if there is a proper model for improving the athlete. The ability to classify and identify the problem is as important as the approach taken to solve it.

The goal of this section is to help individual athletes:

- Achieve and sustain good health

- Manage the load of competition and training

- Encourage adequate rest and recovery

- Fuel sustainable performance

- Recognize the warning signs of overtraining and underrecovery

- Avoid harmful, health-damaging lifestyle habits

- Better understand the main body systems that contribute to health and how to care for them

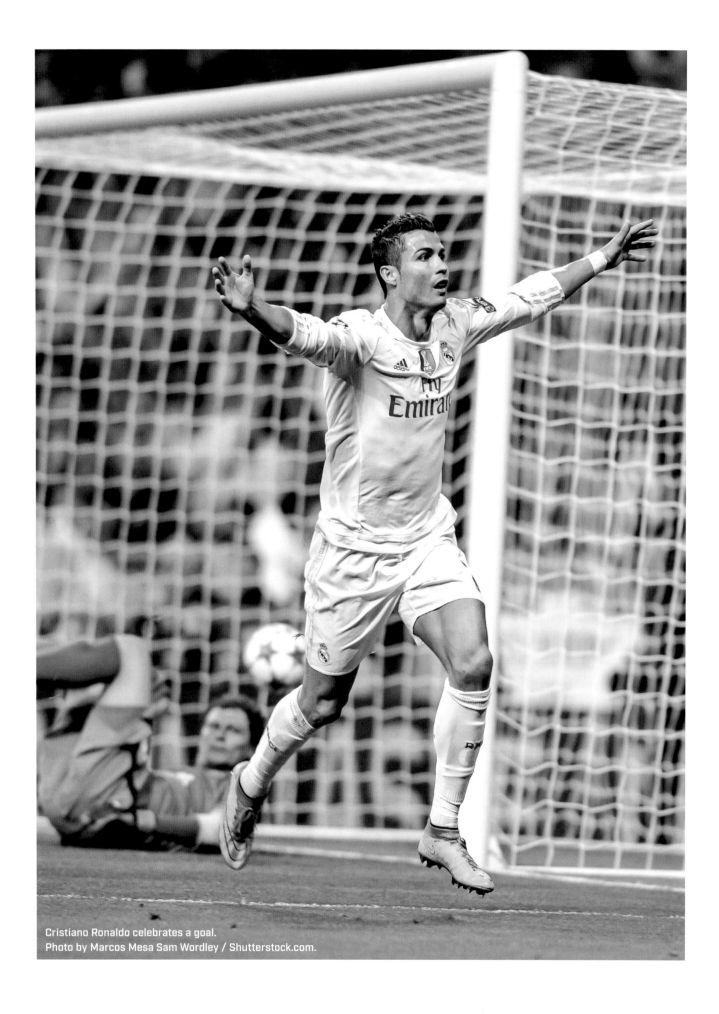

Cristiano Ronaldo celebrates a goal.
Photo by Marcos Mesa Sam Wordley / Shutterstock.com.

FOUR

THE FOUR-COACTIVE MODEL

When it comes to evaluating players and improving their game-day performance, the complexity of competition and the athletes themselves in a team context means that we need a model. In team sports, this is currently lacking, as most teams, even at the elite level, still use a reductionist approach. Another issue is that physical qualities are prized and developed above all else, which we see in the NFL Combine, in sports media discussion of how physiologically athletic players are or aren't, and in the millions of dollars spent on training facilities primarily geared to developing physical attributes.

In this section, you'll see a different way to look at the physiological makeup of a player and how we cannot isolate this but rather need to develop it in concert with the other coactives: psychological, technical, and tactical. All four elements are present to varying degrees in every event in games and during team preparation. We can call them "coactives" because they both complement and rely upon each other.

These four coactives must come together in a synchronized manner to allow the player to execute great actions. They are not independent and cannot exist independently. They are complementary, codependent, and co-reliant.

We can't think about these four alone, though. They all are underpinned by one, more vital, coactive: health. I sometimes call this a "4+1" model—player health is an essential umbrella that affects all four coactives. Without health, none of the other four matter in the long run.

THE TECHNICAL COACTIVE

4.1

We spend so much time trying to maximize players' physical gifts that it's easy to overlook the other coactives that are present in every training session and game. One of these is technical prowess. In the following pages we'll see why coaches need to start paying more attention to decision-making, skill development and execution, and technical context.

JOHN BOYD AND THE EXECUTION OF TECHNICAL SKILLS

4.1.1

American fighter pilot John Boyd has arguably done more to change the way we think about conflict in the past half century than anyone else. One of the greatest thinkers of the period, his ideas were ironically adopted more by the U.S. Marine Corps than the Air Force. One of Boyd's first mental exercises was analyzing why American fighter jets enjoyed superiority over Russian MiGs, even though the latter had comparable, and in some ways better, technology. He deduced that the cockpits in American planes

THE MORPHOCYCLE AND MORPHOLOGICAL PROGRAMMING

The term *morphocycle* refers to the structure and format of a preparation cycle. The preparation (or training) cycle is the flexible period between two games. A morphocycle refers to the units of training and experiences the players are exposed to during that period.

I was first introduced to the term by Vítor Frade, who formalized it in his methodology in soccer preparation, and José Tavares, who is his assistant at Porto FC. It's relevant not just for soccer but for every team sport. The morphocycle is not part of a periodization approach, nor is it an athletic preparation method. (Later, I will explain why the traditional periodization approach is so counterproductive to the preparation of team-sport athletes.)

As is discussed in more detail in "The Preparation," an essential part of the morphocycle as I propose it is *morphological programming*. This refers to the idea that within each morphocycle, there should be a balance of learning experiences that stress volume (the amount of work done), intensity (how rigorous and demanding a session is), density (how many breaks there are within a session), and collision/contact (the amount of vibrational force the athletes absorb).

And as I'll discuss more later in this section, the morphocycle should also be balanced among technical, tactical, physical, and psychological stressors, so players have enough work in each area to prompt adaptation but not so much that they can't recover properly before the next game.

afforded pilots greater visibility, which enabled them to orient themselves more quickly than their Russian adversaries, which in turn enabled them to make faster decisions and perform the desired skill before their opponents could fire. Once again, this text can't do justice to the extent of Boyd's work, but some of his basic principles have been adapted to this four-coactive model.

The U.S. Marine Corps and other elite military units have adopted Boyd's theories and applied them to training and combat with great success. The facet of Boyd's teaching that is most applicable to team sports is the OODA Loop, which consists of four stages:

1. **Observe:** Employ your senses to detect what is going on around you and apply your situational awareness to inform your assessment.

2. **Orient:** Focus your attention on what you've just observed and decide what it means in the context you find yourself in. Here, you make assumptions, judgments, and evaluations based on the available data.

3. **Decide:** Using a combination of what you're experiencing and your prior experiences (experience squared), select the right technical skill movement pattern to achieve your desired aim. This decision can be self-contained, such as a player deciding to move with the ball, or it might involve teammates. The best coaches establish a decentralized decision-making system in which each player is empowered to make their own decisions.

4. **Act:** Keeping your game plan aims in mind, put your decision into action. As soon as this stage of the cycle ends, the first phase begins again.

Another way to refer to the OODA Loop is as an "observation-action cycle," in which observations of what's going on plus prior observations in similar situations inform decision-making. The cycle takes place many, many times in the mind of each player on the field of play or soldier on the battlefield.

I never think about the play or visualize anything. I do what comes to me at that moment. Instinct. It has always been that way.

—Lionel Messi

Looking at the more complex presentation below, you can see the self-improving nature of the loop and the importance of the environment on the decision-making cycle. But again, keep in mind, Boyd's work is far more complex and detailed than can be represented with a four-letter abbreviation. It's an incredibly complex thought system.

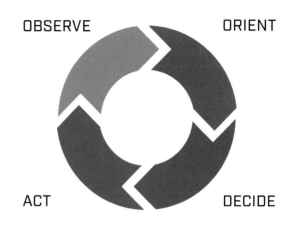

The simplified OODA Loop.

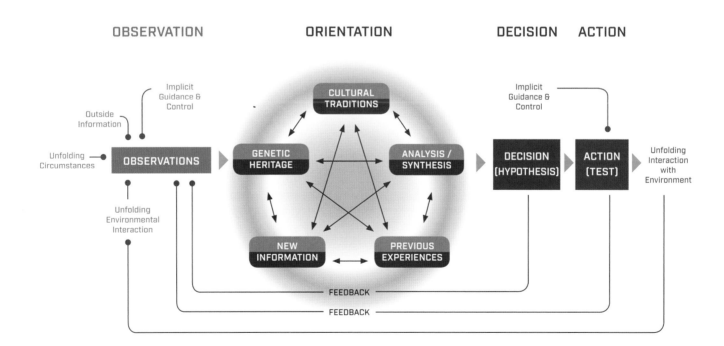

John Boyd's complete OODA Loop.

THE MYTH OF THE PERFECT SKILL

We often hear sports commentators, writers, and talking heads praising certain players for their "textbook" technique. This gives a false impression that there's only one right way to do something in a team sport. Rubbish! There are, of course, players who execute skills in the way coaches often teach them—heeding the cues to keep the elbow in and follow through in shooting a basketball, for example. But the outcome and how sustainable the skill is in the long term are the only two keys when it comes to skill execution. Steph Curry certainly doesn't have a shooting technique that looks "perfect," but the results are self-evident. It's the same with Cristiano Ronaldo's running technique, which so-called experts could pick apart all day long. Meanwhile, Curry keeps breaking records and Ronaldo keeps skinning defenders.

THE IMPORTANCE OF TECHNICAL CONTEXT   4.1.2

If you were on a playground shooting baskets by yourself, you would decide how to alter the way you shoot as you move around the court based on the distance to the basket, the wind, the height of the rim relative to how high you jump, and so on. So there is some decision-making involved. But getting into a game introduces far more complexity into the tactical-technical OODA Loop for each decision.

Even if you put just one more person on the court and the two of you started playing one-on-one, you'd now need to account for the position of your defender, whether they put up a hand to challenge your shot, if they are balanced or imbalanced, if they are trying to body up or hand check you, and so on.

And that's with the addition of just one player. Go into a full game of five-on-five and you've added many more layers. This is why we should never look at the selection or execution of skill—or indeed its outcome—without considering the context.

If you've watched enough games, you'll have likely heard that a basketball player has a "consistent release" on their jump shot or that a quarterback displays "great throwing mechanics" on each pass. But even those players who look like they're exhibiting consistent form in executing a certain skill are doing it slightly differently each time. The variance might be less with closed skills, employed from a consistent place on the court or field in which the opponent cannot do much to apply pressure, like a free throw, but with open skills, many variables dictate how a player needs to perform a skill and how much space and time they have to do so.

Proximity to the target, opponents, and teammates; the position of the ball; and how much pace and spin is on the ball are just a few of the many factors that require players to change how they shoot, pass, or perform any other skill in the moment. Then there are environmental factors, such as weather, crowd noise, and the condition of the playing surface. This is why in a game setting, a skill is never performed the same way twice, nor should coaches expect this. The bottom line is that you cannot learn a skill in isolation and expect it to translate exactly to a team situation during a game.

DECISION   4.1.2.1

The first part of technical ability is choosing the right skill in any given situation, like selecting the right wrench or screwdriver from your toolbox. Correct pattern recall is the precursor to taking effective action. You can't say that a player in any team sport made a "good pass" or a "bad pass" unless you look at the context in which the decision was made. Decision-making is not a stop-and-start thing in any sport but involves a constant feedback loop—the OODA Loop discussed on page 126.

EXECUTION   4.1.2.2

It's not enough to know what to do in a team-sports situation; the athlete must also do it quickly enough and with the right amount of power, precision, direction, and so on to be effective.

We can drill down to know which aspect of the technical OODA Loop we need to emphasize next in practice. Do we focus on the technical dominance of execution or on the decision-making process? The conclusion the coach comes to determines the emphasis placed on the player in practice.

THE TACTICAL COACTIVE

4.2

When it comes to game-day competition, each player's tactical acumen is every bit as important as the physical, technical, and psychological coactives. Let's dive into why this is, how tactics manifest themselves in training and the game itself, and how athletes can better prepare tactically to reach their individual potential while fulfilling their role in the head coach's game plan to achieve the team's primary objectives.

TRAINING THE TACTICAL SYSTEM   4.2.1

When applying the four-coactive model in conjunction with the morphological programming approach, we can't just look at how to ensure physical preparedness by game day but must get athletes tactically ready for competition as well. When assessing performance, coaches often attribute failures in execution to physical shortcomings, but more often than not, elite athletes have more than enough physiological competence to do what is needed and instead lack the requisite tactical know-how.

One element of tactical preparation that's often overlooked is improving athlete decision-making on the field. The exercises, drills, and games coaches come up with should have a desired outcome for an individual, a small group (like the backs in rugby or guards in basketball), or the whole team, but they shouldn't follow a rigid "if this, then that" format in which there's only one correct way to do something. Rather, learning opportunities need to let players make individual choices based on the scenario and their experience, as this is what they have to do in games. It's essential that tactical mini-games and drills occur at or above game speed so that the athletes can execute under pressure on game day.

As well as looking back at the most recent game to learn from past experience, tactical training can prepare the team for the next contest on the calendar. While coaches will want to maintain their principles of play and overall game plan, they might recognize a dominant quality in the opposing team that needs to be taken away, such as the threat of a fast winger in rugby. The scouts might also find a limiting factor in the opposing team that can be exploited, providing further fodder for tactical preparation.

Just like the physical, technical, and psychological coactives, the tactical coactive creates a stress load on the player that is greater cognitively than physiologically. You simply cannot put athletes through high-intensity sessions day after day, or sessions that are dense or have high volume. Otherwise you'll compromise learning outcomes and the players will be worn down going into the next game. This is why the nature of tactical sessions must be balanced within the morphological programming approach.

TACTICAL CONTEXT AND MOMENTS   4.2.2

Just as with the physical, technical, and psychological coactives, athletes' tactical skills need to be developed within the framework of the game model. Tactical acumen that's only theory-based is useless—it's the ability to apply it during competition that truly matters. This is why, when we're trying to improve players' tactical capabilities, we must first look at the four game moments—offensive, defensive, and the two transitional moments. While several things may need attention, we have to pick just one per moment to work on during the upcoming intergame morphocycle.

This targeted approach then informs the mini-games and drills that the head coach and unit and positional assistants create for the week's preparation sessions. Each one must require a specific player (or players) to execute the desired outcome in the relevant game moment. Such action items extend beyond the skills we work on from a technical standpoint, though these must also be performed in a realistic training scenario.

For tactical to-dos, we can again look to the game model and the macro principles of team sport (see section 3.6, starting on page 75, for a refresher). Some tactical competencies that athletes often can improve include ball circulation, player movement, positioning, and the sequencing of all three. The coaching staff can also focus on how they want these applied in each of the game moments, such as advancing the ball quickly in the defense-to-offense transition or applying pressure to the ball handler in the offense-to-defense moment. Tactical training can be used to work on individual players' limiting factors and things that a unit or the team needs to improve as a whole, like positioning to defend a corner in soccer.

TECHNO-TACTICAL SYNERGY 4.2.3

For a team to perform effectively and achieve the objectives of the game plan, it's not enough for each player to have sufficient technical skill or tactical awareness—they must have both. A player might be able to execute the skill of passing beautifully, but if she doesn't have the tactical know-how to predict where a teammate will be, a technically excellent pass will not advance the group's higher aims. Similarly, if a player knows where he needs to be during a play but lacks the technique to do what he's supposed to, the team will fail to score or will lose possession. This is why techno-tactical synergy is crucial.

MACRO PRINCIPLES 4.2.3.1

A key part of the game model relating to technical acumen is the athlete's relationship to the ball and his or her teammates in any given game-day scenario. The position and predicted actions of the opponent are also important here. Cognitive recall and the ability to choose and execute a particular motor pattern are closely linked to all areas of tactical awareness. The understanding of the principles and execution of actions properly with respect to the game principles is critical.

THE PSYCHOLOGICAL COACTIVE
4.3

Having looked at some more bodily coactives, it's now time to turn our attention to the mind. In the next couple of pages we'll examine the importance of a player's emotional, cognitive, and spiritual well-being and the close link between this and overall health on and off the field.

When we profile or assess an athlete from a largely psychological perspective, we see three micro coactives: spiritual, emotional, and cognitive. All three are interlinked and interdependent, but each is a key factor in the performance of the player.

Wer Wissenschaft und Kunst besitzt,
Hat auch Religion;
Wer jene beiden nicht besitzt
Der habe Religion.

He who possesses science and art,
Possesses religion as well;
He who possesses neither of these
Had better have religion.

—Johann Wolfgang von Goethe

SPIRITUALITY
MICRO COACTIVE   4.3.1

For our purposes, the term *spirituality* isn't exclusively about religious belief, although this can be an important part of a player's spiritual makeup. It's also about individuals' roles in society, community, and team or tribe, and their commitment to things they consider bigger and more important than themselves. Awareness of one's self and one's relationships is the fundamental determinant here.

On a professional level, spirituality encompasses how athletes see themselves in the context of the team and organization and their individual relationships with their teammates. From time to time, players who struggle with relationship issues also struggle to relate to others in the locker room or have difficulties interacting with their coaches. This again shows that the boundaries between personal and professional are permeable and can't be dismissed as two distinct entities. One's moral and ethical code underpins the spiritual coactive. While it is fundamentally independent of faith and based in values, these can often be confused.

Many young athletes have yet to understand or find a goal or role for themselves in life. This confusion often affects their ability to identify clear spiritual guidelines early on. Occasionally, this can extend to moral or ethical guidelines, too. The sooner they find this comfort, the easier it is for them to find peace in the perspective and beliefs they hold.

Athletes with a strong spiritual center tend to better understand group dynamics and feel more confident about their role in the organization and in society. Someone who lacks this foundation often struggles in this regard. This doesn't have to be a matter of religious faith; a player may simply be out of sync with the spirit of the team and feel like an outsider who is not involved in the group dynamic.

For players to contribute and feel like part of a team, they must identify clearly a personal reason why they are coming in every day to give their all. This is closely related to the player's needs and identity. There needs to be a connection on a spiritual level—a sense of belonging or a tangible power of togetherness. It's essential that players have the sense that they are invested in the team and that their contributions are valued by the organization, which encourages a sense of responsibility and commitment.

- **Meaning:** Why am I doing this? Why are we doing this? Winning. Love.

- **Connection:** What do I have to offer? What's expected of me? Sense of belonging. Tangible power of togetherness.

- **Control:** How can I positively influence my performance and that of the team? Understand and commit to goals and hard work. Open to learning. Able to contribute.

THE TRIBE   4.3.1.1

John Hoberman, Eric Braverman, Christian Cook, and many others have written at length about how biology—particularly chemicals like serotonin and testosterone—impacts mood, emotions, and, subsequently, actions. This works in reverse, too. Cook even goes as far as to state, "Research indicates mood disturbance as the strongest psychological predictor of mental and physical recovery."[1] In her book *The Mood Cure*, Julia Ross goes into detail about the close links between biology and psychology.

> *I'm more worried about being a good person than being the best football player in the world. When all this is over, what are you left with? When I retire, I hope I am remembered for being a decent guy.*

—Lionel Messi

The actions and moods of the people we're surrounded by can profoundly impact us both physically and psychologically. In a positive sense, being in a supportive, upbeat, and encouraging locker room can heighten players' feel-good hormones and suppress those hormones associated with perceived stress and negative emotions. At the other end of the continuum, the negative impact of tribes on individual psychology becomes evident in the seemingly irrational and inexplicable actions of hooligans. In this case, testosterone runs rampant and results in violence and vandalism. It can also be seen in the slumped shoulders and downward gazes of players whose teams have been playing badly and have become collectively negative and pessimistic.

EMOTION
MICRO COACTIVE   4.3.2

While the terms *emotion* and *feeling* are often used interchangeably, neuroscientist Antonio Damasio says that emotions *originate from* feelings. He suggests that an emotion is the affective response to a stimulus, which is reflected by a set of neural and chemical changes in the state of the body. Therefore, a feeling or an emotion is an idea, perception, or interpretation of a particular object or situation.

Managing emotions on and off the field is an essential prerequisite for high performance and is arguably one of the most impactful components of psychological strength and ability. This is largely because when a player makes a decision in a game and then acts on it, the decision is based on instinct but also on environmental conditions and the actions of the opponent.

A player's decision-making process is partly reliant on past experiences and what she observes going on around her in the moment, but it's also closely tied to emotion. Emotions are the fastest mechanism in the body, so they have a great effect on players' and warrior-athletes' actions and overall performance. In many cases, when a special forces operator enters a room and readies his weapon, it's because he's made not an analytical decision but an instinctual one based on emotional awareness. He has sensed a certain mood in the room and is reacting instinctively to it.

How coaches and players communicate verbally and nonverbally with each other sets the emotional context for each interaction. This is why it's important for the coaching staff to communicate clearly and to try to expose players to only positive experiences during team preparation sessions.

OUT OF CONTROL   4.3.2.1

If players feel secure and believe their needs are being met, they're more likely to be in control of their emotions on and off the field. Lifestyle issues can make athletes feel out of control, and their emotional volatility can manifest itself in disciplinary issues in training and red cards or technical fouls during games. If a player is out of control when around teammates, it's the responsibility of the coaches to make that player understand that she is an important part of the team and that her needs will be best met if she treats those around her better. (I'll get into this topic in more depth in "The Coach.")

Addiction issues can manifest themselves powerfully in a player's emotions. Often, when a player has emotional issues with teammates and coaches—such as irrational outbursts of anger during training exercises or oversensitivity to criticism—the source has little or nothing to do with the team environment.

In many cases, athletes who struggle to make decisions on the field or within the organization have logical decision-making issues away from the game, and those whose emotions frequently boil over during competition have self-control struggles outside of this setting. Daniel Goleman's *Emotional Intelligence* and other books are invaluable references in this area. Goleman's reporting shows how stress can manifest itself in multiple areas of a player's life and wreak havoc on emotions. So if the coaches are trying to help a player emotionally, they should look beyond what goes on during games and practice and dig a little deeper.

EMOTIONAL INTELLIGENCE   4.3.2.2

The ability to be considerate, empathize with others, and be compassionate toward others is essential if an athlete is to function well as part of a team. It's also very important that players understand their own emotions and how these can affect their teammates. Daniel Goleman's landmark text *Emotional Intelligence* is the best reference for more on this topic.

Emotional intelligence is critical for:

- **Self-awareness:** Understanding emotions and being mindful of feelings as they occur

- **Managing emotions:** Handling feelings appropriately

- **Motivation:** Controlling emotions so that we can focus, delay gratification, and limit impulsiveness

- **Empathizing:** Understanding others and recognizing that their emotions are valid

- **Managing relationships:** Developing and maintaining healthy relationships

All of these are critical for the successful development of players and teams and especially for sustainable, dominating teams.

THE CONFIDENCE GAME   4.3.2.3

In any endeavor, there are two types of confidence that someone can develop in themselves and those around them: external and internal. The former can come via feedback from a player's family, the media, fans, and other sources outside the team. The problem with this type of confidence is that it's built on shifting sands. The media can praise an athlete and the team after one game and then slam them after the next. Fans are similarly fickle as the season progresses. Even feedback from family members can vary daily.

The more solid kind of confidence is that which comes from within: you determine the criteria by which you judge yourself and hold yourself to a high standard. How players feel about themselves as people shouldn't change based on the scoreboard or their stats. Nor should they let external forces determine their sense of self-worth. It's certainly important to take constructive criticism from coaches and teammates, but it's equally important *not* listen to praise or derision from anyone else.

John Wooden achieved a level of excellence that few coaches can even dream of, yet he did not believe that who won or lost the game was the ultimate verdict on the team or any individual player (or, for that matter, on his coaching). Victory shouldn't be the only thing to provide validation, Wooden thought; he insisted that instead, "success is peace of mind, which is a direct result of self-satisfaction in knowing you made the effort to become the best of which you are capable."[2]

To put in this best effort in every game, Wooden advised his players to prepare well by giving their all in each practice session, every single day. By trusting in the process he outlined and wholeheartedly dedicating themselves to consistent improvement, the Wizard of Westwood believed, his players would develop the kind of internal confidence needed to succeed on the hardwood.

TRUST IN THE GAME PLAN

Trust in the game plan comes from players' understanding of, and involvement in, the program design. Allowing the players some ownership and commitment to the program encourages trust in the team and what it is doing. If the coach simply dictates the system and does not allow ownership to transition to the players, players will be less committed and involved in the team's success.

PHYSICAL STATURE   4.3.2.4

The way players and coaches carry themselves has a big impact on their own state of mind as well as that of those around them. Posture can set the tone in a room, for good or for ill. To create a positive physical impression:

- Walk and stand tall

- Make an effort to display an in-charge posture—like standing tall and upright—and positive body language—such as smiling and keeping your chin up, literally and figuratively—especially when things aren't going well

- Create and project your own advantage by how you carry yourself at all times; it's within your control

COGNITION
MICRO COACTIVE   4.3.3

Cognition is the athlete's ability to focus, maintain attention, and mentally process what's going on during practice and games. While the cognition micro coactive does not refer to intelligence alone, that is part of it. Howard Gardner has written at length about the various forms of intelligence and the fact intelligence is not a singular factor in *Frames of Mind* and *Multiple Intelligences*. He reminds us that intelligence is specific to tasks and so is essentially a skill. People can have multiple intelligences that they apply in different scenarios—in social situations, in cognitive learning, and in applying their physical gifts. Nonetheless, the ability to process information, go through a logical decision-making process, study and learn, and benefit from individual and team-focused educational experiences is key to improving game-day performance. The ability to think critically is also important.

When I spoke about a player being completely engaged in learning opportunities in order to make the most of them, I didn't mean just running hard or jumping as high as possible. There also needs to be full cognitive commitment and concentration. When employing the morphological programming

approach, it's important to think about the cognitive load that players are experiencing on any given day and to ensure that they're mentally fresh come game day.

Everyone's learning is profoundly impacted by stress and/or disruption to basic health. The ability to engage fully on the training ground, in the film room, and during supplemental learning scenarios and to transfer these experiences to long-term memory is inextricably linked to an athlete's overall well-being.

Conducting a basic psychological profile that takes into account emotion, cognitive learning, and confidence allows us to clarify the areas of greatest need for improvement. Does the player handle stress well? Is he emotionally sound? Are there external issues affecting the player's mental and emotional state? Does she process and learn information properly or fast enough? Does he feel wanted or like part of the team? Does she feel loved here?

HOW WE LEARN   4.3.3.1

We often think of coaching as teaching, and in some ways this is true, but the true role of a coach in a team-preparation setting is to construct situations that expose players to experiences, through which they learn on their own. As psychologist Carl Rogers said, "If it can be taught, it's not worth learning." You could spend hours in front of a blackboard diagramming "when player X moves here, you go there" plays, but until you take these plays to the practice field and have players run them, they're virtually meaningless.

There is a myth that athletes' learning styles (such as learning by exploration or listening) vary, but the reality is that at the elite level, players are largely kinesthetic and visual. This is not because they were born with those learning preferences; rather, these have become the learning methods of choice through training and experience. This means that they learn through moving and, in the case of team-sports athletes, by doing so in a situation that mirrors the game as closely as possible.

As Lynn Kidman explores in her book *Athlete-Centered Coaching: Developing Decision Makers,* the role of the coach is not to tell athletes what to do but to set up learning opportunities that enable them to figure it out for themselves. The more realistic the practice situation, the more seamlessly the players will apply their new habits in games. In her book *The Coaching Process,* Kidman also states, "If athletes spend more time on optimal learning activities they will have a higher success rate." This puts the onus on the coach to plan sessions well so that athletes spend less time listening to instructions and more time doing.[3]

TAPPING INTO THE SUBCONSCIOUS   4.3.3.2

In a team-preparation setting, coaches could tell players everything about the learning experience they're about to have—what it is, why they're doing it, how it will impact their performance in the next game, and so on. But then coaches would miss out on tapping into what New Thought minister Joseph Murphy termed "the power of the subconscious mind."

Athletes must be verbally told certain things in training, so going into detailed explanations about the purpose of games and drills will just use up more of their cognitive capacity. Instead, let them have the experience and figure out what they're supposed to do on their own. This will engage their subconscious and let them figure out the best way to execute the skills that the learning scenario requires, which is far more effective than when coaches have a preconceived idea of how skills should be performed and then stop practice every time an athlete improvises. The next step is to re-create the experience multiple times over different sessions to ingrain the habits that players need to access automatically during games.

As Benjamin Franklin wrote, "Tell me and I forget. Teach me and I remember. Involve me and I learn."

WHAT DO PLAYERS REALLY NEED TO KNOW?   4.3.3.3

If I told you that it's better if a player doesn't know why you're creating a learning experience and, after they've achieved the learning objective, doesn't know what it is they've added to their toolbox, you'd think I'd gone crazy, right? Well, this is actually one of the most effective ways to structure athlete preparation. A basketball player does not need to know that you want her to improve her ability to shoot three-pointers from the left side of the court—she just needs to be able to do it.

As a coach, you're better off spending your time constructing the right learning experience to facilitate such an outcome than explaining at length to the athlete what the goal is, which element it relates to, and so on. All the player needs to know is what to do in that scenario when the next game requires them to do it. The emphasis should be on creating the appropriate exposure and repeating it until a habit is ingrained and accessible in the moment. Don't make the mistake of assuming that players need to know what coaches need to know, because they don't.

KNOWING OR UNDERSTANDING?   4.3.3.4

It's a common misconception that athletes need to fully understand what they do during a game and be able to explain it in detail, like a student reciting an answer on a test. In fact, many of the world's top performers are unable to do so, even at a surface level. Several interviewers have asked Wayne Rooney to explain what he does on the pitch, apparently expecting some kind of revelatory response. No such luck. He told Manchester.com that most of what he does during games is purely instinctual: "You're best when you're on the pitch and you're not even thinking about football, if it doesn't sound too silly. The best things are the ones which just happen. When you think you just overcomplicate it: when the ball comes you just have to do what your body does, what feels right."[4]

Such a response illustrates that players don't have to know what they do between kickoff and the final whistle in terms of being able to recite it—they just have to be able to understand instinctively what to do and then do it.

PERSONALITY AND THE PSYCHE   4.3.4

Sport is a microcosm of society, and just like in a circle of friends or a family, there are many different personalities on a sports team. Players' personalities don't just impact how they act in the locker room but also how they act during practice and in games. Some athletes' off-field demeanors are the same as what they show on the field. I've known plenty of rugby and football players, for example, who are every bit as intimidating away from the game as they are during it. But others seem to have the ability to change personalities and switch personas for the game. When we're looking at how a player's mindset influences her performance, it's important that we take her psyche into account.

BRUCE WAYNE AND BATMAN   4.3.4.1

Some players' game-time personas match their personalities away from sports. Michael Jordan is supposedly just as competitive during card games with friends and on the golf course as he was when leading the Chicago Bulls to six NBA titles, for example. Others can get away with the opposite—being joyous and carefree both on the court and away from it; Steph Curry comes to mind. Yet in some sports and for certain positions, a meek, humble, or fun-loving demeanor just doesn't cut it once the game starts. That's not the right attitude when you're an offensive lineman or rugby prop facing opponents who want to grind you into dust.

So how can an athlete with a laid-back personality become ruthless on the field? By creating an alter ego. Recent examples in sports are Kobe Bryant becoming the Black Mamba as soon as he hit the court and English soccer player Joey Barton being Joey in everyday life and then professional, businesslike Joseph on the pitch. Players who can benefit from a purposefully created second personality need to be encouraged to switch into Superman mode once the game starts and to change back into Clark Kent once the final whistle or buzzer sounds.

The problems start when players who revel in their warrior role during games can't turn it off when the floodlights dim. There have been high-profile players who carried their aggressive and even violent player personas over to real life, with tragic consequences. We cannot in good conscience look at players as athletic commodities; we must treat them as people whose lives are complex and involve much more than what happens on game day. The coaching staff must make it part of their job to be aware of the environments that are molding their athletes away from the team facilities. While they might not be able to halt some players' downward spirals, at least being aware of what goes on in the other eighteen, twenty, or twenty-two hours of each day provides a context to these troubled individuals' actions and can help prevent them from having a detrimental effect on team morale.

THE MORPHOLOGICAL PROGRAMMING APPROACH AND PSYCHOLOGY   4.3.5

The traditional focus in team sports is on developing physical qualities. But the morphological programming approach is more effective because it recognizes that body and brain are one, so it takes into account psychophysiological loads, particularly when it comes to volume, intensity, and density of training. You can have long blocks of concentration that are high in volume, such as a film review session. There are also preparatory and game events that are short but require extremely intense concentration, like a penalty shoot-out. Then there are activities that are psychologically demanding and intensive, like learning new plays. These require greater cognitive recovery than sessions that take less of a mental toll on the players, such as scrimmages.

The cognitive, emotional, and spiritual demands of an athlete's or a team's activity can be very different from the physical load. For example, taking one penalty in a soccer game is not that physically demanding in itself but is widely regarded as being one of the most mentally demanding tasks in team sports. Cerebrally demanding things can also take a tremendous physical toll—consider a stockbroker who dies suddenly of a heart attack. The point is that we can't merely look at the morphological programming profile of an event physiologically without also considering its psychological implications, and vice versa. We need to think about the total stress load on the body and how we can help athletes manage this load.

THE PHYSICAL COACTIVE

———— 4.4

This section concerns a player's physical traits and how they are interrelated with the other coactives of the morphocycle—psychological, tactical, and technical. We'll go over the various components of physical skills and how some of these can be better expressed and developed.

PHYSICAL EXECUTION   4.4.1

When we look at the quality of play on the field from a performance perspective, we focus on three main components of physical execution: biomechanics, bioenergetics, and biodynamics.

BIOMECHANICS   4.4.1.1

Biomechanics refers to the physical structure and movement of the athlete, which is a determined mostly by the structural-anatomical system (see page 174). Biomechanics largely sets the function of the player and how they move. Do they have the appropriate ankle mobility to reach positions of strength? It's related not just to the fixed capabilities of joints and tissues but also to their mobility and ability to coordinate structures and motion segments in movement.

BIOENERGETICS   4.4.1.2

This area concerns the ability of the cardiorespiratory system and energy substrate system (see pages 175 and 176) to fuel an athlete during training and competition. Bioenergetics are also largely determined by the capabilities of the cardiorespiratory

A WORD ABOUT WORDS

The terminology that the head coach and staff use is arguably more important than that used by the team psychologist, nutritionist, or any other specialist, who may all use different terms for similar ideas. For example, "speed" to a strength coach might be "quickness" to a position coach or "reaction time" to a rehab coordinator. The manifestation of a particular quality on the field can have numerous meanings and interpretations. It's the job of the coaching team to absorb and interpret whatever lexicon is used by strength and speed coaches, the medical team, and other specialists, and then to put them into relatable terms for the players.

system to distribute oxygenated blood to execute repeated actions. This is arguably one of the easier areas to identify and improve, but as a result, it's also often accused of being a limiting factor.

BIODYNAMICS   4.4.1.3

Biodynamics refers to the nervous reception and response governed by the nervous macro system (including the central, peripheral, and autonomous nervous systems) and the hormone regulation of the biotransformational system, pituitary-adrenal system, and cortisol-immune system (see pages 166 and 177). We see these systems combining to manifest expressions of speed, power, strength, mobility, and endurance.

The key point here is that these three systems are dependent on each other and complement each other. Careful analysis of players' performance can help identify limiting factors and factors to be emphasized from an individual perspective on the training field or in individual or group/position work.

	QUALITY		MANIFESTATION	DESCRIPTION
PHYSICAL	ALACTIC POWER	ALACTIC POWER	HIGH INTENSITY / SHORT DURATION / ATP-CP / ALACTIC ANAEROBIC SYSTEM	ALACTIC
	ALACTIC CAPACITY	ALACTIC CAPACITY		
	ANAEROBIC POWER	ANAEROBIC POWER	MEDIUM INTENSITY / INTERMEDIATE / LACTIC ANAEROBIC, GLYCOLYTIC / OXYGEN INDEPENDENT / NON-OXIDATIVE GLYCOLYTIC	ANAEROBIC
	ANAEROBIC CAPACTIY	ANAEROBIC CAPACTIY		
	AEROBIC POWER	AEROBIC POWER	LONGER DURATION / AEROBIC / OXIDATIVE / OXYGEN DEPENDENT	AEROBIC
	AEROBIC CAPACITY	AEROBIC CAPACITY		
	EXPLOSIVE STRENGTH	ISOMETRIC	POWER	ISOMETRIC
		ECCENTRIC	DECELERATION	ECCENTRIC
	MAXIMAL STRENGTH			STATIC
	STRENGTH-SPEED	CONCENTRIC	STRENGTH	CONCENTRIC
		RATE FORCE DEVELOPMENT	REPEAT POWER	RATE FORCE DEVELOPMENT
	SPEED-STRENGTH	DYNAMIC STRENGTH-SPEED		DYNAMIC STRENGTH-SPEED
		SPEED-STRENGTH	SPEED	SPEED-STRENGTH
	STRENGTH-ENDURANCE	STIFFNESS		STIFFNESS
		STRENGTH-ENDURANCE	ENDURANCE	STRENGTH-ENDURANCE
	SPEED-ENDURANCE	MUSCULAR ENDURANCE		MUSCULAR ENDURANCE
BIOTRANS-FORMATIONAL	DIGESTIVE		INTAKE, ABSORBTION & GUT HEALTH	
	DETOXIFICATION		LIVER, KIDNEYS & LYMPHATIC	
STRUCTURAL-ANATOMICAL	SIZE, HYPERTROPHY		COLLISION	
	FLEXIBILITY & MOVEMENT		MOBILITY	
	PASSIVE STRUCTURAL		BONES, JOINTS, CARTILAGE, TENDONS, LIGAMENTS	
	INTEGUMENTARY		SKIN, OUTER LAYER/EPIDERMIS	
METABOLIC	METABOLIC ENERGY PROCESSES		ENERGY SUBSTRATES AND METABOLITES	LACTIC ANAEROBIC—ATP, CP, AMMONIA
				LACTIC AEROBIC—GLUCOSE/GLYCOGEN, LACTIC ACID
				AEROBIC—GLYCOGEN, FAT
	CARDIORESPIRATORY		CARDIAC, RESPIRATORY & CIRCULATORY SYSTEMS	
ENDOCRINE	ENDOCRINE, HORMONAL		HYPOTHALAMUS, PITUITARY-ADRENAL SYSTEM	GROWTH HORMONE, TESTOSTERONE, INSULIN, ETC
	CORTISOL-IMMUNE SYSTEM		FUNCTION OF HORMONAL SYSTEM	
NERVOUS	CENTRAL NERVOUS SYSTEM		NEUROTRANSMITTER RESTORATION	
	AUTONOMIC NERVOUS SYSTEM		SYMPATHETIC/PARASYMPATHETIC BALANCE	
	PERIPHERAL NERVOUS SYSTEM		NEUROMUSCULAR SYSTEM	

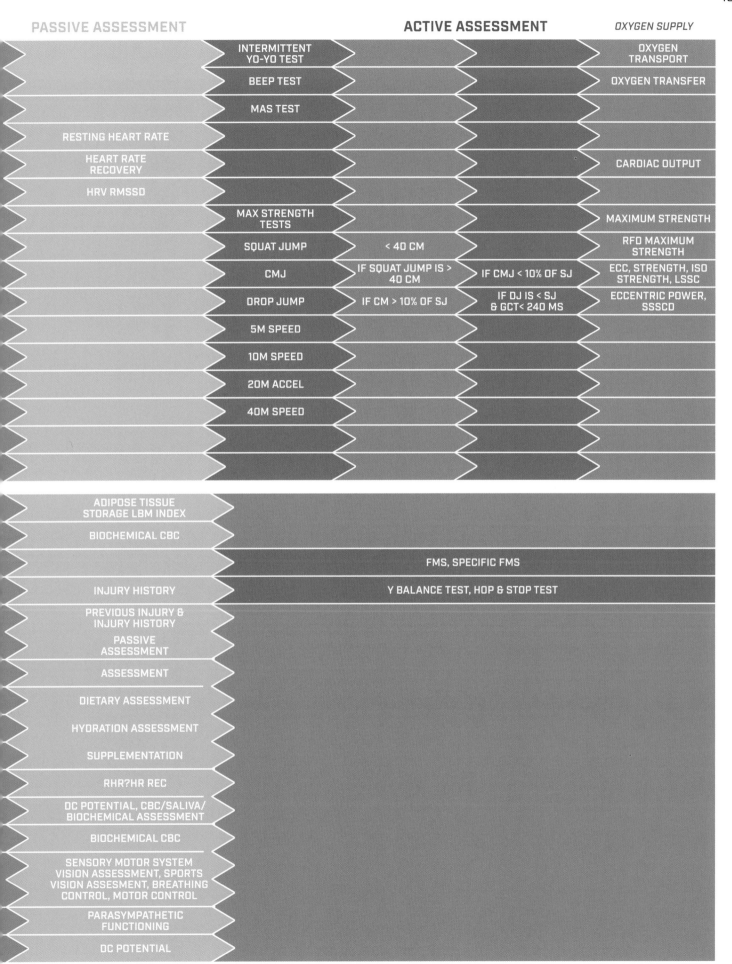

PASSIVE ASSESSMENT

ACTIVE ASSESSMENT

OXYGEN SUPPLY

	INTERMITTENT YO-YO TEST		OXYGEN TRANSPORT
	BEEP TEST		OXYGEN TRANSFER
	MAS TEST		
RESTING HEART RATE			
HEART RATE RECOVERY			CARDIAC OUTPUT
HRV RMSSD			
	MAX STRENGTH TESTS		MAXIMUM STRENGTH
	SQUAT JUMP	< 40 CM	RFD MAXIMUM STRENGTH
	CMJ	IF SQUAT JUMP IS > 40 CM / IF CMJ < 10% OF SJ	ECC, STRENGTH, ISO STRENGTH, LSSC
	DROP JUMP	IF CM > 10% OF SJ / IF DJ IS < SJ & GCT< 240 MS	ECCENTRIC POWER, SSSCD
	5M SPEED		
	10M SPEED		
	20M ACCEL		
	40M SPEED		

ADIPOSE TISSUE STORAGE LBM INDEX	
BIOCHEMICAL CBC	
	FMS, SPECIFIC FMS
INJURY HISTORY	Y BALANCE TEST, HOP & STOP TEST
PREVIOUS INJURY & INJURY HISTORY	
PASSIVE ASSESSMENT	
ASSESSMENT	
DIETARY ASSESSMENT	
HYDRATION ASSESSMENT	
SUPPLEMENTATION	
RHR?HR REC	
DC POTENTIAL, CBC/SALIVA/ BIOCHEMICAL ASSESSMENT	
BIOCHEMICAL CBC	
SENSORY MOTOR SYSTEM VISION ASSESSMENT, SPORTS VISION ASSESMENT, BREATHING CONTROL, MOTOR CONTROL	
PARASYMPATHETIC FUNCTIONING	
DC POTENTIAL	

DESCRIPTION	EXERCISE VARIABLE	METHOD	VARIATION
ALACTIC POWER	ALACTIC POWER DRILLS	ALACTIC POWER GAMES	ALACTIC POWER INTERVALS
ALACTIC CAPACITY	ALACTIC CAPACITY DRILLS	ALACTIC CAPACITY GAMES	ALACTIC CAPACITY INTERVALS
ANAEROBIC POWER	ANAEROBIC POWER DRILLS	ANAEROBIC POWER GAMES	LACTIC POWER INTERVALS
ANAEROBIC CAPACITY	ANAEROBIC CAPACTIY DRILLS	ANAEROBIC CAPACITY GAMES	LACTIC CAPACITY ITERVALS
AEROBIC POWER	AEROBIC POWER DRILLS	AEROBIC POWER GAMES	CARDIAC OUTPUT METHOD
AEROBIC CAPACITY	AEROBIC CAPACITY DRILLS	AEROBIC CAPACITY GAMES	TEMPO METHOD
STRENGTH	EXPLOSIVE STRENGTH	REACTIVE METHODS	PLYOMETRIC
			CONTRAST
	MAXIMAL STRENGTH	SUPRAMAXIMAL	
	STRENGTH-SPEED		
SPEED		MAXIMAL	WEIGHT LIFTING
	SPEED-STRENGTH		ISOMETRIC
POWER		CIRCA MAXIMAL	QUASI-ISOMETRIC
	STRENGTH-ENDURANCE		
ENDURANCE		SUBMAXIMAL	ENDURANCE
	SPEED-ENDURANCE		PYRAMID

DESCRIPTION	EXERCISE VARIABLE	METHOD	VARIATION
DIGESTIVE		PROPERLY PROCESSED FOOD	SUPPLEMENTATION, PERFORMANCE
DETOXIFICATION		FOOD QUALITY	SUPPLEMENTATION, HEALTH
HYPERTROPHY	SIZE	BODYBUILDING	PLATEAU
MOVEMENT	FLEXIBILITY	DYNAMIC	ACTIVE
		STATIC	PASSIVE
PASSIVE STRUCTURAL SYSTEM		REGENERATION PROTOCOLS	STRESS MANAGEMENT
INTEGUMENTARY		HYGIENE	
METABOLIC ENERGY PROCESS		DIET & BASIC SUPPLEMENTATION	CIRCADIAN RHYTHM
			SLEEP QUALITY
			DIGESTIVE HEALTH
CARDIORESPIRATORY		CLEAN FOOD	DETOXIFICATION
ENDOCRINE		REST, RECOVERY & SUPPLEMENTATION	
CORTISOL-IMMUNE SYSTEM		QUALITY DIET & SUPPLEMENTATION	
CENTRAL NERVOUS SYSTEM		DIET & REST BALANCE	FOOD QUALITY & TIMIING
AUTONOMIC NERVOUS SYSTEM		BALANCED DIET	FOOD QUANTITY & CALORIC INTAKE
NEUROMUSCULAR SYSTEM		SLEEP & STRESS REDUCTION	CIRCADIAN RHYTHM

TECHNIQUE

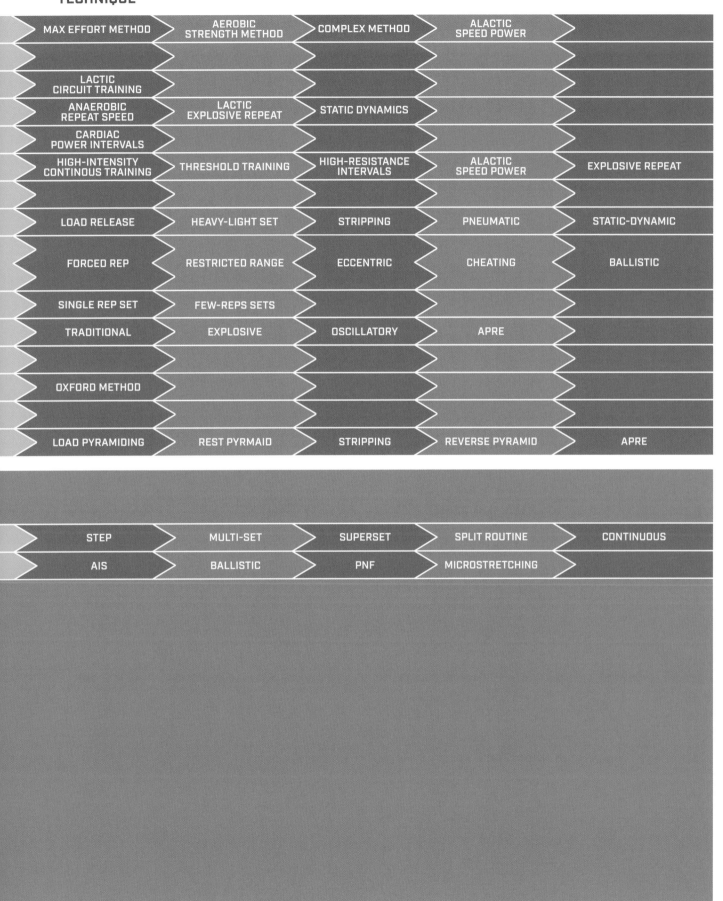

MAX EFFORT METHOD	AEROBIC STRENGTH METHOD	COMPLEX METHOD	ALACTIC SPEED POWER	
LACTIC CIRCUIT TRAINING				
ANAEROBIC REPEAT SPEED	LACTIC EXPLOSIVE REPEAT	STATIC DYNAMICS		
CARDIAC POWER INTERVALS				
HIGH-INTENSITY CONTINOUS TRAINING	THRESHOLD TRAINING	HIGH-RESISTANCE INTERVALS	ALACTIC SPEED POWER	EXPLOSIVE REPEAT
LOAD RELEASE	HEAVY-LIGHT SET	STRIPPING	PNEUMATIC	STATIC-DYNAMIC
FORCED REP	RESTRICTED RANGE	ECCENTRIC	CHEATING	BALLISTIC
SINGLE REP SET	FEW-REPS SETS			
TRADITIONAL	EXPLOSIVE	OSCILLATORY	APRE	
OXFORD METHOD				
LOAD PYRAMIDING	REST PYRMAID	STRIPPING	REVERSE PYRAMID	APRE

STEP	MULTI-SET	SUPERSET	SPLIT ROUTINE	CONTINUOUS
AIS	BALLISTIC	PNF	MICROSTRETCHING	

ANTHROPOMETRICS, SIZE, STRUCTURE, AND SHAPE   4.4.2

The size and proportions of every athlete's body—that is, their anthropometrics—are determined largely by heredity. Height, bone structure, ratio of limb length to torso length, and so on are products of DNA. Heredity also governs body type and shape—whether the athlete is an endomorph, ectomorph, or mesomorph. Body composition can also be manipulated through activity and nutrition, such as by increasing a player's muscle mass or decreasing their body fat percentage.

INTENSITY AND BIOMECHANICS   4.4.2.1

In physiological terms, intensity is the ability to generate sudden force quickly, which is very biomechanically demanding. When looking at how quickly athletes can generate force, we need to focus on how their bodies are structured. Anthropometrics, length of their levers, and joint composition are important. Two athletes can seem to have similar proportions, but their seated height, which is determined by spine length, may be very different. The athlete with the shorter spine will have a lower center of gravity and thus be able to change direction more quickly than a player with a longer spine.

Ben Johnson was very fast out of the starting blocks and accelerated quickly, partly due to his shorter limbs, lower center of gravity, and fast-twitch-dominant muscle profile. Carl Lewis, on the other hand, took longer to get up to full speed but decelerated less once he reached it. Lewis's height, longer limbs, and higher center of gravity influenced his sprinting style. The fact that both were very successful (Johnson's drug abuse notwithstanding) shows that success is not limited to one body type or another.

Orientation—how body structures align—also influences intensity. Mobility work, massage, and chiropractic therapy can help by ensuring that nerves aren't impinged and thus can send messages to the athlete's muscles: a key factor in how much force can be generated and how quickly it can be applied.

MOVEMENT AND MOBILITY   4.4.2.2

To get into and maintain sustainable athletic positions that allow us to generate the required force to perform a skill on the playing field, we need to at least meet mobility baselines, such as 120 degrees of hip flexion when standing. If we lack this capacity, we struggle to stabilize our bodies and start making biomechanical compromises and getting into suboptimal positions that wreak havoc on our soft tissues. In turn, these tissues get tighter, further limiting our mobility and therefore our movement. The solution is to cultivate a daily soft-tissue restoration practice and, per physical therapist and movement expert Kelly Starrett, spend a minimum of ten to fifteen minutes daily on improving mobility.

Yet we can't think about mobility and movement without also considering structure. No wonder Sue Falsone, the first female head athletic trainer in American major league sports, named her company Structure & Function—you can't separate the two. While mobility impacts structure when tight tissues and compromised positions start causing damage and can lead to structural degeneration over time, it's also true that structure impacts mobility. Even someone who has optimal range of motion and motor control will not be able to exceed the natural limits set by their skeleton and joint composition. The key for an athlete is to obtain enough mobility to maximize the potential of their inherited body structure while moving in a sustainable manner that does no harm to this structure.

PHYSICAL QUALITIES   4.4.3

A mistake we often make in team sports is focusing on the quality in which we think a player is weakest, such as maximum strength. We send them off to improve it—such as by doing heavy, low-rep sets of dead lifts and squats in the weight room—and then put them into the next game and expect their performance to magically improve because they're now "stronger."

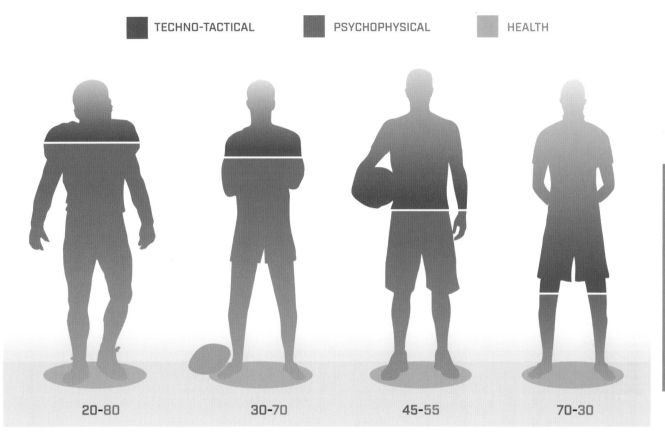

TECHNO-TACTICAL / PSYCHOPHYSICAL DETERMINANTS OF SPORTS

TECHNO-TACTICAL   PSYCHOPHYSICAL   HEALTH

20-80   30-70   45-55   70-30

Different sports have varying degrees of techno-tactical and psychophysical demands.

Instead, we should try to improve a physical quality (or a technical, tactical, or psychological one, for that matter) only if it's a limiting factor in game performance. The quality should also be enhanced in a realistic context that's applicable to competition. This is another example of working backward from the game itself. We also need to determine if the issue is in fact physical or if it's rooted in a limitation of one of the other three coactives. If we find that it is indeed a physiological issue, then it becomes a matter of figuring out what exactly the problem is, determining the best exercise or method to solve it, and then setting aside time during or after practice for the player to work on it. It is also helpful to group several players who are struggling in the same area—

such as with endurance—and have them work on it together. Then they can return to the same learning experiences that the other players in their positions/ units are being exposed to.

THE MORPHOLOGICAL PROGRAMMING APPROACH AND PHYSIOLOGY   4.4.4

If we're going to develop technical ability, we need to manage the four morphological programming dimensions appropriately to improve the learning opportunity and outcome.

PHYSICAL PERFORMANCE QUALITIES

AEROBIC POWER

is the amount of force that a player can exert while running longer distances.

AEROBIC CAPACITY

is commonly just called "endurance." It's how long an athlete is able to go at a sub-maximal level of exertion.

ANAEROBIC CAPACITY

is the ability to exert maximum effort over short distances or for short periods and, in conjunction with the aerobic system, repeat it. It's important, for example, when a rugby winger charges in for a try.

ANAEROBIC POWER

is the bridge between bioenergetics and biodynamics in that it's what fuels the ability to consistently generate power over multiple short distances and durations—for example, a basketball player running back on defense to block a layup, then streaking back down the court to receive a pass on the fast break and dunking.

EXPLOSIVENESS

is the ability to exert power quickly, as in a vertical jump or long jump—in other words, how quickly strength is applied.

ISOMETRIC CONTRACTION

uses muscular force to resist motion, such as when a basketball forward boxes out an opponent and maintains his rebounding position while being pushed.

MAXIMUM STRENGTH

is the ability to generate a maximal singular application of strength, such as for a one-rep dead lift or squat PR. This is usually a concentric (muscle-shortening) movement.

NEURAL POWER

is the nervous system's capacity to produce effort, which is just as important as the muscles' ability to generate force through contraction.

SPEED-ENDURANCE

is the ability to generate speed and either sustain it in a continuous effort or reproduce it several times, as a winger does in rugby.

SPEED-STRENGTH

is an athlete's ability to achieve top speed or close to it and hold it for a short time, as when a soccer player cuts in from the wing and into the box before firing a shot on goal.

STRENGTH-ENDURANCE

is the ability to apply strength over an extended period or several times in quick succession—for example, an offensive lineman holding off a defensive lineman on successive downs.

STRENGTH-SPEED

involves applying strength with a dynamic component, which is often expressed in multiple dimensions. A squat jump is a good example, as strength and speed are combined while going up and down and eccentric strength (muscle lengthening) is required as well as concentric strength (muscle shortening).

VOLUME AND QUANTITY   4.4.4.1

We need to keep volume low when training a new skill in order to maximize learning intensity. A high volume or high number of reps—a "more is better" approach—will undermine the positive impact of most learning experiences. The volume/quantity should be increased only after the player demonstrates the ability to perform the skill with intensity and then density (more on how to balance these later on).

INTENSITY AND QUALITY   4.4.4.2

As learning technical skills is a high-intensity activity, we need to ensure that we prioritize quality above all else. Once a player can do something well a few times, they can do more repetitions to show that they can perform the skill while dealing with acute fatigue.

You can go through this progression by increasing the number of people with whom the athlete has to perform the skill. So in basketball, have them do it first in a one-on-one game, then three-on-three, then a full-sided five-on-five.

NEURAL AND CARDIAC LOADING IN TEAM SPORTS

THE INTENSITY/VOLUME RELATIONSHIP

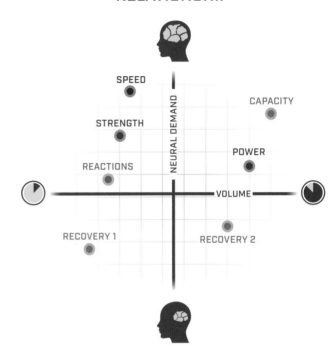

DENSITY AND FREQUENCY   4.4.4.3

Density needs to be kept particularly low when introducing a new skill. In most team sports there are breaks between the times when a player must perform a skill, so it's best to replicate this in practice. It's better for players to focus intently for a few minutes and then take a break so they can replay what they've just learned in their mind. It's also productive to design learning experiences in which the player is forced to perform the required action as frequently as possible.

COLLISION/CONTACT   4.4.4.4

All sports have elements of contact and collision, which affect the amount of vibrational force an athlete absorbs. Contact is more pronounced in some activities than in others. For example, even in sprinting—which few would consider a "contact sport" like rugby, football, or Australian rules football—the impact of runners' feet generates a large amount of force per stride, which takes a collision toll on mus-

cles, bones, ligaments, and tendons that cannot be ignored. If a soccer winger made a lot of long runs into the opponent's half on a pitch that was frozen, that player's contact load would be high.

Collision involves bodily impact and comes into play in true contact sports. So when a cornerback puts a big hit on a wide receiver, both players' bodies are subjected to a high vibrational load due to the violent, explosive force of the CB leaping into the WR as he's running in another direction. Beyond the sheer power generated, such an impact is multi-directional and off-axis, increasing the demands on both players' structures to dissipate the forces created.

We could say a training session that involves sprints or plyometrics for any team-sports athlete ranks high on the contact/collision element of the morphological programming approach. A high-contact rugby practice, for example, would involve scrummaging.

READINESS PREPAREDNESS POTENTIAL

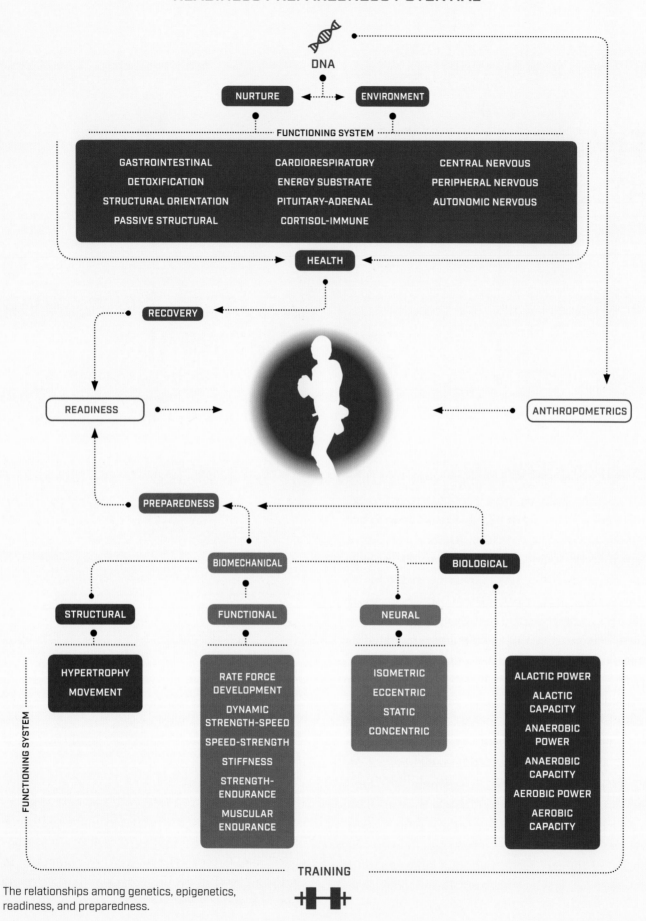

The relationships among genetics, epigenetics, readiness, and preparedness.

FIVE

THE TEAM-SPORT ATHLETE

It might sound strange, but all team-sport athletes are essentially very similar. Every player must have the same qualities to play any team sport, just in varying degrees. Think of a game's requirements (strength, speed, reaction, and so on) as keys on a piano: every tune uses the same keys, but they're played in a different order and with different emphases. So too does each sport require the same attributes of the players, but with different emphases.

Take physical qualities. Strength, power, and speed are all required in soccer, football, rugby, basketball, and other sports, but each sport (and position) needs a different degree of these. Then, as we begin to assess game-time performance and limitations with the four-coactive model, we see that individuals not only vary in how they express physical skills but also bring their own unique combinations of technical, tactical, and psychological capabilities to bear during the game. A particularly high ability in one area can make up for a comparatively low proficiency in another. In this section, we're going to explore how to better evaluate players in this way—recognizing their fundamental similarities while also respecting their differences and ability to compensate for varying competencies.

WHAT IS THE PLAYER EXPERIENCE?

Take any moment in a game and you'll see the interaction of a player and multiple dynamic, complicated systems.

When we look at the complexity of the moment with a systems lens, we see that there are a series of complex microsystems. Cultural, physiological, psychological, technical, tactical, methodological, and strategic subsystems—and many others—all intertwine to form a systems theory for team sports.

Athletes must know where they are in relationship to the ball, their teammates, their opponents, and the boundary lines of the court, field, or pitch. They also must be aware of the best course of action based on the game plan and the goals for them as players, their particular positions, and their units. In addition, they must be cognizant of how much time is left on the clock, both for that particular possession and for the quarter, half, and total duration of the game.

Then technique comes into play. Athletes must select the appropriate skill for a scenario and execute it well enough to achieve the desired outcome. This isn't just a physical matter but also a psychological one, as they need to keep their emotions in check and withstand the pressure applied by the opponent and the moment itself. They also have to possess the physical capability to evade the opposition and get into the correct spot to set up the next action, and then recruit the right muscle fibers and motion segments in sequence, with the correct timing to apply the chosen motor pattern. So four distinct player components—tactical, technical, physical, and psychological—are present at all times.

Every system within the body contributes to the moment as well. The peripheral nervous system and the players' senses gather real-time information. The central and autonomic nervous systems release a cocktail of chemicals that push the body into action. The cardiorespiratory system elevates heart and breathing rates to supply oxygenated blood to the structural system, with the biotransformational system supplying the fuel needed by the energy substrate system to power the required movement. As the brain chooses the right skill and the body applies it, the orientation system provides constant updates on where the body is in time and space as the movement pattern is executed. In short, every system in the body is working together, in sequence, with every tick of the game clock.

Then they must all recover, too.

SHORTSIGHTED ASSESSMENTS OF PERFORMANCE   5.1.1

Imagine a wide receiver poised to catch a pass from his quarterback just in front of the opposing team's end zone. This seems like a fairly small action in the grand scheme of things, but really it's the summation of every experience the receiver has had to this point and challenges each coactive: tactical, technical, physical, and psychological. Does he have the technical ability to make the catch? Is he tactically astute enough to have understood this particular play so that he knows exactly where to be? Do the physical characteristics of speed, strength, and power enable him to get into position, evade, or hold off the cornerback and leap high enough into the air to catch the ball and then keep running into the end zone? And is he mentally tough enough to handle the pressure of

the situation so that he can stay calm enough to execute the required skill at precisely the right moment?

The trouble is that few people think about a point of time in a game in these terms. If the receiver fumbles the ball or mistimes his leap and lets the pass sail out of bounds, a viewer might yell at the TV and make a reductionist assumption based on a perceived shortcoming in one of the four coactives. When it comes to a failed outcome in a game, such an assertion is usually about technical, physical, or psychological factors, not tactical ones. So maybe a fan will yell at a friend, "I told you he can't catch!" as the receiver drops the ball, when in reality the player can catch perfectly well and just misread the play or mistimed his route.

Or in a penalty shoot-out in soccer, we often assume that a player blasted the ball over the crossbar because "she's a choker." Maybe this is correct, but perhaps the athlete sustained a slight strain in her right hamstring that shot pain down her leg just as she planted her foot in readiness to take the shot. A basketball player misses the chance to dunk an alley-oop pass and we throw up our hands and say, "He can't jump anymore." Actually, the player still has a very high vertical leap, but he twisted his ankle three weeks ago when he went up for a dunk and he doesn't yet have 100 percent faith in his rehab, so he hesitated for a moment before takeoff.

Sports professionals have other perspectives. If the player drops a pass, the strength coach thinks the player missed it on physical grounds such as strength, speed, or quickness. The physical therapist sees the failure through a lens that identifies poor mobility and flexibility, the position coach blames poor handling, the psychologist thinks it's due to poor concentration, and the optometrist sees a vision error.

All of these are examples of the myopia of performance in action. We're too shortsighted in our assessment of outcomes or potential outcomes and far too quick to rush to judgment. It's the job of the coaching staff to take a more thoughtful look at what went wrong and to ask the players what they intended and why they think they dropped the attempted catch, missed the decisive penalty, or blew the potentially game-tying dunk.

TEAM SPORT ISN'T LEGOS

As teams have involved more and more specialists in player preparation, we've seen reductionism increase. One of the fallacies of sports science is that you can build the best whole (i.e., successful athletes on a continually improving team) by breaking down the parts of preparation and then reassembling them like a Lego set by the time the game rolls around. Teams are trying to isolate certain elements of training and performance, breaking things down not just into the four coactives but into ever-smaller chunks. So you might have a sports psychologist already working with the team but decide to bring in a mental conditioning coach as well. The physical realm is the greatest culprit when it comes to reductionism, as this is the coactive that's overemphasized most often. There are many excellent directors of performance, strength and conditioning coaches, speed coaches, and other specialists who can contribute to a team's ongoing improvement, but only if they're working within an integrated, holistic, moldable approach that recognizes how all the components of preparation are intertwined.

THE PERSON

Winning is fundamentally a people business, and the business of how people function in groups. Yes, individual players like Messi, Brady, and LeBron make outstanding contributions, but teams of people win games, and exceptional teams dominate.

Great coaches like Jackson, Harbaugh, Walsh, Ferguson, Belichick, Clarkson, Woodward, Henry, and Summit all have been great people managers and possess the emotional intelligence needed to successfully lead teams of men and women. So, before we even discuss winning games or improving players, we must recognize the individuals behind the number, crest, logo, or name. When we're considering the athlete as a person, there are certain biological laws and principles that we need to be aware of and cannot violate if we're to fulfill our duty to

preserve the long-term health of our athletes. In this section, we will look at the nature-versus-nurture argument as it pertains to the origin of great players. We will examine the body as a complex intertwining of systems and present a model for the most efficient development of the athlete. Then we'll progress to the details of athlete development.

In my experience in elite sport, the majority of issues that prevent optimal performance have nothing to do with the sport—they are personal issues. Remember that at the elite end of sport, athletes are good, very good. They didn't suddenly become bad. Some athletes can compartmentalize in order to perform, but many cannot.

We must also appreciate that there are things we cannot measure or prove, but they still can—and should—be modeled. Before we address the player as an athlete, I want to start with our understanding of the person, with their health and mindset as the primary concern.

NATURE AND GENETICS

Like everyone else, athletes are somewhat subject to the constraints and limitations of their DNA. While the effects of nature versus nurture will continue to be debated long after this book is read, in preparing players and teams to win games, we must be cognizant that both play a role in the development of every competitor.

At the most fundamental level, we cannot escape the legacy of our DNA. We inherit certain physical characteristics from our parents and their forebears that are what they are—eye and hair color, limb length, height, and body type (ectomorph, endomorph, or mesomorph). Growing research suggests that our nervous system is determined by genetics. Our parents also pass on certain biological capabilities and limitations that set the ceiling of our athletic performance. You could have Usain Bolt's coach, train six or seven hours a day against his training partners, and eat the same foods, but it's likely you'd never get close to rewriting the sprinting record books, as he did, for one simple reason: your DNA is different from Bolt's.

> *Parts of our genome simply cannot survive a situation where the environment suffers from the full overload of toxins we currently live in.*

—Kat Lahr

Genes affect more than physical qualities. For example, the so-called warrior gene (monoamine oxidase A-L) is associated with increased aggression, suggesting that our DNA also impacts how we think and behave. The warrior gene regulates production of an enzyme that breaks down neurotransmitters such as dopamine, norepinephrine, and serotonin, and how high the level of this enzyme is seems to affect how aggressive people are in response to provocation.

But at the same time, DNA does not mean that fate is predetermined. It simply outlines the ingredients for a recipe; the cooking process can still improve or ruin the final dish.

GENETIC MAPPING   5.2.1.1

When Dr. Francis Collins and his team mapped the human genome in 2003, many sports scientists were convinced that, because we'd completed part of the human body's great jigsaw puzzle, we'd soon unlock every genetic element of athletic potential. Unfortunately, this promise remains largely unfulfilled. Just because you have a map of a country doesn't mean that you understand the history and culture of every town and city on this map, and so it goes with genetic mapping. Though the cost of mapping a person's individual genome has dropped to the point where it might soon be affordable on the consumer market, the usefulness of doing so for athletes hasn't progressed much since the Human Genome Project made its big breakthrough.

Some gene variants related to physical characteristics—like ACTN3 and R577X—have been studied by independent research groups, and inconclusive or contradictory results have been reported. Although there is considerable interest in genetic testing to identify athletic potential, the available knowledge is too limited to justify development and implementation of such a nationwide panel at this point in time. The likelihood of becoming an elite sprinter, for example, is probably influenced by genetic factors, but only a handful of genes have been associated with sprint performance. (One of the most promising candidate genes is ACTN3, which governs the production of a protein that affects fast-twitch muscle fibers.[5])

THE GREAT GENETIC MYTH   5.2.1.2

Once the human genome was sequenced, it became apparent just how big and complex our DNA makeup truly is. The general consensus was, initially, that because we have so many genes, and some are so dominant (like those that control eye color), genes must control everything about us. So a myth quickly grew that still holds sway in many parts of the team-sports performance world: that genetics predetermine sporting fate. However, in the years since the epic Human Genome Project, it has become increasingly clear that we cannot discount the role of the environment when it comes to determining any athlete's potential and that due to our still-limited understanding of genetics, we'd do well not to overestimate the role of heredity.

Consider the above-mentioned warrior gene. While it certainly plays a role in determining the levels of neurotransmitters, these levels are affected by other things as well: they can be altered by exposure to training stresses, nutrition, sleep, and

> *We are survival machines—robot vehicles blindly programmed to preserve the selfish molecules known as genes.*

—Richard Dawkins

performance-enhancing drugs. The warrior gene is just one factor among many that affect behavior in early life.

DNA and Team Chaos   5.2.1.2.1

It's also worth noting that DNA can have a greater or lesser impact on the outcome of a sporting contest based on the number of variables involved. While running one hundred meters is certainly a skill, the task itself is relatively simple and objective: start at the same time as the rest of a group of runners and run to a defined finish line along an even surface over a predetermined distance, without making contact with your opponents and while maintaining a straight course. Since many of the variables are controlled and are the same for each runner, it's easy to see how speed-related genes (such as ACTN3) can have a significant impact on the outcome.

This is not the case for any team sport. Even in sports that involve relatively few players, such as basketball, the number of variables skyrockets when compared to, say, a one-hundred-meter dash. For starters, you have to factor in the relationships: each athlete to his or her teammates, to the ball, and to the opponents trying to stop the athlete from reaching his or her objective. Then there are positional elements relating to the game plan and each athlete's role on the playing surface, plus the fact that for each action the starting and ending points could be almost anywhere within the sideline and end-line boundaries. Once you start to consider variables like an uneven field or pitch, the picture becomes even more complex. This is the same reason analytics and most *Moneyball* concepts have failed to impact dynamic sports like soccer, rugby, and football.

Not only are there far more variables in team sports than in individual disciplines, but a much higher percentage of them are uncontrollable. Technical, tactical, and psychological considerations can't be excluded from running, but they become infinitely more significant in team-sports contests. This is why genetics play a far lesser role in the outcome of a team contest. Simply having the genetic ability to

run faster, jump higher, and last longer is no guarantee—or even a reliable indicator—of success. The most effective Special Forces in the world rely on this as a basic understanding for success. Sadly, some of these lessons were "written with blood."

That being said, we shouldn't completely ignore genetics. My good friend Henk Kraaijenhof made a very important point when he compared our nascent understanding of genetics to what we know about the brain and said that this latter limitation doesn't stop scientists from working on neurology. Kraaijenhof concluded, "I like to work with what we have even if it is a little or not enough." But the second half of his statement was even more telling: "as long as what we have is solid enough for practical application."[6] Remember as well that in elite sports, genetic makeup matters little—the coaches' job is to train the athletes for battle.

Genetic Heritability or
Same Environment?   5.2.1.2.2

Of course, it's impossible to quantify how much genetics really impact on-field performance. Family studies tend to overestimate genetic factors because environment and social structures are also typically shared between family members, making it more challenging to distinguish between genetic and environmental contributions. Twin studies (comparisons of identical and fraternal twins) are often better able to control for environmental effects. In their book *Genetic and Molecular Aspects of Sports Performance,* Claude Buchard and Eric Hoffman cite such research to anchor the suggestion that genetic factors account for 40 to 60 percent of the variation in aerobic performance and cardiac function, 50 to 90 percent of the variation in anaerobic performance, 30 to 70 percent of the variation in muscular fitness, and 20 to 30 percent of the variation in cardiac output.[7] However, there are such a limited number of gene variants related to specific physical traits that, as researchers Lisa Guth and Stephen Roth stated, "these associations are not strong enough to be predictive and the use of genetic testing of these variants in talent selection is premature."[8]

NURTURE AND ENVIRONMENT

5.2.2

While heredity unquestionably plays a part in determining athletes' on-field abilities, too many sports scientists have swung too far in their thinking toward the "nature" side of the nature-nurture continuum. It is becoming increasingly clear that society, community, and family have an enormous influence on athletic development and predisposing certain people to success in sports.

THE MISINTERPRETATION OF ERICSSON

5.2.2.1

If there's one individual from the past fifty years who can easily be singled out as an expert in the study of mastering skills, it's Anders Ericsson. In 1993, this University of Colorado psychology professor published a paper stating that it takes ten thousand hours of practice to master any skill.[9] Others were quick to take note, and a slew of books extrapolating on Ericsson's theory followed, most notably Malcolm Gladwell's *Outliers*. Many of these books misinterpreted his work, however, and because of this Ericsson was motivated to work with writer Robert Pool and correct the mistaken interpretations in his own book, *Peak: Secrets from the New Science of Expertise*.

Yet while *Outliers* makes a solid case for the ten-thousand-hour rule as it applies to expertise in sports, music, and other spheres, the premise is flawed, or at least incomplete. Certainly, greatness is not achieved by accident, and practice is essential in skill development. The mistake is believing that the time input is the *only* environmental factor that affects success. In reality, the quality of the time spent practicing and many other factors are just as important, if not more so, particularly for team-sports athletes.

Exposure to quality coaches who create valuable, applicable learning experiences helps separate great players and teams from good ones. Ten thousand hours spent practicing a skill in a suboptimal or flat-out wrong way would not yield expertise, and nei-

ther would spending all those hours under the tutelage of a novice coach—or even a more experienced one who doesn't get results. Indeed, it'd be better to spend far less time learning in realistic scenarios created by master-level coaches who have proven themselves. Simply racking up robotic practice will not cut it, especially at the elite level.

EPIGENETICS

5.2.2.2

Epigenetics describes biological changes that occur in gene function as a result of exposure to a certain environment—genes are turned on or off based on environmental inputs. These changes are independent of hereditary DNA (i.e., genetics) and instead relate to how the body and brain absorb and are able to act upon survival-relevant "information" from the environment. This supports the notion and theory of the body on every level as one of learning, not simply one of unintelligent biological adaptation. My colleague David Epstein was one of the first popular authors to explore the impact of epigenetics in the context of the ten-thousand-hour rule and other perspectives on athlete development in his book *The Sports Gene*.

While the field of epigenetics is still in its infancy, it's becoming increasingly clear that environment plays a greater role in our continued development than was previously thought. In a team-sports context, this means that each player's family, friendship group, neighborhood, and community contribute not only to his or her emotional and psychological well-being but also to how his or her body withstands and reacts to the stressors of training and competition. The organization can't change how players live but does have the responsibility to educate them on life choices and how these choices can impact their career arc and, on a broader level, their health. This is the thinking behind pro sports initiatives such as the NBA's Rookie Transition Program and the NFL's Rookie Success Program.[10] (Though these initiatives are only partly altruistic. From a business standpoint, it doesn't look good for any league when its players are arrested for drugs, DUIs, or domestic violence.)

THE PLAYER EXPERIENCE 5.2.2.3

The role of epigenetics isn't confined to athletes' upbringing or early development in youth sports—it is a continual factor in their progression in elite sports throughout their career. Athletes, their coaches, and their organizations must be cognizant of the fact that the environment created when preparing for team-sports games impacts not only wins and losses but also the learning, adaptation, and health of the individual and the team as a whole. As such, players must be exposed only to positive and helpfully formative experiences during team preparation.

Player experience is critically important for success, not just for the player but for the team as well. In fact, the success of the team is directly related to the experiences the player is exposed to. These encompass everything from culture to practice.

Traditionally, sports teams have divided players' time into two big blocks: games and training. The focus of the latter has been on improving mainly physical characteristics with specialists, such as strength and conditioning and speed coaches, and dedicated positional or unit coaches, such as a goalkeeping coach in soccer or a backs coach in rugby. The trouble with this old-school approach is that, while sessions with some of the coaching staff and film sessions might pay lip service to tactics, it largely ignores the fact that players are not robots who can simply be exposed to a physical stimulus that they (hopefully) recover from and adapt to. Even the term *training* is misleading. You train animals: they learn to do an action because they're rewarded when they do (or punished when they don't). Players, on the other hand, need to be exposed to *experiences* if we want to elicit instinctual responses during a game.

In reality, every interaction between players and their coaches has a tactical, technical, and psychological coactive, in addition to the physical element. The best coaches create a player experience that affects epigenetics in a manner that elicits a positive consequence or result.

Athletes also progress faster and to a greater degree when they participate in realistic experiences that mirror game-day conditions as closely as possible—as long as they are completely engaged at all times. This is primarily because the experience is incredibly rich and immersive.

THE ECOSYSTEM 5.2.3

No athlete exists in isolation or acts purely with his or her own interests in mind. Rather, athletes (and all people, for that matter) function as part of an ecosystem. Though players have to meet their own basic needs, as long as they feel like a part of their team and are committed to the higher ideals the team is striving toward—both on-field objectives of the game plan and the standards that the head coach has established and the players have committed to—they can be positively impacted by and, in turn, can positively impact group dynamics.

A TRIBE CALLED FAMILY 5.2.3.1

When examining how environment can impact athletes' health and performance, we need to start with the most fundamental tribe: the family unit. Some athletes refer to the team as being like a family, and there's certainly a sense of belonging that comes from striving within a brotherhood or sisterhood toward a championship or other shared goals. But a player's actual family often has an even bigger impact on his or her well-being. (Of course, by "family," I mean whatever the family structure is—the age of the picket fence and 2.4 children is long gone.)

If a player is having problems with a partner or other family member, these issues often manifest themselves at work, where stress reaches extreme levels. External relationship stresses often appear as relationship disruptions in the locker room with teammates or in butting heads with coaches during practice.

Conversely, if an athlete's family environment makes them feel safe, loved, and secure, they're more likely to get along well with members of the team and organization. Another benefit of family stability is that the lack of emotional stress allows players to keep their functional reserve topped up, giving them

> *The coaching team puts a lot of effort into growing us as people, and developing our leadership and decision-making skills. The only way of doing that is by giving us players real power over our own systems and protocols.*
>
> —Richie McCaw

a deeper well to draw from during games and preparation. ("Functional reserve" refers to the remaining capacity of an organism or organ to fulfil its physiological activity; in this context, stress and the energy needed to manage stress and fatigue drain functional reserve.)

TEAM WILDEBEEST   5.2.3.2

Teams competing for titles are driven by tribal instincts and in many ways can be viewed from a primal perspective. Lots of people have studied group behavior in animals and humans, but it's the work of Robert Sapolsky, professor of neurology at Stanford, that best describes how the members of a group sacrifice for a greater good. In one of his case studies, a massive herd of wildebeest was moving across the plains in East Africa and came to a crocodile-infested river. Realizing that it would be suicide to simply plunge headlong into this deadly situation, the wildebeest waited on the bank for a while. After a few minutes, an older animal from the back of the herd was pushed to the front, moved away from the other animals, and threw itself to the crocodiles. As the predators were busy tearing the aged creature apart, the other wildebeest crossed the river unharmed.

Sapolsky contends that the sacrificial lamb (well, wildebeest) in this story was encouraged by the other members of the herd to do what one of them had to do, and that it sacrificed itself because "animals behave in order to maximize the number of copies of genes they leave in the next generation." So to further this end, the older wildebeest was encouraged by those around him to be brave and to distract the crocodiles in the worst possible way.[11]

Now, this is not to say that a team-sports athlete will sacrifice his or her life for the good of the team, but like Sapolsky's wildebeest, teammates can be willing to put the needs of the group above their own. And in certain situations, players can be encouraged to overcome their innate personality and take actions that are out of character to help the team reach its goals.

TEAM CULTURE AND
THE INDIVIDUAL   5.2.3.3

Occasionally, following a team's early exit from the playoffs or an international tournament like the World Cup, we hear tales of dissension among star players, locker room mutiny against the head coach, and all manner of other troubles within the team dynamic off the field that caused them to implode on it. Some teams have widespread personnel issues that lead to more column inches about arrests and other scandals than wins—see, for instance, the Portland "Jail Blazers" team of the early 2000s.

In contrast, some of the best teams are founded on a clear group identity and a strong culture that encourages togetherness and longstanding success. In the NBA, the reserved, businesslike approach of the San Antonio Spurs has led to more than a decade of sixty-plus-win seasons and four titles, and in rugby the strong leadership of coach Clive Woodward and players like Lawrence Dallaglio and Martin Johnson saw England win the Rugby World Cup, rack up twelve successive victories against Southern Hemisphere teams (New Zealand, Australia, and South Africa), and win an improbable forty-one of forty-six games between 2000 and 2003. Woodward was one of the first rugby coaches to apply practical experience from the business world, look to coaches in other sports for best practices, and bring in experts from overseas to give the team a lift.

Clearly, for good or for ill, a team's culture can profoundly impact what happens on the field and in the personal life of each player. That's why it's vital for a coach and the organization to facilitate a culture that values not only wins but also its collective values. Sometimes this means getting rid of talented players who undermine the team's core values, even if there's a short-term cost in the win/loss column. In *The Education of a Coach,* David Halberstam reveals how Bill Belichick did just that, cleaning house at the Patriots and then filling the gaps through informed draft choices and thoughtful trades.

Do not think or let it be suggested that all successful teams are harmonious. Far from it. The great 49ers team led by players like Ronnie Lott, Jerry Rice, Joe Montana, and Keena Turner had a passionate owner in Eddie DeBartolo. He and Bill Walsh had an up-and-down relationship that was often tempestuous, but they shared a unified vision.

THE ORIGIN OF LEGEND

5.3

We get so used to hearing lazy commentary that certain players have reached the top because of natural physical talent that it'd be easy to believe greatness is determined exclusively by nature. But remember, we know from the law of exposure—which states that players and teams consistently exposed to high-performing opponents execute the best under pressure (see page 66)—that nature is only part of the performance equation. The origin stories of some of the most celebrated athletes in team sports history reveal that the environments in which they grew up and learned the game were every bit as important in shaping their excellence as the physical gifts they inherited.

In every one of the following examples, the source of the player's greatness clearly was not DNA alone, and there is little evidence that any of these players had a super combination of genes—in fact, some

5 The Team-Sport Athlete

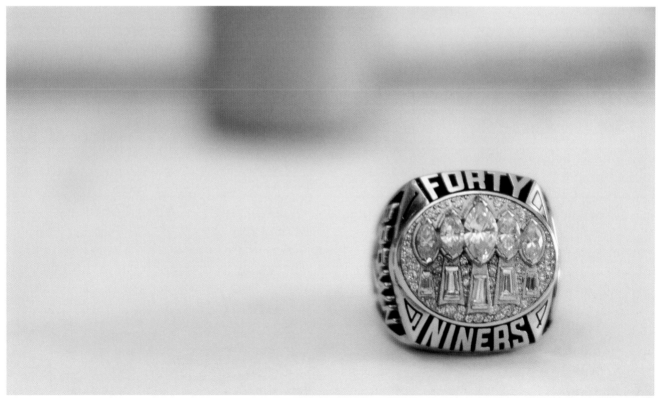

A 49ers Super Bowl ring.

of them were at distinct genetic disadvantages. Environment and terrain played a huge part in every case. Also, each was dominant because their focus on maintaining overall health meant their success was sustainable. Don't be confused by retrospective hype—DNA is a factor, but not the determining one.

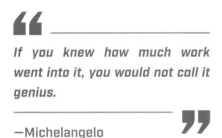

> *If you knew how much work went into it, you would not call it genius.*
>
> —Michelangelo

MICHAEL JORDAN: THE PRODUCT OF COMPETITION

5.3.1

When people talk about the defining factor of Michael Jordan's unparalleled basketball career, they invariably home in on his being cut from his high school varsity team. But the seeds of his competitiveness and will to win were sown far earlier, in his daily battles on his backyard court with his older brother, Larry. Though Michael would come to tower over his five-foot-eight-inch brother, the elder Jordan was a fierce competitor and a fine athlete in his own right. He wouldn't give Michael anything on the court—the younger sibling had to fight and scrap for every point and rebound. In his Hall of Fame induction speech, Michael said that Larry and another older brother, James, "gave me all I could ever ask for as a brother in terms of competition. My brother Larry is an ideal situation where small things come in small packages; this dude fought me every single day."[12]

The man who'd go on to win six NBA titles, six Finals MVP awards, and ten NBA scoring titles later said that he chose the jersey number 23 because he hoped to one day be even half the player that his brother, who wore 45, was.[13] Michael briefly wore Larry's number when he came out of retirement the first time.

Perhaps the greatest basketball player ever focused on overcoming his brother in a similar way to how he later used slights—real and imagined—from opponents to psych himself up before big games. Jordan also attributed his fierce work ethic to his father, who, when he wasn't working as a factory supervisor at General Electric, was usually toiling on projects around the house or working on one of the family's cars in the driveway.[14]

Another mentor was the brilliant University of North Carolina coach Dean Smith, who made an exception to his rule of never starting freshmen when Jordan arrived in Chapel Hill. Unlike the current crop of "one-and-done" players who rush into the NBA after a single college season and often fail to live up to their hype, Jordan spent three years learning from Smith. Beyond the experience of hitting the winning shot for North Carolina in the 1982 NCAA Championship game or winning the John C. Wooden Award and Naismith College Player of the Year award in 1984, Jordan said the most important part of his time at North Carolina was learning from Smith.

TOM BRADY: THE POWER OF HUNGER

5.3.2

When evaluating Tom Brady before picking him in the sixth round of the 2000 NFL draft, Bill Belichick recognized that while the young quarterback might not have the cannonlike arm that most scouts and coaches wanted, he had performed admirably as the key player for one of the most prestigious football programs in the country, playing consistently well in front of a very demanding fan base in a big stadium at Michigan. As David Halberstam put it in *The*

> *If you push me towards something that you think is a weakness, then I will turn that perceived weakness into a strength.*
>
> —Michael Jordan

> *I think that Tom is the type of player that, rather than seeing one thing in his game jump from here to here, you would see ten different things in his game improve incrementally. Then that combination of all of them gives you a little bit better performance in each of those areas.*

—Bill Belichick

Education of a Coach, "Here was a young man who had been caught in an extremely difficult situation, knowing he had a job he could easily lose, and yet he handled the situation with savvy and maturity that went well beyond his years; he had not cracked under pressure, but rather rose to meet the occasion."[15]

The University of Michigan furnace would have burned some players into ash, but it forged Brady and gave him the kind of resilience and mental toughness that he would need to make the cut as an NFL backup. Tom himself would admit that he was only beginning his journey to dominance as he left the Big House. The man selected 199th in the draft was not seen as a future legend by many outside of his own family and circle. But once Drew Bledsoe's injury created an opportunity for Brady to prove himself at the highest level, he showed that he deserved the starter's job and, eventually, regular-season and Super Bowl MVP awards. It's interesting now to look back at Belichick's draft-day assessment of Brady: "He's a good, tough, competitive, smart quarterback that is a good value and how he does and what he'll be able to do, we'll just put him out there with everybody else and let him compete and see what happens."[16]

> *I wasn't naturally gifted in terms of size and speed; everything I did in hockey I worked for.*

—Wayne Gretzky

WAYNE GRETZKY: ALL ODDS STACKED AGAINST HIM   5.3.3

When Wayne Gretzky was learning to play ice hockey, his father, Walter, passed along one of his fundamental principles, which has gone on to become one of the most widely known quotes in all of team sports: "Skate to where the puck is going, not where it has been." Long before Walter's saying became famous, it inspired his son to anticipate what's next, a skill he put to good use in evading opponents who were bigger and stronger. On his way to becoming the most celebrated hockey player in history, the saying that became Gretzky's mantra reminded him constantly of the need to be mentally one step ahead of defenders. This was necessary because, unlike some of his peers growing up and, to a greater degree, the opponents he faced in the pro ranks, Gretzky was diminutive in stature and lacked the raw power that many players harnessed to make their mark on the ice.

Words were not the only way Walter helped his son hone his game. After teaching him to skate on a frozen river near their home in Ontario, he spent thousands of hours putting Wayne through every drill imaginable, so that when his son took the ice for a game, he'd be mentally ready to outmaneuver opponents who could outmuscle him. "When I was five and playing against 11-year-olds, who were bigger, stronger, faster, I just had to figure out a way to play with them," Gretzky said. "When I was 14, I played against 20-year-olds, and when I was 17, I played with men. Basically, I had to play the same style all the way through. I couldn't beat people with my strength; I don't have a hard shot; I'm not the quickest skater in the league. My eyes and my mind have to do most of the work."[17]

LIONEL MESSI: GENETICALLY DISADVANTAGED   5.3.4

Another all-time great who was undersized and out-matched in strength by almost every player assigned to mark him is Lionel Messi. Growing up, Messi was so small that even with growth hormone injections he grew to be only five feet seven inches and 148 pounds. Yet what he lacked in height and bulk, the young man made up for in technical and tactical ability. One of the main reasons for this is that he started his tutelage at Barcelona's famed La Masia youth academy when he was just thirteen years old.

The school's technical director explained how this unassuming, traditional Catalan farmhouse prepares children to follow in the footsteps of their first team idols: "If you want to play the way Barcelona do, you cannot achieve it with lots of big, athletic players. You need small, technical ones, though with some balance in the side. You have to identify the profile of player you need and, from the very start, teach the players everything about that system. It is about creating one philosophy, one mentality, from the bottom of the club to the top."[18]

Messi became the second youngest player to play for Barcelona's first eleven when he took the field against Espanyol as a precocious, floppy-haired seventeen-year-old. Despite his youth, after four years at La Masia "Leo" was more than ready to handle the pressure of wearing the number 10 shirt for his club and, soon enough, his country. Though many regard him as the best soccer player ever to kick a ball, Lionel might not even end up being the best player in his own family. His three-year-old son, Thiago, has already enrolled at the elementary school Barcelona runs, FCBEscola, which is just down the street from La Masia.[19]

RICHIE MCCAW: NARTURE OR NURTURE   5.3.5

As an almost painfully shy farmer's son from New Zealand's rural Hakataramea Valley, Richie McCaw was an excellent student and a hard worker but, in a nation of physical specimens who live and breathe rugby, seemed unlikely to rise to the pinnacle of the sport as he had neither the height nor bulk of many of his contemporaries. Still, his uncle Bigsy saw the strength of character that he believed could help McCaw push past his physical limitations. During a conversation when his nephew was eighteen, Bigsy urged McCaw to outline his goals for the next few years. As the young man vocalized his goals one by one, his uncle wrote them all down on a napkin. McCaw's final goal was to represent the All Blacks in 2004. "You don't just want to be an All Black, you want to be a *great* All Black," Bigsy said. He passed the napkin across the table and gave McCaw the pen. "Sign it 'great All Black,'" he urged. Reluctantly, McCaw did.[20]

Seeing Messi play is like watching a video game. What Messi does on a football field is simply unthinkable. The way he walks from side to side, and once he sees an opportunity, he simply creates magic.

—Victoria Azarenka

> *I think he's probably been the most influential rugby player of all time.*
>
> —Graham Henry

Though signing in such a way ran contrary to his self-deprecating nature, McCaw kept that list of goals to motivate himself as he moved up through the ranks at one of New Zealand's most decorated clubs, Canterbury, and eventually into the national team setup. And quite a mind it is, according to a former professor of McCaw's, who told *The Telegraph* that before he became an international star, the young man wasn't just an "A student—he was an A-plus student."[21] As Gretzky did on the ice, McCaw put his smarts into action on the pitch. He ended up winning his first All Black cap in 2001, three years earlier than he'd hoped. Three years later, he became the captain of his club and his country.

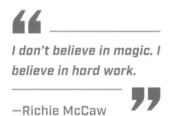

> *I don't believe in magic. I believe in hard work.*
>
> —Richie McCaw

The key lessons McCaw learned at Canterbury concerned not physical prowess but leadership. In his autobiography, *The Real McCaw,* he recalled trailing 29–12 in a cup final against Wellington. Todd Blackadder, who was captaining the side that day, told McCaw and his teammates, "Don't for a minute believe that we're not going to win this." Looking at the scoreboard and the game clock, which showed just fifteen minutes until full time, McCaw had his doubts. Yet Canterbury rallied and won. "That was a big lesson," McCaw wrote. "You've got to believe that it's not over."[22] He would use such a belief to rally his Canterbury and New Zealand teammates time and again.

Humility is another part of what made McCaw so beloved in the locker room. He retired as one of the most decorated players in All Blacks history, having captained his country to two Rugby World Cup trophies and earned 148 caps. Many players would have the number 7 shirt that McCaw wore in New Zealand's 2015 World Cup final win over Australia in a display case for all to see, but while he values the team's colors as much as anyone, McCaw said he isn't sure where the jersey is and that it's "probably in a bag or a cupboard." This is a man who also turned down a knighthood. When asked how he felt about watching New Zealand win its first test match without him, McCaw didn't talk about the glory days but said, "Every opportunity they got, they nailed. That's the great thing about the ABs [All Blacks]. It doesn't matter who you are, the team just moves on."[23]

THE UNDERVALUED ROLE OF HEROES AND ASPIRATION

5.3.6

When we envision sports players, we automatically resort to a form of stereotyping: New Zealand rugby players, Brazilian or Argentinian soccer players, Russian or Canadian ice hockey players. This becomes a somewhat cyclical and self-fulfilling prophecy, especially during lean periods when an organization is enjoying little success.

In his book *The Gold Mine Effect,* Rasmus Ankersen offers an interesting perspective on cultural and social influence on sports. He asks: Why are 137 of the world's 500 best female golfers from South Korea? Why and how does a single track-and-field club in an impoverished part of the world like Kingston, Jamaica, produce most of the world's best sprinters? Why do so many of the world's best middle-distance runners grow up in the same region of Ethiopia? Why do so many of the best soccer players come from Brazil?

> *You inherit your environment just as much as your genes.*

—Johnny Rich

While DNA may be a factor and social economics seem to facilitate development because of more available practice time, role models and aspiration seem to be undervalued as key motivating factors. For example, in Jamaica, Usain Bolt is just the latest in a long line of sprint champions to inspire the next generation, and the high school track-and-field championship is one of the nation's biggest sporting events. In rugby-mad New Zealand, the All Blacks are revered to a degree far beyond any other sports team. Basketball players like John Wall who've made it out of America's crime-ridden inner cities not only give kids in similar areas heroes to emulate on the playgrounds but also the hope of escaping gangs and poverty.

HEALTH

5.4

If there is one central point underpinning sustainable success, it's that athlete health is the most important factor in achieving maximal and sustained performance, for both the individual and the team. Personally, I've never cared for coaches or players saying that their goal is to "win a title." Self-propelling success should be the true goal. We're not concentrating on one win or a single successful season. We're interested in dominating and winning *multiple* championships. And for that, health is essential.

One of the main goals of the four-coactive model is to enable players and their teams to continue making small improvements every day and, ultimately, for such advances to result in more wins. For this to be possible, the overall health of the athlete must be maintained at all times. Just playing better on Saturday, Sunday, or whenever game day falls is not enough. Those contesting the game must also come out unharmed and enjoy a healthy, balanced life.

Physical health is a key factor in its own right—players need to be physically fit to play their best—but it's also generally a precursor to a biochemical and neurochemical balance that leads to a stable mindset. An athlete who leads an imbalanced, unhealthy life might be able to cheat psychophysiology for a time and keep playing at a high level, but after a while, the cracks will widen into a canyon into which the athlete will fall. While it is the responsibility of the athlete to take care of him- or herself, the coaching staff, the medical team, and other members of the organization also have a moral and ethical duty to look after their players. The first step is understanding exactly what we mean when we talk about athlete health.

AN ATHLETE'S DEFINITION OF HEALTH
5.4.1

A major error in coaching is that health is seen as black and white: a player is healthy or unhealthy. This is wrong, as every person's health is on a continuum. The World Health Organization (WHO) states, "Health is a state of complete physical, mental and social well-being and not merely the absence of disease or infirmity."[24] But when it comes to athletes in team sports, the WHO definition typically goes out the window.

Many teams consider their players to be "unhealthy" only if they're sick or injured—though they can even disregard minor illnesses or physical problems if the athlete can push through them and suit up on game day. My contention is that teams can no longer look at player health as simple "sick / not sick," "injured / not injured," and "can't play / can play" binary oppositions. Instead, they owe it to athletes to start thinking about their health holistically and with a broader perspective, rather than just worrying about how many games or practices an individual is going to miss. The corollary is also true: in other words, 99 percent healthy is not 100 percent injured. This mindset is critical for reducing injury and speeding rehabilitation.

THE HOLISTIC ATHLETE MODEL

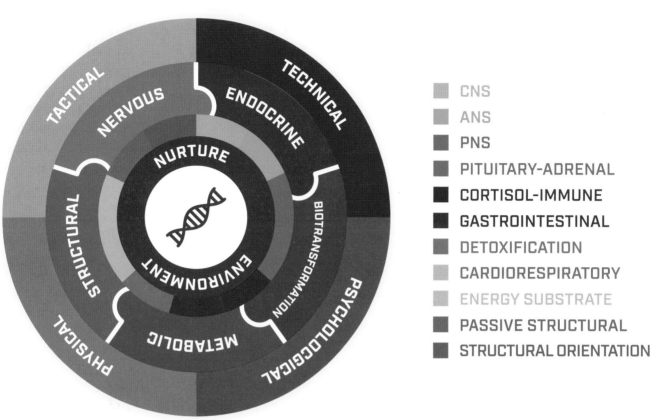

CNS
ANS
PNS
PITUITARY-ADRENAL
CORTISOL-IMMUNE
GASTROINTESTINAL
DETOXIFICATION
CARDIORESPIRATORY
ENERGY SUBSTRATE
PASSIVE STRUCTURAL
STRUCTURAL ORIENTATION

Players, too, need to adopt this mindset. The silo method of trying to keep elements of performance and recovery separate that is encouraged by various departments often transfers to players, who fail to recognize that they are never truly 100 percent healthy. But the players who display the best resilience are those who understand that health is a continuum.

HOW HEALTH UNDERPINS THE FOUR-COACTIVE MODEL   5.4.2

Each element of the four-coactive model—technical, tactical, physical, and psychological—is always present in every game moment and every preparatory learning experience. By viewing the four-coactive model as a whole and managing each component responsibly in each morphocycle, a team and its coaching staff can expose their players to enough stimuli to prompt learning and ensure that athletes have enough time to process what they've learned cognitively and emotionally while also recovering

physically. In this way, the four-coactive model is geared toward continued development of the whole person and respects the overall health of each player. Respecting the fact that volume, intensity, density, and collision/contact stress different body systems to varying degrees and dictate certain recovery durations, the morphocycle approach enables us to introduce sufficient stress to prompt player learning and development without overloading the team physically or cognitively. Instead of delivering immediate benefits, the morphocycle delivers consistent, incremental and continual improvement.

HEALTH AS A LIMITING FACTOR   5.4.3

When evaluating the factors that are either advantages or disadvantages for a player on the field, we shouldn't just use the four-coactive lens. It could be that an athlete has reached the technical, tactical, physical, and psychological minimums to succeed in his or her position and at the required level of play. If the athlete is failing to progress, then it's likely that an element of his or her health is the primary limiting factor. This could be inadequate recovery, substance abuse, a poor diet, or any number of other things. It's important to be aware that the morphological programming approach—which involves balancing volume, intensity, density, and collision/contact to produce continual improvement of the team—will have limited success with an athlete who has a persistent health issue.

FUNCTIONAL RESERVES AND PERFORMANCE   5.4.4

We need to recognize that each bodily system—from the nervous to endocrine to musculoskeletal systems—has a limited capacity for reacting to and recovering from stress that results from lifestyle factors, playing the game, and preparing for competition. In the big picture of athlete health, it's crucial that we also acknowledge that the body has an overall functional reserve that cannot be completely drained if the athlete's well-being is to be preserved. This means that we have only a limited well to draw on when we encounter stressors in any part of our lives, whether they are physical, cognitive, or emotional.

Changing circumstances impact how the body allocates parts of this functional reserve. When you have the flu, for instance, a huge percentage of your overall capacity is dedicated to combating the virus. If you can take your time and recover, your body will typically bounce back in a week or so. But say you're an athlete who has the flu and decides to play in a crucial playoff game. Now you've introduced another stressor that might exceed the total stress load your body is capable of handling. It's now more likely that you'll get injured or your flu gets worse after the game, and you'll have to battle it for two or three weeks instead of the one week it would have taken to recover if you'd rested.

Or perhaps your team has traveled to Europe to play a series of exhibition games and you're exhausted. You go out for a run with a teammate one morning and step off a curb awkwardly. Normally, you'd be well rested enough for your proprioception—your sense of your body's positioning and movement—to give proper feedback about where your foot is in rela-

tion to the pavement. This time, however, fatigue has drained your functional reserve so much that your foot lands awkwardly and you sprain your ankle.

Both examples show that we can't look at performance output in isolation and that players and coaches alike should continually assess their overall functional reserve and identify events and situations that put inordinate stress on one or more systems. They can then scale back the training load as necessary. This will improve the overall health of the player and preempt issues like illness, injury, and burnout.

PSYCHOPHYSIOLOGICAL HEALTH   5.4.5

At the elite level, some teams use sports psychiatrists like Dr. Steve Peters, author of *The Chimp Paradox*, as resources much more than they did a few years ago. Yet if you look at the personnel list for the average team, the ratio of body specialists to mind specialists is at least twenty-five to one. This illustrates that no matter what evidence exists to the contrary, in the world of team sports, we're still convinced that the body alone holds the key to athletic performance.

Not so when it comes to the well-being of our players. The body doesn't operate in isolation but sends signals to and receives instructions from the brain. Beyond this, athletes' psychological, emotional, and spiritual health are key in determining not just the success of their athletic careers but also the quality of life they enjoy during and after their playing days.

As neuropathologist Dr. Bennet Omalu has demonstrated, damage to the body has devastating consequences for the mind as well. Omalu found that the brains of former football players showed evidence of a degenerative disease, chronic traumatic encephalopathy (CTE), that is caused by repeated physical impact—the concussions these football players sustained led to a buildup of proteins in the brain and, over time, progressive degeneration of the brain. The symptoms of CTE include not just physical problems, such as headaches and dizziness, but also behavioral ones: memory loss, poor judgment, erratic behavior, and more. This is yet another example of how we cannot separate psychology and physiology any longer. When it comes to the health of athletes, we must see the body and brain as one. As Socrates puts it, "There is no illness of the body except for the mind."

That said, the most important psychologist is always the "head coach," simply because the coach directs the overall vision, culture, and mood of the team. However, if the coach encounters player issues that are significant, the player needs to be directed to a psychologist or psychiatrist as soon as these issues manifest themselves in the team environment.

HEALTH AND LONGEVITY 5.4.6

When seen through the lens of athlete health, the length of a player's career and the player's longevity after retiring are inseparable. The same habits that a team-sports athlete cultivates to squeeze out every ounce of performance potential while remaining healthy—like getting adequate recovery, dialing in nutrition, and managing stress—also form the core of a long and sustainable life. The athlete might make one-off compromises for success, like trying to play through illness or injury in a cup, playoff, or championship game, but it's the role of the team's coaches and medical staff to weigh such self-sacrifice against the long-term welfare of the players for whom they are responsible. It can be difficult to take the long view when a championship is on the line, but athletes are people whose worth totals far more than what they achieve on the field. The organization has a duty to protect its players so they can enjoy a long, healthy life.

SUSTAINABLE SUCCESS 5.4.7

"The Game" looks at what it takes to better understand how team sports are played so that continual improvement can be obtained. The second component to building a team that is sustainably successful is ensuring the health of each and every player. It's no good to have a couple of überhealthy individuals if the rest of the team falls short in overall wellness. The cracks will start to appear very early in the season and will only lengthen and widen as time goes on. For any team-sports organization to survive and thrive through the rigors of a full fixture list—the travel, the performance highs and lows, the media scrutiny, and so on—there must be total buy-in to the concept of athlete health trumping everything else.

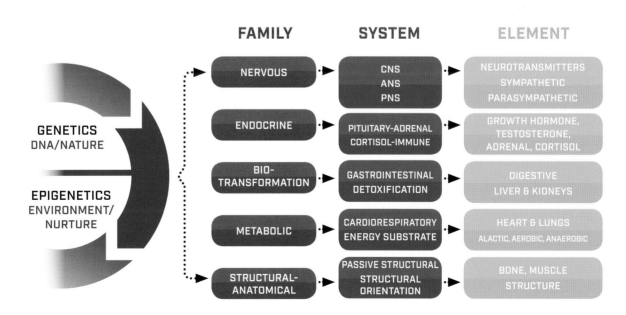

The families, systems, and elements of health.

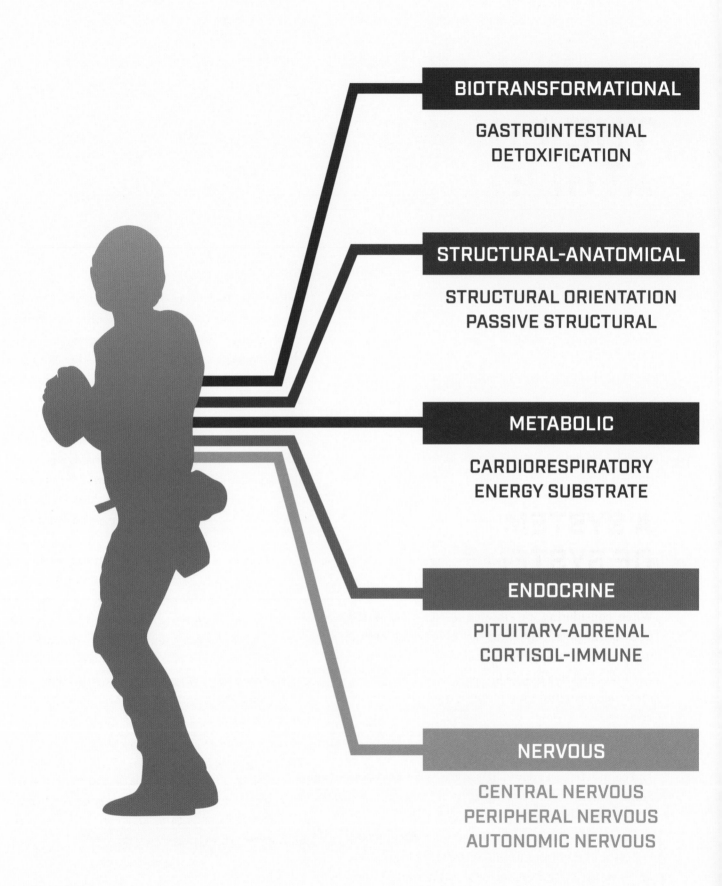

BIOTRANSFORMATIONAL

GASTROINTESTINAL
DETOXIFICATION

STRUCTURAL-ANATOMICAL

STRUCTURAL ORIENTATION
PASSIVE STRUCTURAL

METABOLIC

CARDIORESPIRATORY
ENERGY SUBSTRATE

ENDOCRINE

PITUITARY-ADRENAL
CORTISOL-IMMUNE

NERVOUS

CENTRAL NERVOUS
PERIPHERAL NERVOUS
AUTONOMIC NERVOUS

A system of systems.

SIX

THE HUMAN ATHLETE

The performance of any player is based on the fundamental functioning of the human body and ultimately its health. In order to understand this, we need a model of the athlete's health that allows us to comprehend fundamental performance interactions and how bodily systems function together. Understand that this is not a theoretical, medical, scientific, or physiological model—it's a working performance model. I have used this approach to help simplify the human body for improving performance.

A SYSTEM OF SYSTEMS

6.1

When considering an athlete's health reserve and how it will positively or negatively impact performance, I use a five-system model to profile the player. The main systems in this model are the biotransformational, structural-anatomical, metabolic, endocrine, and nervous macro systems. (We'll examine each macro system in more detail later in this section.) These systems are fundamentally intertwined and cannot be considered in isolation when thinking about athlete health.

Each of these five systems reacts and adapts to stress at different rates. Depending on the morphological programming profile of the training session or game, the systems recover at various speeds, and

without adequate recovery there can be no positive adaptation. Even subsystems of the same system can recover at different rates. For example, the two biotransformational micro systems—digestion and detoxification—take different amounts of time to recharge and adapt following exposure to the stresses of training, competition, and life.

When we come under stress, all of the systems kick into action, although they are engaged at varying speeds and to different degrees and require varying amounts of recovery time. To both maximize and sustain performance, athletes must protect all five systems as much as possible.

In elite sports, for far too long we've overemphasized the physical component of the four-coactive model, spending most of our time concentrating on the impact of training and competition on muscles, ligaments, and tendons—the anatomical structures we mistakenly believe are the main factors that determine performance. The energy systems have gotten plenty of headlines, too, and in recent years we've started paying a bit more attention to mobility, what we eat, and how long we sleep. But by and large, outside of specialties such as physical therapy, nutritional science, and strength and conditioning, we've largely neglected the impact that preparation and game-day competition have on the other three main systems and health, to great cost.

Another shortcoming has been the failure to consider how players' lifestyles affect not only their athletic performance but also the fundamental health that underpins it. Sure, a team might try to get players to track their sleep or follow a certain meal plan, but this random, fragmented, à la carte approach has done little to improve athlete health or even educate athletes on how the choices they make in the eighteen, twenty, or twenty-two hours spent away from the team have a profound impact on their bodies.

HOW WE FUNCTION

6.2

We must protect the five macro systems by making good choices when it comes to lifestyle, stress, recovery, and nutrition. The environment needs to be as low-stress as possible so that athletes are not experiencing additional stress on top of the imposed stressors from training and competition, which they're already having to deal with and adapt to. Athletes need to drink enough fluids and eat the right foods to encourage such adaptations and help their bodies repair themselves before the next training session or game. Recovery practices must be sufficient to allow the body to return to equilibrium from the elevated fight-or-flight state, which is dominant during team and individual learning experiences and competition. Athletes must also minimize the number of toxins in their bodies by avoiding drugs and nicotine, limiting alcohol consumption, and reducing exposure to toxic foods and food additives (including pesticides and antibiotics in nonorganic meat and dairy products).

The healthier each of the body's systems is, the more resilient the athlete will be and the better able to handle environmental pressures and the stress of the technical, tactical, physical, and psychological elements of team preparation and games.

To clearly observe the functioning organism, I look at the following five macro systems:

1. biotransformational
2. structural-anatomical
3. metabolic
4. endocrine
5. nervous

THE BIO-TRANSFORMATIONAL MACRO SYSTEM

6.3

This system manages the energy that we take in and how it's broken down and distributed. The biotransformational system is the one that's arguably compromised most when an athlete's body is experiencing more stress than it can cope with while remaining healthy. This system allows itself to be superseded by other systems to allow the body to handle the immediate threat.

This is one of the most overlooked and underestimated bodily systems, yet it's arguably one of the most important. Only in the past couple of years have researchers started to realize how crucial biotransformation mechanisms are to overall health, and how the microbiome—the collective term for the one hundred trillion microbes that live in the gut, skin, and mouth—contribute to hormone regulation, energy availability, immune system function, and much more.

A chameleon changes color, but never forgets it is a chameleon.

—Vítor Frade

The biotransformational system includes two micro systems, one of which has its own sub-system:

- *Gastrointestinal micro system:* Breaks down, processes, absorbs, and assimilates food.

  - *Enteric nervous system:* This web of neurons in the lining of the gastrointestinal tract controls the intestinal tract and secretes neurotransmitters and hormones.

- *Detoxification micro system:* Excretes toxins and waste. The liver and kidneys are often thought of as the primary detoxing organs, but the skin can also get rid of certain substances and by-products.

THE GASTROINTESTINAL SYSTEM: GETTING TO GRIPS WITH YOUR GUT   6.3.1

This system governs many processes, but for our purposes, its main function is regulating the body's digestion of food and absorption of nutrients and making the resulting energy readily available for activity and recovery. It is a gateway between the external and internal environments and is the mechanism by which the body distinguishes between beneficial nutrients and harmful substances. When this system malfunctions, it can result in indigestion, which can manifest itself in symptoms like diarrhea, gas, and bloating, or more serious conditions, such as celiac disease, Crohn's disease, and acid reflux disease. Any athlete who has had any of these issues can confirm the debilitating psychosomatic impact any kind of performance stress has. These systemic disorders also have been linked to immunodeficiency issues, allergies, and many other complex intrasystem conditions. Over the past fifteen years I've seen many athletes and even more military personnel with gastrointestinal issues and intolerances. Many of these have developed after changes in diet and medication.

GASTRIC ACIDS, ENZYMES, AND NUTRIENT ABSORPTION   6.3.1.1

The body breaks down foods using various enzymes, acids, and proteins. As soon as you smell or see food or drinks, your body kick-starts the gastrointestinal system to increase these substances and get it ready to process what you're about to consume. In the most obvious example, your mouth starts to water as you produce more saliva to start breaking down food. In fact, up to 6 percent of carbohydrate digestion happens in the mouth via oral digestive enzymes. That's why it's important to maintain even the most basic habits, such as chewing food thoroughly rather than wolfing down each meal or snack. Remember, the stomach has no teeth. Hydration is also essential to encourage efficient digestion and nutrient transport.

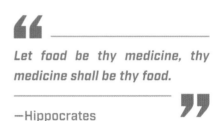

> Let food be thy medicine, thy medicine shall be thy food.
>
> —Hippocrates

Once food makes it to the stomach, other acids, enzymes, and proteins start doing the heavy lifting. Gastric acid is a crucial component of the gastrointestinal system, and when levels are too low, it inhibits digestion and the body's capability to kill harmful microbes and toxins in our food. A normal acidic stomach environment is also very important for breaking down proteins into smaller, more usable chunks. As long as your gastric acid level is in the normal range, proteins are converted into peptides. Pancreatic enzymes then further break down the peptides so that they can be employed in repairing muscle tissue, creating new skin and hair, and many other restorative processes.

Fat absorption is also managed by the gastrointestinal system. Bile, which is produced by the liver and stored in the gallbladder, acts as an emulsifying agent and divides fatty acids into smaller molecules so that they're available for the aerobic energy system, thermic regulation, fat-soluble vitamin assimilation, and dozens of other purposes.

The stomach lining must have sufficient integrity to not only contain corrosive acid but also maintain the health of the cells that release the acid and digestive enzymes. Similarly, should the lining of the small intestine become damaged by a poor diet and other factors, digestion and absorption can be compromised and the athlete can begin suffering from conditions like leaky gut syndrome or IBS.

Gastrointestinal disruption interferes with the absorption of macronutrients—protein, fat, and carbohydrates—and also hampers the body's ability to process micronutrients—vitamins and minerals. An athlete may be taking in enough vitamins and minerals through diet and supplements, but if his or her digestive system is compromised, these nutrients might not be absorbed. Deficiencies can affect hundreds of body processes and leave athletes feeling like they get fatigued quickly and fail to recover properly from training or games. As the body treats the rigors of competition as a stressor, it uses certain vitamins and minerals, such as magnesium, at a much faster rate. So if the digestive system is not making such micronutrients readily available, it inhibits the player's ability to perform as well as deal with the added demands that an active body faces.

> *Digestion, of all the bodily functions, is the one which exercises the greatest influence on the mental state of an individual.*
>
> —Jean-Anthelme Brillat-Savarin

THE ENTERIC NERVOUS SYSTEM: THE "SECOND BRAIN"   6.3.1.2

When we look at the gut through the lens of athlete health, we can't consider it as an isolated entity. The fast-developing field of neurogastroenterology is finding more and more evidence that the gut and the brain are closely related and that the gut is truly a "second brain." The enteric nervous system is a web of around one hundred million neurons located in the lining of the gastrointestinal tract, some of which are responsible for sending signals to the brain from the vagus nerve and regulating the body moving from a fight-flight-freeze state of high arousal into a recovery state. The enteric nervous system operates independently of the brain and spinal cord and controls the motility of the intestinal tract, receives input about its contents and status, and secretes a wide array of neurotransmitters and hormones.

These neurotransmitters and hormones help manage everything from emotional regulation to sleep to muscle repair and growth—in fact, the enteric nervous system produces 80 percent of the feel-good neurotransmitter serotonin.[25] They also help govern stress responses and adaptations, which is why dysfunction in the gastrointestinal system can reduce a warrior-athlete's ability to cope with the rigors of training and battle/competition.

This system also plays a notable role in managing digestion, as it controls the secretion of digestive enzymes. The close relationship between stress, emotions, and conditions such as irritable bowel syndrome is due to the fact that the hormones that govern emotions and stress responses are controlled by the enteric nervous system. Indeed, the term *gut feeling* is more closely related to our actual gut than we've typically acknowledged.

THE DETOXIFICATION SYSTEM

Identifying and removing toxins is the job of another neurogastroenterological system, the detoxification system. It involves the liver and gut from the digestive system but also requires other parts of the body, including the kidneys and the largest organ, the skin. Athletes obviously have a need to detoxify due to the increasing prevalence of manmade toxins and pollutants, the stresses of the hectic and arrhythmic world we live in, which produce an excess of certain chemicals while reducing the level of others, and the ever-higher expectations and stress loads that players are subjected to.

The detoxification system has to also mitigate contaminants and chemicals present in what eat and drink. Some estimate that we process sixty tons of food over our lifetime, and this means that over the span of their careers, athletes—unless they are consuming only organic foods and beverages—are dealing with the bioaccumulation of heavy metals, pesticides, fertilizers, and other contaminants that are rife in our food chain.

Biotransformation is the first stage of detoxification and is predicated on enzymes in the liver breaking down toxins. These enzymes draw in more water to make the toxins more hydrophilic—that is, dissolvable—and oxidize them or subject them to hydrolysis. If the toxins can't be excreted, the liver goes to Plan B, employing transferase enzymes to bind with the substances and help flush them out. If the body still can't get rid of the toxins, the liver releases drug transporters to try to force removal. Sweating can also purge toxins through the skin. Saunas, hot springs, and other forms of hydrotherapy have been used since Roman times to purge the body of heavy metals.

THE SYMPATHETIC SYSTEM: FUEL ON DEMAND

The autonomic nervous system—which we'll discuss in more detail on page 179—is divided into two branches: the sympathetic and the parasympathetic nervous systems. One of the key differences between the two is the speed at which they relay information to and from the brain. Designed for use in stressful and dangerous situations, the sympathetic nervous system sends and receives information incredibly quickly, as if you dial an emergency operator and a fire truck, ambulance, and police car arrive immediately. As a result, it can signal the digestive system to quickly make fuel—primarily carbohydrates—available in order to power rapid and decisive movement.

The elimination of feces and urine is another crucial component of detoxification. One-third of solid stools are toxins, one-third are gut flora bacteria, and the final third is indigestible plant fiber. This is why it's crucial for athletes to get sufficient fruit and vegetables in their diets—the fiber in these plant foods helps the body expel toxins. Excretion of urine and feces is very dehydrating, and the more we eat and get rid of, the more body water levels need topping up.

TO DETOX OR NOT TO DETOX   6.3.2.1

As with every other system in the body, we can either encourage or hinder our ability to detoxify. Ingesting too many toxins or living in an overly toxic environment will not only overload this system but also limit the function of other, interrelated systems.

Four biological factors impact detoxification:

- *Age:* Small children and older people have less ability to process and excrete toxins. This is why we must take extra care to ensure young athletes' exposure to environmental chemicals is limited.

- *Gender + age:* Women have thirty to forty times more detoxification enzymes before menopause than they do after, so older/master female athletes should try to limit their toxin exposure.

- *Genetics:* Hereditary factors can improve or limit an individual's ability to detoxify.

- *Nature of toxin/stress and extent of exposure:* The severity and duration of toxin and stress exposure are arguably the biggest factors in determining how well the body can rebound through detoxification.

The body is in a constant battle to maintain a healthy functioning system, and detoxification is not a retreat but a health system. Athletes can do six things to support optimal detoxification:

- Maintain a diet naturally rich in antioxidants and ensure that as many foods as possible are organic. Cruciferous vegetables and some fruits can aid detoxification, while too much saturated fat can undermine the process. Curcumin, turmeric, parsley, fennel, garlic, and onions can also boost function. Cooking certain oils, vegetables, and fruits at high temperatures can impact the enzymatic and antioxidant content, so it should be avoided when possible.

- Ensure hydration levels are adequate before, during, and after competition and practice.

- Avoid tobacco completely and limit intake of caffeinated and alcoholic beverages.

- Keep body weight stable and prevent sudden loss of weight and/or muscle mass, which releases more toxins into the body.

- Make sure bathroom breaks are regular and that diarrhea and constipation don't become an issue.

- Avoid a low-protein diet, which can lower detoxification capacity.

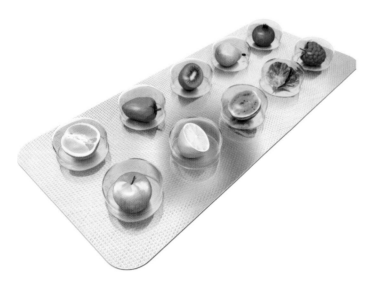

> *Foolish the doctor who despises the knowledge acquired by the ancients.*
>
> —Hippocrates

Make your food your medicine.

THE DANGERS OF TOXINS 6.3.2.2

Toxins in the body can reduce the effectiveness of nutrient breakdown by disrupting the gastrointestinal system. Some chemicals also compromise the body's ability to metabolize glucose and inhibit the absorption of micronutrients. For example, heavy metals such as lead can limit the availability of B vitamins and calcium. Cadmium can interfere with copper levels in the bloodstream. Too much fluoride can act as a poison and affect the body at the cellular level.

Nonsteroidal anti-inflammatory drugs (NSAIDs) can disrupt liver function by reducing the secretion of enzymes that play a crucial part in detoxification. Toxins in plastics can also limit the ability of DNA to repair itself. Liver enzymes can be inhibited by iron deficiency, heavy metals, antidepressants, and antifungal medications. Too much caffeine or alcohol can also adversely affect the detoxification system.

Tests that show elevated blood urea nitrogen and/or bilirubin can indicate a detoxification system that's overworked. Blood testing can also be used to show high levels of heavy metals or solvents. However, tests can be inconclusive, as toxins quickly move from the blood into bodily tissues. For example, the half-life of mercury in the blood is just three days, whereas in soft tissues it's sixty-nine days. Some off-the-shelf substances, such as charcoal, can help with removal of these, but medical chelation therapies are more effective.

THE HEALTH OF THE BIOTRANSFORMATIONAL SYSTEM 6.3.3

In this section, we'll look at how athletes must optimize their nutrition, deal with allergens, and ensure they're not overconsuming medication in order to preserve the health of their biotransformational system.

NUTRITIONAL PRINCIPLES TO SUPPORT DETOXIFICATION AND DIGESTION 6.3.3.1

* *Natural, whole foods* contain vitamins, minerals, and enzymes that are in their purest state and have not been compromised, so the body can extract the greatest amount of nutrients with the least amount of effort and toxin exposure.

* *Organic foods* contain less pesticides and other harmful chemicals than nonorganic options, and sometimes boast higher micronutrient levels.

* *Proportions* are important. We should try to consume fruit, vegetables, unprocessed and whole-grain carbohydrates, heart-healthy fats like olive oil and coconut oil, and protein every day to encourage gut flora biodiversity, adequate detoxification, and enzyme activity.

* *Acid-alkaline balance* is crucial. Disease flourishes if our blood is too acidic but cannot survive if we create a more alkaline environment through a well-balanced diet that includes plenty of vegetables and other alkaline foods. Proteins and starches are acidic, and anaerobic training stresses test our ability to maintain an alkaline-acid equilibrium, leading, in extreme cases, to subclinical acidosis, a buildup of acids in the blood that is more common than many athletes realize. Most fruits and vegetables are alkaline and can help rebalance this scale.

* *Variety* in our diets is uncommon but desirable. We all like to stick to what we know, but it's good to experiment with new foods to provide a full nutrient profile and encourage our bodies to optimally process a broad spectrum of solids and liquids.

* *Unprocessed and raw foods* that are as close to their original form as possible are best, not highly processed foods that have been stripped of many of their original nutrients and contain added artificial ingredients that are difficult for the body to process and detoxify. These substances can include artificial colors and flavorings, high-fructose corn syrup, and other sweeteners.

6 The Human Athlete

- *Nutritional healing* isn't some hippie concept but a very real phenomenon. The body is always trying to heal, repair, and detoxify itself, and we can either help it or hinder it through nutrition. By finding the most potent beneficial foods and incorporating them into their daily diets, athletes can help support regeneration instead of hampering it.

- *Moderation* is another crucial lifestyle habit to cultivate. Eating huge meals or getting into a bingeing-and-depriving cycle can fundamentally disrupt the digestive and detoxification systems and our metabolism.

ALLERGIES AND INTOLERANCES   6.3.3.2

In today's alarmist medical culture of overdiagnosis, we've taken to labeling too many health challenges as "allergies." This is not to minimize the very real discomfort that occurs when you consume a food that doesn't agree with you. But such things rarely fall into the true definition of an allergy, which is a strong and sometimes life-threatening immune reaction to a substance, such as tree nuts. An intolerance, on the other hand, is usually an inability to adequately process a particular food type or a sensitivity to certain properties a type of food contains. Wheat and dairy intolerances often produce stomach discomfort, bloating, and incomplete digestion, effects that can be exaggerated if low stomach acid or enzyme levels are already an issue.

LIFESTYLE FACTORS   6.3.3.3

Negative lifestyle choices can have a profoundly negative impact on the ability to process and absorb nutrients and manage detoxification. Drinking alcohol, smoking, and eating too much junk food cause stress to the digestive system, as do too little or poor-quality sleep and inadequate postexercise recovery.

In contrast, yoga, meditative and spiritual practices, and diaphragmatic (belly) breathing exercises have been shown to not only counter these stress factors but also positively impact digestion. One way these practices work is by encouraging the body to move from its sympathetic alarm state into parasympathetic recovery (these will be explored in more detail on page 179).

OVERMEDICATING AND GASTROINTESTINAL HEALTH   6.3.3.4

The overprescription and overuse of medication—including acid reflux medicine, antibiotics, NSAIDs, and psychiatric drugs—can affect the health of the entire gastrointestinal system.

Many people struggling with low stomach acid mistakenly confuse the symptoms—heartburn, bloating, cramping, and so on—for high acid levels. Even within the medical field, the fact that the symptoms are similar can lead to confusion about the cause. When people with low stomach acid are mistakenly diagnosed with high stomach acid, they start taking medication that is supposed to reduce acid levels, further exacerbating the problem. Spending on the top acid reflux drug has topped $2 billion per year, demonstrating the extent of the problem.[26]

A better solution than taking antacids is combining natural remedies like apple cider vinegar with foods with live active cultures, such as yogurt, sauerkraut, kimchi, and kombucha. The combination of these help "good" gut bacteria to flourish while helping to clear out overgrowth of "bad" bacteria. Prebiotics and probiotics can also improve enzyme activity and the health of the microbiome.

The bacteria *H. pylori* thrives in a low stomach acid environment and actually suppresses the secre-

When diet is wrong, medicine is of no use. When diet is correct, medicine is of no need.

—Ayurvedic proverb

tion of stomach acid.[27] Thus, when stomach acid is low—as it is when someone is on acid-suppressing drugs—*H. pylori* infections become worse. *H. pylori* infections can lead to peptic ulcers by causing inflammation in the stomach lining and disrupting its mucous barrier, exposing the stomach lining to damaging stomach acid. Overuse of NSAIDs can also lead to peptic ulcers because they block an enzyme that protects the stomach lining from stomach acid.

Overuse of antibiotics is also having a detrimental effect on the gut microbiome. In his book *Missing Microbes,* Martin J. Blaser states, "The loss of microbial diversity on and within our bodies is exacting a terrible price." In addition to allowing medication-resistant pathogens to flourish by killing off other bacteria, thus reducing the competition for resources, Blaser writes that using antibiotics destroys microbiota (often called "good bacteria") and "changes development itself, affecting our metabolism, immunity and cognition."[28] One study found that a week-long course of antibiotics disrupted the balance of bacteria in the gut microbiome for up to a year. Study participants also became more drug-resistant than those who didn't take antibiotics, potentially affecting how they responded to future medication.[29] I first saw this many years ago with a rugby team where many players were struggling to gain muscle but at the same time were suffering from intolerances and minor injuries after an overzealous doctor had been prescribing antibiotics for even the most minor illness.

These findings present a challenge for athletes who are, at least at the elite level, quickly issued antibiotic prescriptions by medical teams who want them to get back on the field as soon as possible. It's the job of the health-conscious athlete to try to distinguish between illnesses and infections that need an antibiotic and those that don't and to guard against the temptation to ask for a pharmaceutical remedy immediately upon falling ill.

Athletes must also avoid taking too many NSAIDs, as these too can lower stomach acid, interfere with enzyme activity, and disrupt the microbiome—not to mention putting strain on the liver and kidneys. Steroids, whether taken as performance-enhancing drugs or prescribed by a physician for surgery or injury recovery, also diminish the gastrointestinal and immune systems and should be avoided.

It's not just antibiotics and NSAIDs that can negatively impact gut health. When we consider the impact of psychiatric drugs, we can't just think about what they do in the brain. The twenty neurotransmitters of the enteric nervous system are the same as those in the brain. As all but 5 percent of serotonin is secreted in the gut, increasing the level of this chemical with selective serotonin reuptake inhibitors (SSRIs) also has an impact on digestive tract issues. The two million people who suffer from irritable bowel syndrome typically have surplus serotonin, too. Adam Hadhazy stated in a story for *Scientific American* that this is an example of a "mental illness of the second brain."[30] Interestingly, he noted that a study found that a drug that inhibits serotonin release started reversing the ill effects of osteoporosis. This suggests that the health of the gastrointestinal system and the health of the structural-anatomical system are closely related.

The doctor of the future will give no medication, but will interest his patients in the care of the human frame, diet and in the cause and prevention of disease.

—Thomas Edison

THE STRUCTURAL-ANATOMICAL MACRO SYSTEM

6.4

The structural-anatomical system provides the body with its shape and support structures, including the bones, skeletal muscles, fascia, ligaments, tendons, and other soft tissues. This vital pillar of athlete health is composed of two micro systems:

- *Structural orientation micro system:* Manages the orientation and positioning of joints and insertion points and how structures interact with each other as the body moves through three-dimensional space.

- *Passive structural micro system:* The passive structures of the body that provide its form and generate movement, such as bones, joint structures, muscles, ligaments, and tendons. These are living systems that continue to adapt and change.

There's incredible anatomical variation among individual athletes. In his book *Biochemical Individuality,* Dr. Roger Williams references a Rockefeller Institute study that found incredible differentiation in the weights of organs in 645 rabbits. Subsequent human studies confirmed that organ sizes differ markedly among people, too. This was one of the first ways in which internal medicine showed that we're all as different inside our bodies as we are in outward appearance. In fact, the greatest mistake that authors of anatomy books have unintentionally made is to lead us to believe that we are all the same inside. This isn't the case. Your heart, for example, is located in a slightly different place and orientation from everyone else's. This is why great care must be taken with normative data or drawing conclusions from assessments or screens based on averages.

Proper nutrition is crucial to keep the structural system healthy. The most obvious step is eating properly to get adequate amounts of certain vitamins and minerals that nourish this system: vitamin K, potassium, calcium, and vitamin D. Vitamin K, potassium, and calcium are abundant in dairy products and green vegetables. Vitamin K is also found in fermented products, and other potassium-rich foods include kiwi, broccoli, and bananas. Athletes (and everyone else) should try to get their vitamin D through twenty to thirty minutes of exposure to sunshine a day.

THE STRUCTURAL ORIENTATION MICRO SYSTEM

6.4.1

This micro system governs the makeup of the individual structures within the body—including bones, cartilage, ligaments, and tendons—and how they are aligned in relationship to each other, such as within joints and motion segments. While heredity plays a big role here, we know that certain experiences can change our structural orientation. In collision sports in particular, joints can be repositioned and moved, which affects the structure's orientation and how the athlete subsequently recovers, and if the joint capsule and nerve pathways don't return to their original structure, the athlete may change movement patterns to compensate.

Trauma on or off the field can also alter our structural orientation, such as when a rugby player's collarbone is broken in a tackle. The way we move can also affect structural orientation over time, as our body conforms internally to certain postures. A good example is an office worker whose spine begins to curve after sitting in a slumped position eight hours a day for thirty-five years.

The pathways that nerves follow or are disrupted from in collision sports all affect innervation. Like nerves, fascia (connective tissue) is considered a system of communication within the body. All of these positions and pathways affect how the brain and internal orientation systems consider our positioning in space. In sports, this is obviously critical. When joints become misaligned in a collision, it can greatly affect movement, since origin and insertion points are now in different places with respect to each other.

THE PASSIVE STRUCTURAL MICRO SYSTEM
6.4.2

As we've discovered more about human anatomy and our movement through three-dimensional space, we've come to learn the significance of differing ranges of motion and how this is somewhat dictated by our unique anatomical structures. The anatomical design of various joints varies greatly from person to person, so one athlete's glenohumeral joint (aka the shoulder joint) will likely be different from the next player's. That's why I've often said that there's no such thing as a contraindicated exercise, only contraindicated athletes who can't support the movement or position.

Training can positively impact muscle size, power output, and recruitment (i.e., the number of fibers the body uses to perform a certain movement and how quickly this is achieved through nervous system response). Although the type and structure of an athlete's training influences muscular development, the athlete's potential in this area is largely influenced and somewhat limited by genetics and body type. Ectomorphs are typically very lean and struggle to put on muscle, while an endomorph's body-composition struggles usually center on losing fat. In contrast to both, mesomorphs are quite lean and find it easy to add muscle.

We can't only consider muscle, which is a mistake many trainers and coaches make. The ligaments, tendons, and cartilage are also important. While ligaments and tendons can benefit from strength training, the connections and interplay between these and the soft tissues can also be negatively affected by physical activity. For example, if muscles and fascia become overly stiff, they can start to put undue pressure on a ligament or tendon, which over time predisposes the player to a catastrophic injury. The same can be true of inefficient and suboptimal positioning.

THE METABOLIC MACRO SYSTEM
6.5

This system regulates how energy is derived from food and oxygen, how fuel is distributed around the body, and which pathways are used to do so. It consists of the cardiorespiratory system and the energy substrate system. Together, they determine how the body is fueled for different physical activities and recovery, both with oxygenated blood and with metabolic byproducts like phosphocreatine.

- *Cardiorespiratory micro system:* Composed of the lungs, which add oxygen to and remove carbon dioxide from the blood, and the heart, which pumps the oxygenated blood throughout the body.
- *Energy substrate micro system:* Distributes all the energy allocated by the biotransformational system and is composed of three subsystems:
  - *Alactic:* Very closely related to the central nervous system and the initiation of powerful movements.
  - *Anaerobic:* Enables repeated sudden bouts of effort and muscular movement.
  - *Aerobic:* Enables continuous or intermittent movement over longer periods.

THE CARDIORESPIRATORY MICRO SYSTEM
6.5.1

The cardiorespiratory system is composed of the heart and lungs, and its primary role is to facilitate blood flow and manage the exchange of oxygen and carbon dioxide in the blood. It controls how we consume oxygen and expel and excrete other gases. As an athlete trains and competes, the structure of the heart changes to make the cardiorespiratory system more efficient. For example, endurance training stimulates adaptation in the overall structure of the heart, causing left ventricular hypertrophy and allowing an increase in the volume of blood the heart can pump, while resistance stressors increase the thickness of the myocardium (the heart muscle). Veins, arteries, and capillaries also adapt their structures to the stimuli of exercise, enabling the cardiorespiratory system to shuttle oxygenated blood around the body faster and with more force. Existing blood vessels become more elastic and sometimes larger, and new ones can form, too.

In addition, the metronome that controls circulation—heart rate—changes its tempo. Athletes often have lower resting heart rates than the general population because their hearts can pump blood more efficiently and at a greater volume, so they need fewer pulses to get the job done during everyday activity. The lungs also adapt to physical activity, with increased capillarization to enable greater blood flow, more alveoli to allow greater gas exchange, and increased elasticity of the pleura and alveoli to support faster gas flow. The surrounding muscles of the diaphragm and intercostals also become stronger.

In other words, training changes the structure of the heart, lungs, and blood vessels, and different kinds of training create different kinds of changes. A lot of heavy weight lifting leads to different morphological changes than training to run a marathon.

THE ENERGY SUBSTRATE MICRO SYSTEM
6.5.2

Training also affects the use of energy substrates (ATP, creatine phosphate, etc.) and muscle tissue. The energy substrate micro system processes the sources of energy and is tightly connected to other macro systems: the nervous system assigns the correct energy substrate system for any activity; the digestive system supplies the fuel for the energy substrates to do their job; the cardiorespiratory system is the transport channel for the fuel itself; and the structural-anatomical system is what's put into motion by the energy provided.

The energy substrate system includes the following subsystems:

- *Alactic system:* Has the ability to generate huge amounts of power using ATP (adenosine triphosphate) to power contractions
- *Anaerobic system:* Provides short bursts of energy without using oxygen; consumes large volumes of glycogen (stored glucose)
- *Aerobic system:* Provides sustainable output using oxygen; consumes mostly fats but also glycogen

Most research on energy substrates has been done in sports that rely on one subsystem almost exclusively, but in team sports this is impossible: team-sport athletes use all three together, so many of the findings from this research are misleading. These subsystems are incredibly fluid, and while different sports and positions might emphasize a certain one, every athlete needs to reach certain minimum capacities in each and be able to transition among them efficiently on demand to perform to their potential. The morphocycle is designed to create adaptations in each of the energy substrate subsystems while allowing for ample recovery and regeneration of all three.

THE ENDOCRINE MACRO SYSTEM
6.6

This system responds to the mental and physical demands placed on the neuromuscular system and manages how the body reacts from a hormonal perspective.

The endocrine macro system is made up of two subsystems: the pituitary-adrenal micro system and the cortisol-immune micro system, both of which manage a complex mixture of hormones and receptors.

- *Pituitary-adrenal micro system:* Governs the production of certain hormones within the body and manages the adrenal glands.

- *Cortisol-immune micro system:* Regulates how we respond to bacteria, viruses, and other threats. Cortisol, one of the key stress hormones, is closely linked with this system and the nervous macro system. If cortisol is chronically elevated, it suppresses immune function.

There are many possible ways to look at how these micro systems function and interact. I'm going to focus primarily on their role in helping athletes manage and adapt to stress.

THE PITUITARY-ADRENAL MICRO SYSTEM   6.6.1

This system is responsible for the production of growth hormones and other hormones used for the building and recovery of muscle, mental focus, emotional stability, and many other key functions crucial to athletic performance. When the body encounters a stressor, the pituitary gland and hypothalamus dictate how much testosterone is produced and how this is balanced with other hormones to facilitate growth and repair.

Under ideal circumstances, enough testosterone is produced to prompt muscle restoration and, if appropriate, hypertrophy following training and competition, but if athletes aren't sleeping or recovering well, have taxed other systems, or are exposing themselves to too many endocrine disruptors—such as soy, pesticides in nonorganic foods, toxins in hard plastics, and/or heavy metals, such as those found in poor-quality drinking water—hormone balance can be affected.

To keep hormones well balanced, athletes should avoid such toxic disruptors as best they can, eat organic fruits and vegetables whenever possible, and ensure that they are getting enough rest. It may also be helpful to focus on foods rich in certain vitamins and minerals: magnesium (pumpkin seeds and almonds); B vitamins (seafood, meat, and mushrooms); and omega-3 fatty acids (fish, chia and flax seeds).[31]

We know that the maximization of testosterone and growth hormone involves high-intensity exercise, such as strength training, that stimulates the adaptation and response in the endocrine system. A healthy diet, high in good natural fats and minerals such as zinc and magnesium support optimal hormone regulation. Limiting sugar and excessive stress from all sources also helps significantly.

Some additional supplements may be beneficial, such as D-aspartic acid, vitamin D, and possibly diindolylmethane (DIM). D-aspartic acid is an amino acid that's believed to increase testosterone production. A study published in *Clinical Endocrinology* found that participants with higher levels of vitamin D had significantly higher levels of free testosterone than those with insufficient amounts. And DIM, a substance formed during the digestion of vegetables such as broccoli and cauliflower, may help support a healthy balance of estrogen and testosterone.[32]

THE CORTISOL-IMMUNE MICRO SYSTEM   6.6.2

The cortisol-immune and pituitary-adrenal systems, where cortisol is produced, are closely related. Cortisol is highly significant in immune function—it helps us tolerate high levels of stress, balance inflammation, and deal with viral and bacterial threats.

Cortisol is a stress hormone that is released to mitigate inflammation—a perfectly natural response. But if stress is intense and/or prolonged, too much cortisol can be excreted, which is damaging, can lead to conditions like Addison's disease and can make an athlete more susceptible to illness. If an athlete continually overtaxes a particular system—for instance, by hammering the central nervous system with too much intense interval work or Olympic lifting without allowing for proper recovery—immune system function can be compromised. This means the athlete will be less able to fight off sickness before it sets in and will take longer to bounce back from illness.

To maintain the health of the cortisol-immune micro system, in addition to trying to keep their functional reserve topped up, athletes can consume foods such as green tea, ginger, cruciferous vegetables, elderberries, blackberries, and citrus fruits.

THE NERVOUS MACRO SYSTEM

6.7

This system is composed of the sensory organs, brain, and spinal cord, and the nerves that connect them—basically the body's internal wiring that sends signals to and from the command center of the brain about what we're experiencing and how best to respond. One of the mistakes most sports scientists make is to look at the nervous system from a purely medical perspective. What they need to do is also consider how long each branch of the nervous system (which we'll explore in a moment) takes to recover when subjected to certain stimuli and how the morphocycle should be adjusted accordingly.

The function of the central nervous system is based largely on neurotransmitter function. These chemicals are essential in maintaining good health, as they not only dictate athletes' physical and mental responses to stimuli but also help regulate emotion. In addition, neurotransmitters are in close and regular contact with elements of all the other main bodily systems and the processes they govern. The body is in one sense very much a neurobioelectrical system.

One of the most crucial interactions occurs among the central nervous, enteric nervous, and biotransformational systems. The enteric nervous system has a foot in both the biotransformational and nervous macro systems, but because of its importance in digestive function, it's discussed in detail in the section on the gastrointestinal system—see page 168.

The nervous macro system includes these micro systems:

- *Central nervous micro system:* Made up of the spinal cord, brain, and neurotransmitters, this manages our moods and voluntary actions.

- *Autonomic nervous micro system:* Composed of:

  - *Parasympathetic nervous system:* The oldest branch of the nervous system, this regulates body functions during normal, everyday situations. It's what puts the body into the "rest and digest" state that's needed for recovery, and it creates a metabolic baseline of operation to manage oxygen and nourishment via the blood.

  - *Sympathetic nervous system:* This system, which evolved after the parasympathetic nervous system and has a more sophisticated set of responses, readies the body to respond to dangerous or stressful situations—it initiates the fight-or-flight response. For our ancestors, it increased mobility for hunting, defense, and reproduction by increasing muscle strength, heart rate, and other adaptive responses.

  - *Social engagement system:* This is a more complex emotional and psychological system of communication in social groupings.

- *Peripheral nervous system:* Made up of nerves that connect the central nervous system to the rest of the body, this system is responsible for transmitting instructions from the brain and spinal cord to fire muscles and initiate movement. The peripheral nervous system is also pervasive throughout other types of tissue and connects to all the body's major organs, including the skin. The peripheral nervous system is part of a two-way feedback loop with the central nervous system, both sending and receiving data at lightning speed.

  - *Neuromuscular micro system:* The nerves that run to and from soft tissues throughout the body.

THE CENTRAL NERVOUS MICRO SYSTEM   6.7.1

When we start trying to design and manage morphocycles (preparing athletes for competition by balancing their exposure to volume, intensity, density, and collision/contact in the context of learning experiences and their recovery from each of these—see page 126), it's crucial to recognize how slowly or quickly our bodily systems recover between stimuli. If we introduce another similar load too soon, it will not only minimize the adaptation or cause maladaptation to both stimuli but also overtax our systems. The central nervous system (CNS) takes longer to fully recover than any other system, requiring up to seventy-two hours to adapt to stimuli in some cases.

Plugging this knowledge back into the morphological programming approach, we know that games and preparation sessions that are physically and psychologically intense place the CNS under tremendous strain. So these sessions should be spread out in each morphocycle and interspersed with less-intense sessions. Failure to do so will not only interfere with adaptation and negatively impact game-day performance but also can lead to CNS fatigue, whereby athletes feel chronically tired, struggle to concentrate, and can't fully engage in team learning experiences between games. This is why we need a systems-based model to manage player preparation and game loads.

THE PERIPHERAL NERVOUS MICRO SYSTEM   6.7.2

The peripheral nervous system (PNS) serves two main functions. First, its receptors are continually collecting trillions of bytes of information on the world around us and what we see, hear, touch, taste, and smell. This data is then sent to the brain via dendrites in peripheral nerves. The PNS also is involved in gathering information about where the body is in three-dimensional space—aka kinesthetic proprioception. This impacts the decision-making component of skill execution, which we'll explore in more detail later.

The second role of the PNS comes into play once the brain has received the sensory input, combined it with what it knows from experience, selected a motor program—that is, the physical manifestation of a movement skill—and decided exactly how it will be executed, depending on the unique context in which the skill will be performed. These instructions are sent at high speed from the brain, down the spinal cord, and out to the motor segments that need to move via axons in peripheral nerves.

If an athlete is injured, the PNS can become compromised, altering the quality of the sensory information being collected and skill execution. This is why it's important for some aspect of rehabilitation to focus on reorienting the player and restoring or improving proprioception. Think about the first time you play your sport or run after an injury: you feel imbalanced because your PNS has been thrown off-kilter.

THE AUTONOMIC NERVOUS MICRO SYSTEM   6.7.3

The parasympathetic and sympathetic branches of the autonomic nervous system (ANS) regulate how the body responds to stressors and maintains an equilibrium, also known as *homeostasis.* Athletes are constantly responding to outside events—such as training stimuli and the rigors of game day—that threaten this balanced state, and they must respond biologically. As such, there's a continual cycle between homeostatic disturbance in response to stressors—which the sympathetic nervous system manages—and homeostatic restoration, for which the parasympathetic response is responsible.

When the body is subjected to a threat, the sympathetic nervous system is activated rapidly and starts triggering other bodily systems to respond. To give a few examples: the endocrine system releases hormones, the cardiorespiratory system increases the heart rate, the immune system dispatches proteins called cytokines, the pituitary-adrenal micro system and cortisol-immune micro system deploy various hormones and neurotransmitters (such as dopamine, norepinephrine, and epinephrine), the energy substrate system mobilizes energy stores, and the structural-anatomical system moves the body. The sympathetic response is like a race car driver pressing the accelerator—the car goes to top speed incredibly quickly. The sympathetic-dominant state is commonly known as "fight or flight."

Once the body perceives that the threat has been dealt with, the relaxation response kicks in and the body goes into parasympathetic recovery. The parasympathetic nervous system takes over to try to restore equilibrium—a return to homeostasis. Hormone levels decline, heart rate decreases, metabolism slows, and movement is halted, among many other things. The parasympathetic response, then, is like the race car driver pressing the brake. However, it takes the body a lot longer to ease into the rest-and-digest stage—another term for *homeostasis*—and more bodily processes are dedicated to the sympathetic state. Despite this seeming imbalance, if the athlete can ensure proper recovery through adequate rest, sleep, mobility, and nutrition, the parasympathetic response should be enough to facilitate restoration and adaptation to training stimuli and experiences.

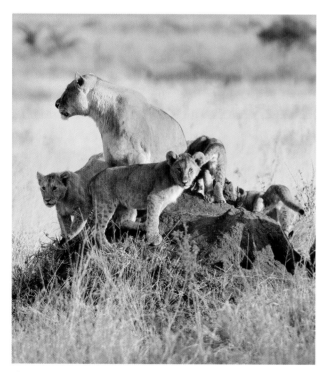

The reptilian and limbic layers of the brain initiate a response to a threat—like a lion—long before the neocortex can reason through what to do. Photo by zixian / Shutterstock.com.

Unfortunately, many athletes fall short in these areas and find themselves in a sympathetic-dominant state in which recovery and adaptation are a daily struggle. Add in external pressures from relationships, finances, and life in general, and it can become increasingly difficult for athletes not only to come out of the fight-or-flight state but also to preserve their overall health.

THE ANIMAL IN ALL OF US   6.7.3.1

As we look at how various systems in the body interact and react to stimuli in athletic contexts and in life, it's important to understand that they act in sequence and that some pathways are faster than others.

The body can be considered an intricate communication network, like the internet. There are two primary ways information is relayed between the brain and body: in hormones and other biochemical markers carried in the blood, and through neurotransmitters and the nerve pathways. The second method is much faster.

The bodily systems that are largely instinctual and that developed to preserve life and safety use neurotransmitters and nerve pathways to kick into gear faster than others when they detect a threat. So if you want to measure a response in an athlete, it's best to look at neural responses first, because by the time you see a response in the blood or biochemistry, it's too late.

Key among the responses to threats are the instinctive responses triggered by the reptilian and limbic layers of the brain. These innate human instincts are what many military trainers attempt to both unlock and manage in order to create an operator who can function in both the world you and I live in and the world they have to work in.

Many things about brain development remain unknown, due to the brain's astounding complexity. Yet scientists such as Paul MacLean have explained that there are three primary layers to the brain: the reptilian, limbic, and neocortex layers. The oldest of these is the reptilian brain, which controls the functions that help keep us alive, such as heartbeat, breathing, and body temperature. The next to develop was the limbic layer, which governs emotional response. It also enables things like maternal bonding and empathy. The neocortex is the newest part of the brain and is responsible for thinking, making judgments, and problem-solving. It's also the slowest part of the brain.

> *I get a feeling about where a teammate is going to be. A lot of times, I can turn and pass without even looking.*
>
> —Wayne Gretzky

When a dangerous situation arises, the reptilian and limbic layers don't wait for the neocortex to think through possible responses. They immediately leap into action to help us survive: the reptilian layer triggers adrenaline and cortisol and raises the heart rate and breathing to get us ready to fight or flee or freeze, while the limbic layer triggers feelings of fear (or possibly anger) and initiates an action, such as pulling your hand back from a hot stove. All this happens before the neocortex may even have consciously registered that there's a threat. If a lion walked into the room, it would be your reptilian and limbic layers that would cue your instinctive fear and trigger the appropriate self-preserving reaction—likely, running away as fast as you could. Of course, in certain professions, such as elite security or firefighters, we want to override this instinct and create different responses.

This is a critical aspect of understanding how elite athletes function. Their quick, instinctive responses to situations and stimuli are not governed by the higher-functioning reasoning of the neocortex and can be developed only through experience. Later I will show you the direct link from nervous system to personality and social skills and how we manage and address fears and perceived threats.

> *The higher nervous system arrangements inhibit (or control) the lower, and thus, when the higher are suddenly rendered functionless, the lower rise in activity.*
>
> —John Hughlings Jackson

THE SOCIAL ENGAGEMENT SYSTEM   6.7.3.2

Stephen Porges's polyvagal theory states that the parasympathetic and sympathetic nervous systems are intertwined with what he calls the social engagement system, which determines how we react to and interact with others. As discussed above, the limbic system is what enables social actions like maternal bonding and helping others, which directly benefit us as well as other people. This is of interest to us because polyvagal theory completely undermines the traditionally fragmented views of the nervous system that have informed how teams prepare players and underlines the importance of the links between athletes and their environment. Traditionally, teams have looked at elements of the various nervous system branches as isolated entities. So they might, for example, look at how stress affects the autonomic nervous system, but not consider its impact on the central nervous system. Or they'll think about the impact of cortisol on anxiety but gloss over how consistently high cortisol levels interfere with the immune system.

THE PERSONALITY
6.8

Players like Messi, Jordan, Brady, and Gretzky all have well-documented examples of having tolerated sustained verbal and physical abuse from players trying to put them off their game. They also had to be able to work with many different people and groups in order to succeed. Together, these facts underline the importance of personality and temperament.

We can't prepare players to win without first acknowledging their personalities. Every person learns in a different manner. Individual athletes also have different tolerance levels for certain stressors, and the recovery rates of their body systems vary. But while many sports teams are comfortable measuring such things from a defined biological marker standpoint, they're often uncomfortable with the imprecise art of evaluating players' personalities. Here's a quick look at how personality impacts performance and, more so, the overall health of the athlete.

THE FOUR TEMPERAMENTS 6.8.1

Taking personality tests has always been popular, both for individuals and for corporate HR departments. These self-administered assessments have remained on the fringe for sports teams, however, which have paid minimal attention to their players' personalities. Some coaches ignore information on personality that could help them create more beneficial learning experiences and tailor their communication to everyone on the roster.

Modern personality tests like Myers-Briggs Type Indicator and Dr. William Marston's DISC Profile trace their origin, method, and results back to Hippocrates, the "father of medicine." Since personality has been observed for thousands of years and the ancient Greeks knew that personality and health were intertwined, it's no surprise that more than two thousand years ago, the Greek physician turned his intellectual powers to unraveling the mystery of human personality. Hippocrates concluded that there are four main personality types or, as he termed them, temperaments:

- *Melancholic* people are typically reserved, thoughtful, and quiet. They sometimes struggle with fear and anxiety, so they need more reassurance than some other personality types. Think of players who struggle with confidence and always seem to be looking for reassurance.

- *Choleric* people are excitable, changeable, and restless. They're typically optimistic but can become aggressive and touchy. These players often have great energy, but they can, sometimes with little provocation, get moody. A calming personal lifestyle and diet can help these players maintain a steady path.

- *Sanguine* people are outgoing and talkative. Though they're usually responsive to direction, their easygoing manner means that they sometimes need to be extrinsically motivated. These players are often the ones who confuse coaches the most, as they are pleasant and talk a lot, which can be distracting. These players can be motivated by competition or having targets to achieve.

- *Phlegmatic* people are calm, even-tempered, and self-controlled. However, their tendency to be cautious means that they can be risk-averse to the point of avoiding new experiences. We all know players who overthink and need to cut loose and just play. Sometimes we confuse their calmness for a lack of concern or passion.

Of course, profiling every player requires work. Nonetheless, there is a lot of value in the management of relationships with key players. Simply acknowledging which of Hippocrates's four temperaments a player fits into allows the coaching staff to know how they can improve the effectiveness of their communication with that player.

Of course, there is also the small issue of the head coach's own personality and self-awareness. Coaches must know how to balance their own temperament with those of their staff and squad.

> ❝
> *All our knowledge has its origin in our perceptions.*
>
> —Leonardo da Vinci ❞

THE FOUR BASIC TEMPERAMENTS

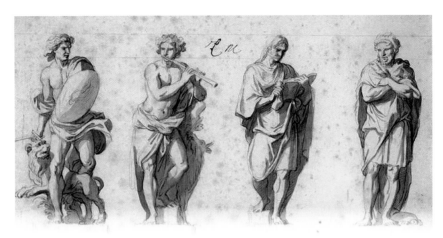

The Four Temperaments, by Charles Le Brun.

	SANGUINE	MELANCHOLIC	CHOLERIC	PHLEGMATIC
	ACTORS	ARTISTS	LEADERS	DIPLOMATS
	SALESMEN	MUSICIANS	PRODUCERS	ACCOUNTANTS
	SPEAKERS	INVENTORS	BUILDERS	TEACHERS
		PHILOSOPHERS		TECHNICIANS
		DOCTORS		
WEAKNESSES	UNDISCIPLINED	MOODY	COLD & UNSYMPATHETIC	UNMOTIVATED
	WEAK-WILLED	NEGATIVE	INSENSITIVE	BIASED
	RESTLESS	CRITICAL	INCONSIDERATE	INDOLENT
	DISORGANIZED	RIGID & LEGALISTIC	HOSTILE & ANGRY	SPECTATOR
	UNPRODUCTIVE	TOUCHY	CRUEL & SARCASTIC	SELFISH
	UNDEPENDABLE	SELF-CENTERED	UNFORGIVING	STUBBORN
	OBNOXIOUS & LOUD	VENGEFUL	SELF-SUFFICIENT	SELF-PROTECTIVE
	EGOCENTRIC	PERSECUTION-PRONE	DOMINEERING	INDECISIVE
	FEARFUL & INSECURE	UNSOCIABLE	PROUD	FEARFUL
		THEORETICAL	OPINIONATED	
		IMPRACTICAL	PREJUDICED	
			CRAFTY	
STRENGTHS	OUTGOING	GIFTED	DETERMINED	CALM & QUIET
	CHARISMATIC	ANALYTICAL	STRONG-WILLED	EASYGOING
	WARM	PERFECTIONIST	INDEPENDENT	LIKABLE
	FRIENDLY	CONSCENTIOUS	PRODUCTIVE	DIPLOMATIC
	RESPONSIVE	AESTHETIC	DECISIVE	EFFICIENT & ORGANIZED
	TALKATIVE	LOYAL	PRACTICAL	DEPENDABLE
	ENTHUSIASTIC	IDEALISTIC	VISIONARY	CONSERVATIVE
	CAREFREE	SENSITIVE	OPTIMISTIC	PRACTICAL
	COMPASSIONATE	SELF-SACRIFICING	COURAGEOUS	RELUCTANT LEADER
	GENEROUS	SELF-DISCIPLINED	SELF-CONFIDENT	DRY HUMOR
			LEADER	
	EXTROVERT		**INTROVERT**	

HIPPOCRATES, PSYCHOLOGY, AND PHYSIOLOGY   6.8.2

In addition to being a pioneer in the study of personality, Hippocrates was among the first influential thinkers to suggest that the mind and body are one. He believed that there were physiological causes and remedies for psychological problems. Hippocrates thought that behavioral instability stemmed from imbalances in the four humors—fluids that the ancient Greeks believed made up the body and influenced both temperament and health—meaning that for Hippocrates, psychology was, at its root, about physiology. Since neurotransmitter function wasn't yet understood at that time, his fluid description was inaccurate, but his principles were not.

He also was correct when it came to the oneness of brain and body. We know that mood—long thought to be exclusive to the realm of the mind—is largely determined by neurotransmitter and hormone levels in the body. When it comes to the psychology of athletes, levels of testosterone, estrogen, dopamine, and other chemicals not only govern the physical impact of game-related and training loads but also impact how players think and feel. As Stanford psychiatry and behavioral sciences professor Robert Malenka puts it, "The brain is what mediates our feelings, thoughts and behaviors."[33] The work of nutritional therapist Julia Ross and others and the discovery of the warrior gene also show how the body's genetic makeup and neurotransmitter balance are affected by diet and can influence how we're predisposed to act in certain ways.

It is a mistake to think that moving fast is the same as actually going somewhere.

—Steve Goodier

OUR MASLOW COMPASS   6.8.3

The reptilian brain and its instinctual nature are directly tied to the foundational layers that form the base of Maslow's hierarchy of needs pyramid, which sets basic needs—food, water, shelter—at the bottom and self-fulfillment needs at the top.

Just like a person in any profession, an athlete is driven by certain intrinsic and extrinsic needs and wants. While a player who has had a successful career and is looking to secure a legacy might be consciously thinking about the self-actualization at the top of Maslow's pyramid—like LeBron James when he returned to Cleveland to win an NBA title—many pro athletes are motivated by the basic need to put food on the table and a roof over their families' heads. The important thing for coaches to appreciate is that the primary motivations of most players are understandable and often, in a sense, primal. These drivers are almost like compasses that are constantly and subliminally orienting us in primal directions. I will discuss this more later when we look at how teams proactively deal with issues regarding discipline and compliance.

First, at a primal level, players are concerned with survival—are they going to live or die? They also have to consider safety and security at the second level of Maslow's pyramid. The retirement of San Francisco 49ers linebacker Chris Borland could be a manifestation of this survival instinct. He described in an interview that, for him, the risk of permanent brain damage that could result from concussions outweighed the rewards of remaining in the NFL.[34]

If a soccer coach meets with the star striker before the start of a new Premier League season and asks him what his motivation is for the upcoming campaign, the player might reply that he wants to lead the league in scoring. But perhaps the athlete is really being fueled by his need to provide fiscal stability for himself and his family—maybe not at the subsistence level but in earning enough to meet the future material needs of his dependents. Or maybe leading the league in scoring is how this player perceives himself achieving financial security.

Topping the goal-scoring chart might well get the striker the security of a better contract and can impact the execution of the coach's game plan, but it's important that both athlete and coach understand the true motivation behind certain expressed desires. This way, if a player is obviously feeling insecure, the coach can reassure him that his needs for fiscal and job security will be met.

The coach also needs to acknowledge that the individual athlete's primal needs would be best served if he knows that his own aims and the team's goals are aligned, so both can reach fulfillment. Fears and needs should not be dismissed but rather acknowledged and redirected. Players don't need to ignore their own needs, but they should recognize that working toward the team's goals will advance their own. The most successful teams are those whose players strive toward a common goal and a higher ideal than the preservation of self.

Acknowledgment of a big team-focused goal also helps satisfy the next level on Maslow's hierarchy: the need for love and belonging. Everyone has a fundamental need to feel like part of a community. As humans evolved from hunter-gatherers into more-organized societies, it became a necessity to fight and possibly die to secure the future of the tribe. This ethos is still reflected in our armed forces, but most of us lack a similar opportunity to be part of a tribal group. For team-sports athletes and personnel, the team is one such tribe.

That's why it's vital to welcome new players and help them assimilate into the locker room, and to remind veterans who are struggling—be it emotionally, behaviorally, or with something more concrete, like a contract dispute—of their role in the tribe and their importance to its continued success. If Sebastian Junger's assertion that "human society has perfected the art of making people not feel necessary" is correct, then every player and coach should take it upon themselves to ensure that no member of the team feels anything *but* necessary and appreciated.[35]

One of the ways in which prayer and mindful meditation are beneficial for athletes is by again committing them to a higher ideal. This can also be help-

THE PHYSIOLOGY OF FAITH

We've explored how physiology—and particularly neurotransmitter levels—can impact mood. It's also important to be aware that your environment and the habits you practice within it also can affect how you feel. There's a growing body of evidence to support the concept that prayer positively affects not only a person's worldview and emotional state but the underlying brain chemistry as well. Andrew Newberg, a neuroscientist at the University of Pennsylvania, has found that prayer increases activity in the frontal lobe while also causing the parietal lobe to go dark, creating a sense of oneness.[36] This is not a new idea. Indeed, one of the seminal texts in this area—William Sadler's *The Physiology of Faith and Fear*—was published in 1912.

ful to the team. If the player is used to acting selflessly and in service to others in their personal life, this may well carry over into how they behave in the team context. Faith in a benevolent higher power also can ease feelings of stress and anxiety, meaning that less of the player's functional reserve is wasted on combating negative thoughts and emotional distress. Making time for daily prayer and contemplation also can have a profound effect on the autonomic nervous system and help trigger the parasympathetic recovery impulse. In addition to helping players manage their egos, faith-based altruism has been shown to increase levels of dopamine and other feel-good neurotransmitters. One major study found that a group who devoted time to volunteerism were 44 percent less likely to die early.[37]

THE RESILIENT PERSON

6.8.4

It's not a stretch to say that most athletes with long, successful careers have proven to be resilient and have a sustainable lifestyle. This doesn't necessarily mean that they have avoided injury and maintained or improved their physicality during their playing days, but rather that the environment they've been in, the habits they've created, and the daily choices they've made have all contributed positively to their overall health and well-being. Their dedication has fostered a persistence that enables them to bounce back from adversity, while their commitment to their overall well-being has enabled them to stay in the game long enough to leave a legacy.

Plenty of people can blaze a trail at the highest level of team sports for a couple of years while partying, abusing alcohol and drugs, and failing to take care of themselves. But rarely do such athletes continue to play at a high level or keep their personal lives on an even keel for long. Eventually there will be a reckoning—physically, psychologically, emotionally, and/or spiritually. This is why the key to helping athletes achieve all they're capable of in sports and in life away from the team is helping them be resilient human beings who are part of a sustainable organization.

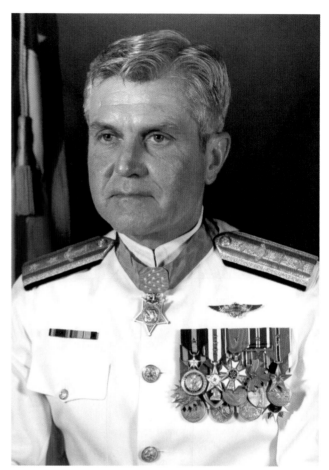

Vice Admiral James Stockdale said Stoicism helped him as a prisoner of war in Vietnam.

> *A Cartesian person would look at a tree and dissect it, but then he would never understand the nature of the tree. A systems thinker would see the seasonal changes between the tree and the earth, between earth and sky. A systems thinker would see the life of the tree only in relation to the life of the entire forest, a habitat for insects and birds.*

—Luís Ribeiro

SEVEN

PLAYER PRINCIPLES

We cannot consider the success of athletes separately from their health, though many coaches choose to ignore players' health and welfare and focus simply on performance. But the better the coaching staff and team specialists understand the overall health of the players, the better able they will be to facilitate the appropriate loading and stimuli that improve game-day performance. In the course of this chapter, we'll look at the qualities that make up each player and how to develop these in a brand-new way. This involves balancing each player's learning and development across each of the four coactives—technical, tactical, physical, and psychological—and doing so in a way that enables the player to apply them together effectively during competition.

THE MACRO PRINCIPLE OF DOMINANCE

7.1

In any given moment and situation, our bodies are monitoring every aspect of our environment and prioritizing and sequencing our bodily systems so that we can do what needs to be done. If you have a cold, your body is dedicating a lot of resources to fighting it. But if you suddenly see someone who's about to be run over by a bus, your body will instantly repriori-

tize and shift all your resources to the task of getting the imperiled person (and yourself) out of harm's way. This is the dominance macro principle—the body creates a systems hierarchy and coordinates resources based on the biggest priority or, in some cases, the most pressing threat. In a sporting context, players may achieve the same things through different means—some players succeed using mostly physical means while others use mostly skill. This is the dominance principle at work: one aspect has dominance, but it is not exclusive.

If your very survival is threatened, your body will initiate the sympathetic fight-or-flight response to keep you alive and unharmed. But if the stimulus is too great or you've drained your battery (aka functional reserve) enough, you will freeze instead. As the body is in one way a closed electrical circuit, it almost always prioritizes the central computer of the brain above all. Organ function also is essential to life, which is why your extremities go numb when you're exposed to extreme cold—your body is shuttling most of your blood flow to your brain and organs to keep you alive.

THE FACILITATION OF FUNCTION

7.2

It's all too easy for coaches to think that their job is to "make" an athlete stronger or "make" them recover better. This is a fallacy. The body will do what it does naturally in anticipation of, in response to, and in recovering from stimuli. The role of the coaching and medical staffs is to facilitate function—whether that's getting stronger, recovering from a game, or learning a new skill. Rather than determine whether the body is doing its job, a coach can help dictate the degree of adaptation or maladaptation.

ASSESSMENT AND PERSPECTIVE

7.3

There are myriad ways to evaluate players outside of a competitive setting, such as with fitness tests, but the only assessment that truly matters is the game itself. And while we can utilize the game model to look at performance in many different ways, at an elemental level we can always come back to two questions:

1. *Is the athlete executing the game tasks properly?* This refers to the outcome and how it fits with the Commander's Intent and the head coach's objectives for each game moment. Simply put, is the player getting the job done? If not, then the coaches can start to narrow down the issue to a technical, tactical, physical, or psychological shortcoming and, if necessary, use active or passive testing outside of the game context to drill deeper into the issue. This will help inform the learning scenarios that the athlete should be exposed to before the next contest.

2. *Is the athlete executing the game tasks efficiently?* We could come up with multiple definitions for efficiency, but in the case of performance assessment, we're trying to see if the way that an ath-

lete is performing skills is safe and sustainable. If the answer is yes, then the athlete should be left alone, but if not, coaches need to help the athlete repattern his or her technique before it causes harm.

Always work backward from the game. If a player is able to execute the tasks required to further the game plan, coaches can allow the player to continue postgame recovery without being subject to the stress of intensive learning experiences that other players who are not executing as well may go through at practice. Fitness-test data don't matter. It's the assessment of the player during game activity that is critical.

THE MACRO PRINCIPLE OF COMPENSATION

7.4

The macro principle of compensation involves how well an athlete is able to mitigate a limitation in one coactive with dominance in one or more of the others.

David Beckham is a prime example. Even during his peak years at Manchester United and Real Madrid, Beckham was not very fast, was not the best in the air, and had one dominant foot. George Best described his abilities more bluntly: "He cannot kick with his left foot, he cannot head a ball, he cannot tackle, and he doesn't score many goals. Apart from that he's all right."[38]

Nonetheless, his superior skill set him apart, whether he was using footwork to create space for a laserlike cross onto the head of a teammate who was bearing down on goal or bending one of his trademark free kicks into the top corner past a helpless goalkeeper. He also understood the game plan and the positioning of his teammates well enough to contribute to an astonishing number of his team's goals as they won the treble (Premier League, FA Cup, and UEFA Champions League) and followed it up by winning the league by eighteen points. Per the principle of functional minimums (more on this later), Beckham had just enough physical capacity to excel at the club and international level and bucketloads of technical skill and tactical awareness, which he leaned on to make himself one of the best players in his sport.

THE MICRO PRINCIPLE OF PERFORMANCE PLASTICITY: THE DIFFERENCE BETWEEN GOOD AND GREAT   7.4.1

If a team-sports athlete is to play at a high level throughout a long career, the need to compensate for limitations becomes more complicated as time goes on. A player with a shorter career might be able to make up for a comparative lack of technical skill with mental strength, at least for a while. But for truly great athletes, the principle of compensation is mutable and, if they continue playing long enough, requires them to master the principle of performance plasticity. This refers to an athlete's ability to continue evolving and progressing throughout their career by developing one of the four coactives—tactical, technical, physiological, or psychological—while maintaining overall well-being.

There's no question that the best example is the greatest basketball player of all time, Michael Jordan. Early in his career, he didn't possess a consistently great jump shot or certain other technical skills, like the ball-handling of Magic Johnson or the passing of Larry Bird. So he compensated with the kind of once-in-a-generation athleticism that earned him his "Air" nickname and defined the first phase of his career. At the same time, though, he worked hard to hone his technical skills.

Like most athletes, Jordan couldn't continue leaping tall buildings in a single bound forever. As his physical gifts diminished, he was able to rely on the skills he'd developed during his überathletic phase, not least an unstoppable fadeaway jumper. During the third and final phase of his career, Jordan's shot didn't get worse per se, but as his physicality continued to decline, he was less able to elevate or get into

space to take his shots of choice. So, after his second comeback, he relied on his tactical acumen to maintain a respectable scoring average against younger opponents, some of whom were almost twenty years his junior. In the second and third stages of his storied career, the impact of his legendary determination and iron will was even more pronounced, too.

Over the course of his career, Jordan was able to become more well-rounded by improving in the psychological, technical, and tactical areas, and he was able apply these abilities only because he stayed in the game for a long time. Though he did lose most of the 1985–86 season to a foot injury, it was Jordan's overall health and durability that made his acquisition of technical skill, tactical astuteness, and psychological strength possible.

An important footnote is the significance of health as the basis for the four-coactive model. Tiger Woods, like his good friend Jordan, also reinvented his game many times, but his poor overall health limited his ability to develop skills in other areas to compensate for his declining physical gifts, which were affected by his knee and back issues.

THE MACRO PRINCIPLE OF LIMITING FACTORS   7.5

By understanding the nature of performance better, we can start to see that some elements are limited and can limit others. Every player has a limiting performance factor in one of the four coactives, and sometimes in two or three. Health, the foundation for all four areas, can prove to be the greatest limiter.

Typically, teams have tried to assess players' capabilities away from competition, usually with physical tests such as end-to-end speed, vertical leap, and one-rep maximums in the weight room. But while such measurements provide a way to compare players in the current stat-happy culture, they mean little when it comes to performance on the field.

An optimal approach is to use the game model to try to better identify and remedy players' limiting factors in the event. In every game moment, all four coactives are on display. If we look at a player's actions in sample offensive, defensive, transition-to-offense, and transition-to-defense moments, it usually becomes readily apparent which areas they are strongest in and which are limiting their effectiveness. Once we've pinpointed one of the four categories, such as technique, we can start to dig a little deeper to see in which of the game moments the player's skillset is letting them down.

If there isn't one clearly identifiable skill that stands out as having room for improvement in terms of technique, we can then look at other factors surrounding selection and execution of the skill. Maybe it's not that the quarterback can't throw a long pass because of inadequate arm strength or poor technique but that he panics when in the pocket or isn't positioning himself in the right way to make sufficient space to throw that long pass.

Once the limiting factor has been identified, you can start trying to reduce its negative impact and improve the player's specific ability in this area. The time and place for this is not during the game itself but in team preparation sessions. So, for example, if you determine that your point guard doesn't finish well around the rim with his left hand, you would set up a drill that requires him to drive down the lane and use his left hand to convert a layup or dunk.

Once a player's primary limiting factor has been identified, it's important not to allow it to have a greater detrimental impact than it already does. So if a basketball player is limited by a comparatively poor vertical jump but is still doing quite well at her level, it's imperative that her vertical does not decline and, indeed, that the training staff help her improve it if possible. Once a limiting factor starts to negatively impact the other components of the four-coactive profile and/or overall health, performance will inevitably suffer. So every player must work to eliminate or reduce such factors. At the same time, all athletes must be encouraged and enabled to maximize their strengths.

THE LIMITING FACTOR CONCEPT

I refuse to use the word *weaknesses* when talking about elite athletes. Rather, I prefer the term *limiting factors* because they are areas that can be developed and improved, and the word *weakness* has a far more negative connotation that might discourage an athlete. In many cases, strong athletes can become infinitely more powerful by simply improving flexibility and mobility and not working directly on power. In this case, poor mobility is hindering the player's ability. You have not made the player better or more powerful per se, but you have removed a limiting factor.

The second reason is that the use of the word *weakness* suggests the player has an inherent deficiency that cannot be changed or controlled. This is not the case: problem areas are simply factors that are limiting the player's improvement. If an athlete had a true weakness, he or she would not be playing the sport.

THE MACRO PRINCIPLE OF FUNCTIONAL MINIMUMS

7.6

Every player has a basic minimum level or degree of competence in each of the four coactives. They need to have this minimum amount of skill simply to play the game effectively. At any position in a team sport, there are baseline levels for technical, tactical, physical, and psychological qualities. If we were to dig deep enough into evaluating the functional minimums for a particular team sport, we could look at every athlete who ever played and say that none of them fell below a certain level and was still successful. In other words, there is a basic minimum level of ability that one must reach to be able to function in the activity.

That's why the language used by sports media outlets concerning the assessment of potential draft picks, transfer targets, and even Hall of Fame ballots is ludicrous. You'll often hear statements like, "She's not a very good athlete" or "He doesn't have a great basketball IQ." On occasion, such blanket criticisms might be accurate, but for the most part, they're uninformed generalities that have little, if anything, to do with these athletes' actual game-time performance.

And really, the primary question isn't whether soccer player X is fast or can jump sky-high or whether rugby player Y is a tactical genius, but whether they are just good enough to perform (in these examples) physically and tactically come game time. The second consideration, which sports radio and TV analysts rarely consider, is how well these players compensate for lower capability in one coactive with superior abilities in the others. An athlete might be among the slowest or tactically challenged at his position, but as long as he's reached a functional minimum in each of the four areas, he should be quite capable of competing effectively.

COACTIVES AND CAREER PROGRESSION

7.7

As explored earlier in this section, good players are able to compensate for limitations in one area by maximizing the positive impact of outstanding capacity in another. Sometimes this is quite pronounced and obvious: even a casual fan may notice when a player makes up for being limited technically, tactically, and psychologically by using their physical gifts to the fullest. In other cases, an athlete's competence might be fairly even across the four coactives, and the need to compensate is much less noticeable. An "all-around" basketball player like Draymond Green is a good example.

Great players are able to adapt such compensations over time as their careers evolve, and we'll look at some case studies of this later on. But for now it's fair to say that if an athlete is to continue their career, they must be able to constantly develop all four coactives. Flipping this upside down, they need to stay in the game to advance in every coactive.

For example, a quarterback needs a minimum level of physical ability and health to be able to stay in the game long enough to develop high scores in the psychological area, and then to be able to spend enough time improving psychologically to then improve technically and tactically. The pattern recognition, decision-making speed, and emotional fortitude needed to win a Super Bowl take time to develop, as shown by the lack of Super Bowl–winning rookie quarterbacks. The same goes for athletes in any team sport. While a young, precocious team can have unexpectedly early success, for this to be sustainable there needs to be a cumulative level of experience that has allowed enough players to get close to their maximum potential in each coactive.

Conversely, as players age, it is their increased technical, tactical, and psychological acumen that enables them to prolong their careers, even as their physical abilities start to erode. It is also essential that they recognize the increased importance of health factors that enable adaptation and recovery, such as sleep and nutrition. Maintaining a solid health foundation will limit the degree to which physical prowess declines and impacts overall performance. Health is also, of course, key to the preservation of technical, tactical, and psychological elements.

It's critical to remember that great technique can also buy time. If you have good technique and are continuing to improve physically, you can do well enough to stay in the game so that your tactical, technical, and physiological abilities can progress. At the highest level, this is really the practical application of a ratchet theory—as time goes on, athletes continue to improve bit by bit until they reach their performance ceiling. Then it's a question of maintaining the coactive and health foundations while continuing to layer on the benefits of experience and expertise. So, in the case of Cam Newton, his physical prowess and health should allow him to stay in the NFL for long enough that his psychological, technical, and tactical abilities skyrocket and he becomes one of the greatest quarterbacks ever.

BEST ADVICE: STAY IN THE GAME   7.7.1

As their playing careers progress, athletes need to address limitations (with help from the coaching staff, using an evaluation of performance during games rather than in training) so that they can negate their impact while also developing their strengths so that they can increase their impact. Continually working at all four elements of performance also means that if competence in one area declines and plateaus, such as physical ability in athletes nearing the end of their career, they can compensate with another, such as mental strength.

It's difficult to create a line of best fit and state categorically which coactives become dominant at which point in athletes' careers because it varies so much. But it is fair to say that athletes must have a foundation of health and then have the baseline physicality to stay in the game long enough to develop the other coactives. How these progress will depend on many variables, including athletes' desire and ability to learn, the amount of playing time, and the quality of the coaching they receive. It's the role of the coaching staff to help players continue their progression no matter what stage of their career they're at, without overemphasizing certain qualities and ignoring or shortchanging others.

MAXIMIZING DOMINANT QUALITIES
7.8

Beyond a certain point, the law of diminishing returns will kick in with any of the coactives. Though sports teams devote so much time and effort to developing players' physical gifts, this area reaches a ceiling more often than technical, tactical, or psychological acumen. For example, is an offensive lineman going to play better because he can squat six hundred pounds instead of five hundred? It's unlikely. It's also possible that being dominant to the extreme in one area can limit ability in another. For example, if players have greatly increased their strength but haven't done enough mobility work, their range of motion might decrease, reducing their overall performance and upping their injury risk. You cannot develop one coactive at the expense of the others without negative consequences.

However, this is not to say that players should ignore their strengths. Rather, they should develop their dominant qualities in ways that are applicable in game scenarios and up to the point of diminishing returns, which coaches can help them identify. And with technical, tactical, and psychological coactives, it's arguable that most players continue improving throughout their careers as they amass experience and are battle-tested in different ways.

ADDRESSING LIMITING FACTORS   7.8.1

Maximizing strengths is one of two ways that players can use the four-coactive model to advance their careers. The other key to staying in and excelling in the game is exposing limiting factors. The first step is to identify these factors in the game context. Film can come in handy here, as it's impossible for players to know what they aren't doing right in the heat of the action (beyond obvious individual failures to execute, like a rugby player's dropping a pass or a soccer player's missing a shot on an open goal).

Similarly, the coach is too involved in the game itself to recognize and make note of areas in which the players need to improve.

Once the coaching staff has had time to review the game film with the four-coactive model in mind and then sit down with each athlete to talk through his or her game experiences, it becomes easier to pinpoint a player's main limiting factor. Though there are always game-to-game variations in even the best players' performances, it's often possible to spot a pattern across multiple games and find something that can be addressed before the next contest.

Perhaps an assistant coach notices that the quarterback isn't completing long passes or is throwing interceptions when attempting passes on third and fourth downs. The next step is to find out which of the four coactive buckets this issue fits into. If we know that the QB has a cannon for a throwing arm and is fast enough to avoid onrushing would-be tacklers, then it's not a physical issue. Similarly, if the player knows the playbook inside and out and is highly experienced, then technical and tactical ele-

ments can be ruled out. That leaves us with a psychological limitation. Knowing the QB got injured in the final game of the previous season when a defensive tackle broke free and sacked him helps the coach identify a possible factor. After talking with the player, the coach realizes that yes, this collision and the resulting damage are still on the QB's mind.

Now it's clear that the QB needs to get past this negative experience. So in the next day's practice, the QB coach tells him to stand in the pocket and throw a long pass to one of two receivers, who go to opposite sides of the field. He does it just fine. Next, the coach increases the complexity by having the QB take a snap, step back into the pocket, and then throw to one of the receivers. He's still nailing pass after pass. To increase the challenge, the coach has a defensive tackle from the practice run at the QB as he's preparing to throw, but without tackling him. In doing so, he's creating a realistic game situation without the risk of aggravating the QB's old injury or causing a new one.

TECHNO-TACTICAL / PSYCHOPHYSICAL DEVELOPMENT OF PLAYERS

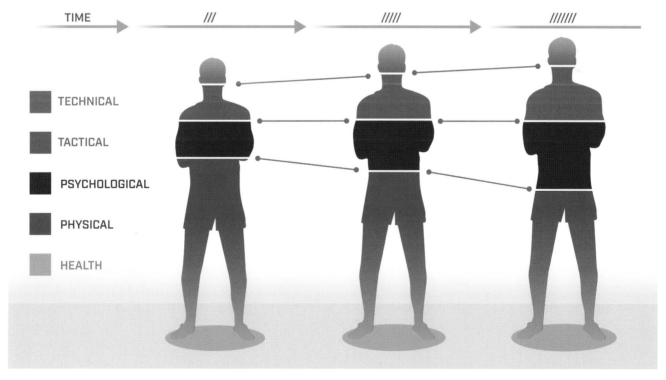

PLAYERS CAN IMPROVE THE BALANCE AND RELATIONSHIP AMONG THE FOUR COACTIVES. THIS GENERALLY HAPPENS AS SKILLS, ESPECIALLY TACTICAL INTELLIGENCE, DEVELOP AS THEY GET OLDER.

The QB hesitates for a split second, and the DT gets to him before he releases the ball. The QB coach pulls him aside and shows him a video of what just happened so he can understand exactly what the issue is. Then they talk about how the QB is fast enough to create space in the pocket and evade the oncoming DT, and strong enough to throw the long pass to a receiver. With this reassurance in his mind, the QB returns to the drill and this time completes the pass before the DT can get to him. Same thing on the next rep. In the next game, he completes all his long passes, with no interceptions. His limiting factor has been eliminated.

This is obviously a best-case hypothetical example. In some cases, it might be impossible to eradicate the limiting factor. But in most cases, it is possible to at least mitigate it and reduce its game-day impact. While you can look for a limiting factor for each player in each of the four game moments, it's best to choose the one that's affecting the player's performance the most and focus on it before the next game. If you try to take on more than one constraint per player, you will have less impact on each one and run the risk of cognitively overloading the athlete.

INJURY IN THE ELITE ATHLETE   7.8.2

In the same way that an elite athlete is a complex dynamic system, the factors that contribute to injury are also complex. We can't just look at mechanics, because mobility and motor control are also factors. The moment the player got hurt can't be highlighted at the exclusion of what led up to the incident, either. A rugby winger who pulls a hamstring likely will have experienced soreness and stiffness in the muscle prior to the game. If we're waiting for pain to show up so the athlete tells the head coach or athletic trainer about it, we're already behind, because pain is a lagging indicator, just as a thirsty player often is already dehydrated. This is why we need to maintain an all-inclusive view of injury rather than an incident- or pain-focused one.

EXPLOITING AN OPPONENT'S LIMITING FACTORS

The concept of limiting factors also can be applied to how a team tailors its preparation for a certain opponent. The head coach will want to maintain the same game plan as always but might adjust certain tactics and elements of strategy to exploit the limiting factors of an opposing team or a particular player. Sometimes this coincides nicely with one of the team's players maximizing his or her dominant qualities. One example was the Cleveland Cavaliers aggressively attacking Steph Curry's defense in the 2016 NBA Finals. They did this not only on a team offense level but also had Kyrie Irving use his devastating quickness off the dribble and ability to finish in traffic to take advantage of Curry on the defensive end.

WHERE SYSTEMS MEET   7.9

Though I've broken down the various bodily macro and micro systems and looked at them from the perspective of sustainable long-term athlete health, we must remember that no system ever functions in isolation. Every action on the field, every learning experience during team preparation, and every occurrence during a player's time off the field involves multiple systems. We also need to be mindful of the fact that the readiness of these systems is constantly peaking and dipping, like soundwaves in a recording studio. The stimuli to which we subject players and their adaptation are impacted not only by how well we balance the load using the morphological programming approach, but by the ever-fluctuating biological and societal cycles—such as public holidays, days of religious observance, and so on—that are continually acting on the athlete.

THE VISION EXAMPLE 7.9.1

The complexity of performance is evident when we look at vision, a bodily process that involves multiple systems. We often think of it as being driven by sight, but sight is only one part of a highly complex, interrelated process. Sight itself is impacted by several factors, such as the athlete's peripheral and central vision capabilities, whether the athlete is colorblind or near- or farsighted, and potential issues like astigmatism. Even an athlete's ability to rotate her head, neck, and torso can affect what she sees on the field or court. Depth, distance, and three-dimensional perception, contrast and color sensitivity, stereoscopic qualities, and the ability to differentiate between objects and patterns all impact the visual information that athletes take in and their ability to process it.

The ability to concentrate visually on certain elements of the game while disregarding others is also crucial. This is a result of years of training in what players should be looking at—like a running back searching for a gap or a point guard reading the defense and his teammates' movements to determine his next pass. So-called game intelligence—that is, how readily and accurately players process the information they're taking in—is also significant.

The brain's prefrontal cortex helps us focus by deciding which visual information is irrelevant and which is important. Once this and other areas of the brain have decided what we're seeing and how it relates to the task at hand, the primary motor cortex selects the appropriate motor pattern and sends this via the central nervous system to the peripheral nervous system.

Beyond vision itself, the limbic brain is involved due to the emotions we instinctively feel when we see certain things. Other regions of the brain get in on the act, too, with the amygdala helping us make sense of what we're seeing based on recent memories and the hippocampus providing additional information from long-term memory. Finally, athletes do what they've been conditioned to do based on the combination of preparation, instinct, experience, and perception. Executing a skill requires the energy substrate and cardiorespiratory systems to team up to supply the designated motor segment with oxygenated blood and fuel. The structural system moves the body in response to what we see and predict what will happen next. Everything an athlete does requires the coordination and sequencing of multiple body systems, so when thinking about athlete health, we have to use a broad, holistic view.

Visual training can improve certain aspects of vision and the speed with which athletes react to visual stimuli, but it tends to do so only in the specific tasks the training system or app serves up, and it's hard to exclude the Hawthorne effect—when people know they're being evaluated, their behavior changes (see page 110 for more on this).[39] So the best way to improve vision with regard to team sports is for athletes to train it in the context of realistic practice and the game itself. This is the same for other abilities—there's no point training them in isolation because that does not mirror a real and applicable game-day scenario.

COLOR AND APPETITE 7.9.1.1

We can use color to influence how we present food to players. For example, bread is normally sold in packaging decorated or tinted with golden or brown tones to promote the idea of home-baked oven freshness. Rarely will you see bread sold in a green wrapper because the color cast onto it would remind buyers of mold. Adding yellow to the wrapper boosts bread sales and gives the product a bright, sunny appeal.[40] In the case of the athlete, a salad bar with brightly colored vegetables might encourage players to make healthier choices in the lunch line.

There's a reason many fast-food chains, including Burger King, McDonald's, and Pizza Hut, use bright colors: they increase appetite. Research has shown that you don't just eat more when exposed to such hues on the logo, menus, and seats; you also eat quicker—fast food indeed! Upscale eateries are just as deliberate in their use of softer shades and muted lighting. They want you to enjoy (and, of course, pay for) a few drinks and a full multicourse meal.[41]

THE QUALITATIVE AND QUANTITATIVE DIMENSIONS

7.10

To sustainably improve performance over the long term, we must work backward from the game itself and from the athlete's performance in it. This means that the coaching staff should assess each player and the team overall in the context of competition. There is simply no other valid assessment than the qualitative one on what takes place on the field. The prehistoric idea that physical qualities alone make an elite athlete is disruptive to the whole concept of winning games.

The coaching staff's four primary tasks as they relate to evaluation are to:

- Identify the player's differentiating qualities. What are the athlete's strengths, and what do the coaches need to do to ensure that those strengths remain his or her key feature?

- Enhance the athlete's ability to develop and apply these dominant qualities. Continue to maximize and develop them.

- Identify the player's primary limiting factor. What is holding him or her back from developing/improving further?

- Make sure the primary limiting factor doesn't get any worse and, if possible, improve it. This should be done in the team context first so that coaches maintain the richness of training experiences. Then, if necessary, isolate the player to stress the mechanism individually.

Many coaches worry only about limiting factors and get sidetracked by focusing on these, rather than ensuring that strengths remain dominant.

MANAGEMENT OF THE HUMAN SYSTEMS

7.11

In this section, we'll look at the weaknesses of traditional training methods like periodization, the relationship between stimulus and adaptation, and the importance of underpinning any program with a solid foundation of athlete health.

IMPORTANCE OF A MORPHOLOGICAL APPROACH

7.11.1

Periodization—systematized training that consists of certain blocks and supposedly prepares an athlete to peak at a certain time (discussed in more detail in 12.3, starting on page 249)—and supercompensation—the post-training phase where the athlete has developed greater capacity than before the program began (discussed in more detail in 12.3.3, page 251)—are theories that have produced great athletes and helped competitors earn numerous Olympic medals, but the environment in which athletes are trained has changed in the fifty-plus years

---

COLOR IN WEIGHT LOSS

If you want to reduce your food intake, replace the normal light bulb in your refrigerator with a blue bulb. The food will look unappetizing, which can help you eat less.[42] The "blue plate special" made famous in the 1930s used this same concept. The color of the plate affects the look of the food and thereby causes the patron to eat less and feel full faster—another dieting tip.

since these approaches were devised. Additionally, advances in science and technology have allowed us to examine each athlete's specific, individualized response to training loads. While anatomy and physiology textbooks used to show how each body system worked in theory and in isolation, we're now better able to explore how these systems function in practice and how they form an interconnected system of systems.

Pioneering research has shown how the body recruits multiple systems simultaneously to spread the load of reacting and responding to stress and recovering from it. This intersystem coordination reduces the physiological cost and leaves athletes with more of their functional reserve, assuming that all systems are healthy and working optimally. That's why we need the morphological programming approach: to ensure that this reserve remains topped up throughout each morphocycle and that the athlete is ready to peak during competition.

PEOPLE-FIRST ATHLETE HEALTH MANAGEMENT   7.11.2

The healthier each of the five systems and their micro-system subsets are, the more stimuli the athlete will be able to handle and the more total stress she will be able to deal with. An individual whose basic health is sound will continue progressing from game to game, helping the team achieve its goal of incremental and sustainable performance improvement.

However, if too many of a player's systems are depleted, overtaxed, or imbalanced, the fundamental health of the player will be compromised and her ability to respond to learning experiences, adapt to stimuli, and recover from training and competition loads will be insufficient. Some ways to avoid this are to encourage recovery with adequate hydration, nutrition, and rest, and to incorporate restorative physical practices such as mobility exercises, breathing exercises, and heat and ice therapy.

It's also crucial that athletes and the team personnel around them take into account scenarios that create added stress on top of the typical day-to-day,

game-to-game, and morphocycle-to-morphocycle pressures. Such factors include illness, extra travel, injury, and personal issues. Contract disputes, team suspensions, and locker room discord can also place players under inordinate amounts of stress, which negatively impacts their well-being. That's why it's vital that teams and particularly the coaching staff think about each player as a person first and an athlete second, as the athlete's health is determined by and, conversely, impacts far more than just athletic performance.

RESPONDING TO STRESS: HOMEOSTASIS AND ALLOSTASIS   7.11.3

Every human body is constantly trying to maintain a sustainable status quo, typically referred to as *homeostasis,* through localized feedback and responses to stimuli. The process that achieves this in the long term is known as *allostasis,* which recruits various systems and mechanisms to respond to stimuli, take the necessary steps to produce adaptation, and then return us to a "normal" baseline.

The trouble is that lighting up the processes that deal with stress over and over again takes its toll and, if the body's five main systems are unable to cope, creates an allostatic load that moves the body's set points and leads to negative changes that can be difficult to reverse or undo.[43] If the load on a player is too great during any team training morphocycle, the desired tactical, technical, physical, and psychological adaptations will not be achieved; in fact, the athlete might regress to lower performance than displayed in the previous game—exactly the opposite of what the team needs to win.

Extended exposure to high stress not only disrupts the athlete's physical responses to training but also reduces the value of each learning experience. Players will not be able to focus as well during team or individual sessions when overstressed, and disrupted sleep will interfere with the brain's processing training experiences, grooving new or improved motor patterns, or moving short-term recollections of what happened that day into long-term memory.[44]

The cost to long-term health can be even more devastating, as a continually high allostatic load has been shown to increase the incidence of disease and chronic conditions. So a series of short-term responses can lead to long-term disruption. Adrenaline and other hormones are released to deal with immediate threats, but over time, the overuse of the pituitary-adrenal micro system without adequate time for recovery can lead to adrenal fatigue, which we commonly call "burnout." Similarly, cortisol (one of the glucocorticoid or steroid hormones) is needed to increase energy production on demand and manage inflammation, but elevating cortisol levels for too long inhibits digestion, encourages fat retention, and disrupts insulin sensitivity.[45]

When the body has more successive stress events than it can buffer, blood pressure and inflammation markers spike, the heart receives thicker, less oxygenated blood, and soft tissues tighten—which increases injury risk. Meanwhile, the immune system becomes less able to fight disease and infection. In addition, prolonged exposure to too much stress reduces levels of the feel-good hormone serotonin, which can contribute to depression. MRIs of patients struggling with high-stress environments have also shown atrophy in certain parts of the brain.[46]

CNS fatigue can be somewhat delayed with branched-chain amino acid (BCAA) supplements, as certain amino acids promote increased secretion of brain chemicals that encourage the body to go into a recovery state and promote better quality sleep. A Swedish study on fatigue in cross-country skiers found that prolonged exercise increases the levels of tryptophan and serotonin in the brain; ingesting BCAAs increases their concentration in blood plasma, which in turn reduces serotonin and tryptophan uptake in the brain.[47] When it's experiencing a high allostatic load, the body also burns through magnesium—which is crucial in regulating the CNS—at a very high rate, so increasing magnesium intake from sources like pumpkin or sunflower seeds, almonds, or a supplement can help limit the impact of CNS fatigue.[48]

To help athletes deal with fatigue better, in addition to certain foods and adequate rest, some research has suggested that the environment can also play a part. In one study, people who were lonely reported feeling fatigue to a greater degree than those who had regular, positive contact with friends and family. Increasing cultural and spiritual awareness was also found to help individuals handle stress and fatigue more effectively, as was the development of coping strategies (see page 185 on the power of prayer and meditation).[49]

It's not just the actual stress that team-sports athletes experience that impacts their overall health. The anticipatory response—how athletes expect a stimulus and subconsciously prime all the systems and processes needed to react to it—is also a contributor to the overall stress load they are subjected to. This can come into play before training and competition and in life events away from the game. If athletes are to maintain their overall health and, particularly, manage stress, they must be aware of the anticipatory and participatory stressors that they have faced and are going to deal with in upcoming contests and preparation morphocycles.

It's also worth noting that just as perceived rate of exertion (PRE) is an important consideration in assessing individual players' responses to each of the morphological programming elements during training, so too can their perceived stress scale scores tell us a lot about how different athletes experience and respond to stress. PRE refers to how hard players feel they worked physically in a game or practice, while the perceived stress scale enables them to gauge the emotional load of the exertion. For example, one player might feel that a double overtime loss was not particularly stressful, while her teammate might be emotionally devastated and physically, mentally, and psychologically exhausted by the game. Such variations should factor into personalized recovery, with athletes playing an important role in honestly assessing how they respond to preparation and game-time scenarios and planning adequate rest and recuperation afterward.

From the standpoint of athlete health, the body and brain are one. The brain wouldn't function correctly without the body gathering and transmitting information about the surrounding environment. On the flip side, the body would not be able to move or do anything if the command center of the brain were taken offline. So we have to look at each system from a comprehensive standpoint that is cognizant of how the brain and body interact and impact athlete health positively or negatively. Just as we must start paying more attention to the technical, tactical, and psychological components of the four-coactive model, so too must we begin to move away from the "body first" approach that has been dominant for decades in sport, from elite athletes down to the amateur ranks.

RECOGNIZING AND MANAGING STRESS

7.12

Everyone can recognize the effects of extreme overload and extreme stress when it's too late: a muscle pull, a completely fatigued athlete, a weak jump, stumble, and awkward landing and a blown-out ACL. The systemic reaction to stress is more hidden, but to understand the athlete as a whole, it's essential to be able to recognize the subtler clues of a body undergoing stress—and how the process can be managed to promote recovery and adaptation. In this section, we'll look at nervous system dominance (how individual players might respond to stress and how this affects training), heart rate variability, central nervous system fatigue, and parasympathetic recovery.

7 Player Principles

STRESS AND ADAPTABILITY

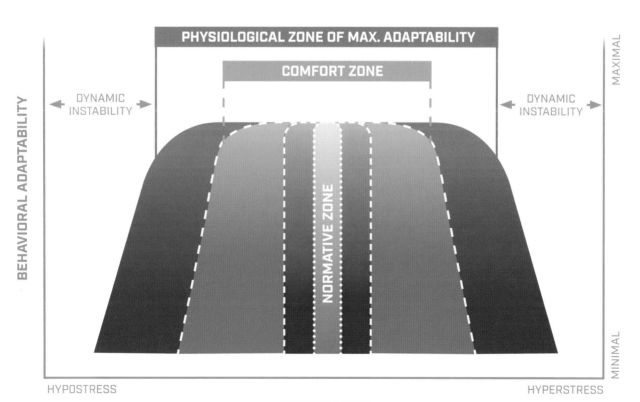

WHEN PARADIGMS COLLIDE: NERVOUS SYSTEM DOMINANCE

7.12.1

The ultimate goal of all teams is to have optimal individual experiences for athletes in an ideal team-sports culture. Classifying athletes as sympathetic-dominant or parasympathetic-dominant can help this by allowing us to individualize warm-ups, cooldowns, recovery and rest, nutrition, and other preparation and performance elements. Understanding a player's autonomic nervous system dominance gives us insight into the athlete's natural, most comfortable preparation style. The basis for this approach can be found in research on overtraining/underrecovering, personality types, and metabolic typing in books like George Watson's *Nutrition and Your Mind* and Roger Williams's *Biochemical Individuality.*

The way I explain the difference between these sympathetic and parasympathetic dominances is with the classic fable "The Tortoise and the Hare." The sympathetic-dominant hare can run himself into the ground, while the parasympathetic-dominant tortoise takes a while to get going but is persistent until the end. But unlike in the story, the hare doesn't have to lose every time if his preparation and recovery are tailored effectively.

For more on how to get the most from tortoises and hares, see the chart at right.

SYMPATHETIC DOMINANCE

7.12.1.1

Sympathetic-dominant athletes are driven, highly motivated, and often irritable. They are more likely to use stimulants to maintain the feeling of high energy that they crave, and they find it difficult to wind down and fall asleep, particularly after the exhilaration of a game. They often crave sugary foods because of the short-term buzz they create. As they can be prone to sudden muscle strains, when warming up, they benefit from slower, more rhythmic movements to help them move to a less hypertonic state before being active at full speed. Sympathetic-dominant players tend to push very hard, but they

are also more likely to develop issues that come to a head with muscle tears or sudden injury. They can be more prone to muscle strains partly due to their strength and power, but again, not exclusively. Sympathetic-dominant players often hate long, slow training because of their inherent makeup. But aerobic development can increase their endurance using interval work such as Tabata sessions or other types of intermittent, high-intensity workouts.

PARASYMPATHETIC DOMINANCE

7.12.1.2

In contrast, parasympathetic-dominant athletes often appear more laid-back and more inclined to rhythmic activity. They typically need more motivation from coaches or other external sources. Unlike their sympathetic-dominant teammates, those on the parasympathetic end of the scale find it easy to switch off and fall asleep. However, they sometimes find it difficult to get going in the morning. Such athletes need a more intense warm-up to increase their excitability and stimulate their bodies so they're ready for practice or competition. They can be more susceptible to Achilles tendon injuries or groin strains. Typically, they can keep going longer than their sympathetic-dominant teammates, but as a result they sometimes grind themselves down. When this happens, it takes them longer to recover from the fast burnout that sympathetic-dominant players often experience. Parasympathetic-dominant athletes are often averse to super-intense sessions, so the coaching staff needs to improve their conditioning with longer duration work.

THE TRUTH ABOUT HRV

7.12.2

There is always a search for a tool or method to understand the level of stress people are under. In recent years, heart rate variability (HRV) has become a widely misused and misunderstood tool for evaluating the autonomic nervous system (ANS) and assessing the functional state of athletes on a daily basis. HRV is, very simply, the variation in time between heartbeats. Although the exploration of biological cybernetics is still in its infancy, obtaining biomarkers like HRV through physical tests can start

MANAGING PSYCHOPHYSIOLOGICAL DOMINANCE		SYMPATHETIC-DOMINANT ATHLETES	PARASYMPATHETIC-DOMINANT ATHLETES
	NUTRITIONAL	Stimulate appetite through alkaline foods (fruit, fresh vegetables) Avoid stimulating substances (coffee, energy drinks) High-density quality foods Snack when needed Low carbs, especially fast carbohydrates Avoid alcohol, caffiene, juices, sugars 70% proteins and fats 30% carbs Avoid large meals to manage blood glucose	Favor acidifying foods (cheese, meat, cake, eggs) Eat protein at most meals Lower fat, lower protein Balanced carb intake Limit fats & oils Easy on nuts & seeds 40% proteins & fats 60% carbs
	ACTIVITY	Slow movements Benefits from relaxing activity	Physical activity
	VISION	Lower levels of light or darkness Relaxing lights and colors Avoid stimulating colors	Bright natural light Stimulating images and colors
	SOUND	Relaxing soft music White noise (e.g., background fan)	Use of intermittent noises Uplifting, energetic music
	TEMPERATURE	Warm bath with essential oils or lavender	Non-humid, comfortable temperature, around 72–75°F (22–24°C)
	SLEEP	Comfortable but cool environment at night to promote sleep Newly made bed, no creases Soft fabrics, e.g., silk	Comfortable temperature at home
	HERBAL TEAS/INFUSIONS	Lavender Rose Floral Valerian root	Eucalyptus Peppermint Cayenne Ginseng
	TRAINING	Benefits from slower steady-state activity No intermittent work Aerobic training suppresses insulin production Avoid maximal training intensities where unnecessary Maximal training intensities increase the insulin response	Benefits from stimulating activity May need longer to activate CNS Power activities preferred
	TACTILE	Relaxing, soft touch	Any intermittent tactile stimulus
	MANUAL THERAPY	Relaxing massage	Intensive massage Active movements
	RECOVERY	Floating in water No sauna Cold showers in the morning, brisk toweling Light and rhythmical exercises	
	BATH	Essential-oil-fragranced bath Lavender Long warm bath	Peppermint Eucalyptus
	SHOWER	Cold showers in the morning	Contrast: alternate hot and cold showers Sauna at medium temperature alternated with cold showers
	SUPPLEMENTATION	B vitamins L-glutamine Melatonin (If trouble getting to sleep)	B vitamins
	STIMULATES	Potassium	Phosporus Calcium
	INHIBITS	Magnesium	
	CLIMATE THERAPY	Moderate ultraviolet irradiation Avoid intense sun	Sea and sea-level altitude optimal Preferred bracing climate

to inform how each player's individualized training and recovery are managed within the morphological programming approach.

THE HOLISTIC THERMOMETER   7.12.2.1

Though it is not the only valuable figure, HRV provides a window for looking into the teeter-totter balancing act between the fight-or-flight and rest-and-digest states of the ANS. In 1963, two researchers, Edward Hon and Stanley Lee, discovered that big changes in RR intervals—the distance between the peaks on an ECG/EKG—preceded fetal death, which brought HRV some media attention in the West.[50] However, Eastern medicine practitioners have focused on the pulse for hundreds of years as they evaluate patients' internal balance. Such assessment was termed "pulse diagnosis" in the foundational text *Mai Ching,* which identified twenty-four different types of pulses. Its author, Wang Shuhe, recognized the negative impact that a poor diet and excessive alcohol consumption can have on the heart and its rhythm. He was also among the first people to realize that there must be some variability in heart rate if a patient is healthy.

When Soviet cosmonaut Yuri Gagarin became the first person to enter outer space, his ship transmitted his breathing rate and electrocardiogram data back to Russian scientists in real time. By measuring these, the Soviets were able to make deductions about the impact of space travel on the heart. It was only natural that this technique would one day make its way to another area of human performance: team sports.

THE DRUMBEAT AND
RHYTHM OF THE BODY   7.12.2.2

HRV measures the beat-to-beat changes of acceleration and deceleration of the heart pump. While greater variability suggests that the parasympathetic response is adequate for adaptation to training stressors, low variability can indicate that an athlete is overtraining, underrecovering, or both. This subject has been simplified here, but it is a critical aspect of human physiology.

If an athlete's preparation isn't systemic, deliberate, and balanced—qualities of the morphological programming approach—then HRV readings can potentially highlight imbalance and excessive training stress. For example, if a player lifted heavy and fast five days in a row or just did interval training all week, the HRV score would likely indicate that the ANS balance was tipped in favor of the sympathetic nervous system activity for quite some time afterward.

Simply put, more variation indicates strong parasympathetic activity while less variation suggests that the sympathetic response is overly dominant.

But even beyond this, we can look closer at the distributions and patterns within the variability again. For example, *high-frequency (HF)* power is associated with the vagal/parasympathetic system, and *low-frequency (LF)* power is associated with both sympathetic and parasympathetic components. The ratio of low- to high-frequency power can suggest relative dominance of either component of the autonomic nervous system: a higher ratio indicates increased sympathetic activity or reduced parasympathetic activity. *Very low frequency (VLF)* power is believed to be influenced by thermoregulation, negative emotions, and the sympathetic response. *Ultra low frequency (ULF)* power typically varies between day and night, and total power reflects the power in all the bands for the twenty-four-hour period and includes ULF, VLF, LF, and HF. A very high *total-power* figure is associated with a greater risk of death from heart attack.

The proper use of HRV in team sports deserves a far more complex treatment than I can give it here, but suffice it to say for now that the majority of writings used by performance specialists are widely inaccurate in their application.

One reason is that HRV is an excellent indicator of stress on the organism but a poor identifier of the exact nature or source of the stress. High HRV, for example, has also been shown to correlate with high VO_2 max output capacity. There also seems to be a

		SYMPATHETIC-DOMINANT ATHLETES	PARASYMPATHETIC-DOMINANT ATHLETES
GUIDELINES TO CORRECT DOMINANCE	STRUCTURAL	Angular face structure	Round face & skull
		Tall & thin	Short, wider build
		Tend to be more explosive athletes	Tend to be more endurance athletes
	PHYSIOLOGICAL	Low or relatively weak appetite	Excessive appetite
		Tendency toward indigestion	Diarrhea
		Tendency toward heartburn	Allergies
		Tendency to sweat a lot	Low blood sugar
		Tendency toward insomnia	Irregular heartbeat
		Tendency toward hypertension	Chronic fatigue
		High blood pressure	Cold sores
		Higher blood sugar	
		Predisposed to infection	
		More frequent bowel movements	
		Adrenal gland dysfunction	
		Cortisol output may rise to abnormal levels	
		Cortisol may cause catabolism	
		High cortisol may also increase insulin levels	
	PSYCHOLOGICAL	Type A personality	Lethargy
		Excellent concentration	Procrastination
		Highly motivated	Slow to anger
		Cool emotionally	Deliberate, cautious
		Irritable	Warm emotionally
		Hyperactive	Outgoing
		Socially withdrawn	
		Tend to wake in the middle of the night	
		Difficulty returning to sleep	
		Elevated cortisol lowers testosterone	
		Elevated cortisol lowers DHEA	
		Prone to anxiety and panic	
	CHEMISTRY	Acidic	Alkaline
	PHYSICAL	High muscle tone	Low muscle tone
		Predisposition to sudden soft-tissue injury	Insidious muscle injury
		Soft-tissue injury	More likely to develop tendon injury
		Variable energy pattern	Can struggle to develop energy at start
		Problem with weight management	Greater need for activation work
		Benefits from longer warm-up	Benefits from proprioceptive warm-up
		Benefits from mobility-inhibition work	May need longer priming period
		Greater tendency to expend energy	May suffer from fatigue
		Hand-eye coordination may deteriorate	
	NUTRITIONAL	Sweet tendency	Slow oxidizer
		Caffiene dependency	Low protein
		Fast oxidizer	Light, lean proteins
		High protein	Low fats & oils
		High fats & oils	Higher fast carbs
		Low fast carbs	

7 Player Principles

relationship between ANS balance and hormone levels. Athletes with low HRV have been shown to have high levels of the stress hormone cortisol and lower testosterone levels. In contrast, athletes with high HRV scores often have higher testosterone and lower cortisol measurements. This suggests that an overactive sympathetic nervous system and underactive parasympathetic response is also related to chronic inflammation (a result of high cortisol) and inadequate muscle growth and recovery (a result of low testosterone).[51] The existence of so many correlations proves HRV is useful but imprecise.

PROMOTING PARASYMPATHETIC RECOVERY
7.12.3

Despite the limitations of HRV analysis, we know that promoting parasympathetic response and dominance leads to longer lives and better health, largely through improving recovery and stress management.

The two fastest techniques to promote parasympathetic activation are slow, controlled breathing and cold water immersion (of the face or body). Another technique is maximizing quality sleep by blocking the stimuli of light and sound and setting the room temperature to between 58 and 65 degrees. In the absence of sleep, a relaxing activity such as reading or meditation can also be helpful. Athletes can also try combining exposure to hot and cold and avoiding exposure to things that will excite the senses, such as loud music and anything on a screen in the two hours before bedtime. During the day, they can also take naps when time allows. It's advisable to avoid prolonged exercise when it's very hot outside and to ensure adequate hydration before, during, and after training.

If the heartbeat gets as steady as the pecking of the woodpecker or as the raindrops on the roof, the patient is going to die within four days.

—Wang Shuhe

OVERTRAINING, UNDERRECOVERING, AND CENTRAL NERVOUS SYSTEM FATIGUE
7.12.4

While it's a positive development that many sports teams have moved away from the "junk" mileage approach and are now recognizing that they need to train at game speed or above to compete at their best, the pendulum has swung too far for some. Now, the challenge isn't grappling with the "more is better" fallacy but rather with the mindset that you need to go hard and fast all the time.

Putting team-sports athletes through too many high-intensity, high-velocity (and sometimes high-contact/collision, too) sessions in a training morphocycle can increase the risk of injury because the structural-anatomical system can't repair the muscles and soft tissues adequately before they are stressed again. Similarly, loading up on this type of training tilts the parasympathetic-sympathetic balance toward a continual fight-or-flight state of heightened awareness, which further impedes recovery.

Inflammation levels then skyrocket due to chronically high cortisol levels, leading to depleted immune function, which can make athletes more susceptible to illness and infection. The biotransformational system is also inhibited, so they don't process food or waste products as effectively, which in turn contributes to suboptimal recovery. Production and balance of hormones and neurotransmitters like serotonin and melatonin are also thrown off, which can cause depression and emotional instability, as well as disrupt the sleep that's so vital to adaptation and performance. Round and round the cycle goes, until the athlete is a physical wreck.

Different types of training stress the body's main systems to varying degrees, and each system has its own unique recovery timeline. The central nervous system (CNS) has one of the longest restoration periods, and after a high-intensity, high-velocity session that requires a lot of large muscle recruitment or high nervous system demand—such as Olympic lifting, all-out sprints, or a long and difficult test like the

SAT or ACT—it can take up to seventy-two hours for the CNS to not only adapt to the stimulus but also be ready for the next one. So another result of overdoing high-intensity, high-velocity training without adequate recovery is CNS fatigue. This is not a one-time phenomenon but rather a condition caused by the accumulated load resulting from athletes hitting the redline for their nervous macro system over and over again.

UNDERMINING TRAINING ADAPTATIONS   7.12.4.1

For the CNS to function well, it needs high-quality information input, which is governed by receptor cells that take in data and neurotransmitters that send it shooting to the brain, like one of those vacuum tubes at your bank's drive-through. When the CNS is exposed to a high degree of stress and isn't allowed to recuperate before the next exposure, both the collection and sending of this data is compromised, as neurons and the sites that produce neurotransmitters are impaired. If the CNS isn't getting good data from the peripheral nervous system, it's not going to make good or rapid decisions, which means that in the next game or training session, that athlete is going to feel cognitively and physically sluggish. CNS fatigue also means that athletes' power output, muscle recruitment ability, and reaction time will be reduced and, due to metabolism disruption, their energy substrate systems will be far less efficient at making fuel available.[52]

In terms of the training and team-preparation environment, athletes whose CNS is fatigued will have lower-quality learning experiences, and their ability to send these from short-term to long-term memory and reinforce positive movement pathways will be diminished. On the physical side, a reduction in growth hormone production resulting from CNS fatigue means that muscles won't repair themselves and grow as they should.

CNS fatigue and the other body system maladaptations associated with going too hard, too fast, and too often are among the reasons it's imperative that we improve the load balancing in our team athlete programming. The morphological programming approach helps ensure that the CNS is stimulated adequately by high-velocity, high-intensity training to produce the desired adaptation while providing enough time for this vital system and interconnected system families to recover fully before the next stimulus.

In addition to limiting the number of CNS-taxing sessions and sequencing these with work that stimulates other systems to allow the nervous macro system to bounce back, it's sensible to ensure the quality of the high-intensity workouts. Rather than prescribe a certain volume of work, like ten sets of one minute fast, one minute slow on the rowing machine, the athlete should stop once speed or intensity declines or form deteriorates. At this point, the athlete has been subjected to at least the minimum required dose to stimulate adaptation, and any further work will lead to a diminishing return—not to mention, given the extreme demands of the session, a greater likelihood of injury.

A more balanced approach to CNS stimulation and recovery not only safeguards this system but also encourages better function by the biotransformational, parasympathetic, cortisol-immune, and pituitary-adrenal systems, and other systems that contribute to adaptation and, most importantly, overall athlete health.

THE ALCOHOL DISADVANTAGE   7.12.4.2

Another way to ensure that the nervous macro system is healthy is to limit environmental and lifestyle factors that can further compromise CNS, PNS, and ANS function. I'm not suggesting that athletes never have a drink again, but drinking alcohol can do far more damage than just making overindulgent players feel terrible the next day.

In the short term, alcohol impacts the CNS by reducing excitatory neurotransmitters while increasing inhibitory neurotransmitter activity. Alcohol can also interfere with muscle growth and repair in several ways, including reducing production of testosterone and other growth-promoting hormones and increasing production of estrogen.[53] It can also prevent the brain from making changes that should result from training and game-related learning expe-

TECHNO-TACTICAL / PSYCHOPHYSICAL DEMANDS ON ATHLETES

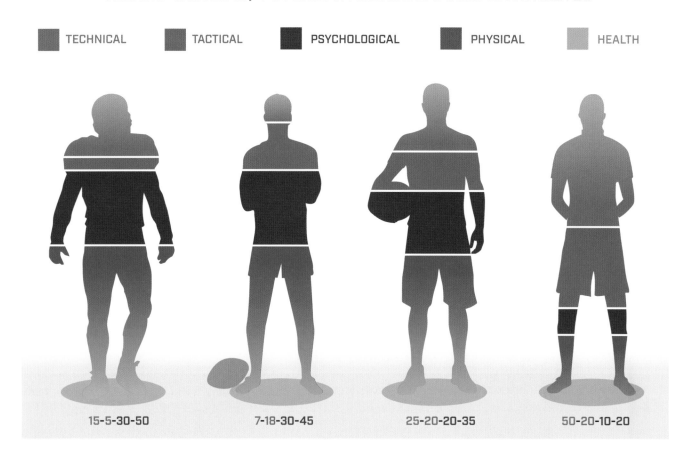

■ TECHNICAL   ■ TACTICAL   ■ PSYCHOLOGICAL   ■ PHYSICAL   ■ HEALTH

15-5-30-50   7-18-30-45   25-20-20-35   50-20-10-20

THE OUTCOMES OF DIFFERENT SPORTING GAMES ARE DETERMINED TO VARYING DEGREES BY THE TECHNICAL, TACTICAL, PHYSICAL, AND PSYCHOLOGICAL COMPONENTS.

riences. And, while the brain is telling you you're happy because alcohol stimulates the release of dopamine, production of emotion-governing hormones is actually being disrupted.[54]

Long-term intake of too much alcohol can more dramatically increase levels of the inhibitory neurotransmitter gamma-aminobutyricacid (GABA), leading to the athlete being less alert and engaged during training and competition. This effect is exaggerated even more because alcohol impedes the release of the excitatory neurotransmitter glutamate. Athletes' reaction times can be reduced, as their receptors become less efficient in sending information to the brain and the brain becomes slower in sending instructions back to the peripheral nervous system.

Over time, drinking can also decrease the activity of adenosine, which plays a vital part in energy transfer and contributes to restful sleep and heart function.[55] It also limits the production of serotonin, which can lead to depression, and profoundly affects the cerebellum, the part of the brain responsible for movement and balance.[56]

To avoid such consequences, athletes should try to stick to low levels of alcohol—typically defined as two drinks or fewer per day—particularly in the hours immediately following training and games, when drinking can lead to dehydration, disrupted sleep, and reduced glycogen replenishment.

THE PERFORMANCE PROFILE

The single greatest difference between my approach and others is that I care about the person first, player second, and athlete last. Most coaches prioritize these parts of a player in reverse and structure team preparation and how they approach athlete health accordingly. But this shortchanges individual learning and development and limits the short- and long-term potential of the entire team. An isolated approach is fundamentally flawed because it fails to respect the complexity of player and team preparation and creates training scenarios that have limited application in competition. Rather than continuing to pursue a reductionist approach, we need to recognize that during every single event that occurs during a team-sports game, the four coactives must coincide.

THE FOUR-COACTIVE PROFILE

When it comes to preparing athletes to compete, the four coactives give us a way to assess each session in the morphocycle and balance it, while we also take the morphological programming profile into account. When it comes to evaluating individual and team performance on the field, we can layer the four coactives over each of the four game moments—offensive, defensive, transition-to-defense, and transition-to-offense—to evaluate how well the game plan objectives are being met in each phase of the game. We can then use the model to identify dominant qualities that need to be maximized and limiting factors that the coaching staff must work on with each player before the next game. Such an assessment can be applied to the opposition, too.

TECHNO-TACTICAL

Assessment of any given player in a team sport involves a complex system. The intervening elements are not only numerous but also interactive. The oppositional relationship between teams varies in different situations or even within a single situation. Every play in a territorial game involves interactions between teammates and opponents, and the player takes these into account in a split second before making the next move.

The members of a team are interdependent, so we need to evaluate individual performance within the team context.[57] Perceptual and motor skills, strategy, tactics, and the overarching Commander's Intent factor into how a player makes decisions and acts in any given situation, which is why we often look at the technical and tactical coactives together. For any player, a combination of skills, prior experiences, and instantaneous evaluation of the specific situation will impact what the athlete picks from their motor program toolbox. Before deciding how to act, the player also considers how each potential application of technical skill fits within the tactics for that particular game.[58]

Technical: In its everyday sense, the term *skill* simply means a technique like shooting, passing, or dribbling. But for our purposes, a skill is a movement on or off the ball that is executed in the context of the game—thus taking tactical considerations into account. Technical ability cannot be assessed or considered outside of a tactical context.

Tactical: Similarly, the phrase *tactical awareness* has traditionally meant how well players grasp the team's tactics and their role within them. But really, tactical awareness involves solving the problems that arise during a game by applying the appropriate skills—thus taking technical considerations into account.[59]

TECHNO-TACTICAL / PSYCHOPHYSICAL POTENTIAL

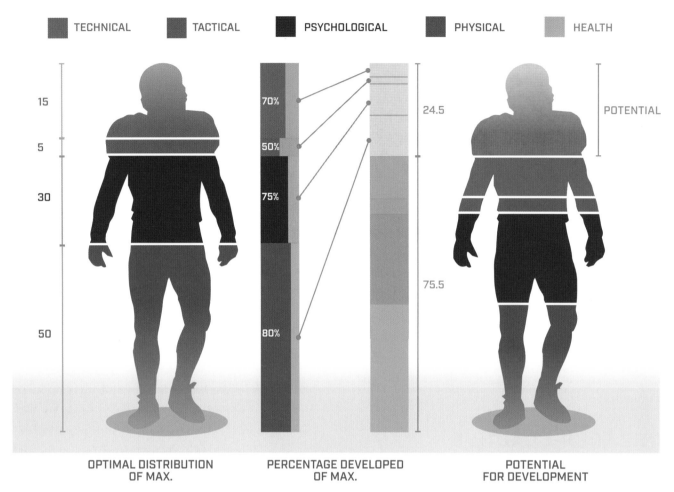

■ TECHNICAL   ■ TACTICAL   ■ PSYCHOLOGICAL   ■ PHYSICAL   ■ HEALTH

OPTIMAL DISTRIBUTION
OF MAX.

PERCENTAGE DEVELOPED
OF MAX.

POTENTIAL
FOR DEVELOPMENT

THESE ARE SUGGESTED DISTRIBUTIONS OF CAPABILITIES, BUT THEY ARE ALSO POTENTIALS—
EVEN WITHIN THESE MODELS, EACH COMPONENT MUST BE MAXIMIZED THROUGH CORRECT TRAINING.

PSYCHOPHYSICAL   7.13.3

As we've discussed in exploring the interdependent relationship between the various bodily systems, the body and brain are one. We cannot put psychology in one box and physiology in another, because they are fundamentally intertwined. There are even certain medical fields, like neurogastroenterology, that look at specific ways that the brain interacts with a bodily system (in this case, the digestive system). This is why we often combine two of the coactives—physical and psychological—into the single term *psychophysical.*

If athletes are to perform at their best, they don't just need the required strength, speed, power, and other physical qualities for their sport and position. They must also be cognitively engaged, in a good place spiritually, balanced psychologically, and able to handle the pressure that the game brings. On the flip side, it's not enough for a player to be psychologically prepared if they're not also physically ready to play. The four-coactive model gives us a way to evaluate players' physiology and psychology and how these coactives are managed during team preparation and manifest themselves during competition.

EIGHT

THE COMPARISON MODEL

It doesn't matter what the sport or level of play is. The five components of the diagram on page 211—tactical, technical, physical, psychological, and health—are common to all athletes, and to people in general. Health is at the center because preserving it is the only way to obtain sustainable success over the long term. The healthier the athlete, the higher loads of physical and psychological stress they will be able to deal with and respond to positively.

While I've chosen to represent technical, tactical, physical, and psychological abilities with distinct zones, the lines between them shouldn't be thought of as immovable walls. They are, rather, interconnected. Also, the degree to which any player applies any element has a certain range and can vary from practice to practice and game to game. Similarly, while there is a baseline of athlete health, a disruption to one or more of the primary health systems—such as if the athlete has a cold or is coming back from injury—can change the health parameters and their impact on performance on any given day.

THE PLAYER COMPARISON

8.1

One of the great misconceptions in sports is the idea that only one method or system can succeed. Greatness can be achieved through many different combinations of technical, tactical, physical, and psychological qualities. The 2015 NFL season had three exceptional quarterbacks on display: Cam Newton, Peyton Manning, and perhaps the greatest quarterback in the history of the game, Tom Brady. The three have many similarities but also many differences.

When comparing Tom Brady's profile to Peyton Manning's, we find many similarities in terms of how they execute the game. Unlike Newton, neither is renowned for his athleticism. We all have seen the YouTube clips of Brady's NFL Combine performance, though this says as much or more about the limitations of this assessment as it does about his physical qualities. But despite their comparatively limited physical gifts, Brady and Manning both have exceptional technical ability and wonderful tactical and game management acumen. Their greatest strength, however, is their determination and psychological calmness under pressure, something Cam Newton has been accused of lacking, for now. Of course, many years in the game and at the elite level helps develop this.

The major difference between Brady and Manning has been Brady's consistently good health, which has enabled him to be more productive on the field, so that he can apply his technical, tactical, physical, and psychological gifts consistently. Yes, Manning's team won the Super Bowl in his final season, but his overall level of play no longer reached the same pinnacle as his archrival's or measured up to the standard he had set earlier in his career. Brady has an almost religious commitment to health and lifestyle that has allowed him to remain at a competitive peak for many years. Cam Newton, like Brady, is committed to a healthy lifestyle, but he also has physical gifts that may exceed those of both Brady and Manning, whose experiences and psychological strengths have enabled them to be prolific for more than a decade.

Brady and Manning overcame their limiting physical factors—and, in the twilight of Manning's career, his health issues—with superior technical and tactical abilities. In Manning's case, he proved to be an expert compensator. As Newton continues to amass more experience and develop technically and tactically, he could reach or even exceed the heights that his two illustrious fellow quarterbacks have scaled—but until that happens, it's simply potential. It could be argued that for now, his limiting factor is mental toughness. If he maintains his physical ability and continues to develop psychological resilience, Newton could one day be considered one of the greatest quarterbacks ever to take the field.

This is just one example of how players can be classified and profiled. Four-coactive profiles of each player allows them to be better integrated into the team—or so you can be better prepared to face them as an opponent.

GAME & POSITIONAL PROFILING

8.2

We need to take into account that every sport has different coactive requirements depending on the nature of the game. This isn't the end of the story, though, as the emphasis on each of the four coactives varies by position, too. While there can be a range for each area within this context—for example, soccer forwards Jamie Vardy and Romelu Lukaku are both successful despite having very different coactive makeups, as are basketball point guards Damian Lillard and Giannis Antetokounmpo—there are still baselines for technical, tactical, physical, and psychological elements in each position.

So, for example, a point guard in basketball must be the most cerebral player on his team and have a rock-solid tactical grasp of the playbook and the game plan. The same goes for a quarterback in football. In contrast, centers and power forwards in basketball and linemen in football generally need to be extremely physically dominant. So when evaluating a player's limiting factors and dominant qualities during a game, it's important to keep the additional context of their position in mind.

But from a scouting perspective, there's a clear identity to a position that indicates if it relies more or less on tactical or technical ability or on aspects of a physical coactive, such as strength or power.

By now, you've surely noted that I haven't given measurements or definitive figures for qualities for any coactive. This is because it is impossible to do so. When we don't know or can't agree on the exact qualities or even the weighting of each, it's impossible to formulate it from the general heuristics I present here.

Profiling and Limiting Factors

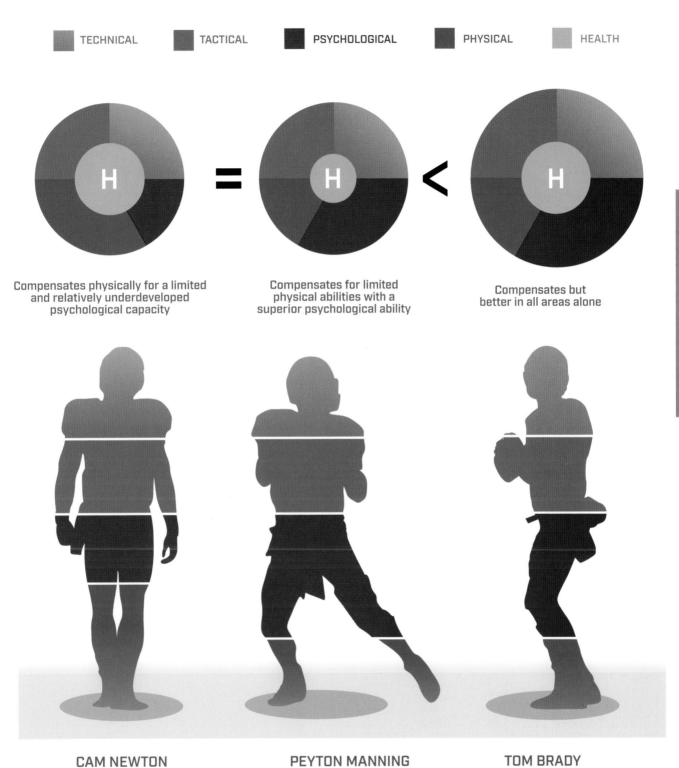

TECHNICAL	TACTICAL	PSYCHOLOGICAL	PHYSICAL	HEALTH

Compensates physically for a limited and relatively underdeveloped psychological capacity

Compensates for limited physical abilities with a superior psychological ability

Compensates but better in all areas alone

CAM NEWTON

PEYTON MANNING

TOM BRADY

8 The Comparison Model

The health of each player is a significant determinant in the resiliency and length of the career each. As we see above, they can all achieve (varying levels of) greatness, but they have different strengths, which determine the manner or method they use to achieve this. The only caveat is that strengths cannot be at the extreme expense of other capabilities and reduce them below a functional minimum. Finally, even though two quarterbacks can achieve similar outcomes with similar profiles, some, like Tom Brady, just do it better than everyone else.

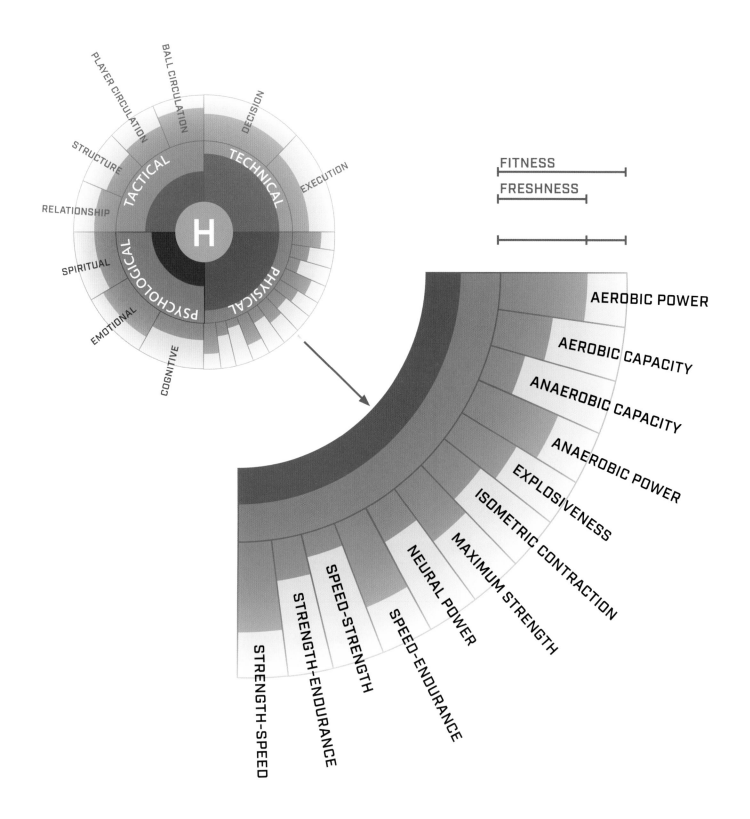

The techno-tactical, psychophysical model and readiness.

NINE

READY FOR GAME DAY

Now let's look at what it takes to get individual players and the team as a whole ready for game day. We'll explore how to evaluate and balance the total load of training and the game itself, the differences between readiness and preparedness, and the vital importance of long-term health superseding individual performances.

READINESS, PREPAREDNESS, AND POTENTIAL

9.1

When we think about getting an athlete ready for game day, we have to look at three areas: readiness, preparedness, and potential. The terms *readiness* and *preparedness* are often used interchangeably in team sports, but in reality there are distinct differences. We also can't ignore how they relate to performance potential on game day.

Readiness refers to a player's physical and psychological state. This takes into account not only what happened during training and education sessions in the week prior to the game—including how well an athlete has recovered from the cumulative load experienced during previous games and the training sessions in the preceding morphocycle—but also recovery from injury and what's going on when the athlete

is not at the practice facilities. Environmental factors, such as family conflict, lack of sleep, or illness, can take a heavy toll on performance, so it's important that the coaching staff is aware of these external issues. Recovery is largely dependent on the athlete's health, which rests on how optimally his or her main health systems are functioning. Nature (DNA) and nurture (environment) both contribute to the health of these systems.

In the context of getting ready for game day, *preparedness* refers to an athlete's grasp of the technical and tactical elements that the coaching staff has covered between games and how physically able a player is to perform at any given time. It's vital that the players have not only learned from their training experiences but can also relate them to the team's core principles and game plan objectives. The level of physical preparedness hinges on how well the team has created and balanced stimuli to prompt adaptations in the body's various systems and how well the player has responded to these stimuli.

An athlete's *potential* to perform in a game is determined by the combination of their readiness and preparedness going into it.

The graph on page 214 shows the relationship between readiness and preparedness as it relates to the season. The goal is for every squad member to be at a high level in both categories right before each game.

PREPAREDNESS VS READINESS

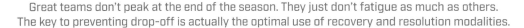

Great teams don't peak at the end of the season. They just don't fatigue as much as others.
The key to preventing drop-off is actually the optimal use of recovery and resolution modalities.

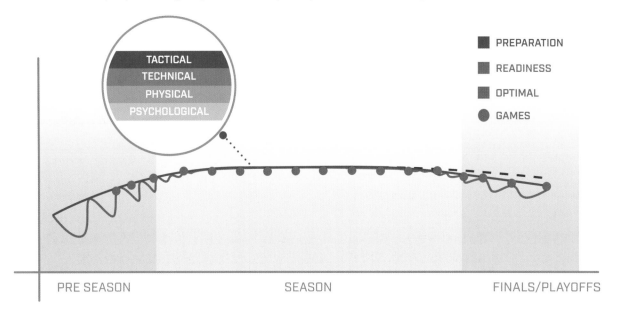

TACTICAL
TECHNICAL
PHYSICAL
PSYCHOLOGICAL

■ PREPARATION
■ READINESS
■ OPTIMAL
● GAMES

PRE SEASON   SEASON   FINALS/PLAYOFFS

UNSUSTAINABLE PREPARATION   9.1.1

Athletes can train hard for a few weeks and see great improvements in physical composition, such as increased muscle mass or reduced body fat and/or weight. Athletes can also get faster and stronger and improve their endurance with a rigorous, intensive exercise regimen. But if the stressors become too great or the athlete doesn't have the foundational health to deal with them, eventually the athlete's body will say enough is enough.

Yes, if you remove the training stimuli, the player will start to backslide in terms of performance (the fear of many coaches at all levels who've been taught that more is better), but if you keep the pedal pushed to the floor, the athlete will not only stop adapting to the stress but also start exhibiting signs of maladaptation. From a cognitive standpoint, he or she will

not develop lasting habits, and this full-bore training cycle may well have stunted the athlete's technical and tactical development.

Inflammation levels will skyrocket because the body is being told to remain on high alert at all times, and injuries will eventually start to creep in. That's why we can't take such a shortsighted, short-term view of training or performance goals for athletes—otherwise we're robbing Peter to pay Paul, and there will be a reckoning in time. If such an approach is extended to an entire team, game-day performance will suffer, as the players will be physically, mentally, and emotionally exhausted by the time they take the field.

Instead, we need to keep in mind an athlete's long-term health when applying the morphological programming and four-coactive approaches to individual and team preparation.

HEALTH >
PERFORMANCE   9.1.2

In the past decade, we've taken giant strides in player performance. The proliferation of information on the internet and across social media has given previously obscure experts the opportunity to share their knowledge with the masses. Such expertise was once confined to hard-to-find, outrageously expensive textbooks or courses at cutting-edge universities but now is readily available to anyone with a web browser.

This accessibility has led to significant advances in team and individual preparation and performance. But all too often, this pursuit has led people to ignore or minimize a simple fact: health has to come before performance. One of the best historical examples is that of the first recorded marathon, in which Pheidippides ran from—you guessed it—Marathon to Athens in 490 BC. The intrepid runner met his performance goal and fulfilled his game plan objective of sharing the news of the Greek army's victory over the Persians. That's the good part. The not-so-good part? He dropped dead immediately afterward.

This is obviously an extreme example, but the lesson still holds true for today's elite athletes. While an athlete's reaching or exceeding individual performance aims and helping the team achieve its goals is fantastic in one sense, it's completely undermined if this athlete is ruined in the process. At all levels of team sports, performance must take a backseat to health. This is essential not only for athletes to have long and productive careers but also for them to live full lives off the field. From a group perspective, the organization will achieve season-to-season success only if most of its players remain healthy.

THE COACH IS
HUMAN, TOO   9.1.3

All the principles we're applying to athlete health also apply to the coaching staff and to every other member of the organization. Though it's undoubtedly rewarding, coaching has to be one of the most demanding professions, not just physically but also cognitively, emotionally, and spiritually. If you were asked to conjure an image of a coach during a game, you'd likely come up with a man or woman either anxiously pacing the touchline or red-faced and yelling like Bobby Knight. But whether a coach displays explosive emotion or sits stoically on the bench, let's not underestimate the difficulty of what coaches are called upon to do.

I'll focus more on the coaching staff in the next section, but suffice it to say for now that if the coaches, and particularly the head coach, aren't living healthy and balanced lives, the potential and long-term success of the team are going to be limited. Simply put, coaches are high performers, too. If a coach isn't fueling well and resting enough, he or she isn't going to create the quality learning experiences that their players need to improve. On game day, a coach's ability to make on-the-spot tactical adjustments and substitutions that can tip the balance between victory and defeat depends on that coach having an adequate functional reserve.

Also, if a head coach who is trying to instill a culture of health doesn't buy into it personally, he or she will undermine the entire initiative. So if a smoothie bar is introduced and the coaching staff makes fun of it, they can do more damage than they would just by failing to start eating better themselves. If you're a coach, try to take a good hard look at your overall health, and if it's lacking in any area, try to address it, for your own good and the good of your team.

PREPARATION AND
PERFORMANCE
QUALITIES

9.2

Here we're going to look at the significance of what the coaching staff members say to each other and the players and how they say it. We will also examine the roles of the back-office staff, the interplay between constraints and synergy, and the importance of getting past looking at athletes as merely disposable commodities.

THE LANGUAGE OF ROLES

As the average size of teams' back-office staff has grown, the number of specialist staff members assigned to each of the four coactives has increased accordingly. Their backgrounds, educations, and experiences in sports often vary greatly and give them different frames of reference. One of the main issues with these disparities is that each discipline has its own language for describing athlete qualities and how they manifest themselves on game day. As quantum physicist Richard Feynman put it, "The real problem in speech is not *precise* language. The problem is *clear* language.…It is only needed to be precise when there is some doubt as to the meaning of a phrase, and then the precision should be put in the place where the doubt exists."[60]

So, to put what Feynman is saying into a team-sports setting, a strength and conditioning coach might talk about a running back's "explosiveness," while the head coach and running back coach say that he is "quick off the line." The speed coach refers to "starting speed." They're all saying the same thing, but the fact that they're doing it in different ways makes it difficult to assess athlete performance during a game and then get every specialist on the same page about how to remedy issues before the next contest. The key is the terms that the head coach and assistants use, as these will dictate the message that is communicated most consistently to the players.

ANALYSIS AND IDENTIFICATION

For a back-office staff to implement the morphocycle correctly and cohesively, they have to speak the same language. It's a good idea for everyone to get around a big conference table before the season starts and define how the staff as a whole is going to label and describe each player quality. This isn't rele-vant just to physical attributes but must also encompass psychological, technical, and tactical elements. Once terminology and usage are nailed down, the staff can identify exercises, drills, and games that can be used to develop players' limiting factors after they've been identified.

CONSTRAINTS THEORY AND SYNERGY

After outlining how to talk about certain qualities and how they become apparent during the game, the next step is to find the main constraint that is limiting each player and construct learning experiences that help players overcome these limitations (for more on this, turn back to "The Macro Principle of Limiting Factors" on page 189). Then you have to test these factors in the only way that matters: the game. This approach has its roots in manufacturing and specifically in Eliyahu Goldratt's theory of constraints, in which a factory worker tries to find the thing that's slowing down the assembly line, changes it, and then sees if the line starts moving more efficiently.

It's vital that you try to identify and work on only one constraint—one limiting factor—per athlete at a time. To use another analogy, a computer programmer who is having trouble with a software program that's running too slowly will change one piece of code and then plug it back in to see if the program runs faster. It would be no use to change three or four code elements and then plug them back into the program, as the programmer wouldn't be able to tell which fix made the difference. (And worse, one of the other changes could introduce a new problem.) It's the same with players' limiting factors and game-day performance.

THE ATHLETE IS A PERSON FIRST   9.2.4

In this section, we've explored why it's necessary to look beyond physical capabilities, which have been the chief obsession of the sports world. When developing athletes, we also need to consider the technical, tactical, and psychological coactives. In addition, we examined the crucial role that environment has in shaping players as athletes and people. While we're on the topic of personhood, I hope I've also convinced you that in order to fulfill our duty to all players, we need to treat them as valuable human beings first and athletes second. There's no point in trying to assess and develop the four coactives without first ensuring that there's a solid foundation of overall health and well-being.

In the next section, we'll look at how we can plug principles for sustainable athlete development into a holistic team preparation model.

By processing information from the environment through the senses, the nervous system continually evaluates risk. I have coined the term neuroception to describe how neural circuits distinguish whether situations or people are safe, dangerous, or life-threatening. Because of our heritage as a species, neuroception takes place in primitive parts of the brain, without our conscious awareness.

—Stephen W. Porges

9 Ready for Game Day

4 THE FOUR-COACTIVE MODEL

1 David A. Shearer et al., "Measuring Recovery in Elite Rugby Players: The Brief Assessment of Mood, Endocrine Changes, and Power," *Research Quarterly for Exercise and Sport* 86, no. 4 (2015): 379–386.

2 John Wooden and Don Yaeger, *A Game Plan for Life: The Power of Mentoring* (New York: Bloomsbury USA, 2009), 23.

3 Lynn Kidman and Stephanie J. Hanrahan, *The Coaching Process* (New York: Routledge, 2011), 83.

4 "The Rooney Files: An Interview with Wayne Rooney," n.d., www.manchester.com/sport/united/rooney-interview.php.

5 THE TEAM-SPORT ATHLETE

5 Yannis Pitsiladis et al., "Genomics of Elite Sporting Performance: What Little We Know and Necessary Advances," *British Journal of Sports Medicine* 47, no. 9 (2013): 550–555; Nir Eynon et al., "Genes for Elite Power and Sprint Performance: ACTN3 Leads the Way," *Sports Medicine* 43, no. 9 (2013): 803–817; Nan Yang et al., "ACTN3 Genotype Is Associated with Human Elite Athletic Performance," *American Journal of Human Genetics* 73, no. 3 (2003): 627–631.

6 Henk Kraaijenhof, "Improving Sprinting Speed: The Three Phases of the Race and How to Train for Them," YouTube video, 8:16, posted by Yosef Johnson, August 4, 2014, www.youtube.com/watch?v=7d7F-2JxUC8.

7 Louis Pérusse, "Role of Genetic Factors in Sports Performance: Evidence from Family Studies," in *Genetic and Molecular Aspects of Sports Performance*, ed. Claude Bouchard and Erich Hoffman, (Hoboken, NJ: Wiley-Blackwell, 2011), 90–101.

8 Lisa M. Guth and Stephen M. Roth, "Genetic Influence on Athletic Performance," *Current Opinions in Pediatrics* 25, no. 6 (December 2013): 653–658.

9   K. Anders Ericsson, "The Role of Deliberate Practice in the Acquisition of Expert Performance," *Psychological Review* 100, no.3 (1993): 363–406.

10   Mark Remme, "Rookie Transition Program Helps Players Adjust to NBA Life," NBA.com, n.d., www.nba.com/timberwolves/news/rookie-transition-program-helps-players-adjust-nba-life.

11   "Transcript: Robert Sapolsky on Behavioral Evolution at Stanford," *Singju Post*, June 22, 2016, singjupost.com/transcript-robert-sapolsky-on-behavioral-evolution-at-stanford/3/.

12   Michael Jordan, "NBA Hall of Fame Enshrinement Speech: Michael Jordan," *Genius*, September 11, 2009, genius.com/Michael-jordan-nba-hall-of-fame-enshrinement-speech-annotated.

13   Joseph Milord, "Had He Been Taller, Michael Jordan's Brother Would Have Been the Greatest Ever," *Elite Daily*, July 31, 2014, elitedaily.com/sports/had-he-been-taller-michael-jordans-brother-would-have-been-the-greatest-ever/691516/.

14   Paul Galloway, "The Driving Force Behind Jordan's Work Ethic Was a Mother Who Cared," *Chicago Tribune*, April 22, 1999; *Michael Jordan: Come Fly With Me*, narrated by Jay Thomas (NBA Hardwood Classics, 1989), VHS.

15   David Halberstam, *The Education of a Coach* (New York: Hachette Books, 2005), 217.

16   Andy Hart, "Flashback: Bill Belichick on Drafting Patriots QB Tom Brady," Patriots.com, April 16, 2016, www.patriots.com/news/2016/04/16/flashback-bill-belichick-drafting-patriots-qb-tom-brady.

17   Vivek Ranadivé and Kevin Maney, *The Two-Second Advantage: How We Succeed by Anticipating the Future—Just Enough* (New York: Crown Publishing, 2011), 4.

18   Rory Smith, "World Cup 2010: Spain's Battle Won on the Playing Fields of Barcelona," *The Telegraph*, July 17, 2010, www.telegraph.co.uk/sport/football/teams/spain/7895208/World-Cup-2010-Spains-battle-won-on-the-playing-fields-of-Barcelona.html.

19   Corey Pellatt, "Lionel Messi's Three-Year-Old Son Has Already Joined Barcelona's Academy," *Complex*, September 7, 2016, uk.complex.com/sports/2016/09/lionel-messi-son-barca-academy.

20   Richie McCaw, *The Real McCaw: The Autobiography* (London: Aurum Press, 2012), 12–13.

21   Oliver Brown, "Richie McCaw: The Quest for Perfection—What Makes the New Zealand Captain the World's Greatest Player," *The Telegraph*, November 7, 2014, www.telegraph.co.uk/sport/rugbyunion/international/newzealand/11214905/Richie-McCaw-The-quest-for-perfection-what-makes-the-New-Zealand-captain-the-worlds-greatest-player.html.

22   McCaw, *The Real McCaw*, 28.

23   Brown, "Richie McCaw: The Quest for Perfection."

24   "About WHO: Constitution of WHO: Principles," World Health Organization, www.who.int/about/mission/en/.

6 THE HUMAN ATHLETE

25   Martin J. Blaser, *Missing Microbes: How the Overuse of Antibiotics Is Fueling Our Modern Plagues* (New York: Henry Holt and Company, 2014), 182.

26   Katie Thomas and Robert Pear, "Medicare Releases Detailed Data on Prescription Drug Spending," *New York Times*, April 30, 2015, https://www.nytimes.com/2015/05/01/business/medicare-releases-detailed-data-on-prescription-drug-spending.html.

27   Chris Kresser, "More Evidence to Support the Theory That GERD Is Caused by Bacterial Overgrowth," *Chris Kresser*, April 2, 2010, chriskresser.com/more-evidence-to-support-the-theory-that-gerd-is-caused-by-bacterial-overgrowth/.

28   Blaser, *Missing Microbes*, 5–6.

29   Julie Beck, "Taking Antibiotics Can Change the Gut Microbiome for Up to a Year," *The Atlantic*, November 16, 2015, www.theatlantic.com/health/archive/2015/11/taking-antibiotics-can-change-the-gut-microbiome-for-up-to-a-year/415875/.

30   Adam Hadhazy, "Think Twice: How the Gut's 'Second Brain' Influences Mood and Well-Being," *Scientific American*, February 12, 2010, www.scientificamerican.com/article/gut-second-brain/.

31   Diane Sanfilippo, "The Real Deal on Adrenal Fatigue," RobbWolf.com, n.d., robbwolf.com/2012/04/09/real-deal-adrenal-fatigue/.

32   Katharina Nimptsch et al., "Association Between Plasma 25-OH Vitamin D and Testosterone Levels in Men," *Clinical Endocrinology* 77, no. 1 (2012): 106–112.

33   Robert Malenka, "Molecular Mechanisms of Reward and Aversion," YouTube video, 6:22, posted by the World Economic Forum, February 19, 2016, www.youtube.com/watch?v=2urguOHfDr8.

34   Mark Fainaru-Wada and Steve Fainaru, "SF's Borland Quits over Safety Issues," ESPN.com, March 17, 2015, www.espn.com/espn/otl/story/_/id/12496480/san-francisco-49ers-linebacker-chris-borland-retires-head-injury-concerns.

35   Sebastian Junger, *Tribe: On Homecoming and Belonging* (New York: Hachette Book Group, 2016), xiv.

36   Barbara Bradley Hagerty, "Prayer May Reshape Your Brain … And Your Reality," *All Things Considered*, NPR, May 20, 2009, www.npr.org/templates/story/story.php?storyId=104310443.

37 Leslie Becker-Phelps, "Altruism Helps Save a Little Girl, and Perhaps You, Too," PsychologyToday.com, April 6, 2010, www.psychologytoday.com/blog/making-change/201004/altruism-helps-save-little-girl-and-perhaps-you-too; Doug Oman, "Volunteerism and Mortality Among the Community-Dwelling Elderly," *Journal of Health Psychology* 4, no. 3 (May 1999): 301–316.

7 PLAYER PRINCIPLES

38 William Langley, "I've Never Been So Insulted," *The Telegraph,* May 20, 2012, www.telegraph.co.uk/news/newstopics/howaboutthat/9276749/Ive-never-been-so-insulted....html.

39 J. Vedelli, "A Study of Revien's Sports-Vision Techniques for Improving Motor Skills," presentation at the convention of the American Alliance for Health, Physical Education, Recreation and Dance, Cincinnati, OH, 1986; J. M. Wood and B. Abernathy, "An Assessment of the Efficacy of Sports Vision Training Programs," *Optometry and Vision Science* 74, no. 8 (August 1997): 646–659.

40 Sarah Rae Smith, "How Color Affects Your Perception of Food," *The Kitchn,* September 23, 2009, www.thekitchn.com/how-color-affects-your-percept-96524.

41 Kate Bratskeir, "6 Not-So-Subtle Ways Fast Food Joints Make You Want to Eat at Their Restaurants," *Huffington Post,* June 16, 2014, www.huffingtonpost.com/2014/06/16/fast-food-marketing_n_5366297.html.

42 Jay Cardiello, "Color Control: Eat Less, Workout More," The Fit List, Shape.com, n.d., www.shape.com/blogs/fit-list-jay-cardiello/color-control-eat-less-workout-more.

43 Bruce S. McEwen, "Allostasis and Allostatic Load: Implications for Neuropsychopharmacology," *Neuropsychopharmacology* 22, no. 2 (February 2000): 108–124.

44 Christopher Bergland, "Chronic Stress Can Damage Brain Structure and Connectivity," PsychologyToday.com, February 12, 2014, www.psychologytoday.com/blog/the-athletes-way/201402/chronic-stress-can-damage-brain-structure-and-connectivity.

45 Dina Aronson, "Cortisol—Its Role in Stress, Inflammation, and Indications for Diet Therapy," *Today's Dietician* 11, no. 11 (November 2009): 38.

46 "Stress and Anxiety: Possible Complications," *New York Times,* January 30, 2013, www.nytimes.com/health/guides/symptoms/stress-and-anxiety/possible-complications.html.

47 Eva Blomstrand, "A Role for Branched Chain Amino Acids in Reducing Central Fatigue," *Journal of Nutrition* 136, no. 2 (February 2006): 544S–547S.

48 Mounir N. Ghabriel and Robert Vink, "Magnesium Transport Across the Blood-Brain Barriers," in *Magnesium in the Central Nervous System,* ed. Robert Vink and Mihai Nechifor (Adelaide, South Australia: University of Adelaid Press, 2011), 73.

49 Judith K. Payne, "A Neuroendocrine-Based Regulatory Model," *Biological Research for Nursing* 6, no. 2 (October 1, 2004): 141–150.

50 Stanley T. Lee and Edward H. Hon, "Electronic Evaluation of the Fetal Heart Rate. VII. Patterns Preceding Fetal Death, Further Observations," *American Journal of Obstetrics and Gynecology* 87, no. 6 (November 15, 1963): 814–826.

51 Antti M. Kiviniemi et al., "Endurance Training Guided Individually by Daily Heart Rate Variability Measurements," *European Journal of Applied Physiology* 101, no. 6 (December 2007): 743–751; J. Mazon et al., "Effects of Training Periodization on Cardiac Autonomic Modulation and Endogenous Stress Markers in Volleyball Players," *Scandinavian Journal of Medicine & Science in Sports* 23, no. 1 (February 2013): 114–120.

52 Eric J. Anish, "Exercise and Its Effects on the Central Nervous System," *Current Sports Medicine Reports* 4, no. 1 (January 2005): 18–23.

53 Doug Dupont, "Alcohol Impairs Hypertrophy and Messes with Your Hormones," *Breaking Muscle,* n.d., breakingmuscle.com/fuel/alcohol-impairs-hypertrophy-and-messes-with-your-hormones.

54 C. Fernando Valenzuela, "Alcohol and Neurotransmitter Interactions," *Alcohol Health & Research World* 21, no. 2 (1997): 144–148.

55 Rueben A. Gonzales and Jason N. Jaworski, "Alcohol and Glutamate," *Alcohol Health & Research World* 21, no. 2 (1997): 120–127.

56 David DiSalvo, "What Alcohol Really Does to Your Brain," *Forbes,* October 16, 2012, www.forbes.com/sites/daviddisalvo/2012/10/16/what-alcohol-really-does-to-your-brain/.

57 Jean-François Richard et al., "The Try-Out of a Team-Sport Assessment Procedure in Elementary and Junior High School PE classes," *Journal of Teaching in Physical Education* 18, no. 3 (April 1999): 336–356.

58 Robin Kirkwood Auld, "The Relationship Between Tactical Knowledge and Tactical Performance for Varying Levels of Expertise," *Master's Theses, Dissertations, Graduate Research and Major Papers Overview,* Rhode Island College, 2006, digitalcommons.ric.edu/cgi/viewcontent.cgi?article=1000&context=etd.

59 Stephen A. Mitchell, Linda L. Griffin, and Judith L. Oslin, "Tactical Awareness as a Developmentally Appropriate Focus for the Teaching of Games in Elementary and Secondary Physical Education," *Physical Educator* 51, no. 1 (March 1994): 21–28.

9 READY FOR GAME DAY

60 Richard P. Feynman, *Perfectly Reasonable Deviations from the Beaten Track* (New York: Basic Books, 2008), 454.

9 Ready for Game Day

PART THREE

THE PREPARATION

It's winter in New Zealand.

A shadow slides slowly along the pavement and climbs up along the outside of the faded metal door. With its dents and rust, it looks like the entrance to any local rugby stadium.

It's just before dawn. The time doesn't matter to anyone. At this hour, only small animals stir. A hooded figure pulls a key from his pocket and puts it in the lock. He turns the key and pulls the door open with a creak.

Halfway down the road, in the shadows under a tree, a thin, hungry fox carefully stalking a rodent stops dead and spins toward the sound of the door as it slams shut. Pausing for a moment and seeing nothing, he resumes his task.

It's just another cold, dark morning for a hungry fox.

It's just another morning training session for Richie McCaw.

The lights flicker on to illuminate the small gym underneath the stadium at Christchurch, home of the Crusaders rugby franchise, one of the most successful club teams in the history of modern club rugby. Its players and coaches formed much of the backbone of the greatest national rugby team ever to play the sport, the New Zealand All Blacks.

The gym lives up to this lofty reputation. It's clean and tidy, but the weights and racks are very old. You'd easily mistake the gym for anything other than an Eastern bloc Soviet gym. Though the equipment is chipped and unvarnished, it's used regularly.

Wearing shorts, a T-shirt, and a gray hoodie, McCaw could be any of the fans who pack the stadium to cheer on his team every Saturday. He eases his stiff body through a series of rhythmic movements, working joints through their range of motion and easing kinks out of his body. The music pumping through his headphones distracts his mind as his muscles start to warm up. He uses the lifts and opening reps and sets to prepare his muscles and joints for the heavier loads and faster movements to come.

Richie McCaw is the greatest rugby player of all time. The simplicity of this statement doesn't take into account the depth of its meaning. He has been so successful for such a long period of time, no other player even enters the debate. McCaw has played more games for his country than any other player and has been captain of the most dominant team in any sport in the world for over a decade. And he did it for the All Blacks, a team that had already set the standard for the game of rugby worldwide. In 148 games, McCaw has been on the losing side only fifteen times. These are accomplishments that will never be surpassed.

Every young rugby player in the world, regardless of position played, has studied McCaw. He is not the biggest player for his position, nor has he ever been regarded as the most skilled. But his ability to influence games and lead his team to victory is unparalleled in modern sports. Given the extreme forces to which every rugby player is subjected, his health has been remarkably stout. He has suffered injuries but has missed very few games over the course of his career. To do this, he has had to play injured. Famously, he played almost a whole World Cup over three weeks with a broken bone in his foot. Unable to train and barely able to walk between games, he declined to get an X-ray until after the tournament, refusing to confirm that anything was broken.

Starting with light, long kettlebell swings, McCaw allows gravity and the pendulum force to take him through slow, smooth arcs that ready his muscles, joints, and nerves for his work sets. Players talk about his strength, but he knows that the secret is simple. Always downplaying his athleticism, McCaw once said that he's "just a typical New Zealand farm boy, really."[1] Like a corn-fed Iowa football player, he's farm strong.

McCaw's physical training has always been very straightforward. Almost all fitness comes from team preparation. The majority of it is honed during small-sided games in practice. In New Zealand, rugby is almost a religion, and children of every age compete in one form or another. They play for something pure: love of the game. McCaw and his teammates throw themselves into training sessions with a similar childlike enthusiasm, whether they're representing the local club franchise or the national team in the next game.

Competing against fellow greats in club practice games every day gets you ready for real games. Players like Reuben Thorne, Brad Thorn, Chris Jack, Dan Carter, Kieran Read, and Sam Whitelock prepare you for international tests. And, as impressive as players' tactical smarts and skill levels are, the mental tests that these teammates bring are invaluable. These intelligent rugby players are constantly thinking of ways to improve on the pitch. But it's not all pressure. The wicked sense of humor of Chris Jack and, more recently, Kieran Read ensures that things never get too serious.

Over the years, between his experiences with the Crusaders and the All Blacks, McCaw has had access to great minds as well as the best physical trainers. Graham Lowe, Nic Gill, and Ashley Jones

(who worked with both teams) all combine a knowledge of physical preparation with an understanding that rugby is a team game that requires both skill and tactical intelligence. All three would deny that a good strength coach can make any player great, but they would likely acknowledge in private that a bad one can do a lot of damage. These coaches have always played games in preseason, and to keep things fresh for the players during this transitional period, they've made a point of not only playing rugby but also using basketball, Gaelic football, and Aussie rules to develop aerobic fitness and hand-eye coordination.

McCaw, holding two dumbbells, steps up onto the plywood box in front of him. Smooth and unrushed, he goes through each rep carefully. He's unconcerned about the actual weight in his hands. For him it's about the effort. He doesn't squat anymore. A sequence of low back injuries over the years outlawed squatting for him. Squats might work for many athletes, but knowing his body as well as he does, McCaw understands that step-ups will maintain the lower body strength he needs.

What most people find incomprehensible is that McCaw, the greatest ever, doesn't regard himself as having any special advantage and doesn't see any specific reason for his success. As far as he is concerned, his "upbringing was very similar to a lot of kids growing up in New Zealand." As such, McCaw has said that he "didn't get given anything special that allowed me to be an All Black."[2]

Many players and coaches have tried to figure out the secrets to McCaw's success. Yet really, everything about this candid player has always been out in the open. One of his only "secrets" has been the fact that he's had little time off between seasons. It seems counterintuitive that this would help him be successful, as most players use the so-called off-season to bulk up or change their training. But because the All Blacks and the Crusaders have always been successful and so had long seasons, one campaign rolls into the next for McCaw. His routine has been very similar week in and week out. So rather than experience troughs and peaks throughout the year, it's easier for him to stay close to a constant peak. He doesn't really have off-seasons or preseasons, and this has actually been a huge help to him in avoiding injury.

Moving to the squat rack, McCaw loads an Olympic bar to prepare for straight-leg Romanian dead lifts. Again, the weight is not the primary concern. McCaw loves how the exercise stretches his hips, lengthens his hamstrings, and loosens his low back. He's a little tired, and he knows that there's no point in pushing too hard and risking injury.

His endurance is kept steady with games almost every weekend. If there is no game and the team has training, small-sided games keep his cardio-respiratory system ticking. If he's on his own, he'll go for a twenty-minute run, and if he's lucky enough to be at home in Christchurch, he has a twelve-minute uphill dirt trail near his house that he runs regularly. He knows every bump and dip of the terrain, and as he's traversing it, he's aware of how his body should feel. If a hill leaves him short of breath, he needs to do some supplementary endurance work in the coming days.

His weekly routine is always the same during the season. Monday, the day after a game, he does a session in the pool and usually gets a massage to help speed his recovery. Tuesday practice follows a video session where the team prepares tactics to work on at full speed. After the meeting, McCaw lifts with his teammates. This session is the strength day, with the focus mainly on the upper body if his legs are still banged up from the rigors of Sunday's game. Wednesday is often a complete rest day, with media interviews sometimes. As captain, interviews are an unavoidable duty for McCaw, though the self-deprecating country boy refuses to get carried away with reporters' praise and always turns the spotlight back on the achievements and hard work of his teammates.

Thursday is the last intense workday of the week. The team practices for about forty-five minutes, hard and fast and at high intensity, followed by a short, power-focused weights session. Friday is a run-through for the upcoming game. Saturday is the "Captains' Run" or "Team Run," when the coaches stand back and let the team leaders take control. Led by McCaw, the captains oversee the short forty-minute practice from start to finish. They run through every scenario they feel they need to the day before the game. Sunday, they win.

Weight training is a staple, but it's secondary to the game. Like most rugby greats, McCaw prides himself on his functional strength. Just as playing the game keeps him fit, it also keeps him strong. The scrummaging, hits, collisions, and tackles all require strength and power. In fact, when it comes to gym strength he is arguably weaker than many of his direct competitors. But this isn't a concern, as everything is secondary to performance on the field. And nobody can argue with McCaw's output, effort, or execution during a game.

Mentally, McCaw is a fox in every sense of the word: sharp, elusive, and relentless. While he's respected as a player on the field, he is also regarded as a master of the gray arts of the game. Rarely punished in games, he plays the game on the edge and right up to the line in the rulebook. Never dirty, but always hard. Constantly talking to referees and either intimidating or befriending them. Whatever it takes to get the win.

Over the years, many physically more impressive players have tried to unseat him, by fair and foul means. Even his face bears testament to this, with a puffy left ear and subtle but visible scars under his chin and in the fat pad above his left eye. Then there are the hidden injuries, which have led to more stitches than he can count in both eyebrows. Standing six feet two inches (188 centimeters) and weighing in at 240 pounds (108 kilograms or 17 stone), McCaw is not the most physically intimidating open side flanker to play the game, but he has dominated opponents at every level. Many opponents have come back each year to face him noticeably bigger and bulkier. McCaw, however, has retained his athletic build, combining power, speed, and endurance.

Games. These are what much of the All Black and Crusader practices revolve around. Small-sided ones with a desired outcome as well as fun ones to keep the players engaged and involved. Watching the faces of McCaw and his teammates switch from concentration to despair and then light up with joy demonstrates the emotional spectrum that games bring and drills don't. Banter and friendly insults flow easily within the safe team atmosphere. There's a constant attempt to play on the edge of the rules. It's almost encouraged, but if you get caught, you run the risk of ridicule.

This is what the All Blacks are so good at. Everything they do revolves around the game. They play the game in every aspect, whether it's trash-talking to put their teammates off, teasing each other, or trying to trick the referee. Everything is competitive and has a slight edge.

McCaw is a master of it, too. Unassuming but firm, he enjoys and partakes in the team's hijinks, but he also maintains a leadership position in the locker room. It's a delicate balance. One of his greatest strengths is his awareness of the team and the individuals within it. This is a trait he inherited from his predecessor in the role of All Blacks captain, the great Tana Umaga.

By this point in his early-morning workout, McCaw is glowing with a layer of sweat. His last two stations beckon, a complex series of core exercises and then a long, slow mobility session. He switches off his iPod now. Taking his time, he concentrates on each rep and his posture throughout the movements. These core exercises have been a staple since he first started playing and have kept his low back and posture strong.

Richie McCaw has a simple on-field job: protecting the ball. This requires being first to every ruck and first to defend it. It means putting his body on the line every time, despite the years of abuse it has suffered.

Northern Hemisphere teams such as England and Wales have frequently attempted to beat New Zealand with superior fitness, power, or strength, but they almost always fail. As McCaw and others have proved time and time again, power is nothing without control and intelligence. The All Blacks focus on playing the game and recognize that it is not won in the gym. Other national teams spend exorbitant sums on exotic foreign training camps that focus on strength and power development at the expense of skills and game sense. The All Blacks, on the other hand, keep a careful balance, knowing that tactics and game intelligence are paramount. The cunning fox will always beat very fit headless chickens.

McCaw slowly gathers his limbs and eases himself up from a patch of sweat on the ground. He will go for a long, hot shower now. Afterward he'll stroll across the road to the café for breakfast. Christchurch sunlight eases in through the high, slim window, brushing across the wall opposite.

The fox is gone.

I directed our focus less to the prize of victory than to the process of improving—obsessing, perhaps, about the quality of our execution and the content of our thinking; that is, our actions and attitude. I knew if I did that, winning would take care of itself, and when it didn't I would seek ways to raise our standard of performance.

—Bill Walsh

As we've seen by looking at the game, the degree to which any team succeeds comes down to its ability to move players through and into space at the correct time in the most efficient way possible. Spatial, tactical, and perceptive ability are the primary cornerstones of all team sports. Technical ability creates space for players when tactical strategies fail. The more efficient the team, the less it needs to rely on individual technical abilities—not to mention that working cohesively as a group is physically less costly. Next are the psychological and psychophysiological components. These serve the players' technotactical abilities or compensate for the absence of them. Recently, physical qualities have been overemphasized at the expense of tactical and technical execution.

Now we explore how to prepare a team to apply technical, tactical, physical, and psychological abilities on game day. Before we look at the plan, let's understand why we need it in the first place.

To prepare the team as well as possible, we need to dive deep into group dynamics, tribal and herd mentalities, and interpersonal relationships. Even the most reclusive players cannot exist in their own little worlds, and while we do need to tailor elements of preparation to the individual, we also must consider how to develop the squad as a whole. This involves rethinking how we approach the preparatory cycle. Teams have long focused most of their attention on the physical coactive, trying to prepare their players and make sure that they're strong, fit, and powerful enough to deliver come game day. But as we've seen, the psychological, tactical, and technical coactives must be developed simultaneously alongside physical capabilities. We need to blow up what we think we know about training and discover a more holistic, all-encompassing model, which is encapsulated in the four-coactive model (explored in "The Player") and the morphological programming approach, which balances the volume, intensity, density, and collision/contact elements of training (explored in more detail on page 238).

Performing complex skills during games cannot be reduced to a "when he goes there, you do this" formula, no matter how good the head coach thinks the plays are. Instead, we need to back up and look at how players truly learn and, as a result, how coaches can create experiences that enable them to discover their own solutions to a problem. Then and only then can we move on to how best to create such learning opportunities through drills and games as part of a balanced morphological programming approach that maximizes players' dominant qualities, minimizes the impact of their limiting factors, and improves the team's technical and tactical execution, all while ensuring that players are fresh for the next game.

We start with planning and scheduling. This is the governing model for all performance and injury prevention. Better understanding the elements that combine and synergize with planning and scheduling can help eliminate unnecessary stressors.

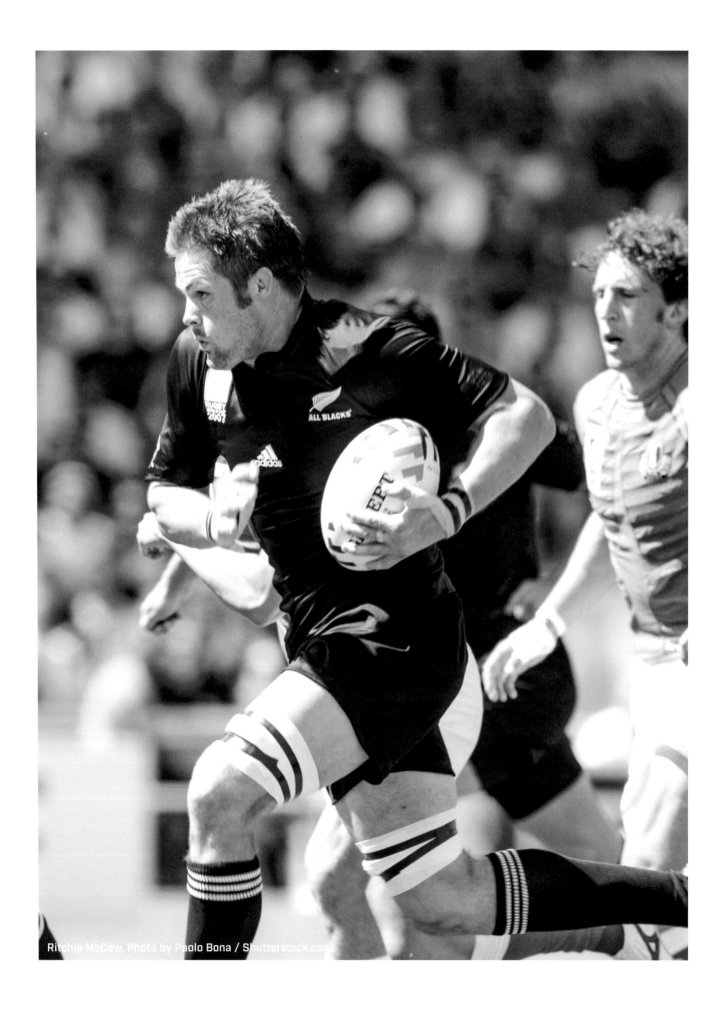

TEN

CREATURES OF HABIT

Sometimes it seems like everyone's actions are random and have little rhyme or reason to them. But while there is day-to-day randomness in our world and we sometimes act inexplicably, most of what we do is a result of the habits and patterns that we create and reinforce and the cycles we find ourselves in.[3] This not only impacts the order in which we perform our daily personal routines—like brushing our teeth, eating breakfast, and making or buying coffee each morning—but also how athletes approach their preparation.

A coach's role is not to condition precise actions that are controlled to the nth degree but rather to help instill positive and sustainable habits in players that enable them to continually learn, grow, and develop. This can best be explained as facilitating experiences for the player—on every level, from a tactical experience that is ingrained to a cellular one

The key is not the will to win. Everybody has that. It is the will to prepare to win that is important.

—Bobby Knight

that resets the body's learned capability after a new personal best in the gym or on the field. All of these are facilitated experiences.

These can be developed from physical habits, like spending ten minutes after practice on mobility work, or cultural ones that reinforce team values, like showing up to practice early. Players don't just have to look at the coach to model such things but can also learn from assimilation by watching the habits and routines of veteran team leaders and how they approach daily preparation. This is particularly important when bringing in new personnel from a draft or via transfer/trade.

SOCIAL RHYTHMS

10.1

Humans function in repeated biological cycles, commonly referred to as circadian rhythms. The most elemental of these is our twenty-four-hour cycle, which is regulated by a "biological clock" in the suprachiasmatic nucleus (part of the hypothalamus in the brain), with daily physiological variations, peaks, and troughs. Our circadian rhythms control body processes across many systems, including sleep-wake cycles, menstrual cycles, mood, hormone balance, heart rate, and blood pressure. Some experts believe that certain diseases and allergies are also subject to biological cycles. Chronopharmacology seeks to use drugs to alter these rhythms if they get out of alignment, while chronotherapy uses techniques like light exposure to reset our internal clock when it gets out of sync.[4]

Our bodies respond to chronological factors biologically—such as by releasing melatonin to promote sleep when the sun goes down. As we're also subject to societal cycles and conventions—for example, the typical workday lasts from nine to six, the typical workweek is Monday through Friday, most children are out of school during the summer—we can expand our thinking to consider circadian rhythms as societal as well as biological. In addition to daily cycles, we have weekly and monthly ones. We're even influenced by religious practices, from daily or weekly observances to significant, once-a-year events like Christmas or Passover. Certain faiths have longer periods of observation, such as Ramadan, the month during which Muslims fast from sunrise to sunset.

The most fundamental aspect of living beings is the one that we most often ignore in sports but has the most impact on the social and familial aspects of the players.

PATTERNS AND ROUTINES

10.1.1

Sustainable-winning sports programs need to respect the influence of society, not on the athletes alone but, just as importantly, on their friends, family, and loved ones, too. These are the people around them 24/7. This is their own personal culture. In most situations, professional athletes are a major influence on the family schedule. If the pattern or schedule they have to adhere to is stochastic in nature, or in direct conflict with the cycles and patterns of everyone else in the family, it can cause conflict.

When family members know that the team has the same day off each week, they can plan around it—even for minor events such as children's birthday parties or family visits. Irregular weekly patterns disrupt family plans and schedules. This may not seem important at first, but players live in the outside world, too, not exclusively as athletes.

Just as it's vital to respect what's going on inside players during and between training sessions, we must also recognize that players exist within the boundaries of society. Sometimes the laws of biology and society overlap. For example, to recover satisfactorily, an athlete must eat and drink several times a day. Societal norms in most cultures respect this biological law with three main meals a day.

In addition, players don't just exist within the team; they're also part of social groups away from the playing and practice facilities. Every player is part of some kind of family, as well as a group of friends, and players' expectations and needs must be considered within the context of such groups. This is one of the reasons that the approach we will present is effective, in that it provides a clear plan for what will happen on each day, so a player knows, for instance, that they can schedule free time with their spouse, significant other, kids, parents, or friends every Monday because Monday is an off day. This may seem insignificant, but in the long, crowded days of a professional athlete, having consistent and repeatable habits is crucial for the family.

By setting expectations in this way and providing a predictable, consistent structure, players, coaches, and staff can live their lives more easily, with less friction and worry. The more regular the pattern and the less unexpected disruption there is, the more likely players are to thrive and perform their best during games. When the team has established familiarity with a system and routine, players expend less physical and psychological effort in adapting to training stimuli, leaving them fresher for competition. This means that a team must have a set of routines—or, as they're referred to in the military, standard operating procedures—for every scenario, such as a three-day road trip, back-to-back home games, and a seven-game playoff series or two-week tournament.

Having routines that respect societal expectations and needs also positively impacts players' physical adaptation to training stimuli. If players know that every Wednesday will include a high-intensity, high-collision Olympic weight-lifting session at 2 p.m., their bodies come to anticipate this stimulus. And then afterward, knowing that a high-protein meal and rest is the next step, the appropriate systems are primed for recovery and restoration by the familiar pattern. Optimization of such patterns means that the team will have deeper physiological reserves to draw on come game day.

There are, of course, instances in which societal factors can encourage and perpetuate negative habits and behavior patterns. An unstable family structure and/or a bad group of friends, for example, can lead to or worsen substance abuse issues in a player. They can also wreak havoc on the player's performance and interactions within the team setting. I'll go into a lot of depth on this topic later on, but suffice it to say for now that team preparation has to take into account how the athletes, coaches, and staff function in view of society's rules, expectations, and conventions, or the absence thereof.

THE IMPACT OF SOCIETY AND CULTURE   10.1.2

When moving to a new team, coaches, players, and staff must educate themselves about the culture of the team and the city, region, and country in which it's located. A team and its players do not exist in a bubble but rather are influenced by their locale.

In his book *Inverting the Pyramid,* Jonathan Wilson explores the origins and impact of the major formations and tactics that have shaped soccer history and the coaches and players who have changed the game. Wilson also examines the profound influence of culture on national and club teams and the style in which they play.

In Ukraine, for example, coach Valeriy Lobanovskyi began using a highly structured game plan at Dynamo Kyiv in the 1970s. He had played with flair, but as a coach, the highly scientific way in which he was educated as an engineer "drove him to a systematic approach, to break soccer into its component tasks," Wilson writes. This is a man who later said that "all life is a number," and that's how he approached his coaching. This was not an individual trait but the result of Russia's obsession with both order and obedience in the Communist years, plus the nation's

fixation on science and technology, which resulted from the space and arms races with the U.S.[5]

Lobanovskyi was also one of the first coaches to use detailed statistics to inform his assessment of his team's performance and that of the opponent. He would then set targets for each player and their unit. "If a midfielder has fulfilled sixty technical and tactical actions in the course of the match, then he has not pulled his weight," the analytically minded Russian coach insisted. "He is obliged to do a hundred or more."[6] While this may sound overly rigid, Lobanovskyi's Kyiv teams did very well, winning multiple league titles, domestic cups, and the 1975 and 1986 UEFA Cup Winners' Cup trophies. His approach suited the mindset of the people and players he was appealing to—but in other cultures he likely would have struggled to get a buy-in.

At the same time in the 1970s, a contrasting style that was the product of a far different culture came to dominate European soccer. Although it was two Englishmen, Jack Reynolds and Vic Buckingham, who laid the foundations for Total Football in the Netherlands, a homegrown coach, Rinus Michels, has become known as "the father of Total Football" and has shaped the modern game more than anyone else, especially through his influence on another dominating figure in European soccer, Johan Cruyff.

Though he was a strict disciplinarian who asserted his absolute authority over his Ajax players at all times, Michels promoted a free-flowing system in which players could slide in and out of multiple positions and move the ball around the pitch so fluidly that their opponents had little chance to get it back. Individual creativity was encouraged, but it had to stay within Michels's carefully organized system. This Total Football approach not only helped Ajax punch above its weight against bigger European powers with deeper pockets and richer traditions of winning, but also came to define the superior ball circulation of the Dutch national team and its talisman (not surprisingly, an Ajax player), Johan Cruyff.

While you could single out Michels and Cruyff as individuals who were key in the achievements of Ajax and Holland, you could also look to the innate creativity and innovation of Dutch culture throughout history. Amsterdam has long been a hub for the arts, and for many years the Dutch were leaders in boatbuilding. They also have a rich architectural heritage. Plus, the 1960s saw a cultural and social revolution sweep the country up in its fast-moving, irreverent current, right before Total Football emerged as one of the most exciting phenomena in the sport's development. Is it any wonder that such an inventive, against-the-grain method of playing "the beautiful game" originated in Holland?[7]

There are many more examples across team sports of how culture impacts not just playing style but also the physical and mental approach to the game, how organizations typically function (or fail to), and how players and fans view their sport and the club at which they ply their trade. These are all important considerations when trying to prepare a team to play its best.

CULTURE, ENVIRONMENT, AND TEAM IDENTITY   10.1.2.1

One of the biggest factors when taking culture into account is determining which cultural traits will prove helpful to the team and so should be promoted among the players, coaches, and staff. Not everything about a culture may prove conducive to the game plan, yet there should be an acknowledgment of its main hallmarks. For example, the San Francisco Bay Area is the home of many fast-paced technology companies and is a hub of innovation. Younger fans might think that the Golden State Warriors began mirroring these traits only in the past few seasons, but in fact the team's up-tempo playing style was representing the culture of its locale as early as 1989, when Tim Hardaway, Chris Mullin, and Mitch Richmond—collectively dubbed "Run TMC"—set NBA scoreboards on fire.

This is not to suggest that head coaches should completely scrap their principles because of culture when they move to a new team and city. Rather, this culture, as well as the history and heritage of the area and the team, should inform the game plan so that it is more widely accepted in the locker room and among the fan base, without the coach's being hostage to them. It is the implementation of this plan and whether the players buy into the coaches' vision that will ultimately determine the long-term success of any team, no matter where it's located, but when a coach is cognizant of the culture, it helps with both.

Another consideration with a new team is how the local environment has shaped the style of play. In cities where streetball is predominant, for example, the run-and-gun style that pervades playgrounds will in some way influence the style and mentality of school and club teams.

Similarly, if you were to coach soccer in Brazil, you'd do well to recognize how the popularity of fast-paced futsal, street games played in close quarters, and beach soccer impact the playing style. Some or most of the current roster may have grown up honing their skills in this way.[8] Just as with culture, incoming personnel must respect environmental factors if the game model and game plan are to be implemented optimally.

BIOLOGICAL RHYTHMS
10.2

As humans, we've always been aware of the rhythms that surround us. We live with the daily ebb and flow of tides and the shift between light and darkness; monthly rhythms of the moon; seasonal rhythms of birth, growth, harvest, and hot and cold; and annual cycles of the sun, migrations, floods, and drought. We have also observed rhythms in our bodies, such as our sleep cycles, daily temperature and blood pressure fluctuations, and the menstrual cycle, which echoes the lunar cycle.

Franz Halberg, the brilliant scientist and founder of modern chronobiology, began his experiments in the 1940s and went on to found the chronobiology laboratory at the University of Minnesota that has since

Biological, Social & Competitive Rhythms

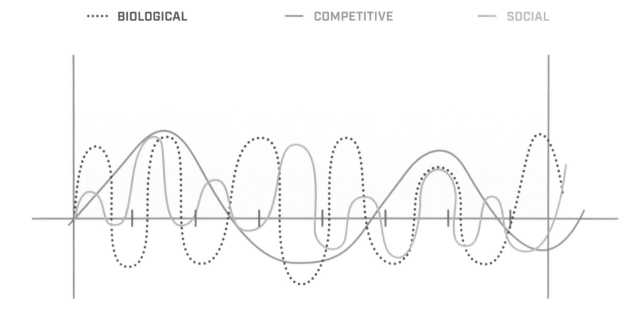

····· BIOLOGICAL   — COMPETITIVE   — SOCIAL

been named for him, the Halberg Chronobiology Center. He offered this rather detailed description of his field:

> Chronobiology is the eminently interdisciplinary science of interactions in time among metabolic, hormonal, and neuronal networks. It involves anatomy, biochemistry, microbiology, physiology, and pharmacology, at the molecular, intracellular, intercellular, and still higher levels of organization. The compounds coordinating a time structure—proteins, steroids, and amino acid derivatives—provide for the scheduling of interactions among membrane, cytoplasmic, and nuclear events in a network involving rhythmic enzyme reactions and other intracellular mechanisms. The integrated temporal features of the processes of induction, repression, transcription, and translation of gene expression remain to be mapped.[9]

Simply put, chronobiology is the study of how living things handle time.

THE SEVEN-DAY CYCLE   10.2.1

The relatively new science of chronobiology has uncovered some unexpected facts about living things, as Susan Perry and Jim Dawson report in their book *The Secrets Our Body Clock Reveal:*

> Weekly rhythms—known in chronobiology as circaseptan rhythms—are one of the most puzzling and fascinating findings of chronobiology. Circaseptan literally means "about seven." Daily and seasonal cycles appear to be connected to the moon. At first glance, it might seem that weekly rhythms developed in response to the seven-day week imposed by human culture thousands of years ago. However, this theory doesn't hold once you realize that plants, insects, and animals other than humans also have weekly cycles.... Biology, therefore, not culture, is probably at the source of our seven-day week.[10]

The modern seven-day week was established by Emperor Constantine in the Roman calendar, first outlined in 321 AD. But as Perry and Dawson note, the origins of a seven-day cycle can be found outside of human society. In his book *Winston Churchill's Afternoon Nap*, Jeremy Campbell gives an account of the centrality of seven-day cycles: "They are of very ancient origin, appearing in primitive one-celled organisms, and are thought to be present even in bacteria, the simplest form of life now existing." In fact, Halberg believed that a seven-day rhythm originated in algae five billion years ago.[11]

So if we accept that the world around and within us is running on a seven-day cycle, it's reasonable to base our method for preparing athletes on a similar time frame. That's one of the reasons I recommend that teams implement the morphocycle approach. Another is that such a cycle respects not only the circadian rhythm of our biology but also the give-and-take between our bodily systems as they continually try to return to a state of equilibrium. Campbell explains, "The two regulatory systems, one imposing sameness in time, the other providing orderly change, are complementary rather than being in conflict. A body function alters in a rhythmic fashion, and homeostasis stabilizes the altered state of that function. The clocks are able to generate regular periodic variations because homeostasis resists random, irrelevant variations."[12]

That's why the morphocycle approach to team preparation stresses focusing on one element—volume, intensity, density, or contact/collision (explained in more detail later in the chapter)—at a time, to encourage the systems engaged in the other elements to recover and regenerate. This enables each athlete's body to return to a state of equilibrium more easily and with a lower energy cost, while still allowing adaptation to the learning that takes place in each session. It also helps reduce injury risk and ensures that athletes are physically and cognitively at their best when the next game rolls around.

LEADERSHIP IN SAPOLSKY'S BABOONS   10.2.2

In "The Player," we looked at neurologist Robert Sapolsky's interpretation of the herd mentality in wildebeests. Now let's revisit his work on another African animal: the baboon. In the mid-1980s, tuberculosis hit a troop of baboons in Kenya, and the alpha males—who were mean and nasty and whose viciousness set the tone for the rest of the group—were claimed by the disease. After their demise, you might expect that strong, aggressive males would take their place. Yet this was not the case. With the alpha males gone, the other baboons became agreeable and amiable. Warfare with other troops was replaced by pacifism, intergroup fighting with grooming, and random acts of violence—like swatting—with displays of affection. Even when the male survivors of the TB outbreak eventually died from other causes, the young baboons that grew up to their place were just as genial. Sapolsky and his wife, Dr. Lisa Share, attribute this to transmittal of the troop's values. "We don't yet understand the mechanism of transmittal," Sapolsky said, "but the jerky new guys are obviously learning, 'We don't do things like that around here.'"[13]

The transformation of the baboon troop from a warmongering group to a peaceable one shows that the personality and actions of leaders greatly influence the rest of the group. We see this same phenomenon in locker rooms. When a team's leaders—whether they are designated captains or just those whom others follow—model certain behaviors and actions, the rest of the squad will do likewise. A coach who is trying to change the team culture needs to look at the influence of the most dominant personalities on the team.

THE BIOLOGY OF BELONGING   10.2.2.1

Sapolsky's long-term study of baboons also reveals that, like humans, these primates suffer from stress-related health issues. Certain personality traits increase the likelihood that a baboon will be depressed or suffer from stress-related illness, Sapolsky said: "Type A baboons are the ones who see stressors that other animals don't." But it's an animal's social integration with the troop that is the biggest predictor of its mental and physical health. "Protection from stress-related disease is most powerfully grounded in social connectedness," Sapolsky continued, noting that socially isolated baboons are most at risk for such disease.[14]

This carries over into the team construct. A player who feels left out of the team for any reason is not only likely to feel depressed but also will undergo profound biological changes that impact state of mind. Sapolsky noted that in baboons, being an outsider has profound effects on the body: "Their reproductive system doesn't work as well, their wounds heal more slowly, they have elevated blood pressure and the anti-anxiety chemicals in their brain, which have a structural similarity to Valium, work differently."[15] To prevent players from developing similar issues, the tribe (i.e., the team) must make an effort to ensure that every member of the squad feels welcome, included, and valued.

BIOLOGICAL RHYTHM AND BIORHYTHMS   10.2.3

Sports physiologist Christian Cook's studies on testosterone and athletic performance were some of the first to show that testosterone isn't just a sex hormone and doesn't impact only muscle growth. For example, BALCO-era baseball players wanted purely physical muscle-building effects, which testosterone creams delivered, but Cook's work—which he has applied in working with the All Blacks, UK Sport, and Bath Rugby—shows that it has other benefits as well. "Obviously, if you put that much testosterone into your body your muscles will grow," Cook told *Wired*. "But within a normal biological range, its main direct role is behavioural. Testosterone gives you more confidence and motivation and that makes you work harder, which indirectly influences muscle growth."[16]

Cook found that testosterone levels are highly individualized, but just like stress hormones in Sapolosky's baboons, testosterone elevation is also partly determined by group dynamics. One factor is whether players are praised or criticized. Cook designed an experiment in which half of a rugby team was given positive feedback by their coach, while the other half received negative feedback. He found that among the positive control group, testosterone levels were 30 percent higher.[17]

Another study, conducted by Peter Totterdell from Sheffield University, evaluated the moods of individual cricket players and the team as a whole. The study concluded that "independent of match events, players could be infected by the mood of their team,

TO REST OR NOT TO REST?

There has been a lot of debate around whether or not players should be rested, most recently in the NBA. When you get past the vague commentary, analysis shows that players or teams who are rested struggle to get back to previous performance levels—they fail to play at their previous speed.

There are multiple reasons for this, but it's largely because complete removal of stimuli (tactical, technical, physical, and psychological) encourages players to fall into a deeper state of recovery, and it takes time for them to return to their previous level. Complete rest disrupts the rhythm of stress and adaptation, and it takes time for players to achieve that rhythm again.

This is why a complete removal of stimuli during the season is risky in most cases. While reduction of volume is not only helpful but necessary, intensity must be maintained to avoid a slump on return.

being particularly likely to catch positive moods." There was also a correlation between good moods and better match play, meaning that when the high spirits of a few players spread to the rest of the group (mood contagion), the team's performance improved.[18] Coaches should bear this in mind when considering how they talk to the team during timeouts and breaks between quarters and halves, especially when the team is losing. If the coach remains positive and upbeat and encourages the squad to keep fighting, it's arguable that the players will be more likely to raise their game and put in the effort needed for a comeback win.

HABITS AND RHYTHM: WHERE SOCIETY AND BIOLOGY COMBINE   10.2.4

We've just seen how biology and psychology can impact behavior. But that's only half of the picture. The reverse is also true: behavior can profoundly influence psychology and biology as well. Psychology professor Ian H. Robertson has demonstrated that one of the three main ways that we dictate our brain chemistry is through the structural-anatomical system. In other words, how we position ourselves and move has an impact on brain chemistry at the cellular level. Indeed, even if coaches don't feel a certain way, they can change their mood by acting a certain way—which will influence their players' feelings, too.

In his book *The Winner Effect*, Robertson refers to an expansive, dominant posture demonstrated by former French prime minister Nicolas Sarkozy in a meeting with King Mohammed VI of Morocco and contrasts this with the typical posture of lower-status junior diplomats, who are more likely to make themselves "physically small—arms folded, legs tight together, heads slightly bowed, shoulders hunched, and so on." He then shares the results of a joint study by Dana Carney and others from Columbia and Harvard Universities in which one group was asked to imitate Sarkozy's "high-power" posture while another was asked to adopt a deferential position. Those in the high-power posture reported feeling more powerful and in charge than the ones imitating slouching, pen-pushing bureaucrats. The impact was also felt at a neurotransmitter level, with the high-power-posture group registering lower levels of the stress hormone cortisol and higher levels of testosterone—results that were reversed in the low-power-posture test subjects.

Robertson writes, "Even tiny, short-lasting changes in the way we hold ourselves can change our bodies and brains in profound ways. . . . No matter what I feel inside, if I *behave as if* I feel the way I want to feel, the feelings will likely follow. Then I might enter a positive feedback loop, where other people respond to me in such a way as to confirm or support these initially faked emotions."[19] This is not to say that coaches should be phony, but rather that they need to pragmatically control how they act in order to impact their own brain chemistry (and therefore mood) and that of their players, depending on the situation. It's clear that attitude follows action, and if we create positive habits, then we can elevate how we feel as well as how we act.

BIOLOGY, COMPETITION, AND CIRCADIAN RHYTHMS   10.2.5

In preparing a team, coaches must realize that their players are human beings who are composed of complicated systems, each of which is constantly trying to maintain a delicate balance to preserve optimal function in any condition. This holistic way of thinking has been dominant in Eastern cultures for hundreds or even thousands of years but lamentably has yet to take hold in the West, where we are still fixated on looking at athletes in a segmented, disconnected way that fails to take into account the totality of their biology.

Every player is subject to continually fluctuating cycles that can be plotted like competing sound waves, the peaks and troughs of each waveform going up and down as the individual is subjected to the varying stimuli of practice, competition, and recovery. We sometimes refer to these periodic cycles or temporal rhythms as *chronobiology,* as they're profoundly influenced by time. Unfortunately, very few sports teams make any effort to understand this area or respect it as they devise and conduct team training.

Too many athletic organizations also fail to acknowledge that while stimuli have definite starting and stopping points, biological systems are constantly at work, even while athletes are sleeping. Practice provides an experience at both the cellular and cognitive levels, with the body receiving and responding to signals across multiple systems, and the morphological programming approach provides a way of categorizing these stimuli so that athletes can respond optimally. Just as the body is continually adapting to physical stress, the brain also never stops learning, creating and reinforcing habits, and putting down layers of experience that it calls upon to inform the observation-action cycles that take place throughout games.

It's unfortunate that in some ways, we mistakenly try to treat athletes as we do machines, not as fluid, complex, and dynamic organisms.

COMPLEX, DYNAMIC, RESPONSIVE, ADAPTIVE, AND SELF-IMPROVING   10.2.6

Athletes are not machines. They are complex, dynamic beings who are responsive, adaptive, and self-improving. So we can't apply cold, logical thinking to the human organism, whether in everyday life or the context of team sports. This is why athletes need to be trained when they are biologically ready, not when an arbitrary, linear schedule says it's time. With human beings, there is no scheduled maintenance. We need to alter how we view our athletes—with their humanity at long last coming first.

Machine learning also goes out the window when it comes to stress responses. Engineers can assess a bridge or tunnel and objectively tell you how much stress it will withstand before collapsing, but assessing human stress is another matter altogether. Almost every warrior-athlete can tolerate a high degree of stress in one area for a short time. If the body perceives a threat, it will draw in every ounce of energy it can from its biological systems to combat or get away from the threat, stabilize itself, and thus preserve life.

For example, if you're thrown into an icy pool, your body will try to keep your core temperature from dropping so low that you cannot continue to function, while simultaneously attempting to find a way out of the pool. But after a certain amount of time, you will become so drained that your systems cannot keep up the fight and will start to shut down one by one.

Another example of stress is what British SAS soldiers experience on an escape-and-evasion exercise in the Brecon Beacons mountain range in Wales. Though in unfamiliar surroundings and under con-stant pressure, many SAS operatives can handle three consecutive days on the run with little to no sleep. While the consequences aren't so dramatic, similar lessons apply to team-sports athletes. A lot of stress concentrated over a day or two will likely be fine, but more than this will quickly start to have negative consequences.

Stressors cannot be thought of in isolation, either. If players aren't sleeping well, this will affect their digestion, inflammation levels, immune system, and more. Or if athletes are sick, their ability to train and recover will be profoundly compromised. If a team member has just one problem area and all other stressors are minimized, he might well be able to cope. But if there are multiple issues, he will soon become overwhelmed and unable to perform at a high level.

WORK BACKWARD FROM THE NEXT MATCH   10.2.7

As we've seen, there are patterns and cycles in life that one has to respect. These have evolved from the laws of nature or society and cannot be ignored, compromised, or broken. An athlete might be able to get away with trying to buck the system for a little while—say, by sacrificing sleep—but the consequences will eventually force them to return to more sustainable habits.

In an attempt to harness these social and biological rhythms, we have to start with the competition cycle and work backward. As such, the only game that matters is the next one. We then design the morphocycle that includes this upcoming match in a way that enables players and staff to respect their physiology, spend time with their families, and have learning experiences that make them physically prepared and cognitively ready to apply the game plan in the next contest.

10 Creatures of Habit

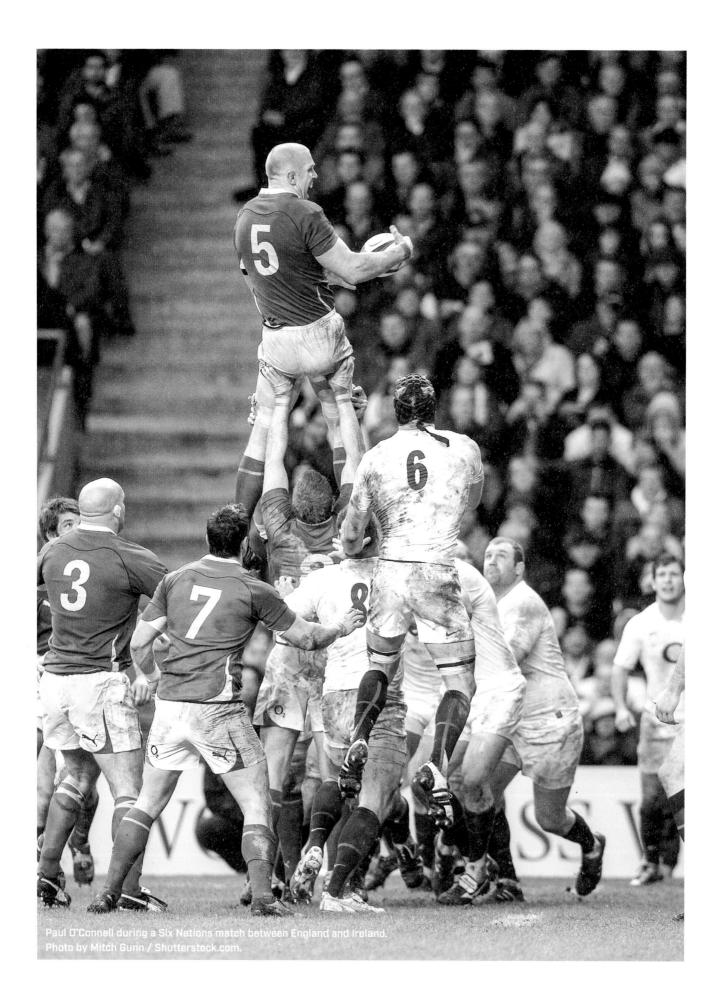

Paul O'Connell during a Six Nations match between England and Ireland.
Photo by Mitch Gunn / Shutterstock.com.

ELEVEN

CREATURES OF STIMULI

Ultimately, everything that affects us or that affects life is a stimulus. How we adapt to a stimulus affects, in turn, how we develop. This is why everything must be considered in totality when it comes to elite athletes. Once this is understood, we need to consider exposure and the dosage of stimuli and how these affect the players.

EXPERIENCE, EXPOSURE, AND EFFECT

11.1

It's important to understand that the experiences players go through expose them to certain stimuli, which in turn produce adaptations. The key to effective programming for sports teams is to deliver such stimuli in a carefully ordered sequence that accommodates the various internal and external cycles that all athletes are subject to. The starting point for each activity and the state of the athlete is important. If you introduce a stimulus too soon after the last one like it, it will blunt adaptation and minimize the learning effect of both experiences.

There's an old Irish fable in which a tourist stops a farmer to ask him, "How do I get to Dublin?" The farmer replies, "Well, I wouldn't start from here." The best training program becomes irrelevant if it doesn't consider the starting point of the players. Fatigued players and rested players respond completely differently to the same program, for example, so the coaching staff needs to think about the physical, emotional, and cognitive status of their players on any given day in the morphocycle and plan the forthcoming sessions accordingly. This involves considering what happened in the preceding days' sessions, what's on the schedule for the following day, and how this affects which morphological programming elements—volume, intensity, density, or collision/contact—to stress and which to allow to recover.

The competitive load is also a crucial factor. If there have been an unusually high number of games—such as during the Christmas period in the Premier League—or a couple of recent contests have gone into overtime, the preparation load will need to be reduced so that the athletes' minds and bodies aren't overwhelmed.

THE ELEMENTS OF MORPHOLOGICAL PROGRAMMING

11.1.1

In sports, the morphological programming approach provides a balance among stressors in order to maximize the player's adaptation and learning. In addition to balancing the four coactives (technical, tactical, physical, and psychological), the morphological programming approach manages four elements of training: volume, intensity, density, and collision/contact. During the morphocycle, the period between games, all these elements are managed so that players aren't overstressed in any area.

VOLUME 11.1.1.1

By "volume" we mean "quantity of work." It can be measured in terms of time, number of reps, time under tension, or space/distance. Think of a one-kilometer race: it has a relatively high volume.

INTENSITY 11.1.1.2

Intensity is the measure of power output and energy; in team sports, it particularly refers to the speed at which work is done. Another way to think of intensity is as a measure of how rigorous a session is. High-intensity work is demanding on neural energy. Think of a hundred-meter race: the volume is lower than in a one-kilometer race, but the intensity is higher.

DENSITY 11.1.1.3

Density measures how often work is done—and, conversely, how many breaks are taken. Ten hundred-meter sprints and a one-kilometer run cover the same distance (they have the same volume), but a measure of density, variability of work, allows us to distinguish between them.

COLLISION/CONTACT 11.1.1.4

All sports have a collision factor. It's a myth that sports like soccer don't. Even completely non-contact sports such as sprinting have it: the impact of the runner's feet on the ground is a form of collision. Collision may best be thought of as a vibrational force that the players absorb.

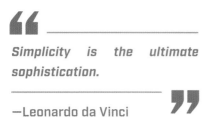

> *Simplicity is the ultimate sophistication.*
>
> —Leonardo da Vinci

MANUFACTURING, TOYOTA, AND WORKING BACKWARD FROM THE GAME 11.1.2

In manufacturing, as in sports, the goal is to deliver a superior product (or performance) on time. In the 1960s and 1970s, Toyota embraced the concept of just-in-time (JIT) production, which enabled the company to adjust to market demands more readily and ensure that they didn't manufacture either too many vehicles, which would increase the number that went unsold, or too few vehicles to meet dealerships' needs. With JIT, they'd also avoid ordering too many costly parts and supplies that might not be needed. By the 1980s, factories in Western Europe and America had recognized the efficiencies that JIT created and started to apply the method to their production processes, too.

The lesson from JIT that we can apply for our purposes is this: once you know how long the effects of all stimuli last, work backward from the game when scheduling a training cycle. Manufacturing lead times are like stimuli. They must be factored in in reverse order for the process to be completed on time. The idea that you can work forward is foolish and yet has been the prevailing mentality in team sports for far too long. Working backward also provides the ability to "program" in real time: to focus on what players are doing from session to session, in contrast to the yearlong blocks in traditional, physically focused periodization (see page 249).

Another reason we should work backward is because it emphasizes that the game itself is the only measuring stick for performance. Unfortunately, many teams still have this backward, placing so much significance on how they structure training that competition becomes almost a secondary consideration.

LEARNING, ADAPTATION, AND HABIT

11.2

If a team repeatedly falls short of its goals during games, it's unacceptable for the head coach to try to justify the shortfall with an excuse like, "They didn't stick to the game plan." A coach cannot simply tell the players what they're supposed to do and then expect them to implement the plan in competition. Rather, before the game, the coach must create learning scenarios that allow the players to experience what it is they're trying to teach. In sports and the military alike, there are no bad teams, only bad leaders.

The learning experiences that a team goes through in each and every morphocycle represent the sum of their stimuli and responses. As such, it's not enough to merely put players through their physical paces—if the squad is to advance during competition, they also must learn technically, tactically, and cognitively during individual, unit, and team training.

THE AIM OF TRAINING IS TO CULTIVATE HABITS

11.2.1

For far too long, sports teams have tried to train athletes to do things the "right way"—that is, in the manner the coach thinks is optimal. But if we're truly trying to create sustained performance improvements on both an individual and a team basis, we need to cultivate and reinforce habits that enable players to achieve the objectives of the game plan in the way that's best for them.

Research by neuroscientists Patrick Haggard and Benjamin Libet shows that when we are exposed to stimuli, we don't just select the appropriate motor skill and then apply it. Rather, our prior experiences and the habits we've cultivated precondition us to respond to stimuli in a certain way. By the time we consciously recognize that we're about to move

SIT OUTSIDE A BARBERSHOP

There's a saying that if you sit long enough outside a barbershop, you'll get a haircut. In sports, exposure to the company of great players and their habits and values will help pass these on to new members of the squad without the coaching staff having to say anything. Elite athletes have so much to learn and remember—particularly in college and pro football—that they don't have much spare capacity. This means that coaches should make it a point to tell them as few additional things as possible. That players should show up to practice ten minutes early or that the team spends extra time on recovery after practice shouldn't be explicitly stated, even to rookies and transfers. Instead, they will learn these things through assimilation just by being around their teammates, particularly the veteran leaders. In this way, it's possible to change their perception of what's acceptable and expected simply by exposing them to the team culture as it exists from day to day.

The single greatest benefit is that in teams with strong cultures, minor things are self-managed by the culture and environment, so coaches need speak only when it's important.

in a certain way, the brain has already decided how it's going to move the body.[20] As the work of military strategist John Boyd shows, faster decision-making can psychologically overwhelm an opponent, and one way to speed the observation-action cycle is to condition our brains by repeating actions until they become instinctive habits.

Ideally, such habits will increase the likelihood that players' actions fulfill the game plan objectives and fit within the coach's preferred style of play. The way to encourage this is to create training exercises that encourage players to problem-solve through trial and error. Repeating the same or similar drills regularly, combined with playing small-sided games, will forge the players' actions into habits that they will then default to during game play. This means that they'll make better and faster decisions—because they've already made those decisions many times over in practice—and this will, in turn, lead to more positive outcomes.

THE RULE OF 100 PERCENT EFFORT   11.2.2

If team preparation is to be effective and all athletes are to progress technically, tactically, physically, and psychologically, so that their play and that of the team keeps getting better, every member of the squad must be totally engaged and committed. Training based on the four-coactive model doesn't just require players to work hard physically, as this will not set them apart when there are many other great athletic specimens on every other team in the league. Rather, it's total effort in all areas—including maintaining concentration, having a positive attitude, and being willing to learn—that will produce noticeable and continuous improvement.

But it's not enough for the players to show up with the intention of giving their all physically, cognitively, and emotionally. The coaching staff must set up training sessions that are conducive to maximum effort.

Coaches like Jim Harbaugh put it upon themselves to devote hours to meticulously planning each and every practice. That way, every drill, every teaching moment, and every second on the clock is used purposefully, and the focus is on quality over quantity. José Mourinho is another who "would fool around with us outside practice, but when the time to work arrived he would be ruthless," said Vítor Baía of Mourinho's highly focused sessions at Porto. "We only practiced for one hour each day, yet those hours were the most intense I've ever seen."[21]

No matter what the drill is, there must be total involvement and immersion in the activity to maximize the experience, not simply because of the need to improve but also so that the players aren't subjected to a suboptimal experience. All great teams, special operations groups, and coaches instinctively know this, having arrived at it through trial and error. This programming and modeling approach simply creates a philosophy for it.

KNOWLEDGE IS NOT POWER   11.2.3

Just because somebody comprehends something or can memorize a piece of information and recite it back to you doesn't mean that they're going to be able to put it into action. You could lecture someone for three hours about the ins and outs of changing a head gasket in a car. But when you put them in front of an engine and ask them to perform this repair, they will likely stare back at you with a blank expression on their face. This is why coaches can't simply explain in practice what they want players to do and then expect them to re-create it on the playing field. No. The athlete needs to be provided with a scenario that encourages them to learn by doing.

A LESSON IN TEAM TEACHING: GIVING ORDERS VS. CREATING EXPERIENCES   11.2.3.1

It's no coincidence that some of the best coaches were also teachers—from UCLA's basketball genius John Wooden, who responded to being called the "Wizard of Westwood" by saying, "I'm no wizard. I'm a teacher," to the man whom the NFL championship trophy is named after, Vince Lombardi.[22] Long before achieving football immortality, Lombardi taught Latin, physics, and chemistry while also coaching basketball at St. Cecilia High School in Englewood, New Jersey. "I wanted to be a teacher more than a coach," Lombardi later explained.[23] It was his ability to teach that made him so effective on the football sideline. Alastair Clarkson, Bill Walsh, and Clive Woodward all trained as teachers initially, too.

As Lombardi and Wooden knew well, developing players' technical and tactical acumen while also preparing them mentally was just as important, if not more so, as enhancing athletes' physical attributes. It's the only way to prepare players so that they're able to do things on their own initiative during competition and problem-solve on the fly as they come up against the frictions of the game.

Therefore, it's imperative that coaches design drills that are focused on furthering their principles within the game plan and *then* on enabling physical elements to fit within this construct. Each player only has to be fast enough and strong enough to execute on their game plan objectives, but the potential for improving technically has virtually no limits and so is a constant work in progress during effective team preparation.

Some of the best coaches—including Wooden and Walsh—were teachers and continued to refer to themselves as such in their capacity as coaches. Yet the real role of a coach is not teaching per se, at least insomuch as it involves the traditional concept of showing someone how to do something. Rather, the role of coach as teacher is to set up scenarios in which players learn by doing, with minimal intervention from the sidelines. It's the experience itself that should do the teaching.

HEN OR PIG: INVOLVED OR COMMITTED
11.2.4

An "Irish fry" usually consists of eggs, sausages, and bacon. There's an old joke people tell about the meal: the hen was involved, but the pig was committed. In the same way, players may all be involved in the team, but not all are fully committed.

The fastest way to teach someone mastery in a skill is to immerse them in an environment where they can fully assimilate it. For example, you can learn French in a classroom or online with Duolingo, and that's a great start. But there's a difference between learning from a book and moving to a small village in the French Pyrenees to learn the language. In addition to correct usage, you'd pick up the local dialect, inflections, tempo, slang, and colloquialisms, which no other experience could give you.

It's the same in team sports. The quickest way to develop players is to fully immerse them in complete experiences that mirror the game as closely as possible. As there are so many elements of elite performance and relatively few great players—too few to provide a good sample size—we can't hope to know everything that's involved in being the best. But what we can do is create an environment that fosters excellence and then get our athletes to commit fully to learning within it.

EMOTION AND INSTINCT
11.3

We like to think that we have conscious control over all our actions, but in reality much of what we do is governed by instinct. In the physiology of the brain,

> *This was how Johan Cruyff worked. He was demanding a lot, but when you got there, and you were in his team, he was an incredible protector. He would push and push you and then he would protect you. He was a master at handling players.*
>
> —Pep Guardiola

instinct and emotion are closely related. The amygdala is our danger sensor and uses fear to trigger evasive or combative action when we perceive a threat in our environment. It is also a long-term memory bank for other emotions, which are recalled to put what we're experiencing into the context of previous experience and determine how we should react to what's going on in the moment.

Then there's the hippocampus, which helps govern how we respond to the emotions that the amygdala serves up. The anterior cingulate cortex also assists in self-control, as well as helping us solve problems and resolve conflicts as they arise. The final piece of the emotion/instinct puzzle is the hypothalamus, which controls the body systems that express emotion, including the structural-anatomical system (which controls body positioning and facial expressions), endocrine system (which is responsible for hormone balance), and autonomic nervous system (which governs heart rate and other involuntary body reactions).

When preparing athletes, coaches should recognize the powerful control that emotions and the resulting instincts exert on skill execution and other aspects of performance. How athletes feel emotionally when they're participating in any learning experience will be just as important to their development as any physical adaptations that result from the stimulus. For this reason, training sessions need to be predominantly positive and give each player the opportunity to feel like they're engaged in something meaningful that's going to improve their game play.

> *Poison is in everything, and no thing is without poison. The dosage makes it either a poison or a remedy.*
>
> —Paracelsus

HOW WILL SCIENCE EXPLAIN THIS?

Teams often want their sports scientists to find scientific studies that will help them predict what's coming next and either hasten that (if what's coming next is winning/improving) or delay or prevent it (if it's injuries). The trouble with this aim is that it's based on a faulty assumption. Science isn't about predicting the future but rather explaining why something has happened and, from that basis, suggesting *possibilities* for the future. Its role in team sports should be to educate us and inform our intuition, not to act as a crystal ball. Science is always subsequent and never first.

It's also worth noting that academic studies are conducted in sanitized and controlled environments. As such, their conditions are the exact opposite of the chaos that exists in the real world of sports. So even though this or that study conducted by a fancy university yielded certain results that the sports scientist finds interesting and believes might be applicable, the true impact on the team might well be different.

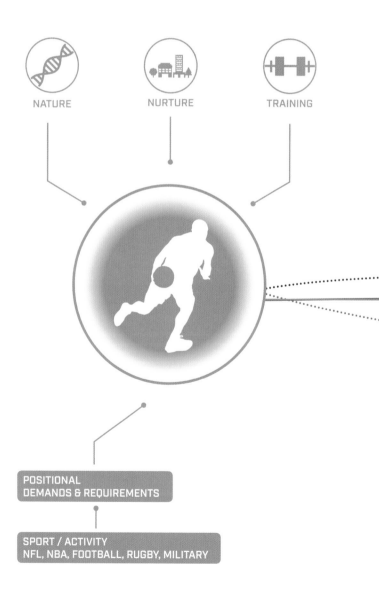

NATURE

NURTURE

TRAINING

POSITIONAL DEMANDS & REQUIREMENTS

SPORT / ACTIVITY
NFL, NBA, FOOTBALL, RUGBY, MILITARY

THE TRAINING RECOVERY MYTH

11.4

One of the most critical perspectives that many people miss is that there is no such thing as full recovery after training; there is simply adaptation to stimuli. The body is always adapting, changing, and learning. There is a delayed and slow recovery of various layers. It is not a simple formula or Lego-type approach. The body will adapt in time, and we can support this process, but it never fully returns to its previous state.

RECOVERY DOES NOT EXIST; ADAPTATION DOES

11.4.1

Trying to separate "training" and "recovery" into two distinct entities is pointless. The athlete's body and brain don't know the difference—all it recognizes is stimuli delivered during learning experiences and the reactions needed to adapt to these stimuli. For example, if you go out for a jog on a summer day, you'll increase the number of capillaries, elevate the efficiency of the cardiorespiratory system, and improve temperature regulation. Taking a hot bath will do many of the same things, just on a much smaller scale. In both situations, your body recognizes that it needs to pump more oxygenated blood and

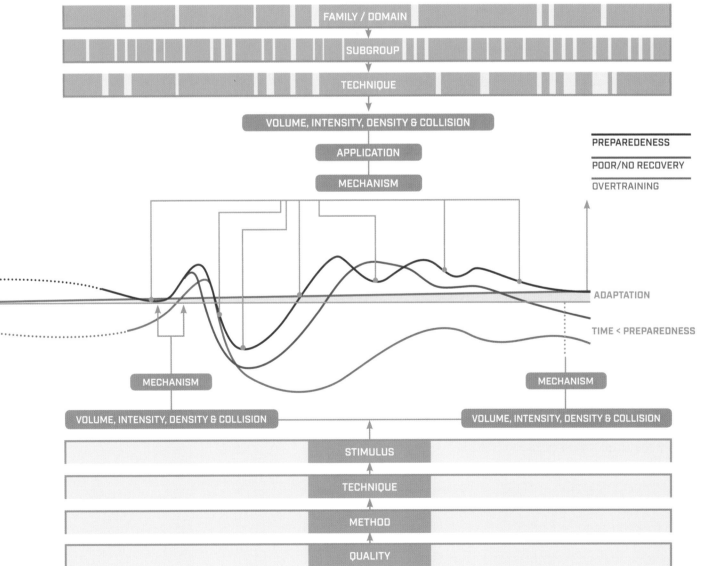

get it to your muscles more efficiently, while also dissipating heat. And the adaptations through which it does this are the same in both scenarios.

As with training stimuli, the timing and dosage of recovery-focused stimuli, like hot and cold therapy, mobility, and nutrition/hydration, are essential. These things never "make" the body recover but can either facilitate or blunt adaptation. The morphocycle approach builds in specific timing and dosage of stimuli to help do the former and prevent the latter, taking into account that each body system recovers at its own rate. Balancing the elements of the morphological programming approach also encourages more complete recovery while preparing the athlete to adapt optimally to each learning experience.

When coaches and players know what to expect each day, they can be more specific and intentional about aiding adaptation. A structured, morphocycle-based system also encourages the formation and reinforcement of beneficial habits, such as getting at least eight hours of good-quality sleep a night and hydrating adequately before, during, and after practices and games.

THE ISOLATION ADAPTATION MISNOMER   11.4.2

Though cells are part of larger bodily systems, they are isolated from the conscious context of team preparation. In other words, what a cell experiences is not the same as what an athlete's mind comprehends, so it cannot differentiate between different types of stimuli or training. What it does know is that it existed in a certain state, was exposed to a stimulus, and must adapt to this stimulus. This adaptation is defined by the stimulus load: its frequency, duration, and intensity.

Such adaptation occurs in a similar way in all types of tissue, whether in the lungs, heart, muscles, or anywhere else in the body. This is why it's impossible to truly focus on one muscle group in isolation. Say you're doing a set of Romanian dead lifts to strengthen hip extensors. In addition to exposing this prime mover to a stimulus, you also involve other muscles as stabilizers, and the antagonist is just as crucial in this movement as the agonist. In addition, the myocardium tissues of the heart will be under load to pump blood to the legs (not to mention the glutes, muscles of the lower back, and abdominals). This is why trying to isolate a muscle group while training is futile. Just as every learning experience involves each element of the four-coactive model and a certain morphological programming profile, so too does a particular stimulus result in cellular adaptation in multiple systems.

SPECIFIC INTELLIGENCE

In our society, we've become too consumed with being book smart and have ignored other forms of intelligence. Never mind that neither Winston Churchill nor Steve Jobs graduated from college—too many of us still think that you need to be clever in the traditional, school-centric sense of the word. Yet examples abound of athletes who have not passed school tests but have aced the practical exam of competition. One of these is the greatest boxer of all time, Muhammad Ali. He had two cracks at a military test because his IQ score (78) was lower than the minimum. "I said I was the greatest, not the smartest," Ali quipped. Yet he was smart enough to beat the finest boxers of his generation and become arguably the most influential sportsman in history. The takeaway is that as long as an athlete knows enough to perform at or above the level that the team needs and the coach expects, they know enough.

THE FITNESS-FRESHNESS BALANCE

One of the main aims of the morphocycle approach is to ensure that the combined load of preparation and competition is not physically, cognitively, or emotionally over-whelming for players. This is why the morphocycle balances multisystem stimuli and recovery rates on each day of the weekly cycle, so that all members of the squad are both ready and prepared when they take the field. They must be not only fit enough but also fresh enough for the game.

In "The Player," I talked about three areas we need to think about when getting an athlete ready for game day: readiness, preparedness, and potential (see page 213). Together, these three areas indicate how well an athlete has recovered from the cumulative load of the preceding morphocycle, how able a player is to perform, in terms of the four coactives, and how well the athlete can perform in a certain game, based on these factors.

FITNESS/PREPAREDNESS & FRESHNESS/READINESS

■ TECHNICAL   ■ TACTICAL   ■ PSYCHOLOGICAL   ■ PHYSICAL

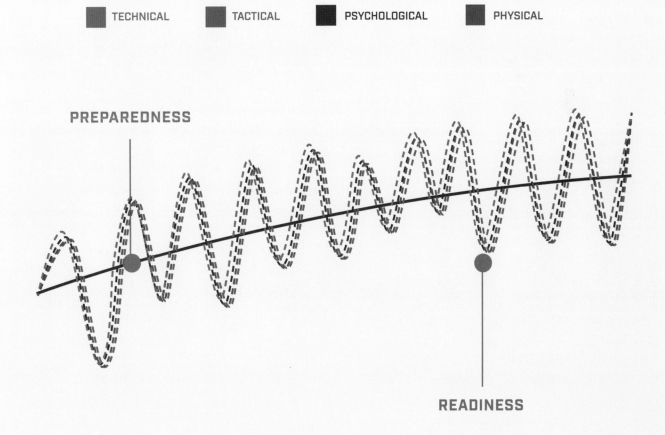

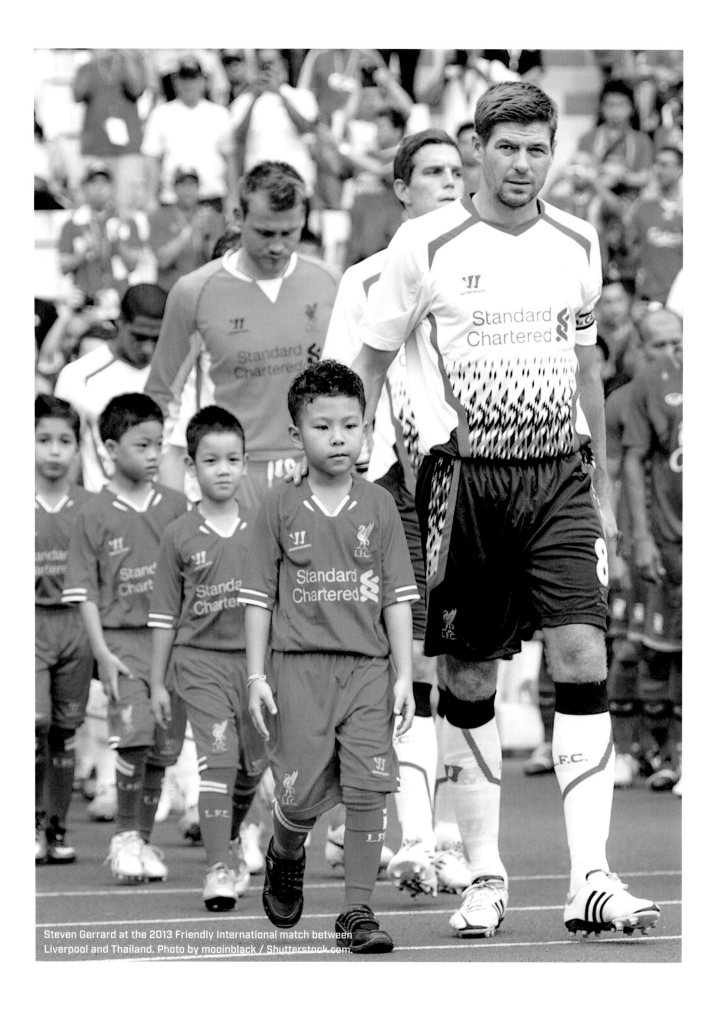

Steven Gerrard at the 2013 Friendly International match between
Liverpool and Thailand. Photo by mooinblack / Shutterstock.com.

TWELVE

THE EVOLUTION OF PREPARATION

In this section, we're going to look at how training approaches have evolved and which, like periodization, have no place on the cutting edge of team-sports performance. We'll also explore how we can incorporate learning theories into our approach and why we need to stop focusing exclusively on physical elements and start paying more attention to developing psychological, technical, and tactical coactives through learning experiences that can be applied in forthcoming games.

WE DON'T LEARN, WE EXPERIENCE

12.1

Before we take a look at the key principles of Russian physiologist Leo Matveyev's periodization approach, we need to back up a bit and explore the theory on which it's based: Hans Selye's general adaptation syndrome model. The Austrian endocrinologist explained the effects of stress and theorized that each exposure to a stressor causes chemical changes in the body. If not managed correctly over time, stress suppresses the immune system and becomes a significant contributor to disease and even early death. "Every stress leaves an indelible scar, and the organism pays for its survival after a stressful situation by becoming a little older," Selye wrote.[24]

This is not simply physical, either; stress leaves an emotional scar that most coaches ignore. This can manifest itself in multiple ways. A previous injury may leave players fearful that they will get hurt again and so make them tentative. The pressure of a potentially game-winning free throw, drop goal, penalty, or field goal is elevated if the player has previously failed to execute. In his book *Waking the Tiger: Healing Trauma,* Peter Levine discusses this in depth, and his research also suggests that when people are already under pressure, their capacity to deal with added stress is diminished.[25]

Selye described the body's neurobiological attempt to deal with stress and maintain equilibrium as general adaptation syndrome, which he defined in 1956 and broke down into three stages:

- *Alarm:* This is the body's immediate, involuntary response to stress, in which the adrenal glands, sympathetic nervous system, and pituitary-adrenal system kick into high gear to address the threat. The brain quickly triggers the release of the stress hormones cortisol, adrenaline, and noradrenaline, which prompt the body to make available fast-acting energy needed to either fight or run—that is, the "fight or flight" response.

- *Resistance:* During this second stress-response stage, when the danger diminishes, the body remains in a state of high alert and is still focusing chemical resources on managing the threat. But as it believes that the initial danger has been somewhat mitigated, the parasympathetic nervous system is simultaneously trying to return the body to its normal homeostasis—that is, a "rest and digest" status.

- *Exhaustion:* If exposure to one or more stressors continues for an extended period, the body's physiological capacity to cope is used up. Now the immune system is depressed, inflammation skyrockets, and, Selye believed, the aging process is accelerated. The body is now less able to deal with additional stress and is more susceptible to disease. This stage is also referred to as *maladaptation.*

THE FITNESS-FATIGUE MODEL

12.2

Another basic theory that informed periodization is the fitness-fatigue model. Though its principles were developed not long after Selye's pioneering work on the general adaptation syndrome model (see page 247), this model was best defined by Vladimir Zatsiorsky in his 1995 book *Science and Practice of Strength Training.* In it, he explains that the duration of the fitness and fatigue resulting from any physical stimulus varies. The key in designing and implementing any training program, then, is to maximize the fitness benefit while giving the body enough time to overcome fatigue so that fitness isn't diminished.

Or, as Zatsiorsky put it: "According to the two-factor theory of training, the time intervals between consecutive training sessions should be selected so that all the negative traces of the preceding workout pass out of existence but the positive fitness gain persists."[26]

SELYE'S GENERAL ADAPTATION SYNDROME

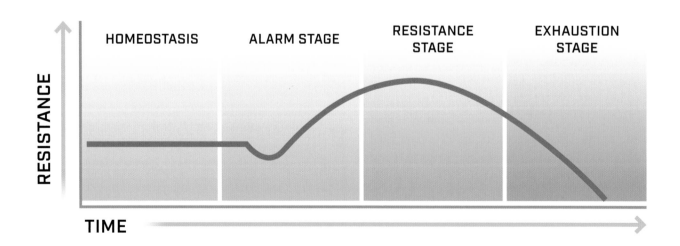

THE PERIODIZATION PARADOX

12.3

In the 1970s, '80s, and '90s, some of the most influential athletic training theories came out of Russia and other Soviet bloc countries. Some of the more individualized elements of Soviet strength and conditioning have become staples in Western gyms and team sports facilities alike, such as Dr. Yuri Verkhoshansky's plyometrics and the kettlebell training that Pavel Tsatsouline popularized. Yet when it comes to team-sports athletes, no method has been so pervasive and impactful on preparation as periodization. As we're about to see, though, its conventional application to team sports is largely ineffective.

WHEN SELYE CORRECTED NIETZSCHE

12.3.1

German philosopher Friedrich Nietzsche famously said, "That which does not kill us makes us stronger." Endocrinologist Hans Selye, however, recognized that it's not the stressor itself that makes you stronger but the recovery from and adaptation to the stressor (or stimulus). So he amended that saying to "It is not stress that kills, but our reaction to it." While this evidently has a negative connotation, a small group of Eastern bloc physiologists recognized that they could manipulate the body's stress response to produce positive adaptations instead of harmful ones. Perhaps, they thought, a training cycle could be created that took into account the stages of general adaptation syndrome and introduced timed doses of physical stimulation that would produce a desired effect, such as increased strength, power, speed, or endurance.

INJURY FACTORS & PATHWAY IN TEAM SPORTS

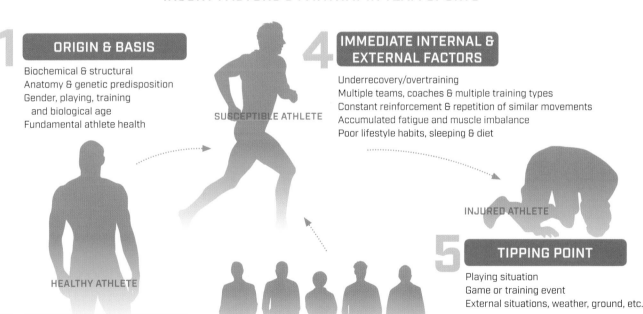

1 ORIGIN & BASIS
Biochemical & structural
Anatomy & genetic predisposition
Gender, playing, training
  and biological age
Fundamental athlete health

SUSCEPTIBLE ATHLETE

4 IMMEDIATE INTERNAL & EXTERNAL FACTORS
Underrecovery/overtraining
Multiple teams, coaches & multiple training types
Constant reinforcement & repetition of similar movements
Accumulated fatigue and muscle imbalance
Poor lifestyle habits, sleeping & diet

INJURED ATHLETE

HEALTHY ATHLETE

5 TIPPING POINT
Playing situation
Game or training event
External situations, weather, ground, etc.

2 ACCUMULATED RISK FACTORS
Accumulated playing, training & biological age
Historical strength training & movement patterns
Injury history
Historical lifestyle, diet & off-field habits
Skill & technical level
Physical fitness

TRAINING COACHES & PROFESSIONALS

3 COACHING & PROFESSIONAL INPUT
Communication among team's coaching professionals
Poor training & preparation practices
Planned & coordinated training
Human factors & input

12 The Evolution of Preparation

The most prominent and influential of these early sports scientists was Leonid Matveyev. His employer, the Moscow Institute of Physical Culture, was charged with improving the performance of Soviet athletes in international competition from the 1952 Helsinki Olympics onward. At the height of the Cold War, this directive also carried an implied subtext: win more medals than capitalist Western nations to show the superiority of communism on the world stage (very Drago versus Rocky, I know).

We now understand that one way Russia and other Soviet nations achieved such a goal was through the state-sponsored use of performance-enhancing drugs. But this dirty truth often obscures the fact that Matveyev and his colleagues also developed new and, for the time, systemic approaches to training. These would form the basis for developing Eastern bloc athletes in the 1960s, 1970s, and 1980s and proved successful in delivering the kind of results the Politburo was looking for.

Using the three stages of Selye's general adaptation syndrome, the fitness-fatigue model, and the stress response theory (how the body responds to acute and chronic stressors) Matveyev started exploring when to introduce certain stimuli and at what dose to promote adaptation without pushing athletes' bodies too far, into maladaptation and a chronic stress/exhaustion state. By using sequential programming that varied the intensity, density, and volume of certain types of training, Matveyev hoped that periodization would deliver continual results by managing the stimulus-adaptation-recovery cycle over the desired period (such as four years for an Olympian). The other aim was to enable the athlete to peak at the required time.[27]

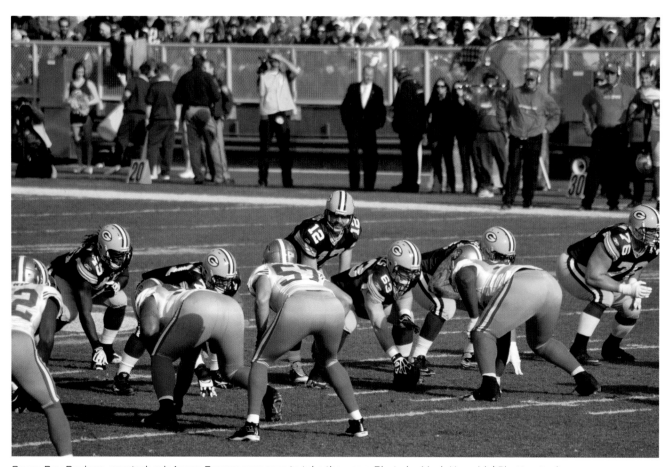

Green Bay Packers quarterback Aaron Rogers prepares to take the snap. Photo by Mark Herreid / Shutterstock.com.

PERIODIZATION AND GENERAL ADAPTATION SYNDROME   12.3.2

Matveyev attempted to sync his new training system with the alarm, resistance, and exhaustion stages of Selye's model. In the alarm phase, the body responds to the training stimulus. During the resistance stage, the body recovers and repairs the damage done during training. Depending on whether the stimuli dose was appropriate and the quality and duration of recovery, the body either returns to its previous state or adapts and goes above this baseline.

This stage, resistance, is the one in which gains in speed, strength, power, and endurance are achieved, Matveyev thought. The third stage, exhaustion, occurs only if the training load was too great, the recovery time and quality insufficient, and/or the next training session conducted too soon and at the wrong density, volume, or intensity.[28]

COMPENSATION, SUPERCOMPENSATION, OVERTRAINING, AND CUMULATIVE EFFECT   12.3.3

One of the key elements of periodization—and the most valid for team-sports athletes—is the timing of the training stimulus. Matveyev was one of the first sports scientists to recognize the essential role of recovery in promoting physical adaptation in athletes. If an athlete is exposed to the right amount of stimulation/stress at the correct effort level and allowed to recover adequately, there is not just compensation for an individual stimulus but supercompensation for multiple stimuli introduced throughout the morphocycle, which results in even greater gains. However, if the next training stimulus is introduced too early, supercompensation does not occur.

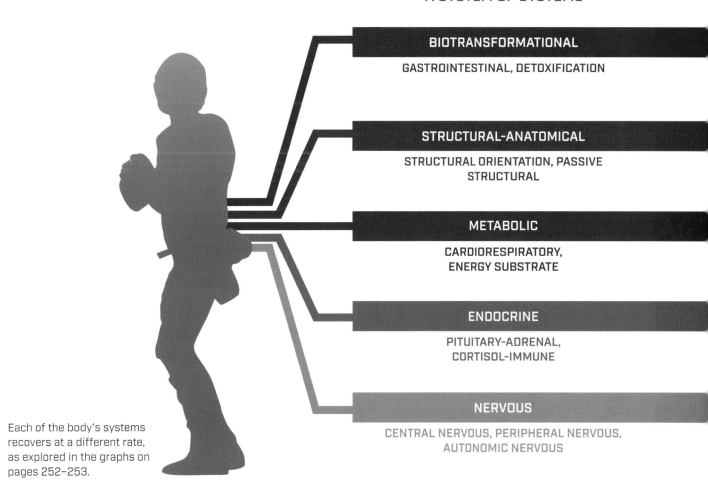

A SYSTEM OF SYSTEMS

BIOTRANSFORMATIONAL
GASTROINTESTINAL, DETOXIFICATION

STRUCTURAL-ANATOMICAL
STRUCTURAL ORIENTATION, PASSIVE STRUCTURAL

METABOLIC
CARDIORESPIRATORY, ENERGY SUBSTRATE

ENDOCRINE
PITUITARY-ADRENAL, CORTISOL-IMMUNE

NERVOUS
CENTRAL NERVOUS, PERIPHERAL NERVOUS, AUTONOMIC NERVOUS

Each of the body's systems recovers at a different rate, as explored in the graphs on pages 252–253.

MULTIFACTORAL RECOVERY MODEL

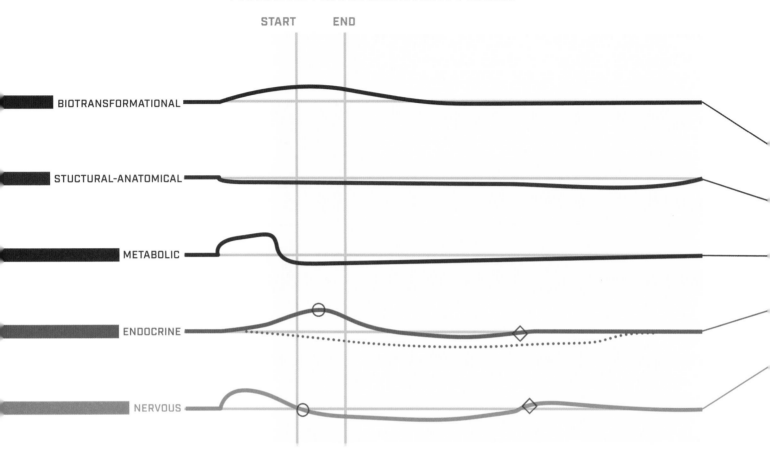

In this case, the training effect of the previous session is minimized and the athlete's accumulated fatigue will hinder performance during this second session and adaptation. Over time, the individual would be hampered by the negative impact of overtraining, leading to chronic fatigue, injury, and poor results in competition. This issue can also rear its head if there's insufficient variety.

It's not just training too much that can lead to suboptimal adaptation, periodization devotees insist. Failing to introduce a new stimulus soon enough can also compromise the effectiveness of the program. If there isn't great enough frequency, the response to previous sessions is blunted and "de-training" occurs. This concept is part of the stimulus-fatigue-recovery-adaptation theory, which covers the relationship between each of these phases and shows why we cannot consider any single one of them in isolation when programming for our players.[29]

THE GREAT PERIODIZATION MISINTERPRETATION   12.3.4

Matveyev and other Russian and Eastern European periodization pioneers initially designed their systems with individual athletes and Olympic medals in mind. Though Matveyev's books The *Problem of Periodization in Sports Training* (1964) and *The Fundamentals of Training* (1965) reached some early adopters in the West, it was Scottish national track and field coach Frank Dick's 1975 translation of Matveyev's system that introduced a large audience outside the Soviet Union to periodization.[30] This exposure grew with the 1983 publication of Tudor Bompa's popular book *Periodization: Theory and Methodology of Training*.[31]

It wasn't long until sports teams discovered periodization and tried to apply it to preparing their squads for game-day performance. Almost inevita-

PLAYING SQUAD: MULTISYSTEM EXCITATION & FATIGUE

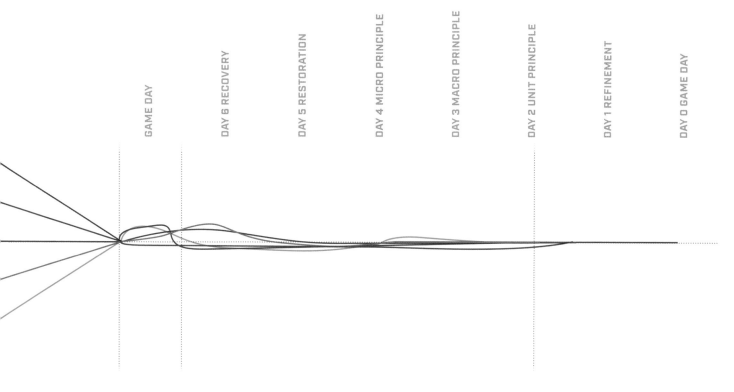

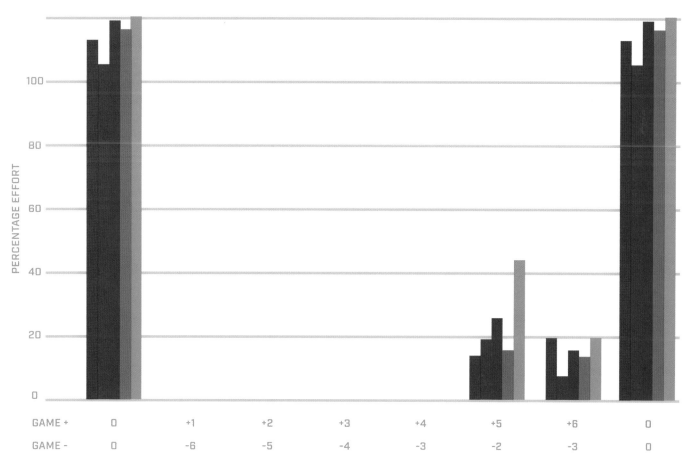

	GAME DAY	DAY 6 RECOVERY	DAY 5 RESTORATION	DAY 4 MICRO PRINCIPLE	DAY 3 MACRO PRINCIPLE	DAY 2 UNIT PRINCIPLE	DAY 1 REFINEMENT	DAY 0 GAME DAY
GAME +	0	+1	+2	+3	+4	+5	+6	0
GAME −	0	−6	−5	−4	−3	−2	−3	0

PERCENTAGE EFFORT

bly, the teams that first adopted this new systemic method were those in Soviet countries. Periodization had quickly delivered on its promises in individual competition, so there was no surprise when club and national teams decided to implement it in an effort to gain similar results. However, this linear approach did not translate to Soviet team sports, though some were successful, such as the Red Army, Anatoli Tarasov's great ice hockey team.

THE REDUCTIONIST PERIODIZATION FAILURE

12.3.5

Matveyev's periodization model and its derivatives have proven very effective when used to train Olympic athletes and other competitors who are tar-

geting optimal performance at a single event that occurs only every few years (even though the concept of peaking is flawed in multiple ways). And although many contemporary detractors dismiss periodization wholesale, many of the core elements—including supercompensation, accumulated load, oscillating recovery cycles, varying stressors to avoid overtraining, and promoting long-term development of the athlete—are very useful in the preparation of sports teams.

The trouble comes when we try to extrapolate rigid, compartmentalized periodization methods to team sports chapter and verse. A lack of sequencing and integration of training factors will result in high levels of fatigue, reduced potential for optimizing performance, and a greater risk of injury. There is little evidence that old-school periodization is effective when applied to team-sports athletes, and

ADAPTATION & RESIDUAL FATIGUE

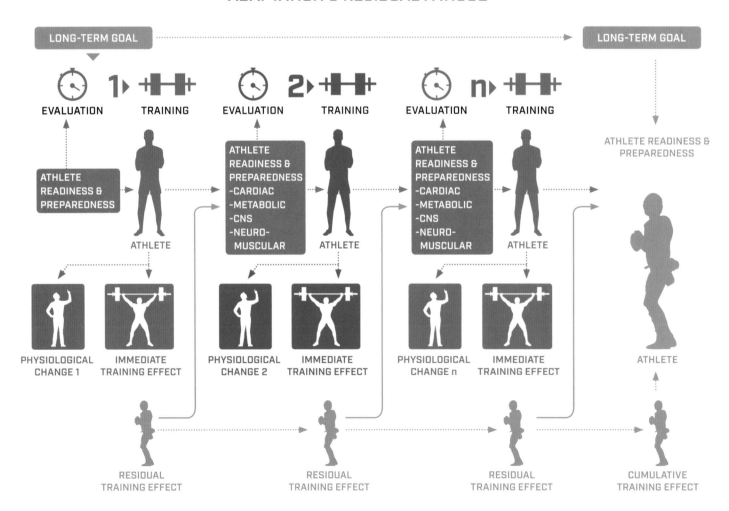

where studies have been conducted, they've made the same mistake as many periodization practitioners in looking at the impact on only one physical element. Another limitation of the literature is that most research has not centered on elite athletes but rather on beginners and intermediate athletes, who would respond rapidly to almost any systematized training approach.[32]

INDIVIDUAL SPORTS VS. TEAM SPORTS: DIFFERENT NEEDS   12.3.5.1

Individual and team sports have different preparation requirements. Though competing in track and field, tennis, or any other predominantly solo discipline does require some degree of tactics, this element is far more complex in team sports. This means that more time must be devoted to it and that the learning and mastery of a game plan is every bit as impactful as what players are physically capable of. With its core focus on physical elements, traditional periodization falls short of what's required to help teams and the athletes that compose them succeed from a tactical standpoint.

Then there are the discrepancies between the individual disciplines that periodization was initially designed for and team sports. The very nature of the competitive season in American football, soccer, rugby, and other team sports is fundamentally different from that of individual disciplines. Though athletes in track and field, swimming, and other such sports do compete more than once a season and have to negotiate national team selection trials, they are ultimately targeting an Olympiad, world championship, or other singular event and focusing all their training and preparation on it. This is why periodization can be effective, even though its impact in Eastern bloc countries may have been exaggerated by the fact that national sporting bodies dominated every aspect of their athletes' lives.[33]

In contrast, team-sports athletes usually play at least one game a week, and often two or more every seven days. In addition to club duties, they may have national team commitments that extend their season even longer.[34] Yes, team-sports athletes may be chasing a championship and, in certain sports and leagues, making the playoffs immediately beforehand, but to achieve these goals they must perform optimally week in and week out, not on just one day.

Periodization typically fails to meet this need for consistent performance, particularly when looking at every member of a team-sports squad. As Matveyev's countryman and fellow physiologist Yuri Verkhoshansky rightly wrote, "Coaches still following the outdated elements of periodization find it extremely difficult to keep their athletes in top form throughout the competition season."[35] And in fact, applying periodization to team sports can be detrimental and even damaging to athletes' health and performance.

THE PROBLEM WITH PEAKING   12.3.5.2

Sport scientist Vladimir V. Issurin writes that periodization often "leads to dramatic reductions in lean body mass, maximal strength, maximal aerobic power, and even maximal speed." He adds that for sports teams, "the generalized concepts of peaking and tapering make no sense."[36]

From a sports science perspective, the very idea of "peaking" is, as Issurin writes, inapplicable. The media-created notion of a team coasting through the regular season and then flicking a switch come playoff time is a myth. Coaches may well rest certain key players periodically and, in sports like basketball, pull their starters once they've built up an insurmountable lead in order to conserve energy, but rare is the team that's able to go from mediocrity to greatness between the regular season and postseason like a car changing gears.

THE FOCUS ON THE PHYSICAL   12.3.5.3

Another problem with a sports team rigidly following a periodization approach is its overemphasis on physical training. Certainly, every athlete must have a baseline of speed, strength, endurance, and other physical qualities depending on the sport, position, and level of competition. Then there are anthropomorphic factors to consider—you're not going to see a 120-pound lineman playing in the NFL, and neither are there any 325-pound forwards in soccer.

And yet physical traits are only one component of athlete performance in a team-sports setting. We must also consider the technical, tactical, and psychological elements. Technique and skill are important in individual sports, but their context is different within a team setting, as athletes must be able to apply them in relation to their teammates.

Similarly, athletes in individual sports must employ tactics—such as a runner pacing a marathon correctly. But the need for tactical awareness in team sports is elevated, as players must take into account the Commander's Intent and sub-objectives of the game plan in each of the four game moments.

José Mourinho is quick to dismiss the old approach of just preparing players physically: "I have no idea where the physical aspect ends and the tactical/psychological aspect begins, but football encaptures both. I can't separate the two, but what I can say is that football is not all about the physical aspect, it's about much more than that. In the grand scheme of things, the physical aspect is probably the least important element. Without organization and a talent in exploring the different tactical models of the game, your weaknesses quickly become apparent, regardless of how fit you are."[37]

We also cannot ignore the psychological demands that team sports place on every competitor. This facet of preparation not only involves the emotional and cognitive load (and the fatigue that results) during the game itself but must also encompass the impact of training and what happens when the player isn't at team facilities. And when it comes to game day, according to multi–Super Bowl–winning coach Bill Walsh, "Those who are able to perform best are those who are able to remove tension, anxiety and fear from their minds."[38] This isn't automatic but must be conditioned by the coaching staff's creating gamelike scenarios in practice and empowering each team member to improve his or her performance during intrasquad competition.

Despite these facts, many sports teams continue to overemphasize the physical element of team preparation and rely on periodization to structure practices. Furthermore, this reductionist approach fragments physical elements—such as strength training, mobility, and speed work—and then attempts to put them all together come game day. This simply does not work and manifests itself in suboptimal performance, increased injuries, and, ultimately, shorter careers.

Prioritizing physical training at the expense of the other three elements of team preparation—technical, tactical, and psychological—also manifests itself on game day. While there was an age in which teams could get away with "power basketball," putting their five biggest, strongest, and fastest basketball players on the court and so on, advances in technique and tactics across all team sports have rendered such an approach obsolete, particularly at the elite level.

Does it help to have big, strong, and fast players who can run all day? Absolutely. But without the proper tactics, technique, and psychological preparation, such athletes will be unable to apply their physical gifts over the long term and will ultimately be overcome by teams composed of more well rounded players who are cognitively, technically, and tactically advanced. It's also a misconception that old-school periodization doesn't recognize physical training, particularly strength work, as having a skill component.

When athletes improve their squat or dead lift, it's not just that they've physically adapted or undergone cell-level advances—they've become better at the skills of squatting and deadlifting. They've increased muscle recruitment, executed a motor pattern more quickly, and improved their efficiency. And it's only by continuing to refine their skills and movement quality that they will keep progressing. So even regarding physical training as purely about muscular development is a faulty premise.

TRAINING BY THE CALENDAR   12.3.5.4

Another limitation of traditional linear periodization as it has traditionally been applied to team sports is its separation of athlete's physical development into distinct, cut-and-dried phases, including familiarization, preparation, control, competition, maintenance, and restoration. The issue is that team sports are not linear, and it's simply ineffective to train athletes in a way that emphasizes certain stimuli in individual phases of the season, post-season, off-season, and preseason and then leaves them untouched for the rest of the year.

One example is how American football and rugby teams typically approached strength training. As soon as the last game of the season ended, the coaches would tell their players to get in the weight room. The goal seemed to be to get as strong and powerful as possible in the off-season and show up to pre-season training in tip-top shape. In the periodization system, this stage of off-season strength training would be known as the *preparatory period.*

Only when it was time for preseason camps to open would the emphasis be switched to the technical and tactical elements of the game (psychological preparation is largely ignored in periodization). During this "transition period" before the competitive season, strength training would be put on the back burner as the team transitioned from preseason to the competitive season, as it was thought that athletes were "strong enough" by this time and that lifting weights before and between games would overtax them and increase injury risk. Once the season was over, there'd be another short transition period of active rest before players got back to bench pressing and squatting their hearts out.

Coaches hoped that such a model would allow athletes to steadily improve throughout the season and peak for the playoffs and championship games. The reality was far different. In fact, the moment the players cut back or stopped their strength training, they started losing the gains they had spent all summer achieving. So essentially they got weaker and less explosive with every game.

Then there were the adverse effects of neglecting the other components of preparation. The athletes regressed technically and tactically in the off-season as they focused all their efforts on getting stronger, so that they were ill prepared by the time the first game rolled around. And because of the frenetic nature of the competitive season, there was no time to play catch-up.

This example might seem outdated, but the philosophy of favoring physical training above all else and breaking preparation down into disparate silos that are emphasized or neglected depending on the competitive calendar is still widespread across all team sports. An unintended consequence of trying to focus on separate elements of team preparation is that the more you break things down, the more gaps you create.

Any math teacher will tell you that when you divide something, you actually create three entities—two numbers and one gap. And the more gaps there are, the less your preparation will come together during competition. Think about jigsaw puzzles: one with fifty pieces is a lot easier to complete than one with five hundred.

ISOLATING THE FOUR COACTIVES   12.3.5.5

There is little doubt that the specialists involved in preparing team-sports athletes—strength and conditioning coaches, psychologists, physical therapists, and so on—have all advanced their craft since Matveyev's periodization model became popular in the mid to late 1960s, but within many organizations they are still isolated and functioning within the constraints of an outdated overall approach to team preparation.

Development of physical attributes such as power, strength, and speed has existed in a vacuum for too long. To be useful once the players take the field, each of these attributes must be developed with sport-specific application in mind. Otherwise, the team preparation will be for its own sake rather than targeting real-world performance improvements. It's not about how big, strong, and fast each member of the team is but rather how effectively their physical attributes can be applied with respect to technique, tactics, and strategy during competition.

Teams need to start recognizing that skills don't develop in the same way as physical characteristics and must come to realize that while technical and tactical acumen are harder to assess than physical benchmarks, they're equally important, if not more so. Unfortunately, most organizations have yet to arrive at this conclusion.

As physiologist Jay R. Hoffman wrote, "Although tremendous growth has been seen in strength and conditioning programs in American football for the past 25 years, the utilization of sport science to maximize the performance ability of American football players is still lacking."[39] Such a judgment of isolated, periodized preparation is not confined to American football or strength and conditioning but applies to all team sports and the specialties that prepare their athletes when they try to follow a siloed, linear approach.

Another part of the problem is that sports science itself remains largely fragmented. Many team-sports organizations have one group focusing on research-driven studies that can impact how the coaches prepare players physically. Then, down the hall, a second group is concentrating on statistics and objective game-day outcomes. Unfortunately, the reality is that there's little harmony or collaboration between these two factions, meaning that they're often pulling the coaches in two (or sometimes many more) different directions.

The experts in each area quite often do wonderful work, but the lack of integration means that their insights are of limited value, particularly during the hectic atmosphere of the competitive season. This is another reason that within the world of team sports, the promise of sports science remains largely unfulfilled.

Perfection is not attainable. But if we chase perfection, we can catch excellence.

—Vince Lombardi

THE ALWAYS-ON WORLD OF TEAM SPORTS   12.3.5.6

There have also been significant changes in team sports scheduling that further reduce the usefulness of periodization. For example, soccer teams in the Premier League have multiple preseason friendlies. During the Premier League season itself, they also compete in the FA and Football League Cup. If the club finishes high enough in the league, it will host and travel abroad for additional Champions League or Europa Cup games.

Then there's the possibility of the World Club Championship. In addition, the best players also represent their countries in the European Championships, African Nations Cup, Copa America, and the World Cup, plus all the qualifying matches and international friendlies. Players in rugby, basketball, and many other team sports also have playing duties for their countries to add to their club responsibilities.

The result is that in some ways, the competitive season never really ends, and even if there is an "off-season," it is extremely short and leaves little time for the kind of preparatory training that is so essential to the periodization model—so even if the model itself were effective in the first place, it's not feasible in this environment. And for members of the military, there are tours of duty, but they could be called into action at any time, so they must stay in a constant state of readiness and preparedness. Such stark realities also eliminate the possibility of tapering—that is, reducing the intensity of practices right before competition.

Simply put, team-sports organizations must recognize the limited effectiveness of a periodization approach that favors physicality above all. A more comprehensive, all-inclusive model is needed if teams and athletes are to improve not just physically but also technically, tactically, and psychologically as well. Only with such a model will they be able to reach their potential and improve their winning record in the long term. And in team sports, as Vince Lombardi drilled into every football team he coached from day one, "winning isn't everything, it's the only thing."[40]

WHY PERIODIZATION DOESN'T EXIST

▬▬▬▬▬▬▬▬▬▬▬ 12.4

When Russian sports scientists came up with the original principles of periodization, they were trying to prepare runners to perform their best in an Olympic final—a single event with a four-year run-up. The challenge, then, with trying to apply their approach to team-sports athletes is twofold. The first is the nature of the discipline. Running and other individual sports, like Olympic lifting, do of course have a skill component, but they are nowhere near as technically and tactically complex as team sports. Second, team-sports athletes never have a singular moment in time four years in the future to build toward—they typically have to perform at least once a week.

According to Vítor Frade, traditional periodization is not applicable: "The Tactical Periodization training is a methodology whose greatest concern in the game aims to produce a team in the competition. That is why the Game Model and tactical dimension are assumed to guide the whole process of training."[41] In other words, we can't make the mistake of traditional periodization and focus only on the physical elements. In contrast, tactical periodization includes technical, psychological, and, as the name suggests, tactical coactives, which must be developed simultaneously in a morphocycle approach that works backward from the game.

Another reason that old-school periodization doesn't work in team sports is that there's a very short off-season, which means that the preparatory block is virtually nonexistent. Between duties for club and country, a player must maintain continual readiness and preparedness year-round. In many sports, not least Premier League rugby and soccer, teams are also playing in several competitions simultaneously, further invalidating periodization's focus on a single event.

For example, a player for Manchester City might look at his game calendar for the next six weeks and see five Premier League games, an international friendly, two Champions League games, and a domestic cup fixture. If a team is to compete for a title, it must maintain a high standard of play throughout the season. Even in sports like basketball that have a playoff system, playoffs consist of seven-game series, which eliminates the possibility of building toward a single performance event, as traditional block-focused models do. This is why, for the team-sports player, Soviet-style periodization, or what it is now interpreted as, does not exist.

THE PRINCIPLE OF VERTICAL INTEGRATION

▬▬▬▬▬▬▬▬▬▬▬ 12.5

While we've looked into the limitations of applying traditional periodization to the preparation of team sports athletes, a variation of this methodology that came from individual sports is more useful and relevant for our purposes.

Though he will always be unfairly tainted by the doping scandal that swirled around his premier athlete, Ben Johnson, during the 1988 Seoul Olympics, coach Charlie Francis revolutionized how sprinters are trained before, during, and after the competitive season. From the 1960s on, almost every coach applied Matveyev's method to track and field. During his own time as a world-class sprinter and then as a coach, Francis realized that this system failed on multiple levels, including the fact that his athletes couldn't just peak once for a big championship final—they also needed to perform optimally at all the elite IAAF events like the Weltklasse in Zurich, as well as the increasingly competitive trials for the Olympics and World Championships.

So he borrowed a business term, *vertical integration,* which refers to the process whereby a company combines two or more stages of production rather than specializing in one stage and outsourcing the others, and used it to create a more nuanced and inclusive periodization model that took into account the need for continually improving times on the track, the individual biology and strengths of each athlete, and a more detailed understanding of how training impacts body systems such as the central nervous system. By sequencing high-intensity sessions that put a big load on the CNS—like Olympic lifting—and low-intensity ones—say, longer, less-intense track sessions—Francis recognized that his athletes would recover more quickly. The impact on the CNS was determined, he realized, by the relationship between intensity and volume (see the graphic below).

As he prioritized one element of training—such as volume—Francis dialed back another that had been recently emphasized—like intensity. And yet all components—volume, intensity, density, and collision—were present at all times, throughout the year. In addition, quality was paramount, even on higher-volume days. As Francis himself put it, "If your workout deteriorates, stop the workout!"[42] He was a big believer in exposing his training group to the minimum required stimulus to make change, saying, "Do all that you need to do to make an athlete better and nothing more."[43]

Such thinking shook the sprinting world, as it had been previously believed that tapering before big events was essential, that explosive training should

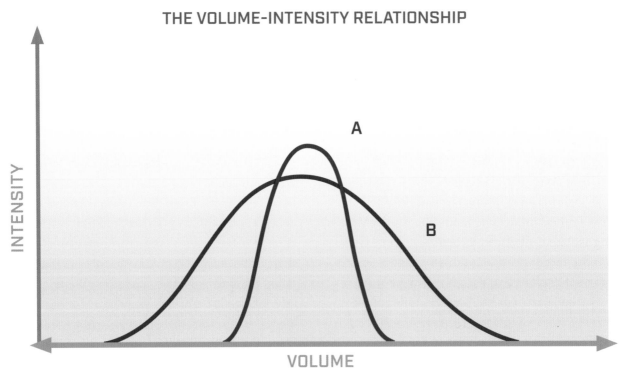

THE VOLUME-INTENSITY RELATIONSHIP

CNS RECOVERY

As Charlie Francis reminds us, the impact on the CNS is determined by INTENSITY X VOLUME, so that in the diagram above, the impact of Example A is less than the impact of Example B, even though the intensity of Example A is higher.

be avoided during the competitive season, and that sprinters could and should be exposed to isolated stimuli that targeted only one quality (speed, reaction time off the blocks, etc.). The old approach also bought into Matveyev's belief that big blocks of certain types of training should be used exclusively at set times of the competitive year/cycle.

Francis blew up all this outdated methodology. His integrative approach enabled his athletes to recover more fully, achieve more consistent and sustainable improvements, and avoid overtraining by ditching the old "more is better" philosophy that for years ran sprinters into the ground (pun intended). By the time he passed away in 2010, Francis's system had been fully validated, with his training group combining for nine Olympic medals, twenty-three world records, and more than 250 Canadian records.[44]

Francis's vertical integration approach isn't valid only for individual competitors such as track and field athletes but can also be applied to sports teams.

THE MORPHOCYCLE AND WEEKLY RHYTHM

12.6

The concept of long-term planning looks excellent in books, but the reality is that these offer good guidelines at best. With modern team sports, the most effective basis for all planning is a weekly pattern.

Charlie Francis influenced many coaches by transforming isolated, physicality-focused periodization into a more integrated, adaptable type of programming for sprinting. He also identified intensity as the key variable, not volume. Several other pioneers have since gone even further in creating an effective, sustainable model for preparing athletes and teams for continual improvement in competition.

The morphocycle, the weekly pattern model that we're going to explore in depth in this section, is largely based on the pioneering work of people like soccer coaches Carlos Queiroz and Rinus Michels,

football coach Bill Walsh, powerlifting coach Louie Simmons, and professors José Guilherme Oliveira and Vítor Frade. This morphocycle approach combines traditional tactical periodization with the European model of functional health, vertical integration, and Western periodization principles.

In the mid-1990s, Frade, a professor at the University of Porto, devised the tactical periodization approach to preparing soccer teams. This is the approach that first established the four game moments (discussed in "The Game") and the elements of the four-coactive model (discussed in "The

THE SEVEN ELEMENTS OF VERTICAL INTEGRATION TRAINING

Charlie Francis suggested that each of the following seven variables should be present in every practice, for every athlete, throughout the year. Each is emphasized or de-emphasized, depending on the composition of other recent training sessions, to encourage full recovery.

1. Bioenergetics / biodynamics / biomotor abilities
2. Intensity
3. Volume
4. Density
5. Frequency
6. Method
7. Means (exercise)

We adapt these concepts specifically with Vítor Frade's morphocycle approach to team sport and combine them in a holistic approach.

Training your team is the most important part of being a successful football manager—it is the difference between winning leagues and failing.

—José Mourinho

Player"). Unsurprisingly, given the proximity of the two organizations, Frade's ideas made their way from the university to FC Porto, where the system profoundly impacted the methods of José Mourinho, André Villas-Boas, and Aitor Karanka. The methodology was implemented in soccer, but over the years I've successfully integrated these principles of tactical periodization into a holistic model and made them applicable to American football, basketball, rugby, and other team sports, with huge success.

As the name of Frade's system suggests, the tactical dimension was the primary consideration for the coaching staff at Porto, as this is what determines how the team plays the game and meets the aims of the game plan. That being said, the other three elements of the four-coactive model—technical, psychological, and physical—are still very important in tactical periodization, and their advancement is essential if the team's application of tactical principles is to progress.

Within the tactical periodization approach, each week (or whatever the period is between games) takes the form of a morphocycle in which learning experiences involving all four coactives are balanced in a way that facilitates certain outcomes and resulting adaptations in players, yet also allows for adequate recovery between stimuli. The morphocycle also achieves harmony among the morphological programming elements, which are emphasized or de-emphasized in relation to what has come before, what's coming next, and, most importantly, each day's relationship to the next game.

By varying the composition of the morphocycle but keeping its basic structure—including the length of training sessions and the timing of practice—consistent, the team stabilizes its performance, leading to a continually high level of play. Using such a model also has the benefit of giving the coaching staff a way to plan and program that respects the biological and societal rhythms the athlete experiences and puts the game itself at the center of everything the team does.[45]

This approach is based on winning science and using sports science the way it should be. Dismantling the reductionism that has dominated science for centuries and replacing its stiffness with both flexibility and stability gives us a more holistic approach to learning and development.[46]

RECONNECTING THE GAME AND TRAINING   12.6.1

Because the game is inherently complex and nonlinear and training must mirror the game if it's to be effective, training too should be complex and nonlinear. This is not to say that players' experiences should seem difficult or hard to grasp—in fact, quite the opposite. By structuring practices in a multifaceted way that takes into account tactical, technical, physical, and psychological elements, coaches can simplify player education by breaking it down into parts. In the four-coactives approach that I adopted from Vítor Frade, training mirrors the game as closely as possible, so the ball is used a lot more than in some traditional systems that overemphasize the physical component of play.

Within many sports organizations, team preparation has remained ineffective because it involves a series of isolated, abstract concepts that hopefully come together on game day. In contrast, tactical periodization aims to prepare players for the situations they'll face playing against the next opponent, and so works backward from the game itself. As José Guilherme Oliveira, former Porto youth coach and one of Frade's fellow professors in the University of Porto's sports department, writes, "It takes from the game that which is most important and transports it for training, which is constructed by actions of the game itself."[47] In other words, there's no disconnect between what happens in the practice facility and what the coaches want their players to achieve during competition.

The term *tactical periodization* is a misnomer, as it implies that the approach is purely about tactics, which in soccer is critical. But while it certainly incorporates tactical elements, the model also stresses including the four-coactives approach in each team and individual practice session, as this best re-creates the game experience. Perhaps Portuguese soccer television and radio analyst Luís Freitas Lobo describes it best when he says that in training, this approach "never separates the physical, the tactical, the technical—the skills—and the mental in the work. Physical preparation doesn't exist by itself for Portuguese coaches. It's integrated with the tactical game. You don't do any physical exercises without transferring them to the game."[48]

If César Luis Menotti, coach of the 1978 World Cup–winning Argentina side, is correct in saying, "A team above all is an idea," then tactical periodization is the blueprint for instilling such an idea in a team. By the time a coach is yelling from the sidelines during a game, it's too late to communicate key principles. Instead, they must be introduced, encouraged, and reinforced during team preparation so that individual players' habits are conditioned with the team game plan and its objectives in mind. That way, when it comes time to react to a game-time situation, the automatic response will be more likely to further the team's aims in a tactical context. The goal is not to remove individuality or creativity but rather to encourage it to flourish within a systematized methodology.[49]

A weekly programming framework enables us to take the new way of viewing and analyzing the game that we developed in "The Game" and integrate it with our training approach. So learning experiences created for the athletes are now devised and executed within the context of the four game moments: offensive, defensive, transition-to-defense, and transition-to-offense. Implementing tactical periodization means that every exercise or drill conducted in practice is relevant to how the head coach wants the players to act collectively during the game. So if, for example, a coach wants her team to spread the ball wide a lot during the offensive moment, she will construct learning experiences that encourage this.

As one visiting coach observed while watching FC Porto's junior teams train, "The physical, technical, tactical, and psychological elements are never worked on a separate way. Everything is included while the main concern of every exercise is to organize the team for one of the four moments of the game. This way of working trains the team to react automatically to every moment."[50]

The athlete is seen in a holistic manner, from a unique process of teaching and training. Reinforcing this idea, you cannot separate the athlete from the person, who cannot be considered as a performance machine but must be seen as a human being, with all the complexity that entails.

At any club, coaches should prepare the first team in the same way as the youth and reserve squads. Employing tactical periodization in an academy from the time kids can kick a ball ensures that there

GREAT MINDS THINK ALIKE

Great coaches in various sports from around the world have come to similar conclusions about how to best prepare their athletes and work backward from the game in doing so. For example, the philosophy that Jim Harbaugh has used at Stanford, with the San Francisco 49ers, and at the University of Michigan has many similarities to the principles Graham Henry used with the All Blacks. There are also many commonalities among the coaching philosophies of José Mourinho, Alex Ferguson, Bill Belichick, Gregg Popovich, and many more of the most successful coaches in team sports.

is continuity throughout the organization, and if players work their way into the first team, they're already familiar with how it prepares and plays. The positive impact of teams using the same morphological approach and tactical periodization that are employed by the senior team in their youth academies is self-evident: clubs managed by Portuguese coaches utilizing this approach have won their domestic league multiple times, as well as the top leagues in Greece, Switzerland, Russia, Egypt, and Mexico.[51] And despite a blip during the 2015–16 season, Mourinho led Chelsea to three Premier League titles, Real Madrid to the summit of La Liga, Inter Milan to two Serie A titles, the Italian Cup, and the Champions League, and, fittingly, Porto to two league titles, two cup wins, and a first Champions League trophy. The key here is congruity and coherence among every age group involved in the club. Youth players who make it to the next level are already grounded in the principles of tactical periodization and so are well prepared to progress as they move up to the Under-15s, Under-19s, and Under-21s, and into the senior squad.

MORPHOLOGICAL PROGRAMMING

12.7

Periodization had too many negative associations and conclusions to be relevant for team sports. In contrast, programming is an approach to help plan team-sport training. It refers to short-term, reactive planning that is based on the immediate status of the athlete, with consideration to the overall plan for the next game. My morphological programming approach gives primacy to winning through tactics, regulating the collective organization, and developing the physical, technical, and psychological coactives alongside tactics. This process focuses on the recognition of patterns in the game, achieved through the operation of the principles of a game model, therefore being specific training. This is the basis for organizing the week. It is essential to develop a new way of training that transcends the conventional fragmented, reductionist theory: a more unified, tactical periodization system, based on the new way of seeing the game that was discussed in "The Game."

Programming, which can be defined as adapting management principles to the reality in which we find ourselves, is a much better approach.[52] Compared to rigid, unyielding periodization, programming is much more flexible and responsive and can determine strategies of action much faster in shorter time frames. The cohesiveness of the approach is managed by the framework of a game model, which is based on a full, holistic understanding of the sport. Programming involves not only exploiting adaptation principles but also taking into account how individual athletes respond psychophysiologically to the cumulative effects of training. There are many advantages to programming over a periodization approach, not least of which is that it balances the level and timing of competitive activity more accurately. Programming also uses real-time information, even when it's incomplete, to make nimbler and more efficient adjustments.

> *Water [H₂O] is an essential means to extinguish the fire. However, if we separate its components—hydrogen and oxygen—then instead of putting out the fire, it glows even more.*
>
> —Ricardo Carvalho

THIRTEEN

FACILITATING EXPERIENCES

As we've discussed, the role of a coach is to facilitate a learning experience, not enforce a lesson. This is why we use a weekly cycle as the core of all team preparation. Some coaches, like Raymond Verheijen, advocate the use of a biweekly cycle, and this too can be utilized somewhat effectively, but at the elite end in professional sports, a weekly pattern is ideal, since this is how society as a whole functions. This helps with habit development. For athletes to develop positive long-term habits, coaches need to create optimal conditions for habit acquisition in the team environment.

THE LAW OF INDIVISIBILITY

13.1

One of the primary errors in current team-training approaches is that we attempt to isolate each of the four coactives, as well as their constituent parts, and train them separately. So we attempt to have players work on their physical qualities in the weight room or at the track and confine tactical elements to team training. Then we have the players go away and practice a technical skill—like shooting free throws in basketball or kicking drop goals in rugby—without incorporating any of the conditions they will face in a game. In an effort to develop athletes cognitively, we send them to sports psychologists. Then we attempt to put all these pieces back together in time for the

next game, believing that because we've checked all the boxes, performance will naturally improve.

Unfortunately, it simply doesn't work like that. The factors of preparation are indivisible. Rather than trying to boil down player education into separate elements, we need to develop technical, tactical, physical, and psychological qualities at the same time. This needs to be done with the goals for each game moment in mind, with all of these contributing to the achievement of the Commander's Intent.

Two more things that cannot be divided are preparation and competition. You may have heard the adage "Train slow, play slow." This appears to be a cliché, but it's also true. Athletes cannot prepare one way and play another. Everything that's done in practice should relate to the game plan in some way, and the conditions of each exercise should be as close as possible to those that players will experience in the game.[53]

IT TAKES MORE THAN TWO RIGHTS TO RIGHT A WRONG

13.1.1

Imagine you're a world-class golfer and you perfect your swing. Then one day you go to practice and you forget your best clubs. On this one crazy day you decide to swing for an hour with clubs that are the wrong size for you. How much damage does this do to your motor memory and golf swing?

A similar principle applies when preparing team-sports players. If the morphocycle calls for a high-intensity session, it's no use having athletes do it four times at 90 percent effort and then three times at 50 percent. This will condition their body to lower its excitation level and to put forth a suboptimal level of exertion in future sessions. Instead, if the session is meant to be demanding, it needs to be demanding every time. This is not to say that a coach won't sometimes back off on the number of sets or the speed if the competition cycle has ramped up and the athlete is going to be playing an unusually high number of games. But even in such a scenario, the player must fully participate at top effort. Every sub-par experience has an effect on the brain, and when your goal is excellence, that cannot be tolerated.

FOCUSING ON FUNDAMENTALS

13.2

When introducing children to team sports, it's no surprise that most coaches focus on the basics so that the kids get a solid foundation upon which to build. But once they've gotten through the first couple of years, it's amazing how little time many coaches spend continuing to hone these players' technical skills. The mindset seems to be, "Well, they know how to shoot/pass/dribble by now."

This means that an inordinate number of team-sports athletes start to move away from core competencies and begin relying on physical gifts to get them through school, college, and even professional play. Yet some elite coaches recognize the problems that neglecting skill work can present, even at the highest level. When working out a comprehensive plan that would transform the England rugby team from perennial underachievers into the number-one side on the planet going into the 2003 Rugby World Cup in Australia, Sir Clive Woodward decided that his squad had to get back to basics.

If they could pass and tackle well, they would be better able to implement the tactics and strategy of his game plan. Similarly, if they hoped to beat not only home nation and European rivals but also the Southern Hemisphere powerhouses that had dominated the sport for so long, they would have to improve their skills and timing in scrummaging and lineouts. So they did, honing their fundamentals so that they passed more quickly and tackled more cleanly while working with specialist coaches on lineouts, scrums, and kicking.[54]

Another component of England's success under Woodward—they not only lifted the Webb Ellis Cup and Five Nations (later the Six Nations) titles but at one point won an astounding forty-one of forty-six games—was that unlike many other coaches at his level, Woodward was determined that his squad would not spend what little time they had together working on physical preparedness. At their very first team meeting, Woodward said, "We won't be spending time building fitness during these sessions. That will be done by you and us outside this environment. I fully expect you to be in the best physical condition possible, ready to play your best rugby, when you show up here. If you don't, you'll soon find yourself off the mailing list."[55]

In making this radical decision, Woodward gave his players and coaching staff more time to work on skills, tactics, and psychological preparation. It was their improvement in these key elements of the morphological programming approach framework that enabled England to exceed expectations. Their improvement took six years to complete, but in the end, Woodward's meticulous preparation crystallized in Jonny Wilkinson's last-minute drop goal in 2003, which sank the home side and gave England its first Rugby World Cup trophy.

One of the most influential minds in basketball, Dr. Jack Ramsay, echoed Woodward in the way he advised coaches to prepare their teams, starting with the basics: "Basketball, like all sports, is predicated on the execution of fundamentals. The coach is a teacher. His subject: fundamentals."

Working on fundamentals is only going to be beneficial for more-experienced athletes if these skills are performed at a gamelike speed in a practice scenario that closely mirrors competition. When a fellow coach asked Steve Belichick, father of multiple Super Bowl winner Bill and a man known by his admiring peers as a "coach's coach," what he should do about a punter who was amazingly accurate in practice but performed poorly in games, Steve asked how the misfiring punter practiced. "Well, he punts and punts and punts, one after another," came the reply. "Have him practice the way he kicks in a game," Belichick suggested. "Have him punt, then take a fifteen-minute break, and then punt, and then take another break." The other coach followed Belichick's advice, and the punter began replicating his practice-field accuracy in games.[56]

It's the same in any sport: for skill work to be effective in competition, it needs to be honed under pressure and in real-world conditions. A basketball player can't improve her passing by throwing a ball against a wall for an hour.

PREPARING TO WIN
13.3

A key directive in the overall approach to preparation is that the goal is always to win. Form follows function. The style of game play is secondary to the aim of the operation—to win games.

THE END DICTATES THE MEANS
13.3.1

If you spend any length of time working with sports teams, you'll see how easy it is to get caught up in the means—how the team practices, what exercises the players do in the weight room, and so on. But this is really a backward approach to preparation. It is an extension of the same mistake the Philadelphia 76ers, under the misguidance of Sam Hinkie, made with the now-debunked phrase "Trust the Process." Trusting the process is always secondary to getting the win. Winning and the ability to make or find a way is very different from following a path for its own sake.

History has shown that turning this method on its head and letting the end dictate the means yields far better results. Think about the military for a moment. Commanders don't sit around a table debating what their tactics are going to be for a particular mission before they know what the mission and its objectives are. They wait to find out what needs to be done—like rescuing a hostage or clearing a neighborhood of hostiles—and then figure out how they're going to do it. We apply the same intentional, goal-focused decision-making to preparing sports teams for competition.

We believe the best athletes are those who know the most about their sport and as such arrive on game day more prepared than their opponents.

—Sir Clive Woodward

THE POWER OF HABITS AND ROUTINES
13.3.2

Team-sports coaches and military commanders use repetition to create habits that their warrior-athletes can access on demand without thinking, enabling them to conserve functional reserve capacity—their overall ability to deal with stress in any form—to handle the randomness and chaos of battle and sporting competition. As baseball great Yogi Berra said, "You can't think and hit the ball at the same time." The way to approach this is to create a state of calm, alert readiness. Ivan Pavlov's classical conditioning experiments have a lot of useful lessons, but his best-known experiments, such as training dogs to salivate when they hear a dinner bell, are not applicable to human beings in general, and particularly not athletes.

When trying to design training experiences that will help players better apply the game plan principles during competition, it's important to keep in mind what the end goal is: to win games. Then we can work backward to develop a training strategy to achieve that goal. The game model provides the structure on which the game plan is built, and the complexity of the game must be reflected in the way team preparation is designed. After the primary goal of winning, the coaching staff should outline and agree on objectives for each player.

Coach Wooden offers a definitive statement on what's needed for a team to achieve its ultimate goal of winning: "You must define success as making the complete effort to maximize your abilities, skill, and potential in whatever circumstances present themselves…. The score will take care of itself when you take care of the effort that precedes the score."[57]

EVERYTHING MATTERS   13.3.3

If a few players disrespect assistant coaches, cut corners during team training, and cheat on rep counts in the weight room, these aren't merely isolated discipline problems but also indicators that the players are not fully committed to the team and its principles. Eventually, these same players will let you down during a crucial game.

From a training perspective, every rep should be performed to the best of a player's ability. They may not be perfect every time, but reps performed with half-hearted effort undermine not just the good reps but the entire learning experience. The coaching staff must also take responsibility for designing sessions that focus on the right things while eliminating elements that are negative or irrelevant in reaching the desired outcome. Coaches need to make training as realistic as possible to ensure that the lessons are experienced properly by the players—even if it means replicating discipline consequences. We must take extreme care to understand what our aims are during any team preparation exercise and how this dictates the design of the learning experience.

Beyond team preparation, the phrase "Everything matters" also applies to team culture. In the military, special operatives learn early on that they don't exist in isolation but depend on support staff. One British Special Forces general explained to me that he and his fellow officers stayed with the men they were training in the jungle even when offered better accommodation by local royalty. While he was halfway through this story, the general paused to turn around and thank the service lady who brought us tea while looking her in the eye.

This furthered his point—that athletes and soldiers alike should treat everyone in the organization with respect. This is true whether players are training at home, visiting an opposing team's arena, going on a foreign tour, or staying in a hotel. Sure, some successful players do act dismissively or disrespectfully to others, but they're examples of how it's possible to be a champion but still a loser. There's obviously a practical benefit to being nice to airline staff, hotel desk staff, and other support personnel: they'll treat you better if you come back. But beyond this,

A head coach should measure success in terms of how well he is able to carry out his responsibilities relative to what he feels coaching is all about. As such, he can place greater emphasis on developing his players to take advantage of their full potential, and on developing a proper foundation for the team to perform well in the future, than on whatever actions might otherwise emanate from a 'win-now-or-else' approach.

—Bill Walsh

how players conduct themselves and interact with others impacts the success of the team. If they're respectful and courteous to strangers, they're likely to treat teammates, coaches, and fans better. A willingness to be grateful to the video intern will carry over into gratitude to family members and friends. This is why coaches like Clive Woodward went out of their way to get players to buy into a behavioral code that's applicable in any setting and scenario. Even if you're an amateur athlete, act like a professional who considers demeanor and treatment of others to be an important part of that professionalism. It's an example of how everything really is everything. You can't isolate elements of performance even if you want to.

> **Earn the right to be proud and confident.**
>
> —John Wooden

THE FREEDOM TO BE FREE   13.3.4

Game principles are simultaneously open and closed. Tactics are open to the myriad changing circumstances that each preparation session and game presents, but underlying, guiding principles are closed in that they provide a structure of framework to fall back on when such circumstances occur. Principles do not determine the way that an athlete will act in a given situation, but they do predetermine the choices that an athlete has.

Jocko Willink and Leif Babin wrote in *Extreme Ownership* about the standard operating procedures (SOPs) their Navy SEALs unit followed:

> We standardized the way we loaded vehicles. We standardized the way we "broke out" (or exited) from buildings. We standardized the way we got head counts to ensure we had all of our troops.... There was a disciplined methodology to just about everything we did.

But there was, and is, a dichotomy in the strict discipline we followed. Instead of making us more rigid and unable to improvise, this discipline actually made us more flexible, more adaptable, and more efficient. It allowed us to be creative.... When things went wrong and the fog of war set in, we fell back on our disciplined procedures to carry us through the toughest challenges on the battlefield.[58]

The same holds true for athletes: a clear game plan gives players a structure within which to be creative and adapt to changing circumstances. The best coaches recognize that every player is a person first, not a robot that can be controlled. The athlete should be free to act...without acting freely. SOPs outline the operating system just as a game plan outlines the game model; just as military tactics are changed minimally in combat according to the situation, so are tactics changed during a game to fit the situation. But even when a tactical change is needed, the core principles of the team must remain intact.

CONSCIOUS AND UNCONSCIOUS DILEMMAS   13.3.5

All decision-making represents in some ways a conflict between prior intentions, established before encountering a situation, and the intentions present during a specific situation. For the athlete, "prior intentions" can be articulated by consciously wondering, "What has the coach asked me to do in this situation/game moment?" The intention during an act, however, is subconscious and concerns what the player is used to doing in such situations—not what she has consciously decided to do. Habit formation develops a balance between the two, in which the athlete creates a consistent way of doing things that enables them to act intuitively during the game while still being cognizant of the game plan objectives.

PRESENTING THE GAME MODEL 13.3.6

No matter what a coach is saying to players about the game model or any of its principles, he or she should speak with utter confidence and conviction. This attitude is relayed not only in the content of the message but also in tone of voice, gestures, and posture. You can't give a command performance unless you act like you're in command.

It's within the head coach's control to create an advantage and protect it no matter what the result of the game is. The score doesn't validate or invalidate the model and shouldn't affect how the coach continues to communicate and reinforce it. When things aren't going well, the coach must work even harder to look confident, walk tall, and use positive verbal and body language (more on this on page 399). As soon as the leader drops their head, the players will follow.

RETHINKING TEAM SESSIONS: PREPARATION VS. TRAINING 13.3.7

Preparing athletes to play games shouldn't be thought of as "training" in the classical sense. Yes, we have used this word interchangeably with "preparing" (time for a self-administered slap on the wrist), but we're not trying to program a robot to act in a certain way when we're getting athletes ready for competition. Instead, team-sports preparation should focus on providing players with contextualized, guided experiences that result in the acquisition of certain learning, knowledge, and competencies. In other words, it's the responsibility of the coaches to point the way for their athletes, and it's the job of those players to be fully engaged in learning. They are prepared with a style of play in mind, but through their experiences, behaviors, and expressions, they form, to some extent, their own style of play.

A morphocycle is intended to create a weekly pattern of logical experiences through which players acquire and develop specific knowledge, technical skills, and tactical acumen. Simultaneously, the coaching staff is creating a sustainable relationship between work and recovery, which encourages the creation of patterns of action. For the team to progress, the tactical dimension must come first in coordinating and modeling the operational process of team preparation. This is a 180-degree turn from the traditional physical-first approach.

THE MORPHOCYCLE 13.4

Adaptive and responsive organisms—that is, athletes—must be prepared with a similarly adaptive and responsive system. The morphological programming approach, which balances volume, intensity, density, and collision/contact, and the four-coactive system of developing tactical, technical, physical, and psychological qualities in players are executed simultaneously to form the optimal approach for preparing teams to win in modern team sports. One of the primary limitations of traditional periodization is its inflexibility and rigidity. In contrast, the fluidity of the morphocycle enables the coaching staff to change the team's preparation schedule based on the changing conditions of the competitive calendar.

These include the availability of the squad (always a big challenge for international teams), the rigors of games played close together during a season with a packed schedule, and team travel. The coaches can also change the morphocycle to take into account upcoming playoffs, the start or end of the competitive season, and league-mandated breaks, such as All-Star Weekend in the NBA and the winter break in many European soccer leagues.

The Morphocycle

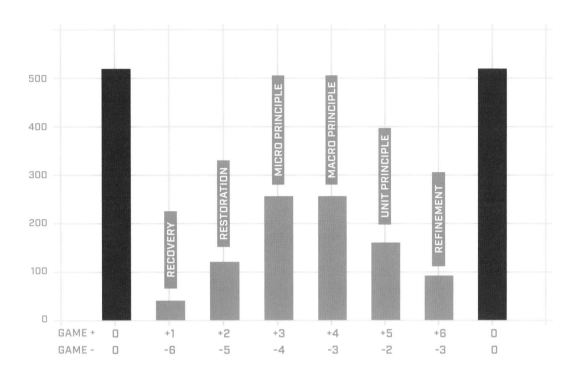

WHY A MORPHOCYCLE? 13.4.1

As the "morph" part of the name implies, the morphocycle can be changed and adapted as needed, based on the best possible information available at any given time. As Vítor Frade explained it to me, it is by nature agile, so it can contract or expand to accommodate the variables the team faces. In some ways, then, morphocycle programming has combined the best characteristics of object-oriented programming, just-in-time production, chaos theory, and the "scrum" method of project management, which involves each member of a team reporting on their progress daily and working together toward defined goals. Like a company employing the scrum, a team implementing the morphocycle is able to move fast and adapt on the fly to further the ultimate aim: winning more games.

Regardless of how each morphocycle shapes up, volume, intensity, density, and collision/contact are all present to some degree, and we're enhancing tactical, technical, physical, and psychological traits at once by exposing players to learning experienc-

es designed to improve decision-making and execution in the next game. When there are shorter breaks between games, players have less time to recover and coaches have fewer days to prepare. In such situations, when the morphocycle is contracted, the head coach should prioritize technical and tactical improvements, though there may be little time to do anything revolutionary before the next game.

In contrast, when there is more time between games, there is a greater opportunity to work with the squad on psychological and physical factors that will, if the morphological programming approach is designed and deployed correctly, improve the team's performance in upcoming games. The team's principles and game plan objectives also remain consistent throughout any and every morphocycle.

No matter how the length and composition of the morphocycle varies throughout the year, it remains a systematic, thoughtful, and deliberate system that aims to create incremental improvements on game day as the season progresses. And though the approach may seem complex, its main goal is devastatingly simple. As Super Bowl–winning coach Bill Walsh put it, "The bottom line in professional sports

13 Facilitating Experiences

is winning. Everything has to focus on that product: winning football games. Other offshoots—the public relations, the merchandising, the high-sounding philosophical approach—mean little compared with being successful on the playing field."[59]

EXPERIENCE AND RATE OF IMPROVEMENT   13.4.1.1

We often think of expertise as the potent combination of skill and knowledge. These are certainly two of its main components, but there's a third: experience. University of North Texas professor Katherine Thomas suggests that this can be defined as "the interaction of skill, knowledge and the psychological variables." In other words, an athlete's application of technical skill depends on what her brain has done before in practice and competition, which helps inform how she applies her tactical acumen and technical ability.[60]

For a long time, researchers believed that skills developed at a slower rate than knowledge and decision-making, but this assumption has since been turned on its head. Still, most studies agree that amassing greater experience helps decision-making, knowledge, and skills to progress. This shows that we cannot evaluate players' performance one-dimensionally but should instead consider how the technical, tactical, physical, and psychological coactives all impact what happens during competition. It also furthers the idea that players can continue to progress only if they acquire more playing experience and stay in their sport. This is a telling lesson for coaches considering the development curve of the younger members of their squad.[61]

Nature has provided man with the possibility to enhance his abilities in extreme situations, and we need to utilize it in the training of the high-class athlete.

—Yuri Verkhoshansky

THE PRINCIPLE OF EXECUTION

13.5

The beginning of the competitive season is too late for players to start putting the habits they're forming during preparation cycles into practice. Players need to regularly participate in competition in order to become used to executing successfully in games. They need to be tested in competition at least once a week throughout the year, ideally every day. Competition can take the form of intersquad scrimmages, exhibition games, or any other competitive situation. Players just need to get used to delivering when it counts. As the saying goes, "Train hard, fight easy."

THE PRINCIPLE OF COMPLEX PROGRESSION

13.6

Before players can grasp the micro principles of the game plan, they must comprehend its main principles. Only when the squad understands the general idea of how the head coach wants them to play the game can the coaching staff start adding in more complexity. The more time the athletes spend on the team, the more they're exposed to deeper layers of the game plan. As their understanding progresses, so too will their ability to put the principles into action and, hopefully, achieve the objectives for each game moment.

While the term *complex progression* implies regular advancement, the journey is not always linear. If, when assessing game performance, the coach sees that players are failing to adhere to macro principles, the coach may have to dial back the complexity to address these more fundamental issues.[62]

THE PRINCIPLE OF PROPENSITIES

In any game moment, the coach wants a particular player, unit, and the entire team to act in a certain way. However, this cannot simply be dictated like a military commander giving a subordinate a direct order. Rather, the coaching staff should create contexts of experience and allow athletes to figure out how to perform the task on their own. A player's prior experiences, preferences, and acumen in each of the four coactives will determine exactly how they respond in any given situation. Their learning style will also have an impact. They have to be creative and show ingenuity during the game because of the many variables involved, so learning opportunities should also allow a degree of originality and interpretation. Then habits can be created through repetition. As long as the players keep in mind the principles of play and the game plan objectives, how they express and achieve these should be up to them.[63]

THE PRINCIPLE OF PERFORMANCE STABILIZATION

13.8

A lot of factors in team sports change daily. Some players are hurt, others are ill, and some bring the burdens of family problems and addictions to the training ground. Then there are all the external forces that are brought to bear on a team, including media scrutiny, contract negotiations, and so on. Once game time arrives, environmental factors like rain and wind, a poor-quality field, and injury take their toll. This means that performance is unlikely to follow a flat, constant line.

However, one of the main benefits of using the morphological programming approach is that it offers a stabilizing effect amid the chaos. The balance among volume, intensity, density, and collision that the coach's weekly plan brings is one aspect of this. Another is the recovery that is built into each iteration of the morphocycle. Then there is the familiarity of the players' knowing what to expect on certain days—from the day off after the game, to the recap of the week's learning experiences two days before the game, to the final walk-through before kickoff/tipoff. Such routines provide comfort and reduce anxiety, further contributing to performance stabilization.[64]

THE PRINCIPLE OF PERPETUAL IMPROVEMENT

13.9

As I've discussed, one of the reasons conventional, physically focused periodization doesn't work for sports teams is that its programming is aimed toward an athlete peaking at a certain point in time. This isn't possible in team sports because, unlike Olympic athletes in individual disciplines, there is no single event that can be planned for four years in advance. Rather, players must perform at a high level every week. The morphological programming approach holds that as players improve technically, tactically, psychologically, and physically within the construct of the game plan, that improvement will continue over the course of the season. And unlike the physical improvement, which is the focus of traditional periodization, all four of these qualities will advance simultaneously.

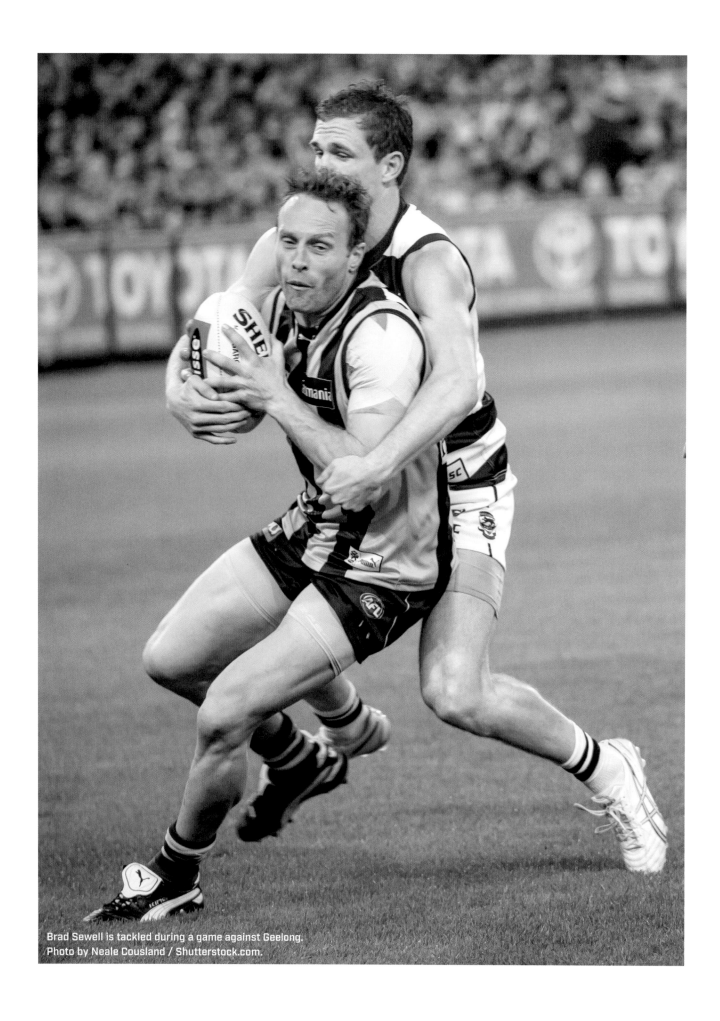

Brad Sewell is tackled during a game against Geelong.
Photo by Neale Cousland / Shutterstock.com.

FOURTEEN

THE METHODOLOGY

In this section, we'll look at how to improve player performance by scheduling carefully planned learning experiences within the weekly morphocycle. In addition, we'll take a deep dive into psychophysiological principles, introduce a few examples of weekly preparation cycles, and look at macro-level implementation.

MACRO EXPERIENCES OF THE MORPHOCYCLE

14.1

The morphocycle approach involves creating a weekly cycle for players that is holistic, all-inclusive, and macroscopic in nature. As the week unfolds, the coaching staff oversees the players as they work their way through four distinct morphocycles, one for each of the four coactives: technical, tactical, physical, and psychological. Within each of these subcycles, the four elements of the overarching morphocycle—volume, intensity, density, and contact/ collision—are all present to some degree. They are emphasized or de-emphasized throughout the week to allow players to recover from certain exposures and learning experiences, even as they're being stimulated by others.

THE TACTICAL MORPHOCYCLE

14.1.1

The tactical morphocycle concerns the development of strategy, which is based on achieving certain objectives within each of the four game moments as part of the game plan. It also covers the tactics that players will use to express the strategy on game day. These will vary depending on the opponent and should aim to both maximize the strengths of your team and exploit the opposition's known weaknesses.

DEVELOPING STRATEGY AND TACTICS

14.1.1.1

When you watch a game, you see a style of play. This style consists of tactics employed with certain goals in mind. A tactic is deployed to achieve an objective, not simply for its own sake. Despite the way the sports media praises the tactical innovation of certain coaches whose methods bring their teams short-term success, tactics are rarely unique or new. Rather, most tactical innovations involve progressions of things that have been used before but went out of vogue for a time. High pressing in soccer is an example. It isn't a new phenomenon. During the 1960s, Victor Maslov was the coach of Dynamo Kyiv, and it was there that he introduced the concept of pressing the opposition to the European game. But while pressing isn't a new concept, it has certainly become more technically advanced in recent years as coaches have become more aware of the intricate mechanisms that have to be put in place to press effectively.

Tactics that are adopted or copied without a clear understanding of the objective they're to be used for end up as simply an exercise. The best example in soccer is tiki-taka. By 2013, what had originated with Ajax and was later advanced at Barcelona as a fluid, dynamic attacking movement consisting of short, quick passes and endless running had become a byword for conservative, low-risk possession football. That's not the fault of Guardiola or Barcelona but of the handbook ideologues who slavishly copied them. Without the genius of players like Xavi and Iniesta, tiki-taka can turn into passing for passing's sake.

When looking at the tactics of other, more successful teams, a coach should not just try to copy the tactics chapter and verse. As U.S. Marine Corps general Alfred M. Gray rightly said, "In tactics, the most important thing is not whether you go left or right, but why you go left or right."[65] So if a coach is intrigued by a certain tactic that another team is using, she should first try to find out how it is helping the team achieve a certain objective and whether the tactic fits with her existing game plan. If not, she should look elsewhere for tactical inspiration. Tactics have to be purposeful and work with the talents of the available personnel.

Practice doesn't make perfect. Perfect practice does.

—Red Holzman

THE THREE PHASES OF TEAM PREPARATION   14.1.1.2

One way to look at what coaches should focus on in preparing their teams between games is to use the three phases below. When there's less time available because of a crowded calendar, phase 2 can be minimized or skipped:

1. *Individual correction and recovery* from the previous game

2. *Acquisition of learning experiences* that improve tactics and further game plan objectives

3. *Rehearsal of patterns* before facing the next opponent

These phases are not rigid but rather must be adapted depending on the schedule. I've often heard coaches say, "You should spend X amount of time on…" but such assumptions are all too often based on the illusion of ideal situations in which every player is healthy and there's a lot of time between games. The reality is that there are no ideal situations in team sports, so you have to work as effectively as possible in any given scenario.

If there are at least seventy-two hours between games, it's safe to assume that most players will be able to recover all their systems to at least 90 percent, but in back-to-back game situations, they won't. Regardless, the main aim has to be for the athletes and the team to play the next game at their best, individually and collectively. This doesn't necessarily mean being faster or stronger than they were the last time they took the field, but it does mean an improvement in performance—which can just as easily come from improved decision-making, skill execution, and tactical application.

In an article on the limitations of the NFL Combine, writer Greg Bishop noted that the starters on Stanford's college football team under Jim Harbaugh had only missed a combined total of sixty-seven games in three seasons. One of the reasons? "Stanford trains its team to play football, not to bench-press or to win 40-yard dashes."[66] In other words, the psychological, tactical, and technical elements of team preparation are just as important in winning team-sports games as physical factors, and in fact, emphasizing these other three factors may not only boost performance but also limit injuries from overtraining. People often ask, "How strong do you need to be to play in this or that league?" I'd change that up and ask, "What's the *least* amount of strength you need to play in the league?"

Now, certain sports and positions require more strength, speed, or endurance than others. Yet even in power positions, such as a rugby prop or a lineman in American football, once you cross certain physical baselines, extra strength, speed, or power is practically worthless—the law of diminishing returns applies on the game field, too. This is because once a player is strong, fast, or powerful enough, continuing to improve these qualities requires more input than justified by the little-to-no output this will yield on the field. A lineman who can do twenty-four reps of 225 pounds in the bench press will not be a better player than he was when he could only do twenty-two reps, no matter what the NFL Combine might want us to believe. Also, such a player would be better off directing his time towards improving his psychological skills, technical acumen, or tactical ability, which *would* improve his game-day performance. A player in any sport and at any position can never have too much technical or tactical knowledge or be too psychologically prepared. That's why it's vital that we develop *all* our team-sports athletes in these areas.

DESIGNING THE EXPERIENCE   14.1.1.3

As we know, a game can be considered a complex, multifactorial phenomenon with a set of interacting elements that create something entirely different than the sum of its parts. That's why we need a structured model that gives us a systems-based approach to address the complexity of sports games.

In keeping with the concept of fractals, which we looked at in "The Game," every experience that a player has in practice should accurately represent some facet of the game itself. Such an experience cannot focus only on the execution of a motor skill—that is to say, to merely try to develop the player technically. Nor can it require the player to make a decision based just on his comprehension of the team's strategy—that is, a tactical choice. The player must do both, because this is what will be required in the game.[67]

Affordances and Signifiers   14.1.1.3.1

When we design experiences for players, we should try to do so from the perspective of affordance. In his book *The Design of Everyday Things,* Don Norman states, "The term *affordance* refers to the relationship between a physical object and a person (or for that matter, any interacting agent, whether animal or human, or even machines and robots)."[68] Essentially, this refers to the qualities that the person interacting could experience. So, for example, a door affords the opportunity to open it, close it, or knock on it—each possibility is an affordance.

Signifiers are the clues someone sees that make affordances clearer, just like surfaces and gaps in maneuver warfare. So if a door had a "Push here" sign on it, this would signify that it could be pushed, whereas if it had a sign saying "Pull," the implication would be that pushing the door wouldn't open it. A sign is just one example of a signifier. It could also be a sound, a gap, or any number of other indicators.[69] This is what players learn to see and observe during practice experiences. There are so many signifiers in a sport that it's impossible to re-create them artificially. This is the nirvana that virtual reality is chasing.

Imagine a simple practice experience where a player must run with a ball past some teammates. He sees a pattern of opponents in front of him. The coach has instructed four defenders to try to tackle the ballcarrier. All are equally spaced except for one player, whom he has asked to leave a wider gap. The ballcarrier notices two gaps that offer limited options for running through, but he also sees a third that is marginally larger than the others. He runs through this one. The design of the experience created a signifier—the proximity of the four players to one another—and an affordance—the player's ability to run through a gap. The learning experience was intuitive and complete, and the player with the ball learned to identify an opportunity without the coach needing to say anything.

DEVELOPING TRUST AND PATIENCE 14.1.1.4

Great teams, like the New England Patriots, Barcelona, Anatoli Tarasov's great Soviet ice hockey team of the 1970s, and, during Peyton Manning's prime, the Indianapolis Colts, express a patience and smoothness that comes from players' familiarity with and trust in the game plan and teammates. One of the most fundamental aspects of Barcelona's play is a calm, methodical approach to build-up play. In contrast, young and inexperienced teams typically have a herky-jerky, arrhythmic style in which they make frequent mistakes and struggle to maintain possession or establish a consistent tempo.

When a team plays in a coordinated fashion in accordance with predefined goals, it provides stability and order on both sides of the ball that can counteract the chaos that unfolds during every game. As I outlined in section 1.2.4 on the micro principle of dynamic stability, the problems that athletes face individually and as a team cannot be predicted or truly controlled, but when they play with organization and a spirit of cooperation, these problems are easier to solve.[70]

INDIVIDUAL EXPOSURE 14.1.1.5

At certain times in each morphocycle, most often early in the week, individual players have the exposure to work on maximizing their dominant qualities and improving those things that are limiting their performance. This could involve refining a technique or a small tactical element. However, the individual work should not be done in isolation or in an abstract setting but rather in a manner that's similar to the game itself.

MICRO UNIT COHESION 14.1.1.6

Sometimes coaches might need to improve how teammates in a unit, group, or line (for example, the offensive line in football) relate to each other in one or more of the game moments. So in rugby, for example, the backs might need to spread the ball better coming out of the scrum. Or in basketball, the guards might not be communicating well enough on fast breaks.

MACRO UNIT COHESION 14.1.1.7

When working on macro unit cohesion, the coaching staff is typically trying to improve defensive or offensive timing, structure, or sequencing. Very often this is tied to positional awareness and relational movement. So perhaps an offensive coordinator in football would spend time with his players as an offensive unit trying to improve how they handle the pressure of an opponent's blitz.

COLLECTIVE COHESION 14.1.1.8

Collective cohesion involves improving how the entire team acts as a whole in a certain situation, transitioning and moving from sequence to sequence. This often involves team structure after restarts, for out-of-bounds plays, and for set pieces. So a basketball coach might concentrate on a couple of inbounds plays for when the ball is passed in from under the opponent's basket, while a soccer team might want to improve how it sets up to defend corners.

INDIVIDUAL INITIATIVE IN A TEAM BRAIN 14.1.1.9

Even in elite military units, in which orders need to be followed for missions to be successful, commanders have come to recognize that while they need to train soldiers to develop certain habits that they can immediately access during combat, they must also develop independent thinkers. In his book *Smarter Faster Better*, Charles Duhigg shares a case study about how this played out during a training exercise in the U.S. Marine Corps.

During their final challenge in basic training, prospective marines had to cross a large pit as a team within a certain time limit, without touching the floor. Each recruit was wearing a gas mask, and they were told that none of them could act unless they heard the team leader give a direct order. The trouble was that nobody could hear the leader because of the gas masks. They eventually figured out how to cross the obstacle by moving synchronously in a line using the planks and ropes provided by their officers.

"Technically, we could send them back to start over because each person didn't hear a direct verbal command from the team leader," the drill sergeant said later. "But that's the point of the exercise. We know they can't hear anything with the gas masks on. The only way to get across the pit is to figure out some workaround. We're trying to teach them that you can't just obey orders. You have to take control and figure things out for yourself."[71]

The same goes for team-sports preparation. No matter how well the head coach can make strategic changes during a game, the athletes are still the ones out there playing against an opponent whose main aim is to beat them. Each and every player, whether they play for twenty seconds or ninety minutes, will be forced to make decisions very quickly, any of which could positively or negatively impact the final score. So it's the job of the coaching staff to avoid merely issuing orders that they expect to be carried out to the letter, and instead prepare the team in a way that helps them become better leaders and independent thinkers.

THE TECHNICAL MORPHOCYCLE   14.1.2

Although a coach might have a desired outcome in mind for a certain player, I've explained the importance of the techno-tactical relationship and allowing the athlete to select the right skill based on the situation and previous experience and execute it as they choose. For the longest time in team sports (and most individual ones, for that matter), coaches have obsessed over teaching athletes perfect form—whether that's throwing a spiral just so in American football, shooting a free throw in basketball, or kicking a drop goal in rugby—without teaching them to self-regulate and critically learn, especially since there is no perfect form, only perfect principles.

In team preparation and scrimmaging, the coaches' focus should instead be on setting up scenarios for players to make decisions and execute habits on their own initiative, with whatever form they choose to get the job done. This will translate to effective decision-making and instinctive execution come game day.

BERNSTEIN'S BLACKSMITH AND SKILL SPECIFICITY   14.1.2.1

When Russian neurophysiologist Nikolai Bernstein conducted his pioneering movement studies on how manual laborers perform daily tasks, one of his subjects was a blacksmith. Bernstein observed this highly skilled craftsman striking his hammer hundreds of times. There was no coach standing over his shoulder saying, "That one was wrong," and correcting his motor pattern. The blacksmith had likely been at one time the apprentice to an experienced master who showed him what to do and then let him prove himself. What Bernstein observed was that while the blacksmith held the hammer the same way and swung it in a similar manner each time, every repetition was slightly different. And yet the man achieved the results he was looking for with his metalwork.[72]

For team-sports players, the same principles apply, and their elite technical ability is both self-correcting and constantly developing. Though the best in any game have consistent form that coaches idealize and kids imitate (see Michael Jordan's fadeaway jumper or his driving to the basket complete with his tongue out), their skill execution has inherent variability and changes depending on the infinite number of possibilities that each game presents. If a defender is closing quickly, the wind is blowing a certain way at a certain speed, or the ball takes an odd bounce, players simply cannot execute the skill they select precisely as they would if one or all of these variables were different. It's up to the individual to use his observation of the moment and his prior experience to adapt the skill and make minute adjustments so that it has the desired impact—creativity and ingenuity at work.

Therefore, during team preparation, coaches at any level should not concern themselves with a player's form—whether it's passing, shooting, dribbling, or any other skill. Rather, they should concentrate on creating experiences that encourage a certain outcome but leave it up to the players to decide how to achieve it. Repetition of certain drills can help players make autonomous choices during competition, but variation within team exercises will help facilitate continued learning and skill improvement that can be applied when it counts.

As Bernstein's blacksmith research showed, skill execution is not static but rather is constantly changing and evolving. As athletes amass more game experiences, they will refine and improve how they perform certain skills and will be able to apply them effectively in a broader range of situations. If the coaches review film and see that one of the players is shooting in a new way, they should not attempt to "correct" this change unless the outcome is unsuccessful or a potentially harmful movement pattern is putting the player at risk. The athlete will typically find the expression of a skill that bests suits them and the situations in which they find themselves.

MICRO PRINCIPLE OF AFFORDANCE
14.1.2.2

The best players can select the appropriate skill and execute it so quickly and effectively that their opponents cannot prevent the intended result—like intercepting a pass or blocking a shot. This decision never happens for its own sake but rather in a tactical context that changes every time based on the game moment; the player's proximity to the ball, teammates, opponents, and the goal; and the time in the game. The tactical and technical elements aren't the only considerations; the decision also depends on the physical and psychological coactives.

CONTEXTUAL EXECUTION
14.1.2.3

Practicing any sports skill by itself provides limited benefits. If a tennis player hits a ball off a wall over and over again, for instance, he might improve his footwork and reaction skills. But this practice is only superficial because he doesn't have to contend with the net or, more importantly, an opponent trying to hit the ball away from him after he has completed his stroke. So hitting a forehand, backhand, or any variation against a static object is not really executing the true skill but rather a poor-quality photocopy of it.

When it comes to team sports, such practice is of even less value due to the need to perform skills with both teammates and opponents in mind. Athletes need to add the element of perception to their movement to develop their skillset and make it more applicable to an actual game. This can sometimes be scaled up or down in complexity, with playing surface size, number of teammates, and the amount of movement varied by the coach.[73]

WHAT ABOUT SCORING?
14.1.2.4

While scoring is in some ways the most high-impact part of the offensive moment in any sport, it is also the one that should receive the least attention during preparation morphocycles. If you emphasize scoring in practice, it places more stress on players and will make them think too much about shooting, which slows decision-making and negatively impacts skill execution. Instead, coaches should spend more time on creating scoring opportunities through improved build-up play.

Just as in golf or for a sniper, there must be a level of acceptance before the final action takes place. This comes only after there has been proper preparation through structure and routine, which prevents players from being distracted as they process information. It helps them manage the unexpected, as a strategy the player believes will work is in place. Routine is a structure to work from. Acceptance is the last part—an action doesn't need to be perfect. Rather than overthinking, the sniper has to pull the trigger upon deciding to act, just as the soccer player who has freed herself from her marker in the penalty box now has to take her shot on goal.[74]

THE TECHNO-TACTICAL SYNTHESIS
14.1.3

As I've highlighted several times, it is impossible to isolate the elements of performance, so they must be managed in a holistic manner. Even the process of describing these elements runs the risk of creating the perception of separation, but the reality is that you cannot separate technical and tactical actions, training, or experiences. As such, we need to evaluate and develop technical skill execution within the tactical framework of the game plan. Hue Jackson arguably best described the techno-tactical process that an elite quarterback goes through in trying to process information and execute a play:

> Imagine this. A guy has 11 seconds to get the play from me [over the headset]: He has to understand the formation, the play and sometimes an alert. Then he has to tell that play to the offensive team. Then he has to think through the defense. He has to make sure he communicates with [the other offensive players] through words and hand signals. Say it's *Trips Right Lizzy Left Quanzi.* He's got to get the play. Then give the play.
>
> Now he has to decipher what the defense is doing [at the line of scrimmage]: Personnel, front, coverage. Who's the Mike [middle linebacker]? Now you think you figured it out. Then you say "Set-Hut." Now the processor is rolling: You've gotta decide in milliseconds, "Where do I go [with the ball]? What do I do?" There's a pre-snap thought and a post-snap thought. Now you got all those dudes on the other side—they're trying to hurt you, they're growling, talking [expletive] to you. You've gotta handle all that. And now, under those conditions, you're paid to make plays. And if you don't? Well, you've got to repeat the process right away.... And how do you deal with the stress of missing the play?[75]

This incredibly involved sequence of decisions and actions has to be performed quickly and precisely, with tens of thousands of people in the stands yelling, screaming, and critiquing every move. So the player has to be not only competent enough cognitively to consider his or her skill selection and execution within the framework of the game plan, but also sufficiently emotionally resilient to handle the pressure of the moment. Then there are the player's teammates to consider. In team sports, decisions and isolations happen within a social setting, so the individual must know where his or her teammates are and where they're going to make best use of the ball before passing it, for example.[76]

It's not enough for players to possess high-level technical skills. They also need to be able to express these as part of their real-time solutions to the challenges and problems that arise during every game, and to do so with the Commander's Intent and sub-objectives in mind. The ability to match a skill to a particular issue and apply it at just the right time is often what elevates players into the elite echelon of team sports. This is possible only when they're able to combine previous experiences and a quick, accurate assessment of current game conditions to select and apply the right technical movement.[77]

THE PSYCHOLOGICAL MORPHOCYCLE

The fourth coactive that is incorporated into the morphocycle is psychological. We break down this domain into three elements and need to consider the individual and total load on them in each weekly morphocycle. These elements are emotion, cognition, and spirituality. Mental toughness and team identity play a role, too.

THE PSYCHOLOGICAL PROFILE

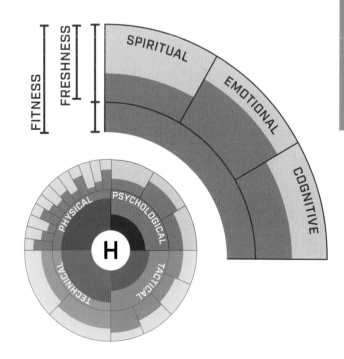

EMOTION   14.1.4.1

Emotion governs the way athletes express themselves in words and deeds. It is also responsible for mood and how well players relate to teammates, coaches, and other members of the organization. Emotion is also an expression of a player's personality.

As a rule, the emotional load on the team should be kept as low as possible during the week. The game itself exerts such a large emotional load on players that they need the intensity in this area to be dialed down later in the week. The only exception is if a player has checked out and her level of excitation, alertness, or arousal is too low. In this case, the coach might want to up the emotional ante by introducing a real or imagined threat.

Good coaches keep the emotional load low by ensuring that there is emotional control in every session they manage. Rich Ohrnberger, a New England Patriots lineman, described the emotional environment that Bill Belichick creates: "That's not the easiest environment to be in. It was stressful. It separated you sometimes from your immediate family, but you felt an obligation to this organization to really give your all. At any other place there was a focus on football and winning but never quite to the level of New England. And it really was attributed to how Bill ran the show over there." Rick Venturi added, "If he has a motivational style, I'd say that it's constant emotional discomfort. That's why his teams never flatline."[78] As I learned from Jack Harbaugh, emotional alertness prevents complacency, and complacency is lethal for any coach.

COGNITION   14.1.4.2

This element of the psychological morphocycle involves structural analysis and processing learning experience stimuli like verbal and auditory cues. It's also the area responsible for grasping strategic and tactical concepts and their subsets, like set plays. As players need to be mentally fresh come game day, most of the cognitive learning load should be concentrated in the first few days of the morphocycle, at least in terms of conscious learning. Later in the week, the focus can switch to more subconscious experiential learning.

If a player gets emotionally imbalanced or has a spiritual issue, cognitive learning often suffers, and the quality of preparation experiences will decline. Similarly, if the cognitive load is too great, an athlete can suffer spiritually and emotionally—all three dimensions of the psychological morphocycle are intertwined. The key is keeping each dimension in the yellow stage, without any or all going into the red.

SPIRITUALITY   14.1.4.3

The spiritual element involves a player's place in the team and the wider world. It concerns self-focused questions like, "Who am I?", "What am I doing here?", and "Why is this game meaningful?" as well as outward-facing considerations like the importance of teammates and coaches. The ability to find meaning or feel like they are contributing to a worthy process is important to all individuals. The key thing is that the team unity, culture, or spirit is constant in practice just as on game day.

Remember, the basis of someone's psychological perspective is their belief system. This is the player's fundamental and conscious understanding of the world. People can change their belief structure, but it is difficult, slow, and beyond the scope of this book. A player's belief structure is often forged by the influences and mentors she's had in life. The belief system is also influenced by faith, life experience, education, and the culture the person has been exposed to. These cross-pollinate. From this basic understanding of life and our role in it, we all form a set of values that we act upon in daily life. The belief system educates the value system.

From these two come our attitudes toward various events and actions. When it comes to athletes' psychology, we cannot think of them only as players. They are also part of a family, part of a culture, and part of a tribe (i.e., the team). The environment they're exposed to at home, at the team facilities, and with friends and the wider community have a significant impact on their state of mind, for good or ill. From the team perspective, it's important that players feel a sense of unity. This can be threatened by different scenarios that present themselves between games. Let's look at two examples.

When one player is elevated to the starting line-up, a teammate has to drop down to the bench. Depending on the scenario, this can create discord and disconnection, so some head coaches defuse this by explaining their reasoning to both players, making them realize that the decision is not personal but for the good of the team. It's imperative that newly benched players are reassured that they're important to the team and that they feel secure in the knowledge that they have a future with the organization. How this is communicated depends on the coach's preference.

A contrasting situation is when one player performs exceptionally well and receives a lot of positive media attention. Almost every player likes this to some degree, and who can blame them? But they must be reminded that they're only in this position because of their teammates, so that they remain humble and remember their responsibilities to the tribe. A great example of this was Steph Curry's attitude during the press conference for his second MVP award.

When asked what it takes to be a great teammate, Curry said, "You've got to be unselfish, know that the team is bigger than individual success. You've got to have that trust in each other. You've got to care about each other and be committed to whatever your goal is as a team. Everybody has a role and everybody has a part in the team's success. So we are a great testament of that, all 15 guys on this stage. We understand what it means to be a collective unit and to have fun doing what you do and playing for each other. Good things usually happen when you have that mindset."[79]

The coaches need to maintain a constant state of involvement in the spiritual state of the team. This should stay consistent throughout the morphocycle, although, as it's also subject to exterior forces like relationships with family and friends, this can take continual effort.

MENTAL TOUGHNESS   14.1.4.4

Performing consistently at the highest level is no easy task. In addition to their own expectations, athletes must deal with the cheers and jeers of the crowd, media scrutiny, the hopes of family and friends, the demands of teammates and coaches, and many other factors.

This means that cultivating mental strength is every bit as important as developing physical strength. The six key areas of mental toughness are concentration and focus, self-efficacy, tolerance for frustration, self-confidence, determination, and persistence.[80] These traits should be encouraged every day during team preparation, and mental toughness should become a cultural value that every member of the squad recognizes and embraces.

TEAM MENTAL TOUGHNESS   14.1.4.5

Though the example of a star player can be contagious in the locker room, it's not enough for a single individual or a couple of athletes to exhibit mental toughness. The entire squad must become mentally strong and resilient as a group. There are plenty of team-sports athletes who find it easy to believe in their own ability to overcome adversity and perform under pressure, but the true test is developing such trust in one's teammates as well. The level of trust in the last guy or gal at the end of the bench has to become the same as the confidence in the perennial All-Star, because you never know when this benchwarmer will be called upon in a crucial moment that could define the team's entire season. Such trust has to be earned by every player's demonstrating their full effort and commitment.

Some teams resort to looking outside the organization for guidance on mental toughness. The trouble is that, like skill and tactical acumen, mental toughness is situational. This is not to say that lessons cannot be gleaned from them, but in sports, psychological resilience is specific to the task at hand and must be developed during competition and game-like preparation experiences.

Culture and Collective Identity   14.1.4.5.1

It's not enough for a team to develop a style of play that defines and distinguishes it. It must also create an identifiable culture anchored by unshakeable beliefs and values (which I'll cover in more depth in "The Coach") and a collective identity. For example, while leading Butler to two successive national championship games in the NCAA Tournament, Brad Stevens decided that the team would not only emphasize the Butler Way (which "demands commitment, denies selfishness, accepts reality, yet seeks improvement every day while putting the team above self," per the school's mission statement) but also be known as an excellent defensive team.[81]

In addition, the coaching staff should create individual "intentions"—in other words, individual goals for players or units like the backs in rugby, defensive linemen in football, midfielders in soccer or guards in basketball—related to the "collective identity," without loss (and, actually, with gain) of individuality. This means that each player's and each unit's game-time objectives further the team's main aims. Finally, the team needs to reconcile its previous aims with present and future objectives in action—that is, the head coach needs to construct a game model that represents the team's culture and collective identity, which will make it resonate at the individual and collective level.

THE PHYSICAL MORPHOCYCLE   14.1.5

If players are to implement the tactical and technical elements of the game plan in competition, they must be physically prepared to do so. Unfortunately, it's common for teams to focus so intently on developing speed, strength, power, endurance, and other physical qualities during individual and team preparation that players become overloaded and break down. The physical morphocycle seeks to upend this approach.

The first way it does so is by understanding expressions of speed (like sprinting), power (say, jumping), strength (weight lifting), and other physical elements as skills, which I will explore in more depth in a moment. As part of this skill-centric mindset, we don't just think about the muscles involved in the activity and the stimulation and adaptation of them. Instead, we recognize that each instance of a physical skill also has a technical, tactical, and psychological component.

In addition, the morphocycle takes other body systems into account, recognizing that from a biological standpoint, there is far more involved in any physical activity than muscles alone. Taking the load on these other systems into account, we create each week's morphocycle around a minimum-effective-dose approach that places just enough stress on athletes' bodies during learning experiences to produce adaptation while ensuring that they're ready to apply their physiology to its fullest potential on game day.

PHYSICAL EXPRESSION IS A SKILL   14.1.5.1

Take the improvement of any physical skill and coaches and players will inevitably say that the player got faster or stronger. The trouble is that they're focused on the outcome and looking at the improvement from a purely physical perspective. Really, the reason that someone runs the forty-yard dash quicker is because they got better at the skill of running, and the reason they added forty pounds to their bench press max is because they improved the skill of bench-pressing. These are neural improvements and technical mastery, with physical adaptations that we see afterward. It's *not* because we just "got stronger." The term *muscle memory* is a little misleading, because when we improve the execution of a skill, we are accessing a familiar pattern that allows us to recruit more resources, most of all neural and metabolic, at a higher speed or with greater efficiency than the previous time we did it. Adaptation takes place after we perform the skill, not during it, which is why the morphocycle takes into account the varying recovery rates of bodily systems as well as the sequencing of stimuli.

Now let's look at the three main elements of the physical morphocycle.

BIOMECHANICAL 14.1.5.2

This element involves the structural-anatomical system. Performing any physical activity doesn't just create microtears in muscle fibers but also stresses bones, ligaments, tendons, fascia, and other structures. Most injuries happen when we attempt to isolate muscles and discount the roles of these other structures. The biomechanical dimension is largely impacted by total volume. It usually recovers within forty-eight hours of being exposed to a stimulus.

NEURAL 14.1.5.3

In keeping with the psychophysiological approach, we cannot exclude the brain when we train the body. When we lift more weight, run faster, jump higher, and so on, we're not just using muscles that have become larger through previous stimuli; we're also using an upgraded neural pathway. This is one of the most overlooked elements of physical preparation and arguably the most important, as the neural system is responsible for two-way communication with the structural-anatomical system and recruits more resources (muscle fibers, fuel from the energy substrates, etc.) to enable us to perform the skill more efficiently. It's also what we rely on for perception and awareness and is closely tied to the psychological coactive. As a result, the neural element takes the longest to recover, sometimes up to seventy-two hours.

BIOLOGICAL 14.1.5.4

The biological element concerns the transport of gases (like oxygen and carbon dioxide in breathing), liquids (blood and water), and fuel from the energy substrates around the body. Of the three physical coactives, the biological one usually recovers the fastest, often within twenty-four hours. That being said, such a time frame can be extended by the nature and duration of the load to which the body is exposed, and, like the other two physical ele-

ments, its recovery can be undermined by environmental factors such as poor nutrition, dehydration, emotional stress, and inadequate sleep. Energy substrates in particular may take longer to recover.

THE PSYCHO-PHYSIOLOGICAL MACRO MODEL

14.2

Elite athletes need not only well-developed physiological and technical characteristics but certain cognitive characteristics, too.[82] The greatest error of traditional periodization is to assume that psychology is anything more than unsolved physiology. Matveyev's periodization methods did prescribe variations in volume or intensity, but only as they related to physical training. To effectively prepare a sports team, we need to consider other elements—namely technical, tactical, and psychological—that impact game-day performance. If we're going to evaluate the game itself holistically through the game model, we must approach team preparation (as well as athlete health) in a similarly all-encompassing way.

For any sports team to reach its potential on the field, neither physical development nor any other element of preparation can be isolated. Physical attributes are not applied by themselves during games, and neither are tactical, technical, or psychological qualities. Every action, event, and moment in a game involves all four attributes in some measure, regardless of whether one, several, or all of the players are involved. So we must prepare teams in the practice facilities in a realistic gamelike manner.

Otherwise, what happens between matches will have little bearing on what goes on during the game itself. Plus, you can't spend weeks focusing on developing just one physical trait—speed, strength, endurance, and so on—because in reality, all are present in any training activity. This is another reason that traditional linear periodization just doesn't cut it when it comes to preparing team-sports athletes.

Instead, I advise combining the morphological programming approach elements and four coactives into a single, unified morphocycle approach that takes into account the physiological and psychological impact of every type of team preparation and balances them, so that as some bodily systems are highly stimulated to produce adaptation, others are de-emphasized to promote recovery. In contrast to linear periodization, in which coaches try to isolate certain elements of physicality during long blocks at certain times of year, the morphological programming approach, like Charlie Francis's vertical integration, seeks to develop all four elements simultaneously throughout the year, with one goal in mind: delivering incrementally better competitive performances on a progression curve that is sustained throughout the season.

As you watch a game, you see that the tactical, technical, physiological, and psychological elements are never executed independently. Everything is involved at every moment. The tactical dimension assumes the lead in this training method, as we believe that if we conduct all our training sessions respecting our principles of play, we can make our players better in all other coactives (physical, psychological, and technical) as well.

HOLISTIC STRESSORS   14.2.1

Each preparation day is easily ranked according to how much the session will tax the players in terms of volume, intensity, density, and collision/contact. During each cycle, be it one, two, or four weeks long, the head coach and staff should aim to create only enough stimulation in each of these areas to trig-

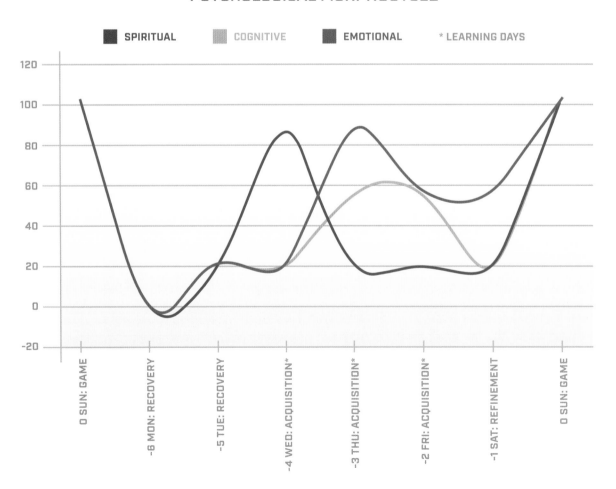

PSYCHOLOGICAL MORPHOCYCLE

ger the required adaptation, while empowering each player's body and brain to recover sufficiently that the players can perform their best in the next game.

When planning the upcoming cycle, days should be balanced so that the cumulative load is manageable in each area and when taken as a sum total across all four. This total should always be lower than that of any competitive game; in fact, preparation load should never exceed 50 percent of game-day demands (except for the practice/reserve squad, whose morphological programming loads can be higher, as it doesn't have the additional stimuli of games to cope with). The coaching and medical staffs should also consider the combined effects of games plus training. Sometimes they mistakenly believe that a morphocycle has not been too stressful, only for the added demands of the next game to push several players to a breaking point.

The focus in each of the four squares on the morphological programming quadrant should be on quality, not quantity. This load balancing is of even greater importance in sports that have more games and less rest and recovery between them. In such scenarios, players have not only a reduced capacity to handle physical load but also less cognitive ability to absorb tactical and technical changes, as discussed in "The Game."

By responsibly and thoughtfully juggling each morphological programming component across the morphocycle, the coaching staff can optimize the learning experiences they create for their players and maximize the adaptation to each stimulus. This will lead to the highest possible degree of advancement from one game to the next, assuming that every member of the squad puts in 100 percent effort at all times. The game, then, becomes a qualitative assessment of the learning experiences that the team has been exposed to up to that point and a gauge for how effective preparation was in the preceding morphocycle—not to mention an opportunity for the coaches to look at how effective their programming has been and in which areas it can be improved.

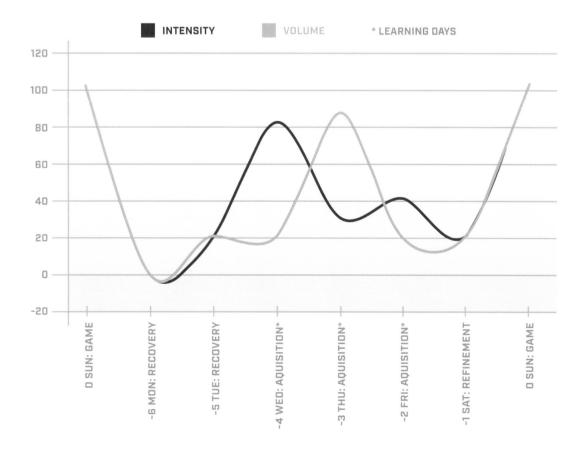

Emotional involvement and being in a state of high alertness and awareness will invariably enhance the quality of learning experiences during training. Habits formed in the off-season and preseason will carry over to the regular season, so it's important that players are equally dedicated in their preparation for exhibition games as they are for derby contests against their fiercest rivals.

As former Swansea soccer coach Brendan Rogers said about his arrival at the Welsh club, which he guided to promotion into the Premier League before leaving to take the reins at Liverpool: "When I first came in I said to the players, we will push ourselves in every element of training, so it's reflective of the real game, so I don't have to go on about intensity all the time because that is an obligation."[83]

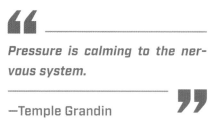

Pressure is calming to the nervous system.

—Temple Grandin

COGNITIVE, PSYCHOLOGICAL & EMOTIONAL MORPHOCYCLE

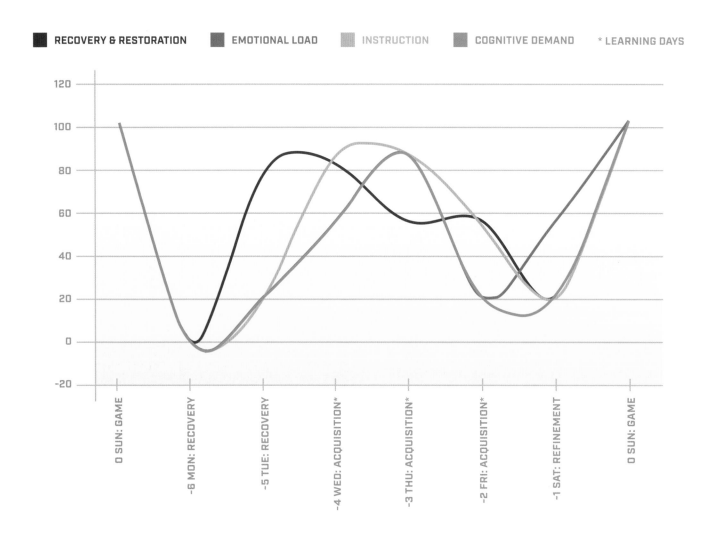

BALANCING ELEMENTS OF THE MORPHOLOGICAL PROGRAMMING APPROACH   14.2.1.1

It's essential to take into account the varying recovery times for training that focus on each morphological programming component. For example, high-intensity work that's also high-collision typically places more stress on the central nervous system, which requires more recovery than certain other body systems. As with other aspects of recovery, the amount of time it takes for the CNS to fully regenerate increases with accumulated load.

One consideration is the load that each type of day has on three body systems:

1. Metabolic (heart, lungs, and blood flow)

2. Structural-anatomical (muscles, soft tissues, fascia, and bones)

3. Neural (the central and peripheral nervous systems)

The effects on all three systems also factor into recovery time. No day should rank as "high" for more than two of the four morphological programming parts, or the athletes will be physically, cognitively, and emotionally overloaded and will not adapt positively to the stimuli they're subjected to. One or two days of this can jeopardize the positive potential of an entire morphocycle.

So Tuesday and Wednesday, say, should not both involve sprint work or Olympic lifting. It would be better to schedule these sessions at least two days apart, such as on Tuesday and Friday. While the coaches wouldn't want to stack too much endurance work, it typically requires less recovery, so practice days with greater volume can be closer together.

It is possible to vary how training sessions are performed so that they score differently on the morphological programming quadrant. For example, if the head coach had the players run ten one-hundred-meter sprints at high speed with one minute of rest after each max-effort piece, the session would be high in intensity, medium in collision, medium in volume, and low to medium in density.

However, if the players ran each one-hundred-meter sprint at a low-to-medium pace and the rest time between pieces was increased to four minutes, then the session would be low to medium in intensity, medium in volume, low in density, and medium to high in collision. The reason for the higher collision score is that the athletes' feet would be in contact with the ground longer than in the faster variation of the session, so they would absorb more vertical force. A coach might use the first option the day after the players experienced high volume and the second option after a medium-intensity, low-volume day.

WORKING ON A TIGHT SCHEDULE   14.2.1.2

It's more likely that a team will be effective if the players understand the game plan and its principles and can easily and consistently execute game to game, rather than having a constantly changing plan that the coaching staff thinks is brilliant but the players struggle to grasp. As LeBron James wrote while leading his Cleveland Cavaliers to the best record in the NBA's Eastern Conference during the 2015–16 season, "Structure and consistency create perfection."[84]

Implementing a straightforward blueprint that has been rehearsed so often that it has created instinctive patterns that are accessed faster than the opposition can react becomes crucial when there is limited opportunity for preparation. So with only a few days between games, the coaches should reiterate core principles for each of the four game moments (offensive, defensive, transition-to-offense, and transition-to-defense). They should emphasize only a couple of additional tactical points that will enable the team to fix the mistakes from the last game, capitalize on its strengths, and disrupt the upcoming opponent's game plan.

Regardless of how often a team competes, though, the overriding goal of preparation is always the same: improving performance during the game so that the team gets progressively better and wins more often. As such, the coaching/training staff should avoid emphasizing any one of the four elements on back-to-back days—even if there's a long break before the next game.

VOLUME EXPOSURE AND EFFECT

14.2.2

Volume is the amount of work done. High-volume work is typically performed at a lower intensity and is often high density, as frequent breaks are not required. Volume-heavy days are also usually low on the collision scale. For days with longer duration, the muscles are under tension for more time but with a lower load. It's typical for a team to have high-volume physical training on days that also feature a high cognitive load, with film breakdown and macro-level tactical discussions. Such days are often followed by a lower-volume, lower-density day that features higher collision and intensity.

In the early years of team-sports preparation, athletes typically follow a higher-volume plan, which is necessary to develop training/work capacity. However, over time this need diminishes and increasing intensity becomes more of a priority. As athletes age, they become less able to handle high volume in combination with high intensity, and it's better to sacrifice some of the former in favor of optimizing the training effects of the latter, as the diagram below shows.

INTENSITY EXPOSURE AND EFFECT

14.2.3

Intensity refers to how rigorous and demanding the day's practice session is. High-intensity sessions often require frequent breaks, even if they are short, so they are often low density. In addition, high-density work often goes hand in hand with high-collision workouts. As it's impossible to sustain high intensity for very long due to the structural and neurological load (think of the rigors of a set

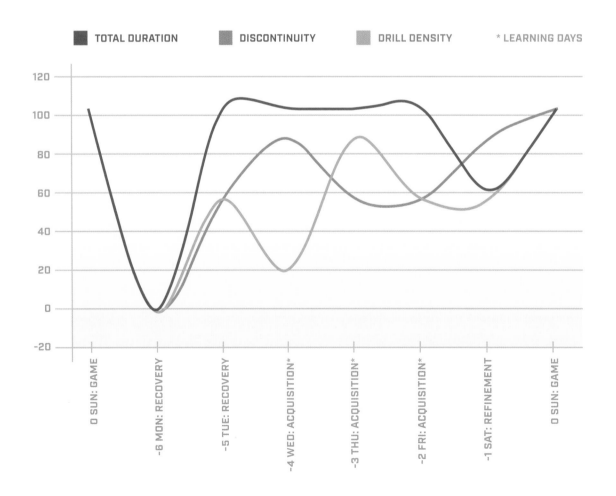

of lung-busting Tabata intervals), the impact of such days is often offset by low volume.

DENSITY EXPOSURE AND EFFECT
14.2.4

In a team-preparation context, *density* refers to how many breaks there are within a day's training. Though high volume can be paired with high density, high intensity necessitates more frequent rest periods so that the players' bodies and minds can recover and refocus. There is a higher overall accumulated load on the muscles during high-density sessions.

CONTACT EXPOSURE AND EFFECT
14.2.5

Contact is synonymous with collision. Within the realm of contact-heavy team sports, days that are high collision can involve quite a bit of work with full-contact practices and the use of tackle bags, scrum simulators, and more. The higher injury risk associated with high-collision days, which are often also high intensity and cause the body to absorb a lot of vibration, requires volume to be lower and recovery time to be longer. Such sessions are also typically broken up with plenty of rest/active recovery intermissions. As with high-intensity sessions, the muscles are under high load but for a short time.

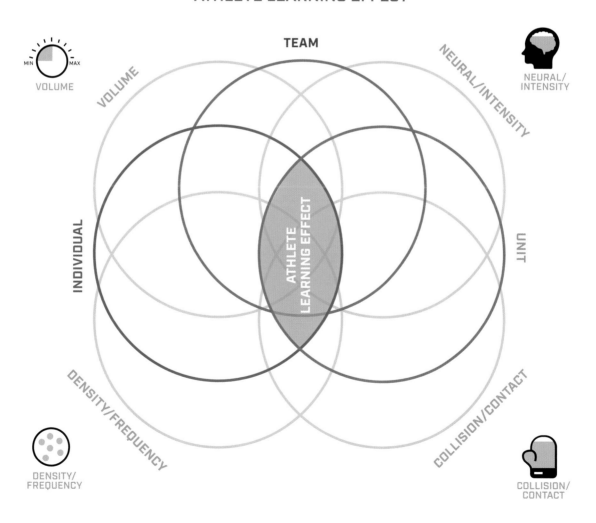

ATHLETE LEARNING EFFECT

MUSCULAR DEMANDS   14.2.5.1

We've already explored the need to vary the stimulation of neural and metabolic systems. Now let's turn our attention to another category of stimulus: muscular. Each morphological programming element places different demands on athletes' muscles and other soft tissues, including ligaments, tendons, and fascia. To ensure that athletes adapt and recover optimally across the morphocycle and that these soft tissues completely regenerate by game day, the coaching staff must vary the stresses placed on them and make sure that the cumulative load is not excessive.

SEQUENCING OF STIMULI   14.2.6

When game day comes around, the goal is for each of the bodily systems to have been emphasized and de-emphasized throughout the previous week's morphocycle so that each is now fully rejuvenated. Different sports have different requirements, and this impacts how stimuli are sequenced during preparation. In rugby and football, for example, strength and power are paramount during a game. This means that it's best to train these elements early in the week so that the affected bodily systems have as long as possible to recharge before they're called on to apply strength and power in competition.

Certain other elements don't take as long to recover from and don't degenerate as quickly as strength and power, with endurance being the primary example. Speed is somewhere in between. We usually stress speed early in the morphocycle and then top it up in lower volume as the week progresses. From a psychological standpoint, technically and tactically intensive sessions place a great strain on the nervous system, just as Olympic lifting does. As the neural system can take up to three days to fully adapt and reboot, we want to schedule the most demanding tactical and technical lessons for earlier in the week, too.

COMBINATION AND SUMMATION   14.2.7

A core aim of the morphological programming approach is that players be relaxed and ready come game day and not held back by inhibiting factors resulting from overtraining or underrecovery, such as:

* Volume: Players are worn down and have "heavy legs."

* Intensity: The squad is mentally exhausted by the high cognitive load of intense sessions.

* Density: Players may not have slept or eaten well enough to recover from dense sessions.

* Collision/Contact: Athletes have knocks and bruises.

A simple way to look at the potentially adverse effects of placing too much emphasis on a single morphological programming approach element is to imagine each element as a cup. What I've discovered over years of working with college, professional, and national teams is that elite athletes can and will compensate adequately if two of these cups are full. But if three or all four are overflowing, they will fail to perform adequately, be unable to meet their coaches' game plan objectives, and/or get injured. The trouble with traditional periodization is that it fails to heed the warning signs in each area, let alone consider the ramifications of cumulative overload in all four elements. In contrast, the morphocycle method seeks to maintain a reasonable level in all morphological programming elements so that none of the cups are ever more than half full when game day arrives.

DRILL & GAME CLASSIFICATION

VOLUME   NEURAL/INTENSITY   DENSITY/FREQUENCY   COLLISION/CONTACT

VOLUME   NEURAL/INTENSITY   DENSITY/FREQUENCY   COLLISION/CONTACT

CONDITIONING DRILLS

- Non-cognitive (no thinking needed)
- No decision-making
- Non-technical
- Non-tactical

RUDIMENT DRILLS

- Basic movement skill
- Isolated action
- Simplistic (noncomplex)
- Repetition of a learned and perfected movement
- No player contact
- No cognitive involvement

VOLUME   NEURAL/INTENSITY   DENSITY/FREQUENCY   COLLISION/CONTACT

VOLUME   NEURAL/INTENSITY   DENSITY/FREQUENCY   COLLISION/CONTACT

TECHNICAL DRILLS

- Basic movement skill
- Integrated technical action
- Isolated context
- But can be a series of combined technical skills
- Complex actions and execution of a learned technical movement
- May involve another player
- Limited cognitive involvement

TACTICAL DRILLS

- Repetition of a single game movement pattern
- Integrated technical & movement actions
- Isolated tactical context
- Low-level decision making
- Repetition of a learned tactical movement
- Multiple-player involvement & interaction
- Cognitive involvement

VOLUME   NEURAL/INTENSITY   DENSITY/FREQUENCY   COLLISION/CONTACT

VOLUME   NEURAL/INTENSITY   DENSITY/FREQUENCY   COLLISION/CONTACT

TACTICAL GAME

- Integrated tactical movements in specific decision-making contexts
- Games designed to elicit specific tactical and technical actions
- Replication of specific game scenarios and decision-making in context
- High cognitive demand
- High decision-making demand
- Position-specific
- Can be opponent-specific

SMALL-SIDED GAME

- General technical and tactical demand
- High-level decision-making
- High technical demand
- High cognitive involvement
- Technical actions in a nonspecific tactical context
- Nonposition- and nonopponent-specific
- Games designed to elicit nonspecific tactical and nonspecific technical actions

ENERGY SYSTEM CYCLING

Within the framework of the morphological programming approach is energy system–specific team preparation. These three systems are aerobic, anaerobic, and alactic.

AEROBIC

Aerobic training relies on the utilization of oxygen. It is characterized by higher-duration, low- to medium-speed sessions that are either continuous or composed of fairly long intervals. These sessions produce lactic acid and other by-products that athletes must flush out through a cooldown, post-session mobility work, and active recovery. Generally, the coaching staff will emphasize aerobic training on a day that is high volume, low intensity, medium to high density, and low collision/contact. As the aerobic system recovers the fastest of the three energy systems, it can be stimulated closer to game day without interfering with the team's physical readiness. It's also used earlier in the cycle in conjunction with lower-intensity, longer-duration player education and film sessions.

ANAEROBIC

Also known as the anaerobic lactic system, this energy system does not require oxygen but does produce lactic acid. Work periods are short and intense and necessitate longer active recovery/rest periods than alactic intervals, so that the body can flush out or recycle the lactic acid before the next work period.

Anaerobic sessions are typically performed at the point in the morphocycle when the coaches are going for low volume, high intensity, low density (lots of short breaks), and medium to high collision. Anaerobic sessions are typically performed in the middle of a morphocycle to give athletes ample recovery time before game day.

ALACTIC

The alactic system is a subset of the anaerobic one and recruits fast- and slow-twitch muscle fibers for rapid actions that are short in nature. Alactic sessions do not result in the accumulation of a significant amount of lactic acid.

BALANCING THE ENERGY SYSTEMS

Just like the four morphological programming components, each of these three systems is present at all times in every team preparation session, but only one is dominant on any particular day. A single drill may have a different characteristic, but overall, the energy system emphasized for the day must be in keeping with the main morphological programming element at that stage in the morphocycle. This will ensure that a satisfactory stimulus is created to produce adaptation without compromising game deliverables.

ENERGY SYSTEM DRILL DESIGN

It's possible, and often desirable, for strength and conditioning coaches to help players develop their energy systems in the weight room and gym. Yet the coaching staff can also design drills that assist this work on the training ground. At right are some guidelines for structuring such drills.

THE PRINCIPLE OF HOLISTIC SUMMATION

The adaptations of a cell, fiber, or person are not the result of a single exposure to a stimulus but of the combination of all the stimuli they've experienced. The game is the litmus test for the holistic summation that has occurred during the morphocycle and provides insight into the overall load that the players have been subjected to and the recovery that follows. As there is a limited amount of time between games and a finite amount of summation that any player can respond to and still be fresh for game day, the coaches must settle on a short list of critical objectives and then prioritize them.

DRILL/GAME DEMANDS

VOLUME NEURAL/ INTENSITY   DENSITY/ FREQUENCY   COLLISION/ CONTACT

VOLUME NEURAL/ INTENSITY   DENSITY/ FREQUENCY   COLLISION/ CONTACT

AEROBIC POWER DRILL RULES

- Medium duration of physical actions (between 120 and 480 seconds' work)

- Submaximal efforts: 80% effort in every movement

- Medium rest periods to allow full recovery & submaximal efforts in each drill

- Aerobic work:rest = 1:1 -> 1:2

AEROBIC CAPACITY DRILL RULES

- Long duration of physical actions (120+ seconds' work)

- Submaximal efforts: 75% effort

- Short rest periods, incomplete recovery in each drill

- Aerobic work:rest = 1:1 and below

VOLUME NEURAL/ INTENSITY   DENSITY/ FREQUENCY   COLLISION/ CONTACT

VOLUME NEURAL/ INTENSITY   DENSITY/ FREQUENCY   COLLISION/ CONTACT

ANAEROBIC POWER DRILL RULES

- Short duration of physical actions (less than 45 seconds' work)

- Intense, maximal efforts: full 100% effort in every movement

- Medium rest periods to allow full recovery & maximal efforts in each drill

- Anaerobic work:rest = 1:3

ANAEROBIC CAPACITY DRILL RULES

- Medium duration of physical actions (between 60 and 120 seconds' work)

- Intense, maximal efforts: full 100% effort in every drill

- Medium rest periods, incomplete recovery in each drill

- Anaerobic work:rest = 1:2

VOLUME NEURAL/ INTENSITY   DENSITY/ FREQUENCY   COLLISION/ CONTACT

ALACTIC DRILL RULES

- Very short duration of physical actions (less than 7 seconds' work)

- Intense, maximal efforts: full 100% effort in every movement

- Long rest periods to allow full recovery & maximal efforts in each drill

- Alactic work:rest = 1:5+

14 The Methodology

SUMMATION OF EFFECT

14.2.10

When planning the next day's training session, the coaches must think about more than just the physical load that emphasizing and de-emphasizing certain morphological programming elements will have on the player. They also need to consider what the emotional and cognitive impact will be and then evaluate whether the summation of effect is sufficient to promote learning and advancement while not being too great for the players' bodies and minds to respond optimally.

If I asked a player to perform a maximal vertical jump, gave him some very bad news or involved him in some kind of charged argument or debate, and then asked him to make another attempt, his second leap would almost certainly be lower. This isn't because he's been physically drained by the first repetition but because I've placed an emotional burden on him. If we only consider the physical load on the player, we are not accounting for the change in performance caused by the emotional stressors.

BIOLOGICAL SYSTEM STIMULUS, ADAPTATION, AND RECOVERY   14.2.10.1

Sprint coach Charlie Francis was one of the first sports professionals to take into account the impact of various stimuli on the central nervous system and factored its restoration into his vertical integration preparation approach. When getting today's team-sports athletes ready for competition, we also need to consider the stimulus, adaptation, and recovery of the peripheral nervous system (PNS), cardiorespiratory system, autonomic nervous system (ANS), and structural-anatomical system, as well as the metabolic system. Again, this needs to be done within the context of the morphological programming approach.

SESSION STRUCTURE AND DESIGN: SPEED, STRENGTH, CAPACITY, AND REACTION   14.2.10.2

In addition to developing the three primary energy systems—alactic, aerobic, and anaerobic (see page 294)—coaches should structure team preparation sessions to develop four additional components: speed, strength, capacity, and reaction. Like selecting the energy systems for each day in the morphocycle, choosing one of these four components should adhere to the prescription of the morphological programming elements emphasized and de-emphasized.

TRAINING DRILL CLASSIFICATION   14.2.10.3

Just as it's vital to classify and distinguish primarily physical sessions, it's also beneficial to stratify sessions that involve the technical, tactical, and psychological coactives as they relate to team preparation.

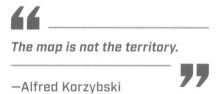

The map is not the territory.

—Alfred Korzybski

DRILL/GAME DEMANDS

VOLUME   NEURAL/INTENSITY   DENSITY/FREQUENCY   COLLISION/CONTACT

VOLUME   NEURAL/INTENSITY   DENSITY/FREQUENCY   COLLISION/CONTACT

AEROBIC POWER GAME RULES

- Medium duration of physical actions (between 120 and 480 seconds' work)

- Intense effort and work rate: full 100% effort in every game

- Medium rest periods to allow full recovery & maximal efforts in each drill

- Aerobic power work:rest = 1:1 or less

AEROBIC CAPACITY GAME RULES

- Long duration of physical actions (180+ seconds' work)

- Intense effort and work rate: full 100% effort in every game

- Short rest periods, incomplete recovery in each drill

- Aerobic work:rest = 1:1 and below

VOLUME   NEURAL/INTENSITY   DENSITY/FREQUENCY   COLLISION/CONTACT

VOLUME   NEURAL/INTENSITY   DENSITY/FREQUENCY   COLLISION/CONTACT

ANAEROBIC POWER GAME RULES

- Short duration of physical work (90 seconds' work and less)

- Intense effort and work rate: full 100% effort in every game

- Medium rest periods to allow full recovery & maximal efforts in each drill

- Anaerobic work:rest = 1:2

ANAEROBIC CAPACITY GAME RULES

- Medium duration of physical actions (between 120 and 240 seconds' work)

- Intense effort and work rate: full 100% effort in every game

- Medium rest periods, incomplete recovery in each drill

- Anaerobic work:rest = 1:1

VOLUME   NEURAL/INTENSITY   DENSITY/FREQUENCY   COLLISION/CONTACT

ALACTIC GAME RULES

- Short duration of physical work (90 seconds' work and less)

- Intense effort and work rate: full 100% effort in every game

- Medium rest periods to allow full recovery & maximal efforts in each drill

- Alactic work:rest = 1:2

14 The Methodology

THE PRINCIPLE OF SUSPENSION OR AMPLIFICATION

14.3

When we observe some recovery strategies, often we are really seeing are coaches and athletes trying to suspend the physiological reaction to certain stimuli. Use of water, temperature, icing, and cryotherapy are perfect examples. Players apply ice to reduce pain and inflammation, and in the short term, it often does what they want it to. But as we know from Gabe Mirkin—the inventor of the RICE (Rest, Ice, Compression, Elevation) protocol for acute injury treatment—applying ice actually delays injury recovery.[85]

While an athlete might want or need to blunt the body's normal reaction to stimulus in extreme circumstances—such as when a star player gets hurt in game six of the NBA Finals and does whatever needs to be done to play in the deciding game seven—the morphocycle approach typically seeks to avoid such suspension of a reaction. In contrast, there are situations in which the coaching staff might want to amplify a stimulus or training effect.

Timing is everything when it comes to amplification. If players drink coffee before a game, it can sharpen their focus. Consuming caffeine after a game has a different impact, improving replenishment of the glycogen stores that were depleted during competition. So it's important that coaches and athletes alike consider when a stimulus is administered and what impact it will have on amplification or suspension.

Here are some examples, focusing primarily on amplification.

Amplification or Suspension of Volume Effect: You can amplify the effects of volume in several ways. One is to add running or some other kind of aerobic work at the end of practice. Another is to minimize the recovery between sessions or parts of a session.

Amplification or Suspension of Intensity Effect: Say you have four players who performed poorly in the last game because of a clear physical quality, such as failure to recover fast enough, or ability to maintain focus, and you identify that their anaerobic conditioning is the root of the issue. Instead of making them run sprints, have them go through drills and small-sided games for the first half of practice, then pull them out for a certain period to do some anaerobic work. While they're still fatigued, put them back into realistic gamelike situations, thus amplifying the effect of intensity. This applies most often to intensity of concentration and intensity of skill execution in game situations.

Amplification or Suspension of Density Effect: One of the best ways to amplify density is to have athletes perform skills and drills with little to no rest time in between. In the weight room, creating supersets of two or more exercises can also provide amplification.

Amplification or Suspension of Contact Effect: We rarely want to amplify the signals that result from collision. But there is a need to, as Jim Harbaugh reminds his players, "build a callus" and get used to the stress. This particularly applies to full-contact sports like rugby, football, and Australian rules football, in which collisions can injure athletes. To suspend the effects of contact, coaches could prescribe more rest, cryotherapy, and foods that reduce inflammation, like berries, oats, and coconut oil.

THE RECOVERY STIMULUS PARADOX

14.3.1

As with the morphological programming approach elements—volume, intensity, density, and collision—we can also amplify or suspend recovery. It's a myth that you can force recovery through nutrition, hydration, mobility, sleep, or anything else. But you can either hinder or facilitate it, and again, timing and dosage are key. For example, taking fish oil right after a lifting session will certainly reduce an athlete's inflammation markers, but it will also blunt the signal that the body receives from such inflammation, which can have the effect of reducing muscle repair. However, if the athlete waits a few hours to take the fish oil, the body will have received the initial signal that these muscles are torn down and need to be restored, and as the resulting reparation has begun, the fish oil will have its intended benefits without interfering with recovery.[86]

In addition, we need to acknowledge that the body is unable to differentiate between training and recovery (or, indeed, education)—they're just different types of stimuli, delivered in different doses at different times to elicit a desired response or adaptation. So if a player elevates her heart rate with thermic cycling (such as taking a steam sauna and then jumping in an icy plunge pool), her body doesn't recognize that this is any different from a physical practice session—all it knows is that it's been exposed to a stimulus, and it reacts accordingly.

RECOVERY: HELPING OR HINDERING ADAPTATION   14.3.1.1

Every player has a unique recovery and adaptation rates for each of the body's many systems, and every player can process different amounts of stimuli. Players also have differing overall functional reserves—that is, the total load that they can handle and recover from collectively across all biological systems. This means that to be both physiologically and psychologically ready for game day (as well as tactically and technically prepared), each player's preparation and recovery need to be somewhat individualized.

Despite the individual variations needed in player preparation and the absence of absolutes that cover every athlete, it's necessary to establish baselines and guidelines for the entire team. One crucial consideration is the typical time it takes each bodily system to recover from a stimulus, which impacts the sum toll that each component of morphological programming preparation and the game has over the course of every week and morphocycle.

Here are some illustrations and charts that show how recovery/therapy can be balanced before and after team preparation in a sample morphocycle to encourage adaptation and optimize regeneration.

It's a false premise to think of recovery as merely techniques and modalities that we use to force the body to respond to stimuli with adaptation. In reality, the body will recover eventually, with or without external intervention. The only question is whether we introduce additional stimuli (mobility, electrical stimulation, hydrating fluids, etc.) appropriately to either help or hinder the inevitable adaptation. Do it right and you get faster, more complete recovery, but do it wrong and you get slower, minimized restoration—effectively maladaptation. You can't stop the body from adapting in some way to stimuli, but you certainly can assist or interfere with the degree to which it does so.

The only time you want to interfere with the body's natural stimulus response is when you're trying to promote another kind of adaptation or you need to intervene to protect the athlete. For example, if a basketball player rolls her ankle just before halftime in a championship game but insists on playing in the second half, the medical staff will take measures at halftime that blunt the natural swelling response and enable her to continue. However, it's worth noting that such intervention will have consequences later, as the body resumes or even heightens its typical adaptation/response.

Therefore, when considering the balance between the morphological programming components, we also need to take into account the "dose" of recovery-stimulating techniques that athletes receive, when they receive it, and how it will combine with other stimuli to either promote or obstruct adaptation. After all, the only difference between medicine and poison is the timing, the amount administered, and substance interaction.

For example, exposing an athlete to cold water before a game can act as a stimulus, but it is more often used after the final whistle blows to reset the nervous system and encourage parasympathetic recovery. It's worth noting that where a player starts is an important consideration. If you drink a double espresso thirty minutes after downing your first double shot, you may become jittery or get stomach cramps. But if that's your first dose of caffeine for the day, you'll probably be fine.

The same goes for training. If a team is doing its first endurance session for the week, it'll likely be fresh and the session will be effective. But if it's the second time that day that an old-school coach has made the players run laps, they're going to be fried afterward. That's why the balanced, all-inclusive approach to team preparation encouraged by the morphocycle is so crucial in ensuring sufficient recovery—it provides the correct starting point for each day's stimuli.

Though there are no absolutes, as every player recovers at slightly different rates, the graph below gives a guide for the time required by each biological system to recharge, which the coaching staff can take into account when planning both morphocycles and athlete recovery. The good thing is that the morphological programming approach recognizes the differing restoration periods and encourages full recovery of each system by elevating and relegating

them depending on which technical, tactical, physical, and psychological elements have already been taxed during the week and which will be predominant later in the week.

In this way, the integrated approach to team preparation and recovery respects the fundamental, inviolable laws of biology, prompting players' bodies and brains to adapt to training stimuli, allowing ample time for each system to recover, and avoiding overtraining and burnout. On the other hand, periodization pays no heed to the constant fluctuations of our biological systems and the way they adapt or fail to adapt based on chronobiology, so it invariably falls short of expectations in the long run.

PLAYING SQUAD: Recovery Periodization, 1 Game Week

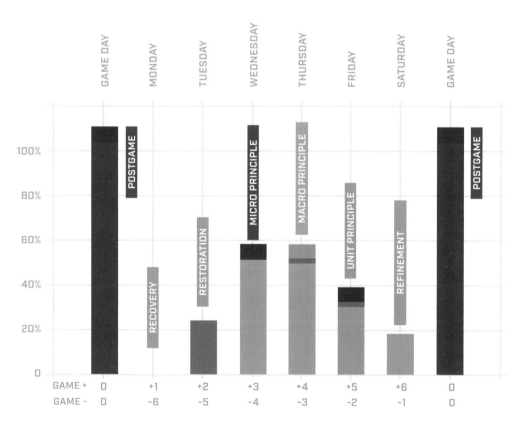

POSTGAME
Cold recovery
Compression clothing, carbohydrates, and protein drinks encouraged

RECOVERY 1
Day off
Self-recovery massage or flush suggested

RECOVERY 2
Low intensity: 70% of max
Spaces
Straight line open-stride pace

STRENGTH RECOVERY
Supplementation and stimulating
Cold exposure or flush
High-anti-inflammatory diet
Massage encouraged

CAPACITY RECOVERY
Supplementation, carbohydrate supplementation, contrast flush
Slow cooldown
Massage & mobility encouraged

SPEED RECOVERY
Carbs & protein
Supplementation
Stimulating cold exposure or flush
High-anti-inflammatory diet
Massage encouraged

REACTIONS RECOVERY
Carbs & protein
Supplementation, flexibility, and massage encouraged

FACILITATION OF MORPHOLOGICAL ADAPTATION   14.3.1.2

Another aspect of team preparation that typically makes great improvements with the morphological programming approach is nutrition. It used to be that even the best nutritionists set up meal plans and guidelines for what players should eat and drink and when, with a catchall mindset that assumed each practice day would be similar. But when a team transitions to the morphological programming methodology, it quickly becomes apparent that no two days of team preparation are the same, so neither are the nutritional and hydration demands.

As nutritionists now have advance warning for what stimuli each day will emphasize, they can better tailor meal plans/guidelines to suit the players' specific recovery and restoration needs after each session in the morphocycle. A nutritionist might also tailor meal plans for individuals who are trying to change body composition, gain muscle, or lose weight. If a player is having game-day performance issues, such as cramping or physically fading late in games, the nutritionist can be called on to intervene. The same is true of athletes' recovery from injury and illness.

PLAYING SQUAD: Periodization Programming, 1 Game Week

The Morphocycle

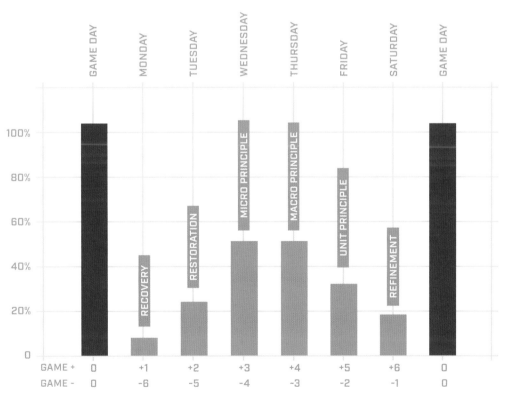

RECOVERY 1
Football specific: jog, stretch, dynamics, pool
25 mins
125–140 bpm

RECOVERY 2
Low intensity, 70% of max
Spaces
Straight line open-stride pace

STRENGTH
High intensity, 90–100% of max
Space, numbers, eccentric loading, acceleration, deceleration, multidirectional (e.g., 1v1s)

CAPACITY
Moderate intensity, 80% of max
Space, numbers, long lactate components of game (e.g.,transition, overlap runs)

SPEED
Intermediate intensity
Game-related speed
Repetitions, quickness, quantity, quality

REACTIONS
Low intensity
Reactive speed and match preparation
Repetitions

14 The Methodology

Even if the team does not have the resources to retain a nutritionist, the players and coaches can follow some basic principles that guide how they eat and drink at different points in the preparatory cycle to maximize adaptation and recovery. So they'll come to know that, for example, they need more protein on a high-intensity day. The emphasis should not be on creating dictatorial policies but rather on giving players the best available information on the percentages of macronutrients (carbs, fat, and protein) they should be ingesting according to the morphological programming profile for the day and then trusting them to make good decisions about their own nutrition.

Similarly, players must make their own decisions about portion sizes based on their body composition and metabolism, which can vary greatly among teammates. For example, a 180-pound point guard is probably going to need smaller helpings than a 275-pound center, but he may need to eat more often to keep his energy levels up.

If players are not heeding the nutritional breakdowns and are eating more or less than they need to for adequate adaptation and restoration, this will manifest itself in below-par performance and biomarker/body composition red flags during team testing. It's also worth letting players know that nutrition can impact recovery for up to forty-eight hours

PLAYING SQUAD: Periodization Programming, 1 Game Week

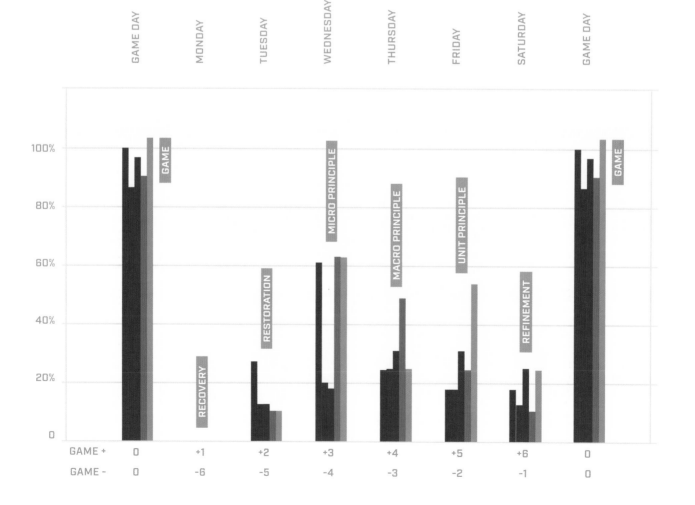

after a training stimulus, so just getting enough protein, replenishing glycogen stores, and rehydrating immediately after a session (the acute recovery period) is not going to be enough.

As with massage, cold-water immersion, electrical stimulation, and other recovery modalities, teams need to recognize that there is no real difference between the nutrition aspect of restoration and the stimulus that preceded it. The goal with both is to prompt adaptation in the individual, which leads to improved team performance when it matters most.

MULTIPHASIC EFFECT   14.3.2

The theories that underpin periodization attempted to show the body's reaction to and recovery from exposure to load as a simple up-and-down, stimulus-and-adaptation curve. This is an oversimplification, as the effect is multiphasic and nonlinear. My Glo, Slo, Flo model for recovery offers a way of looking at this: In the Slo phase, the body is winding down to recover from a stimulus, but this doesn't happen immediately after training. It takes a while for an athlete's excitation level to drop, which is why I say that there is a Glo phase first. Finally comes the Flo stage, when the body has adapted to the stressor and is ready to respond to more stimuli.

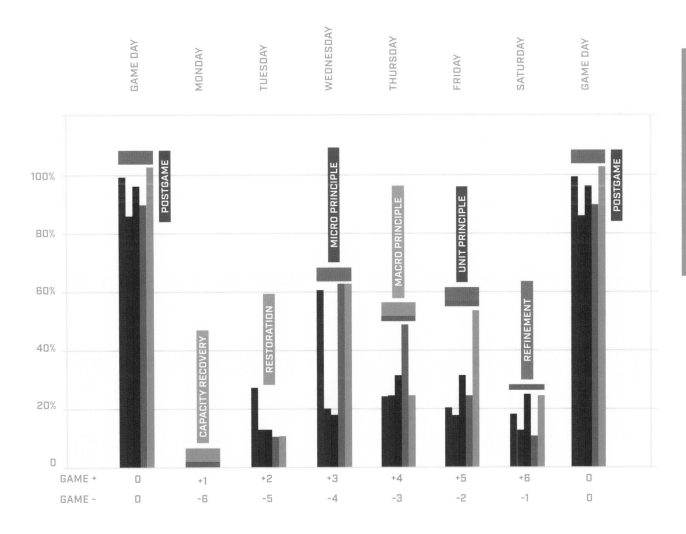

PLAYING SQUAD: Multisystem Excitation & Fatigue

PLAYING SQUAD
Management of Therapy, Game Week: Parasympathetic-Dominant Athlete

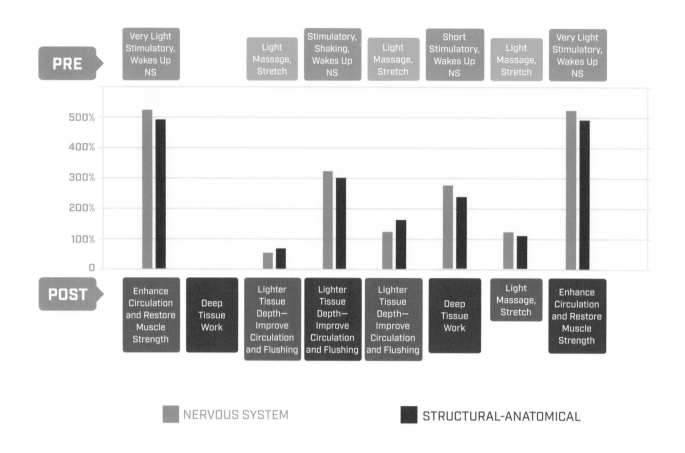

PRE

| Very Light Stimulatory, Wakes Up NS | | Light Massage, Stretch | Stimulatory, Shaking, Wakes Up NS | Light Massage, Stretch | Short Stimulatory, Wakes Up NS | Light Massage, Stretch | Very Light Stimulatory, Wakes Up NS |

POST

| Enhance Circulation and Restore Muscle Strength | Deep Tissue Work | Lighter Tissue Depth— Improve Circulation and Flushing | Lighter Tissue Depth— Improve Circulation and Flushing | Lighter Tissue Depth— Improve Circulation and Flushing | Deep Tissue Work | Light Massage, Stretch | Enhance Circulation and Restore Muscle Strength |

■ NERVOUS SYSTEM   ■ STRUCTURAL-ANATOMICAL

PRINCIPLES OF MORPHOCYCLE DESIGN

14.4

Say you're the coach of an NBA team that's going to face Steph Curry and the Warriors in your next game. You don't need a scouting report to know that Curry can fire and hit a three-pointer from anywhere once he crosses midcourt. So in practice, you may have three of your guards rotate into Curry's role and then back into guarding the player who's imitating Golden State's sharpshooter. You instruct the three-point shooter to shoot as he sees fit once he has crossed midcourt. This forces at least one and preferably two defenders to close him down immediately and not sag back to leave the shot uncontested. In this way, the offensive player is exposing the defense to a realistic experience that will look very much like what they'll see from Curry in the next game. The coaching staff hasn't had to explain anything to the defense, other than perhaps not to allow an uncontested shot.

This is an example of designing practice experiences to imitate the game, a principle that holds true in virtually any practice drill in any sport and for all four game moments. Whether you're trying to

PLAYING SQUAD
Management of Therapy, Game Week: Sympathetic-Dominant Athlete

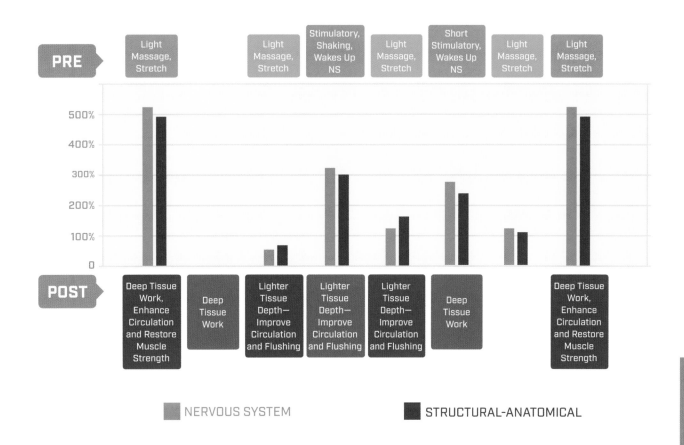

reinforce a principle of play that applies to all opponents or trying to take away the main strength of a particular player or unit, you can use your athletes on one side of the ball to expose their teammates on the other side to a learning opportunity that's directly transferable to the upcoming contest. Remember, you have a game model and game plan, and the alterations should be minimal.

This section outlines the tactical and technical structure for morphocycle programming. Space prevents outlining the exact protocols, but the philosophy outlined here explains the principles of constriction. And, as ever, we're working backward from the game.

To switch effectively from defense to social engagement strategies, the nervous system must do two things: [1] assess risk, and [2] if the environment looks safe, inhibit the primitive defensive reactions to fight, flight or freeze.

—Stephen W. Porges

14 The Methodology

DAY 0: EXECUTION   14.4.1

Game day is the ultimate test of players' preparation and grasp of the game plan and the effectiveness of the prior week's learning experiences. The focus right before the game should be mental preparation. As former England rugby coach Clive Woodward wrote several times in his autobiography, "it's what's between the ears" that wins games. Ideally, the dress rehearsal should be as realistic as possible so that players take the field/court/pitch confident in what's expected of them and their ability to implement the game plan and handle the frictions of the game.

The coaching staff should briefly walk and talk the players through as many game-time scenarios as possible so that they're prepared for the most likely scenarios, both good and bad. As Bill Walsh once told an interviewer, "You need to have a plan even for the worst scenario. It doesn't mean that it will always work; it doesn't mean that you will always be successful. But you will always be prepared and at your best."[87] At this stage, though it's about delivery, the time for talking and thinking is over, and we move to allowing instinct to take over.

When exploring positive and negative situations, it's not enough to state what could go wrong or right; the coaches must also advise the team how to respond, in keeping with the key principles. This isn't just a coach's monologue but rather a two-way exchange of ideas between the coaching staff and their athletes, to ensure they are taking control of the decision-making. There is going to be a large emotional load on the player, so the management's role is to ensure they don't exacerbate or add to it.

In many ways, this is the day on which the head coach has least impact. The idea here is to allow the players to express the key objectives and ensure that they have control of the process. The less the coach says, the more ownership the players have. The goal is to remove all possible frictions of the game so that the players themselves can function in the fog of the game and maximize spare mental capacity.

This day is designed to allow the greatest recruitment of resources across all spectrums. Little recovery is done postgame unless a player is injured or a performance is needed the following day. Natural recovery is facilitated and the game experience is maximized with coach-driven feedback.

DAY 0: EXECUTION

On Day Zero, performance is in the control of the players. The key objective is that nothing new interrupts their ability to recall, focus, and perform. Everything, apart from the actual opponent, should be as familiar as possible to the players to preserve the spare mental capacity and problem-solving ability for execution. Food, meals, hydration strategies, warm-ups, travel timing, and so on should all be the same and familiar to allow the players to relax before the game. This allows the coach to observe players in the same conditions long before game time and gently "tune" players who need to reach the optimal state of mind pregame.

Allowing the players, especially leaders and captains, to rehearse and walk through the game, principles, and objectives without the coach's intervention helps translate into player ownership and leadership during the game.

DAY MINUS 1: REFINEMENT

14.4.2

The day before a game marks something of a hand-over from the coaching staff to the team. In rugby, for example, the captains often run the practice. Team preparation on this day is about refinement. It emphasizes the players' ability to recall information, execute skills, and get into structural formations seamlessly.

From a physiological perspective, it seems like a "speed" day, when the coaches get the players and the ball moving as fast as possible. But the reality is that the speed is primarily from the shoulders up. Decision-making sharpness is critical to the whole process. By playing game-type scenarios that anticipate the decisions they will face and going through drills at game speed, the players will be better able to handle the pace of competition.

This day gives the coaches the opportunity to recap the key technical and tactical lessons they've covered since the previous competition and to make sure that the team is prepared to adapt its aims for each of the four game moments to take the upcoming opponent's preferences into account. This day also provides the coaching staff with the opportunity to bring together all the components from earlier in the cycle.

The key here is that the players feel mentally alert and aware of the goals and plan for the game. This is also the point where the team talks through every possible scenario, such as if it gets a big lead early. What if it concedes scores early? What is the response? The players need to be prepared cognitively to handle good and bad and identify the appropriate tactical, technical, and psychological responses.

The goal is to make sure that each team member is stimulated just enough while still being refreshed for the game tomorrow. The day focuses on ball speed more than player speed, and on decision-making. We also want to limit the number of players in the drills, reduce the game duration, and restrict the playing space so that there are fewer maximum-speed efforts and lots of rest between them. The main focus is on perceptive and decision-making speed. There's no deceleration; drills are performed at 100 percent, with a long work-to-rest ratio. Volume should be low, intensity high, and density in the medium range, with no collision/contact or eccentric work. Minimal recovery should be needed, but if anything more significant is required, any amplification of stressors should be prevented.

DAY -1: REFINEMENT			
LIFESTYLE & NUTRITIONAL	**PSYCHO-PHYSIOLOGICAL**	**TECHNO-TACTICAL**	**OPERATIONAL**
Higher focus on recovery options. Adaptation is delayed. The goal of the day is to make sure that each player is stimulated just enough while still being refreshed for the game tomorrow.	Relaxation and reflection. Minimal loading. Ease of travel and rehearsal are key elements in helping players get a good sleep on the last night.	Final rehearsal pregame. From physiological perspective, it is a "speed" day—for the ball. Speed for players is primarily "from the shoulders up."	Player demands are paramount, second only to coaches and families. Families of players and coaches must be a major focus so that players can focus on what they need to and not be distracted.

DAY MINUS 2: UNIT PRINCIPLES

14.4.3

This is the day to put all the previous work together tactically and technically. Issues from days minus 5 and minus 6 (see pages 312 and 314) will have been corrected at this point. Corrective work has been done with individuals and then the macro unit. Now we use the whole field.

This day is also the only one on which we use games exclusively, maximizing decision-making and transitioning to instinctual performance. It's easy to do too much on this day, as players are sharp and fast, but the secret is to put all the pieces together. On days like this, the scout team or second-string team is invaluable. Intensity is at maximum, volume is medium, and density is very low. Collision is also low.

Technical drills that demand speed are used between games. At this stage, everything has a decision-making aspect. It's important to avoid eccentric load today. Instead, load the concentric phases and develop power. On this day, the highest accelerations and limb velocities are experienced, but not for long distances. Once again, everything is at maximum effort.

More speed can be added to the program to maximize the stimulus if some players don't get the requisite loading. Again, it is easy to overload, so this should be added to the program carefully. By playing small-sided games and going through drills at game speed, the players will be better able to handle the pace of competition. This day also gives the coaches the opportunity to recap the key technical and tactical lessons they've covered since the previous game and to make sure that the team is prepared to adapt its aims for each of the four game moments to take the upcoming opponent's preferences into account. If the team is playing away, this might be the day they travel, in which case the available time can be spent getting the players' circulation going and ensuring that they're physically and psychologically ready for the upcoming game.

Drills and games need to have a reduced number of players and shorter efforts, and they need to take place in a restricted space, so that the game intensity can be maintained. This way, there are more opportunities for speed efforts and more rest between them. Limit deceleration to reduce unnecessary load. Notice the focus is on the correct execution of game principles, not on physical variables, not on GPS measures or force plate data.

DAY -2: UNIT PRINCIPLES			
LIFESTYLE & NUTRITIONAL	**PSYCHO-PHYSIOLOGICAL**	**TECHNO-TACTICAL**	**OPERATIONAL**
Higher carbohydrate intake, low fat. Managed hydration to ensure electrolyte intake. Recovery is prioritized today.	Today is the only day on which we use games exclusively, maximizing decision-making and transitioning to instinctual performance.	This day puts all the previous work together tactically and technically. Speed is increased in games to maximize the stimulus.	Travel day. Efforts are always made to ensure this is seamless for the players and coaches. Advance parties and groups are essential.

DAY MINUS 3: MACRO PRINCIPLES

Due to the high intensity and high collision/contact of the previous day (see page 311), this day should have the opposite characteristics. Another reason to go with high volume at this point in the week-long morphocycle is that the body is typically able to recover faster from high volume than from the other three elements of the morphological programming approach. Collision/contact and intensity should be low on this day, and density can be medium to high. This is the last day that the coaches should stress players' physical capacity before the next game.

From a physical perspective, the play takes place in larger spaces to introduce more peripheral variables into the learning experience. We also move to larger spaces to integrate with the team's various units, such as an offensive line in football, the guards in basketball, or a striker partnership in soccer. The focus is on the macro units and micro principles. Here we focus on capacity.

It is arguably the most important day because it's the only one on which we can afford to introduce a volumetric load. From experience, volume is a dangerous stressor. Volume is the riskiest element for team-sports players, but on the macro principle day we can go to maximum distances and have the unit work as a whole on some full-size aspects of the field.

This day can also be the one on which the team focuses on making tactical adjustments for the next opponent. Within such sessions, the coaching staff can distill a few simple points about what they want the team as a whole and its units and individual players to focus on with regard to the other team's tendencies in each of the four game moments.

Games and drills are performed with maximum commitment, as on every other day. Here the focus is not on ball and player movement but primarily on the relationship and sequencing between the two. This is because the spacing and timing must be exact. If anything, you want to keep the regular width of the playing area and limit the length, but it depends on the positional requirements.

Players can also be given the chance to assess their performance in the previous game. Only if the coaches ask them about the choices they made in certain situations and the players consequently relive these experiences can they recognize what they did right or wrong. This is a prerequisite to making adjustments for the next game. The focus should be on the player self-correcting within the game plan guidelines—coaches shouldn't be giving orders about what needs to change or how skills should be better executed.

Capacity and structural loads can be amplified on this day. We aim to develop every aspect of the cardiorespiratory system by stressing the limiting systems that need development. We can do so by amplifying specific stressors.

As the players practice, the coaches are always watching the cumulative loads on the player, paying attention to cues such as reaction times, errors under pressure, and correct positioning. Another cue is time under tension (TUT), first introduced as a strength-training concept by Ian King but popularized by Charles Poliquin. This is one possible method to amplify the volumetric effect on the athletes and their structural tissues, and it was the basis of a pioneering technique used by Craig White in the 1990s with many rugby teams and with huge success. Should bounding or plyometrics be needed, it can be added here, but in many cases it's not necessary. The profile of this day is medium intensity, high volume, and medium to high density. Collision is quite low.

There should be more players in each tactical drill than on the previous day, with more space for each exercise and a longer duration in each small-sided game and overall. The intensity should be like that of a game but with plenty of rest between reps. In soccer, for example, games might be contested in five-on-five, six-on-six, seven-on-seven, and eight-on-eight games in more space than yesterday.

This will result in a greater number of medium-intensity runs and more long ones. There will be fewer high-intensity efforts and a little more vertical stress, since the players will get closer to max speeds but will perform fewer accelerations. Bigger spaces mean more running and more use of spatial intelligence.

This is a perfect day to make notes on nervous system dominance. On days like this, players who are parasympathetic-dominant can potentially overstress themselves. One further point is that while intensity is low, we know that if volume is kept high for a period of time, the intensity effect starts to rise also—even though that element is not being targeted. You can consider this to be the "tuning fork" day, on which you know what the team looks like as a whole on the field and can see whether the communication between teammates is adequate or needs more work.

It's not important how we play. If you have a Ferrari and I have a small car, to beat you in a race I have to break your wheel or put sugar in your tank.

—José Mourniho

DAY -3: MACRO PRINCIPLES			
LIFESTYLE & NUTRITIONAL	**PSYCHO-PHYSIOLOGICAL**	**TECHNO-TACTICAL**	**OPERATIONAL**
Greater carbohydrate and hydration intake due to increased volumes and loads. More distances are covered, but less time under tension.	Greater group and team unit (mental) reflection. Communication is very important on this day for clarity of role. Less contact and collision.	From a physical perspective, the play takes place in larger spaces to introduce more peripheral and team variables into the learning experience.	There should be more players in each tactical drill than on the previous day, with more space for each exercise and a longer duration in each small-sided game and overall.

DAY MINUS 4: MICRO PRINCIPLES

On this day, we begin to improve micro principles of play and improve the cohesion of the micro unit, the smallest unit of play. To do so, the coaches design games and drills that emphasize the tactical and technical stressors the players find themselves under during the game and improve them in the unit or small group they work in (like the backs in rugby or the guards in basketball).

From a tactical and technical perspective, this day can be spent distilling the macro lessons from earlier in the week into smaller chunks. This day often sees the players working with skill and unit coaches to address issues from the previous game and build on what went right. Younger players often need more discovery learning, in which they can physically and cognitively act out the tactical lessons that the coaches are trying to convey. Conversely, older players sometimes benefit more from classroom-based learning that is less experiential, as they have accumulated more game-time observations throughout their careers. Simply playing film is often enough for them to point out where they excelled or fell short of expectations.

The players move between multiple games and drills on this day. The focus here should be working on drills specific to what the team and unit need to improve on during the game itself. The stress needs to be in the drill and allow recovery opportunities during small-sided games. We primarily use such games on this day to develop tactical and technical abilities. Players can be subjected to eccentric loads, as long as the coaches monitor them.

As players might need to work with multiple specialists on this technically/tactically focused day, each session might be quite short in duration but high in intensity. This should be mirrored in the team's physical activity, which is focused primarily on strength and power today. On the field, there can be some contact and collision, too. To balance this out, the sessions should be low volume and low density (i.e., shorter total duration and frequent breaks).

This is a relatively high-intensity day, with medium to low volume and low density. This allows muscular time under tension to be maximized and strength qualities to be stimulated, but with plenty of rest to maximize efforts. Collision/contact is highest today.

DAY -4: MICRO PRINCIPLES			
LIFESTYLE & NUTRITIONAL	**PSYCHO-PHYSIOLOGICAL**	**TECHNO-TACTICAL**	**OPERATIONAL**
Higher protein and fat intake. Supplementation is focused on anabolic optimization. Strength loading and individualized energy system can be applied.	This day is optimal for any applied personal reflection, mindfulness, and mental training. Focus is on personal and individual learning. Higher level of contact expected.	Individualized technical games preferred to re-create contexts for individual improvements. Distill macro lessons from later in the week into smaller chunks.	High level of preparation for focus on the individual drills and games. For this reason, this day often has the greatest number of external consultants and specialists on-site.

The rationale is to maximize strength early in the week, with 100 percent effort and maximum time to recover. The nature of the games has meant that there has been a large concentric force but also a large eccentric force (the largest of the week), so this must be respected should we choose to amplify any strength work.

When we design drills and games, we try to ensure that they follow some guidelines from a technical/tactical standpoint. Each exercise involves a reduced number of players within a smaller space. The total duration is low also, but the game and effort intensity is high. So, for example, we might train in drills or games of one-on-one, two-on-two, three-on-three, and four-on-four, which generate short, explosive, powerful movements within the context of the tactical design. Expect to see a greater number of jumping efforts, decelerations, and changes of direction. There will be more explosive and short movements, which result in a greater number of physical contacts and collisions.

LONGEVITY

As a side note, people often assume that some players stay in the game for a long time because of their technical and tactical abilities, but in fact, this is often backward. Remaining active in a sport is what often enables players to develop technically and tactically over time. Such advanced capabilities enable older athletes to compensate for declining physical skills—think of Peyton Manning in his final Super Bowl–winning campaign in the 2015–16 NFL season. The longevity principle also applies to coaches—Sir Alex Ferguson never would have developed into a manager capable of winning thirty-eight titles with Manchester United had the organization fired him during a disastrous spell in 1990. (For more on this idea, see section 6 in "The Player.")

After practice, we can add to the player load with weight or strength training to maximize the stimulus. However, this is always secondary to tactical or technical development—not only philosophically but also psychologically. On days like this, techniques used by Olympic weight-lifting coaches or power lifters such as Louie Simmons and the coaches at Westside Barbell Club are appropriate, as they maximize and amplify the stimulus on the body for that day. Again, though, the technique is not as important as understanding the effect on the player.

Depending on the players and their physical needs, the lifting can be on one of two ends of the strength-power spectrum. Often jumps and medicine ball work are added to this day to maximize power and force generation, but again, this is player-specific.

DAY MINUS 5: RESTORATION

14.4.6

While this is "day minus 5" when we're working backward from the game, it's important to also think of it as the second day after a game. Players' bodies are still recovering from the exertion of competition. Of particular concern are the neural demands, which we cannot be completely sure of. Movement is a skill that taxes the CNS, as is decision-making. Elite athletes can access these resources better and to a greater degree than normal people, but they also appear to have the potential to exhaust themselves more.

Therefore, it's best to open the day with learning sessions in which the coaches break down what went right and what went wrong during the game and how this will shape preparation for the next contest. It's essential that the head coach also present the result in a constructive, positive light in this initial session, whether the game was won, lost, or tied.

The team's mental approach must remain unchanged, and it must stay committed to core principles no matter what, so it's the job of the head coach to hit the psychological reset button. In the wake of defeat, this involves avoiding blame, picking out positives ("We executed to the game plan"), and objectively assessing areas for potential improvement. Conversely, if the team routed its last opponent, the coach needs to counter complacency and reinstill determination to build on the win. Perhaps the team played poorly and was lucky to win, in which case the coaching staff must point out this reality rather than allow players to develop false confidence based on a poor performance. As these sessions can be lengthy and require prolonged attention, they can be mirrored by medium- to high-duration physical sessions.

Any recovery facilitation done on a day like this must use the same stimulus that was used to cause the fatigue: movement patterns and skills. This also means that we are developing skills and not wasting any time. In observing the drill, you may think the effort is submaximal, but in reality the effort is maximal from the perspective of where the players are at that moment. One underlying theory is that you condition the body to recover in this shorter period.

On this day, the work-to-rest ratio should mirror that of the game. There is a very low emotional load, and forty-five to sixty minutes' total duration is plenty. Tactically and technically, the drills and games on this day are focused on putting the players in situations where they develop a skill that is regarded as a limiting factor in their game. This could be something like center backs in soccer volleying the ball or props in rugby and defensive backs in football catching and handling the ball to develop intercepting skills. This is a medium-volume day, but very low intensity and low density, with no contact or collision.

DAY -5: RESTORATION			
LIFETYLE & NUTRITIONAL	**PSYCHO-PHYSIOLOGICAL**	**TECHNO-TACTICAL**	**OPERATIONAL**
Provision of passive recovery options (hydrotherapy can be used) after active options. Physical loading is in the same manner as the game (same physical loading patterns).	Presentation of game assessments. Critique of performance presented in clear, clinical manner to avoid emotional stress. Errors are critiqued, not people.	Reintroduction of training. Light movements. Technical development is ideal. Focus on personal improvement.	Clear communication of week ahead, processes, and options for players and families. "Housekeeping" day; no other day is used for non-sport activities.

14 The Methodology

DAY MINUS 6: RECOVERY

14.4.7

The day after the previous game—working backward from the initial game on day 0, this is day minus 6—is most often a rest day. Some teams and coaches do group recovery sessions, and some schedule early-morning training to prevent players from staying out too late after a game. Dutch soccer coach Raymond Verheijen prefers to make the second day after a game day (in our terminology, day minus 5) the team's day off. However, I've found it more beneficial for players' emotional states if they take the first day (day minus 6) off.

As I've already touched on, game day is extraordinarily taxing, so it requires as much physical and cognitive recovery and restoration as possible. Giving players a day off immediately after competition serves three main purposes. First, it gives their systems a rest and a chance to reset, which respects biological laws. Second, a rest day respects the laws of society by giving athletes time to spend with friends and family. And third, taking the day after the game off gives the coaching staff the opportunity to evaluate the team's performance during the game, find limiting factors, and plan for how to reduce their impact before the next game.

This twenty-four-hour break also gives the coaches the chance to study the upcoming opponent's habits and draft key education points for the players that will influence tactical and strategic adjustments.

Educated and driven players should be encouraged to do some fun recovery work in a pool with their kids or friends, which will be beneficial physiologically and much less onerous than the methods they use at "the office" (the team's facilities).

DAY -6: RECOVERY			
LIFESTYLE & NUTRITIONAL	**PSYCHO-PHYSIOLOGICAL**	**TECHNO-TACTICAL**	**OPERATIONAL**
Replacement of fluids and energy substrates is the priority. Easily digestible foods, lightly cooked, to reduce the stress on the digestive system. Low in fat.	Spending time away from work. Allow mental recovery. Family time, away from the game and environment. Allow mental stressors to be removed.	Light, rhythmical movements. As little load-bearing as possible. Stress can be applied, but only in systems not in state of alarm.	Ensure players are protected from commercial demands or unecessary requests. Protection of each person's privacy on this day is essential. No unnecessary communication.

APPLICATION OF THE PRINCIPLES 14.4.8

The attitude, effort, and execution that athletes bring to practice each day is only part of the challenge when it comes to preparing effectively between games. Another vital factor is how well the coaching staff has planned each session in the morphocycle and every exercise therein. There should never be anything accidental in a training session. Every activity must be geared toward the accomplishment of a specific goal or set of goals focused on improved understanding and implementation of the game plan principles in the next game and subsequent ones.

Each weekly (or shorter, depending on how close together the team's games are) morphocycle has to be put together in a thoughtful and logical way. As the time spent with players is limited and the athletes can take on only so much cognitively and physically, prioritizing is one of the head coach's most important tasks. Even if the coach identifies a long list of objectives that the team is failing to meet, the focus must be on the areas of potential improvement that will yield the biggest dividends and correct the most limiting errors.[88]

Dominant qualities and limiting factors cannot be examined through the lens of the previous game alone. The coaching staff must also consider how these will likely affect play for good or for ill against the upcoming opponent and reshuffle strategic and tactical priorities accordingly. For example, if a football team defended the running game poorly in a recent loss, defensive adjustments are obviously needed. But if the following weekend's opponent derives most of its offensive yards from the passing of a prolific quarterback and is generally poor on the ground, then perhaps correcting the biggest defensive flaw from that defeat can wait until the next morphocycle.[89]

In addition to working on tactical and strategic modifications the head coach deems necessary for effective play against the next opponent, the team should spend some time working on drills and small-sided games that reinforce its immutable style of play. The main objective for each game moment should never change, and these should be reinforced by working on macro or micro principles connected to each one. This way, the team will continue to progress in how well it executes the game plan every game, even as it makes minor adaptations for each opponent.[90]

It's easy to confuse strategy and tactics. One way to make this distinction is to think of strategy as the overarching plan for the game and tactics as methods of achieving this aim. Tactics need to be varied depending on what worked and what didn't in the previous game and the predilections and tendencies of the opponent in the next one. Such knowledge is one aspect of successful strategic planning from week to week. Another main consideration is the plot of the upcoming game, which means taking into account the opponent's recent form, the implications for the game's result, and how the head coach wants players to react in certain situations. The team also needs to plan for the circumstances of the forthcoming game, including travel and accommodation requirements, the differences between home and away contests, and the potential impact of weather. Keeping these variables in mind, the coaching staff can adjust the team's preparation as needed.[91]

SEVEN-DAY MORPHOCYCLE 14.4.9

I recognize that not every sports team plays just one game per week, nor do they play all their games on a Sunday. Remember that the morphocycle is like an accordion in that it can be expanded or contracted as needed.

As a comprehensive seven-day cycle is based on a long interim between games, the team has more of a chance to be exposed to all four morphological programming elements in a way that stimulates adaptation and progression in each area.

> *You have no choices about how you lose, but you do have a choice about how you come back and prepare to win again.*
>
> —Pat Riley

THE LEARNING EXPERIENCE

14.5

For too long, teams have tried to create training drills to improve a skill or player attribute in isolation, focusing on the inputs, the sets, reps, training plans. This perspective is fundamentally wrong. These drills bear little or no relation to what goes on in the game, and coaches often fail to recognize that all elements of performance are intrinsically related and indivisible. Other mistakes the coaching staff can make are telling players they're going to perform a skill in a certain way, rather than designing an experience that players can learn from, and designing training exercises from their own perspective, not the player's. All training should be considered from the player's viewpoint.

In this section, we'll explore a radically different approach that takes the lessons of the previous game and uses them to inform learning experiences that will help individual players, units, and the team as a whole perform better in the next contest. We'll also see how to approach learning holistically so that it takes technical, tactical, physical, and psychological coactives into account, and how players should be allowed to explore and problem-solve to come up with their own solutions rather than being given precise, my-way-or-the-highway instructions.

THE MACRO PRINCIPLE OF SPECIFICITY

14.5.1

One of the most important parts of the weekly morphocyclical programming philosophy is specificity: everything the coaches have the players do in practice must further the expression of game plan goals.

So if a basketball coach has the objective of getting the ball over the half-court line as fast as possible in the transition-to-offense moment, he should design drills that encourage this. The principle of specificity also states that the coaching staff should limit their interventions and let players figure out how best to perform the desired actions. For any drill to be effective, players must also focus intently. Another aspect of specificity is that all drills and small-sided games in practice must be performed at game speed, so that scenarios are as close as possible to what happens during competition. This way, the players can apply what they've learned without dissonance.[92]

THE MACRO PRINCIPLE OF DISASSEMBLY

14.5.2

Even the most intelligent players can handle only a certain level of complexity. In highly structured sports like football, just learning the playbook so that athletes can run a certain play in practice and in games without thinking is a sizable task in memorization and cognitive processing. To introduce the game plan so that it's understandable and actionable, the coaching staff must break it into smaller chunks—in other words, they must disassemble it. You sometimes hear commentators saying that this player has a "high basketball IQ." Effective disassembly must make sub-principles and sub-sub-principles understandable to the player who is on the extreme opposite end of the scale. Otherwise, implementing the game plan is going to prove impossible.[93]

THE MACRO PRINCIPLE OF HIERARCHICAL ORGANIZATION   14.5.3

Every principle of play is vital to the execution of the game plan. But at the risk of lapsing into cliché, if everything is a priority, then nothing is a priority. The head coach must rank each of the objectives for each game moment and then focus most of the team's time and effort on the top one or two. Another reason for doing this is that players have a limited capacity to retain and act on information. If a principle is not being applied properly, the coaching staff might shuffle and reorder these priorities so that they can mitigate a limiting factor on an individual, unit, or team basis.[94]

THE PRINCIPLE OF INVOLVEMENT   14.5.4

When Daniel Coyle was researching his book *The Talent Code,* he asked expert musicians and athletes to describe the nature of their most productive practice sessions. Focus was one of the frequently mentioned characteristics of what he calls "Deep Practice."[95] If a training session is to be deep rather than superficial, the players must be fully involved. One of the best methods for encouraging such engagement is to design drills in a way that forces players to make their own decisions about how, when, and in what context they select and execute a skill. This is far more effective from a learning perspective than providing the answers for them in advance.

THE PRINCIPLE OF GUIDED DISCOVERY   14.5.5

One of the most effective ways athletes learn is by working in a scenario that encourages them to achieve a certain outcome but enables them to figure out their own path to this destination. In such guided discovery, coaches don't tell them what the target is for the drill or what steps they should take to reach it; instead, the athletes have to explore, experiment, and find their own way. As the authors of one study put it, "Allowing learners to interact with materials, manipulate variables, explore phenomena, and attempt to apply principles affords them with opportunities to notice patterns, discover underlying causalities, and learn in ways that are seemingly more robust."[96]

During such guided discovery, intervention from the coaching staff should be minimal, brief, and highly purposeful. This lesson comes directly from John Wooden, who told a high school coach he was mentoring, "Corrections should be no more than 10 seconds if possible, the player should be addressed by first name, nothing should be mentioned that would discourage the player, and the correction should be packed with practical information the player needed to make the change. 'Kyle. Make your cut at the right time. It was a little early. Wait a second and see what happens. Try it again.'" Wooden also told the young coach to minimize the number of "coaching statements" he made during practice so that there would be less time spent on talking and more on doing.[97]

TACTICAL CONSIDERATIONS AND DESIGN   14.5.6

Because the tactical coactive determines implementation of the game plan, each drill should be purposeful and deliver a tactical experience with a defined learning outcome. For example, if you recognized that your defense needed to maintain its shape better when trying to thwart counterattacks, you could use a floating player in a five-on-five small-sided game. Having a sixth player on offense will force the defense to improve its communication and organization. You could also be more granular and stipulate that the extra player can only attack down the right or left side. Or if you wanted the offense to improve how well it retained possession while under defensive pressure, you'd switch the floating player to the other side.

TECHNICAL CONSIDERATIONS AND DESIGN
14.5.7

Cones can be used to create no-go zones that players can't move into. For example, if you know an upcoming opponent has a player who's a potent attacking threat on the left side of the field, you could design drills that cut off this area and force the person role-playing to come into the middle. You can also create drills that exaggerate certain situations, like having two or three tight ends to encourage the quarterback to throw more to one side.

PSYCHOLOGICAL CONSIDERATIONS AND DESIGN
14.5.8

Depending on how close you are to the next game and how involved the players are, you might want to increase or decrease the psychological load on them. This can be manipulated by either talking to them or not before practice, inviting families to watch a scrimmage and creating a heightened level of competition between players in a certain position. It's worth noting that increasing psychological load should rarely be done the day before a game, as it cannot be sustained for long and needs to have an element of surprise to be effective.

PHYSICAL CONSIDERATIONS AND DESIGN
14.5.9

Two of the simplest ways to vary the physical load on the squad is to increase or decrease the numbers of players involved in small-sided games and drills and to alter the size of the playing area. You can also change up work-to-rest ratios and tinker with the duration of practice.

MORPHOLOGICAL CONSIDERATIONS
14.6

As we know, many games are not simply weekly events. NBA games, for instance, happen far more frequently—perhaps far too frequently! Regardless, the principles of the morphocycle remain the same, whether it's stretched or shortened to suit the competition cycle. How we adapt and manipulate the morphocycle is very important so that we can ensure the integrity of the player experience.

THE PRINCIPLE OF PRESERVATION
14.6.1

The demands on players' metabolic, cardiorespiratory, central nervous, and other systems vary from day to day depending on the morphological programming profile for any particular day. Coaches sometimes sense fatigue and are tempted to completely change the morphocycle approach. In these instances the coach should stick to the same morphocycle and not drastically alter team practices, apart from changing the overall volume (duration)—the intensity should be maintained.

Coaches should maintain a consistent focus on realistic scenarios that are highly relevant to the game-day situations players will soon find themselves in. It's also vital that athletes prepare at or above game speed (creating overload to result in adaptation). Former NBA All-Star, Hall of Famer, and MVP Bill Walton said of the team sessions run by college coach John Wooden, "Practices at UCLA were nonstop, electric, supercharged, intense, demanding, with Coach pacing the sidelines like a caged tiger, barking instructions, positive reinforcement and maxims: 'Be quick, don't hurry.' He constantly changed drills and scrimmages, exhorting us to 'move quickly, hurry up.' Games seemed like they happened in a slower gear."[98]

One effective way for coaches to train teams effectively on multiple days in each morphocycle is with small-sided games. A day that requires a soccer team to prepare using low volume, high intensity, low density, and medium to high collision could involve five-a-side practice in a restricted area that's just a portion of a full-sized pitch.

If the next day dictates higher volume, low intensity, high density, and low to medium collision, the coach doesn't need to blow up the practice method but rather change just one variable: the size of the playing area. Simply increasing the size of the field will result in all these changes to the morphological programming elements. Other factors that could be altered include the number of players on each side, the number of touches players are required to make, the duration of the game, and the number and length of breaks.

SPORTS SCIENCE, TECHNOLOGY, AND EVALUATING PREPARATION   14.6.2

Teams with bigger budgets and better facilities can enhance their assessment of individual and collective preparation with monitoring that includes measuring heart rate variability (HRV), inflammation markers, and lactate and hormone levels (the presence of stress hormones like cortisol indicates chronic overtraining and/or underrecovery). Organizations can also employ advanced analytical technology, including GPS, motion sensors, and electromyography (EMG) monitoring.

Regardless of how complex and advanced some of the most high-tech performance-monitoring tools are, their use should not complicate team preparation for the players. Athletes need to focus all their efforts on training and recovery; the last thing they need is the unwelcome distraction of too much technology or the cognitive overload of spreadsheets full of numbers.

For simplicity's sake, particularly in the early days of transitioning to the morphological programming approach, it might be best to choose just one measurement to evaluate how each session and recovery from its stimuli rank in all four morphological

programming areas. For teams with access to blood testing and heart rate monitors, this could involve:

- *Volume:* Cortisol, time, total number of reps, GPS distance
- *Intensity:* HRV, max rep lifted, max number of sprint efforts, max speed
- *Density:* Resting heart rate, work-to-rest ratio, total number of rests, reps/session
- *Collision/Contact:* Creatine kinase, number of contacts

If a team has fewer resources, it can use simpler, subjective measurements to determine the morphological programming profile for each day of the upcoming cycle, such as:

- *Volume:* Total duration of sessions
- *Intensity:* Combination of coaches' and players' perception of effort
- *Density:* Total volume minus total time of rest periods
- *Collision/Contact:* RPE, stiffness vs soreness

Physiological metrics do not indicate the ability of a player to play the game, and there is limited evidence that these are even able to assess fatigue.

If the longest session a coach will ever conduct is two hours long, this can be used as a 100 percent marker, which enables the coach to score all shorter sessions as a percentage. Similarly, if 100 percent of intensity in a speed session is ten one-hundred-meter sprints, then the coaching staff can work backward from this marker in planning the intensity of all other sessions. For density, 100 percent might be the maximum practice time (deducting breaks / active recovery periods) of eighty minutes. A full-contact football or rugby scrimmage would be considered 100 percent on the contact/collision scale. Obviously, due to the risk of injury, such a maximal session, even for short periods, would be used sparingly.

Just like appraisals of competitive performances using the game model, assessments of the morphological programming elements during preparation should combine objective, quantifiable measurements with subjective judgments. In evaluating sessions, it's not just coaches and specialists who should give their input. Coaches might believe that a certain day's training will be manageable based on their assessment, but due to a combination of factors—such as the stage of the season, the nature of recent games, and the stress of travel—some or all of their players might come away with a far different impression.

Therefore, it's important to get daily player feedback and make use of the insights that can come from what we call rate of perceived exertion (RPE). Even if a player's biomarkers or fitness-tracking numbers indicate that a session has been too taxing, this is rarely a problem if they don't *feel* overworked. Though blood testing often does a good job of show-

DECISION-MAKING DESIGN

The understanding of how interactive decision-making truly is has been explored by economists such as John von Neumann, Robert Aumann, and Thomas Schelling. Game theory and interactive decision theory demonstrate that an individual's decision-making influences the way other people anticipate the effects of this decision and from there make their own choices. We see this play out on the sporting field, too. Watch any game and you'll see players trying to anticipate what their opponents are going to do and attempting to influence that decision, perhaps by showing them space to move into or giving them their weak side. This is why we need small-sided games in practice: to encompass the totality of the experience.

ing the physical impact of team practices on each player, it fails to take into account the cognitive or emotional impact. Anyone who thinks that the game is not emotionally draining for players should carefully consider what Antonio Damasio said: "When we talk about emotion, we really talk about a collection of behaviors that are produced by the brain. You can look at a person in the throes of an emotion and observe changes in the face, in the body posture, in the coloration of the skin and so on."[99]

THE TACTICAL OPERATOR   14.6.2.1

Of course these same principles apply to the tactical operator. The difference is that in many cases there is less opportunity for planning. In special operations groups where they still use traditional Soviet periodization approaches, there is a slightly different demand for physical fitness. That said, the morphological approach is an infinitely smarter way to develop the tactical athlete because there is less variation in loads and injury risk is much reduced. Development of technical and tactical qualities are synced with the development of physical qualities.

WHY SCRIMMAGE AND GAMES ARE CRITICAL   14.6.3

A complex system like any team sport is not simply the sum of its parts; it's governed by the relationships established among all its elements, which make the system behave in a certain way. The game is an indivisible unit: it's not divided into offense and defense; rather, these are two sides of one coin. Each player is a functional, holistic unit: more than simply piec-

He who can handle the quickest rate of change survives.

—John Boyd

es of physical, tactical, technical, and psychological elements. The priority is always the game, the interaction of the elements and operation of the whole system. Therefore, the only way we can develop all elements is to do so concurrently, in a scrimmage that echoes real-world scenarios.

The way individuals perceive and interpret the data they're bombarded with in a game depends on their experience, values, skills, needs, and expectations. It is important to note that the expression of the game model in scrimmage is not just organization in space and a breakdown of specific tasks by the players but the existence of a unitary concept to develop the game. The game is a living, breathing expression in its own right. In other words, the game model is a general theme that allows players to establish a common language among themselves.

By making changes to the smaller elements, the training games and drills, the coaching staff creates variety to maintain players' engagement and interest level while allowing the squad to work on its core game plan principles in a manner directly related to competitive play. At the same time, maintaining a similar day-to-day structure reduces player anxiety and removes the burden of coming up with dramatically different practices from the head coach. This approach also allows coaches to stick to the prescribed morphological programming approach loads for each day in the morphocycle.

THE IMPORTANCE OF TIME WITH THE BALL AND OTHER PLAYERS 14.6.3.1

Another key consideration in scrimmages is getting players as much time with the ball as possible. Too many coaches are wasting time putting players through unrealistic drills that have little to no relevance to what happens on game day. There are also too many instances in which coaches have players working individually on skills in drills that are of little use when facing another team, as they're not conducted with simulated pressure that resembles what the players will face in league play.

Returning to ball-focused, team-centric exercises will lead to higher-quality preparation, a more thor-

ough grasp of tactics and strategy, and the elimination of wasted time. Here's José Mourinho's take on why preparing with the ball is of such great benefit: "My training sessions aren't long, they're dynamic and incredibly time-efficient. I like my team to learn to love the ball, and to know what to do with it once they win it back. Three-hour training sessions will only serve to bore the players. They would quickly fall out of love with the ball."[100]

PERCEPTION IS REALITY, ANTICIPATION IS ACTION: FACILITATING DECISION-MAKING 14.6.4

Decision-making can often seem random, and there have even been books written on this premise. But in reality, the way players perceive what's going on around them and anticipate what's going to happen next guides the skill they decide to choose and execute. A successful game model gives players the freedom to make decisions but also guides them into good decisions through repetition in practice.

The principles that the coaching staff instills and reinforces on a daily basis help their team members to better contextualize each situation that unfolds during the game and create a set of beliefs that aid their decision-making. Such principles improve individuals' decisions within the context of the team and its overarching group goals.

There is no such thing as a disembodied mind. The mind is implanted in the brain, and the brain is implanted in the body.

—Antonio Damasio

BASIC INSTINCT   14.6.4.1

It takes half a second or less for players to observe what's going on around them, select the best skill for the situation, and put it into action. This incredibly brief time frame shows that there is little if any time to think consciously about the best way to proceed. Rather, decision-making is instinctual. (See page 180 on how the reptile and limbic parts of the brain respond to threats faster than the conscious mind.) If athletes can learn to better anticipate what's going to happen next in the events unfolding around them, they can reduce the time it takes to assess and act to a fifth of a second or less. This increase in anticipation and, therefore, action comes from the experience of being in a similar situation in the past.[101]

Almost everything we do, we do unconsciously. When learning to do something for the first time, we feel insecure and are conscious of many details of the action. However, with practice, we act in an increasingly unconscious fashion. This means that we can perform faster and use fewer resources while doing so, giving us spare mental capacity for other things. So this has to become one of the primary goals for any coach: to create experiences that allow players to create positive habits so that they can react without thinking in a game.

SPARE MENTAL CAPACITY   14.6.4.2

When a player is deciding what action to take, her mind creates a simulation of possible actions and reactions, running through representations and models of the actions to create the possibility of its realization—all at warp speed. The brain then uses memories of previous similar experiences to predict the results of different possible actions and opts for the one that has the most positive effects or the least chance of failure. The brain only has the capacity to focus on a certain number things at once, and very often coaches consume the players' brains with so many thoughts and messages that there is no spare mental capacity left for things that matter, such as concentration and focus.

Each experience of taking action, then, becomes part of the memories you draw on to anticipate the results of decisions the next time a similar situation comes about. Neuroscientist Antonio Damasio showed that the result of an experience helps determine future actions through the use of emotional states. Emotional states also become tied to memories of past actions, which can be positive or negative. So when you're deciding what to do, you're more likely to subconsciously choose an action that made you feel good the last time you performed it, which is usually the result of a successful outcome.

HABITS AND PRACTICE DESIGN   14.6.4.3

Every training session has to be planned and designed to match the Commander's Intent and sub-objectives of the head coach's game model. Systematic repetition of the tactical principles with maximum involvement should eventually enable players to transform match-play patterns from training experiences into habits that can be applied subconsciously on game day. This is the ultimate goal

People who are great thinkers, in science or in art, people who are great performers, have to have that kind of capacity. Without that kind of capacity, it's extremely difficult to manage a high level of performance because you're going to get a lot of extraneous material chipping away at the finery of your thinking or the finery of your motor execution.

—Antonio Damasio

in preparing the team.[102] Our brain prepares us to respond to our environment long before we actually move our body, and the more that players learn about their teammates' preferences and tendencies, the better they can anticipate what's coming next. This is something I see firsthand in practice with Jim Harbaugh on a daily basis.

Of course, the question of fatigue comes into play. The intensity of play that observers see may be different from day to day, as the complexity of training sessions varies, but the "player experience" should not—they should still be giving maximum effort. If a team has played on Sunday, no player is fully recovered physically, mentally, or emotionally on Monday or Tuesday.

Athletes should always play with full concentration, but the level of concentration available to them is relative to their recovery and readiness to train. The higher the levels of concentration during preparation sessions, the less chance there is that players will make mistakes and waste training time.

The main factors that influence the psychological progression and learning complexity in scrimmages are:

1. Complexity and principles

2. Dynamic complexity

3. Number of players

4. Space

5. Duration of the exercise

These factors are directly related, and time of the competitive season should be taken into consideration, as it will directly affect the emotional as well as physical load on the players.

Energy Systems in Drill & Game Design

ENERGY SYSTEM	DRILL/GAME	WORK	WORK:REST	EFFORT	NEURAL	VOLUME	RECOVERY
ALACTIC	DRILLS	< 7 SECS	1:5+	100%	HIGH	LOW	FULL
	GAMES	< 7 SECS	1:5+	100%	HIGH	LOW	FULL
ANAEROBIC POWER	DRILLS	< 45 SECS	1:3	100%	HIGH	MEDIUM	FULL
	GAMES	< 90 SECS	1:2	100%	HIGH	MEDIUM	FULL
AEROBIC POWER	DRILLS	480 -> 120 SECS	1:1 -> 1:2	80%	LOW	MEDIUM	FULL
	GAMES	480 -> 120 SECS	1:1 -> 1:2	80%	LOW	MEDIUM	INCOMPLETE
ANAEROBIC CAPACITY	DRILLS	120 -> 80 SECS	1:2	100%	HIGH	MEDIUM	INCOMPLETE
	GAMES	120 -> 80 SECS	1:2	100%	HIGH	MEDIUM	INCOMPLETE
AEROBIC CAPACITY	DRILLS	120 SECS	1:1	75%	LOW	HIGH	INCOMPLETE
	GAMES	120 SECS	1:1	75%	LOW	HIGH	INCOMPLETE

14 The Methodology

USE OF DRILLS & GAMES IN TEAM SPORT PHASES

	EARLY PRESEASON	LATE PRESEASON	NONPLAYING	IN SEASON
CONDITIONING DRILLS	✓✓✓	✓	✓	✗✗✗
RUDIMENT DRILLS	✓	✓	✓	✗
TECHNICAL DRILLS	✓✓	✓✓	✓✓	✓
TACTICAL DRILLS	✗	✓	✓✓	✓✓✓
TACTICAL GAMES	✗	✓	✓✓	✓✓✓
SMALL-SIDED GAMES	✓✓	✓✓✓	✓✓✓	✓✓✓

✓ Activty has limited use.   ✓✓✓ Activity is strongly encouraged.

✗ Activity is rarely used.   ✗✗✗ Activity is not used.

[Johan Cruyff] was the most courageous coach and manager I ever met. When he smells the talent it doesn't matter if the age is 16 or 17 because he believed in, what in Spain we call, the efecto mariposa [butterfly effect]. For him one good pass at the beginning could create absolutely everything....Cruyff loved mathematics because it helped him think in new ways about formations and finding space in football—just as other sports such as basketball and, in particular, baseball, opened his mind.[103]

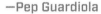

—Pep Guardiola

JOHN BOYD'S OODA LOOP   14.6.4.4

In "The Game" and "The Player," I discussed the OODA (Observe, Orient, Decide, Act) Loop, the four-stage model that former fighter pilot John Boyd devised to explain how combatants make decisions and act during combat. In terms of team preparation, coaches should try to improve the speed at which the team moves through Boyd's cycle by devising drills that require them to make decisions in gamelike conditions. Since decision-making in the game is impacted by the movements of others and the ball, small-sided games with certain constraints—such as restricting field size or having the attacking or defending unit add another player—can improve the effectiveness with which players move through the four stages of the OODA Loop.

With every fractal-like player incident, the aim is to, as Boyd might say, get inside their decision-making cycle and disrupt it. To make them think. If they think, they stop, and if they stop, they are dead.

CORRECT DESIGN AND IMPACT OF GAMES AND DRILLS   14.6.5

As we construct the player experience, we need to bear in mind some important aspects of drills and games. As much as possible, we want to use games to create the experience, not drills. Drills are only used when a learning experience is in its very early stages or there's no possible way to recreate the experience in a game or small-sided game. Here are some important considerations when designing drills:

Central Nervous System and Learning Fatigue: It's not just physical activity that tires out the CNS but also cognitive load. This is why high-intensity sessions should be limited in duration: so that the team doesn't experience learning fatigue and fail to benefit from the learning opportunity.

Complexity of Principles: When trying to avoid learning fatigue, we need to recognize that the intensity of the players' concentration is directly related to how simple or complex the principles are that they're trying to master. The greater the complexity, the more concentration is required.

Complexity of Dynamics: Another consideration is that the complexity of dynamics is bound to the rules and objectives of the exercise. The more rules there are, the more difficult it is for players to focus and get to the intended learning outcome. This is why simplicity is often the best way forward when creating drills.

Number of Players: How many players each team has in small-sided games is directly related to the variables of decision-making. The greater the number of players, the higher the complexity of the principles the coaching staff wants to see unfold.

Space Game: The speed of each player's decision-making correlates with the size of the space available. This also impacts physiology, as smaller spaces require players to change direction more sharply and frequently, leading to more eccentric muscle contractions.

Playing Time: This concept is related to exercise type, the number of players, and the main principles being explored. To create intense learning experiences, decrease the time of each rep and overall duration of the session to stabilize performance and ensure optimal quality of the player experience.

THE IMPORTANCE OF VOLUME   14.6.6

Volume is generated through systematic repetition. Repeating exercises over and over again so that the players implement desired behaviors unconsciously. In short, volume intensifies learning. But volume also is the most dangerous variable in that it can cause overtraining and increase injury risk. Too much volume, whether in the form of time, space, or distance, leads to increased loading, TUT, and repeated movements. Therefore we try to monitor the volume, but we never attempt to reduce the intensity. We indirectly manage intensity by manipulating the volume.

LARGER PITCH/FIELD/COURT DRILLS AND GAMES   14.6.6.1

Generally, as the size of the playing area increases, so does the rate of perceived exertion (RPE) and intensity. Drills on the full playing field should be used primarily for development of aerobic fitness early in the training program. There is less lateral movement and less eccentric stress in games on longer pitches, so these can be introduced earlier in the week, switching to smaller-sided games as the game nears. Depth perception is needed more in larger pitches, particularly when the play is lengthwise.

If we run away at full speed, we will do a great intensity. However, if we make the same distance with a tray of filled glasses—and if we made that journey with the utmost speed possible without the cups falling—then this second action, despite being slower, is more intense because it requires more concentration.

—Vítor Frade

14 The Methodology

SMALL PITCH/FIELD/COURT DRILLS AND GAMES   14.6.6.2

For adaptation purposes and to minimize injury risk, the size of the playing field should not change by more than 20 percent. Smaller pitches (combined with appropriate work-to-rest ratios) are best suited for developing anaerobic qualities and intensive endurance. With large squads, this means multiple games. Smaller pitches require far greater decision-making and are more mentally demanding, with greater ball-handling skills and more peripheral vision required. A smaller playing area will invariably increase the number of touches for and passes made by each player. In soccer, a smaller ball can be used to improve control and touch.[104]

IMPROVING DECISION-MAKING   14.6.6.3

One of the simplest ways to enhance decision-making in players is to switch from one playing direction to another (from lengthwise to across the width of the field or vice versa). The pitch area remains the same, but the focus shifts from depth perception challenges to peripheral vision challenges.

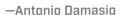

We are not thinking machines that feel; rather, we are feeling machines that think.

—Antonio Damasio

There has been plenty of discussion by people in a variety of roles on decision-making, but with great teams, the most intense training scenarios have produced the great decision-makers in competition, whether in elite military units or in sports. As Greg Roman, former offensive coordinator with the San Francisco 49ers, points out, such decisions often have to take place in the context of very complex tactical concepts:

People's brains are different. In the preseason, [the opposing] defense might play three things. Well, you can process three things. In the regular season, though, now they might do six things while disguising all of them before the ball is snapped. Can you process them *this fast*?

Try this: "Hey, it's second-and-5, we're in Tiger, they just played Cover 3, so let's go *Flank Right 2-Jet Z-Sail F-Drive.*" Tiger is a personnel group. Flank Right is the formation. 2-Jet is the protection. Z-Sail and F-Drive are two route combinations. And that is the simplest play, and formation, I could call: A two-receiver route and [another] two-receiver route, and the first one I said, you wanna start your eyes there. Or the play could end in the word "alert," which means if we get a certain look, be alert to audible for a specific play that we memorized during the week. Now, are they in nickel? Are they treating this as three wides or are they staying in base? Oh, they're matching, say, Richard Sherman on [Charles] Clay...you need to be aware of that. So you've got a pre-snap read, then a drop read and a set read. On your drop, you're reading something—you have a primary receiver, or a primary route combination—then once your back foot hits and you don't throw the No. 1 read, then you're into your set read, and now you're getting through a progression: *Ding ding ding ding ding.* Meanwhile somebody's trying to hold you up and clothesline you. And you have to do all this in maybe two seconds.[105]

The ability to master such complicated tactical matters doesn't come automatically, and such a level of complexity can only be understood and acted upon with consistently great work in team practices over time. As there is always a limit on practice time before the law of diminishing returns sets in and players get physically and cognitively overloaded, the head coach and staff have to carefully choose the tactical elements they think are most important for the team to grasp.

TEAM SELECTION   14.6.6.4

Usually teams are best split up evenly by fitness and position. However, teams can be divided between fit and unfit players during the competitive season, with the unfit ones on the side with fewer players, so they need to work harder and have the opportunity to improve their fitness.

FLOATING PLAYER   14.6.6.5

Floating players switch sides depending on possession and/or direction of play. They will sprint more and cover more distance if used properly in a game. The floating player can be used in most small-sided games, though in those of more than four-on-four they might be lost in the action or can hide. The floating player is often one who needs more fitness work, particularly anaerobic effort.

USE OF CONCURRENT OR
INTERMITTENT TIMING   14.6.6.6

During games in which there are intermittent work-to-rest periods, there is an increase in the distances spent at higher speeds. In games of a continuous nature, rate of perceived exertion and average maximum heart rate percentage goes up.

WORK-TO-REST RATIOS   14.6.6.7

Blocking the games in to one- to four-minute periods with ninety seconds to two minutes of rest or active recovery blocks in between will help elevate the quality level of the session. It will also allow players to train at a higher skill level and enable decision-makers to execute plays with a higher success rate, leading to an increased standard of play. The coaches should either decrease the work blocks and/or increase the rest periods.

INCREASING INTENSITY   14.6.6.8

To up the work rate in games, the duration must be kept short, to between one and three minutes, depending on the time of the season. To increase the aerobic load, the rest can be decreased gradually. Once the number of players increases beyond seven or eight for soccer and American football, ten or eleven for rugby and Australian rules football, and three or four for basketball, intensity usually slips below matchlike levels.

GENERAL GUIDELINES
FOR SMALL-SIDED GAMES   14.6.6.9

In a moment I'm going to dive into how to design small-sided games (SSGs) for several different team sports. But first, here are some universal guidelines:

1. Keep work blocks short in small-sided games. Intensity is kept very high.

2. Rest periods are more frequent. Fatigue can set in faster than in full-sided games.

3. Keep the players moving quickly. End the session if plodding sets in. Submaximal effort will only reinforce bad habits and means that player work rates are dropping off.

4. Contact must be included in other training blocks in the week, as it is limited in SSGs. Collision is the greatest fatiguing element for the players.

5. Ensure that player effort is maintained and use verbal encouragement to prevent players from hiding. Some athletes tend to sit back and avoid working hard in the organized chaos of SSGs.

6. Ensure that explosive, power-based movements are continued through the whole SSG block. Because SSGs are intense, players never recover fully, so more rest periods must be used to maintain quality of work and explosiveness.

7. Reduce risk of injury by conducting games on smaller pitches before moving to bigger pitches, especially if players have performed weight training during the same morning.

8. Ensure that there is no repetitive submaximal work, which can be especially detrimental to explosive athletes. Control rest periods to minimize it.

9. Rest periods get shorter as a block progresses. Rest is longer at the beginning and is gradually reduced over a number of weeks and/or sessions.

10. The most important thing in all SSGs is to maintain the intensity of action (meaning the totality of the four coactives, not simply physical elements). When intensity is maintained, development is continued and performance excellence is refined.

11. You cannot use SSGs to develop "skill under fatigue." We address this by either (a) limiting fatigue or (b) improving overall skill levels. This means that fatigue develops later and the skill is performed for longer, or more frequently for a longer period, at the high level of intensity.

EXTENSIVE VS. INTENSIVE SMALL-SIDED GAMES   14.6.7

Any small-sided game will use all energy systems—alactic, anaerobic, and aerobic—but we can better classify them as either extensive (aerobic) or intensive (anaerobic lactic or anaerobic alactic).

Extensive Small-Sided Games

- Performed at between 60 and 80 percent of maximum heart rate or between 65 and 85 percent of maximal effort.

- Often used to enhance the ability to recover among players and occasionally to improve endurance.

- Should ideally be undertaken once sufficient aerobic and anaerobic qualities are in place.

- Should be performed early in the session to achieve best effort, with work periods of between five and ten minutes (eventually) and rest periods of between one and two minutes.

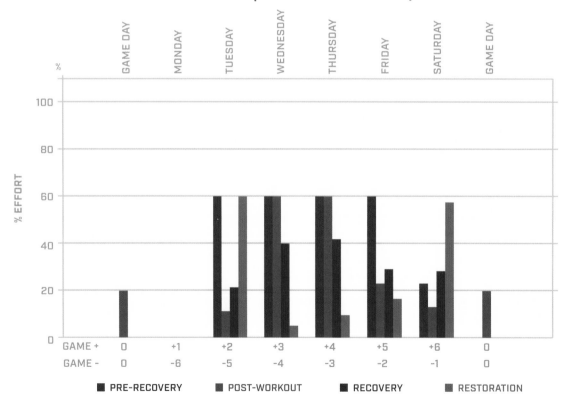

PLAYING SQUAD PROGRAMMING
In Season | Weeks 1–8 Recovery

Intensive Small-Sided Games

- Performed at 80 to 90 percent of maximum heart rate or greater than 85 to 95 percent of maximal effort.

- Must also sometimes be performed at 90 to 100 percent. The work blocks are shorter for these more intense sessions, with work periods of thirty seconds to two minutes and rest periods of one to two minutes. Or a one-to-one or one-to-two work-to-rest ratio can be used.

- Can be undertaken after stressing anaerobic capacity has been completed and are used primarily to improve game-related agility and anaerobic qualities.

Following are two charts showing how to structure intensive and two-stage extensive SSGs using the approach of coach Raymond Verheijen, one of the most influential figures in the world-renowned Dutch soccer academy structure. His principles for SSGs are also applicable to American football, rugby, Australian rules football, and other team sports.

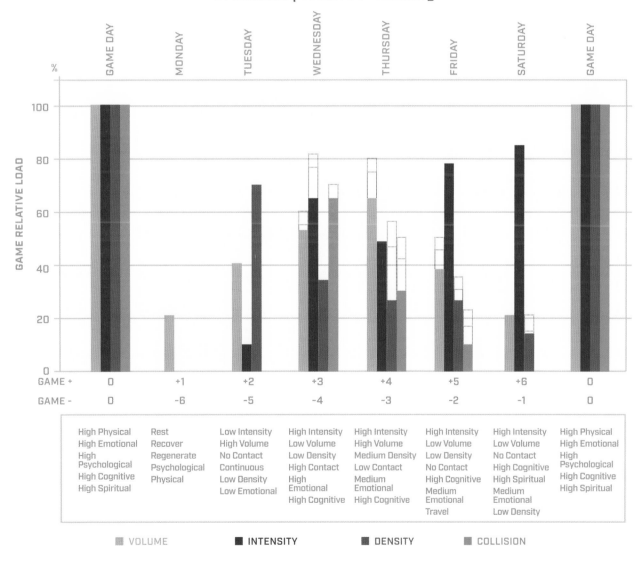

PLAYING SQUAD PROGRAMMING
In Season | Week 14+ Loading

	GAME DAY	MONDAY	TUESDAY	WEDNESDAY	THURSDAY	FRIDAY	SATURDAY	GAME DAY
GAME +	0	+1	+2	+3	+4	+5	+6	0
GAME −	0	−6	−5	−4	−3	−2	−1	0
	High Physical High Emotional High Psychological High Cognitive High Spiritual	Rest Recover Regenerate Psychological Physical	Low Intensity High Volume No Contact Continuous Low Density Low Emotional	High Intensity Low Volume Low Density High Contact High Emotional High Cognitive	High Intensity High Volume Medium Density Low Contact Medium Emotional High Cognitive	High Intensity Low Volume Low Density No Contact High Cognitive Medium Emotional Travel	High Intensity Low Volume No Contact High Cognitive High Spiritual Medium Emotional Low Density	High Physical High Emotional High Psychological High Cognitive High Spiritual

VOLUME   INTENSITY   DENSITY   COLLISION

14 The Methodology

OPTIMAL GAME SELECTION FOR APPROPRIATE PLAYER EXPERIENCE

GAME OPTION 1

GAME OPTION 2

GAME OPTION 3

GAME OPTION X...

WHAT DO WE GET FROM THE GAME?

IS IT A PHYSICAL TRAINING SESSION?

IS THIS A SKILL-FOCUSED SESSION?

WHAT ARE OUR PRIORITIES?

WHAT IS THE PHYSICAL OUTCOME?

1. AEROBIC-ENDURANCE-VOLUME

2. ANAEROBIC-INTENSITY-WORK RATE

3. ALACTIC-POWER-STRENGTH-SPEED

4. IS THERE CONTACT? COLLISION?

WHAT TECHNICAL ELEMENT ARE WE ADDRESSING?

KICKING? CATCHING? ONE-HANDED PASSING?

OVER-HEAD CONTROL? HANDLING AT SPEED?

IS THERE A TACTICAL ELEMENT WE WANT TO ADDRESS?

IS IT A PHYSICAL TRAINING SESSION?

IS THIS A SKILL-FOCUSED SESSION?

WHAT ARE OUR PRIORITIES?

WHAT TYPE OF EQUIPMENT DO WE NEED?

IS IT A PHYSICAL TRAINING SESSION?

IS THIS A SKILL-FOCUSED SESSION?

WHAT ARE OUR PRIORITIES?

SELECT GAME

SELECT GAME

GAME TYPE

- GAME TYPE A
- GAME TYPE B
- GAME TYPE C
- GAME TYPE D

SCORE

- 3 CONES
- SCORING GATES
- SCORING SPACE
- TIME
- SHOT CLOCK

PHYSICAL

- ENERGY SYSTEM
- PHYSICAL
- ALACTIC
- DOWN UPS
- ANAEROBIC
- CONTACT
- AEROBIC

STRUCTURE

- STATIONS
- STATIONS
- STATIONS
- CONTINUOUS
- WORK/REST
- CEREBRAL
- TWO HALVES
- ROTATING TEAMS
- TECHNICAL SKILL
- FULL REST
- CONTACT
- ACTIVE
- TACTICAL

SPATIAL

- NORTH, SOUTH, EAST, WEST
- DEAD ZONES
- PITCH SIZE

TECHNICAL

- KICKING/CATCHING
- FORWARD/BACKWARD
- ONE-HANDED

DURATION

- KICKING/CATCHING
- FORWARD/BACKWARD

SPORT-SPECIFIC PREPARATION

14.7

The preparation of a team at any level of any team sport can be optimized by employing the morphological programming approach and recognizing that all four elements are present in every session, just as they are during a game. This being said, the game-day demands of American football, basketball, rugby, soccer, Australian rules football, and all other team sports vary considerably, so their preparation must be tailored accordingly.

MACRO INCREMENTATION

14.8

The most successful teams are those who can continuously produce winning results. They consistently develop and improve, learning from challenges and growing. This development needs to be done slowly and purposely. There needs to be a reinforcement of key principles and gradual rate of improvement.

THE ANNUAL PLAN
14.8.1

Using this holistic approach, there is still an annual plan with a preseason and postseason, but to all intents and purposes there is no variation in the weekly schedule. The single greatest difference is the speed of execution through the year.

Yes, volume increases through the preseason to develop capacity, while spaces and decision-making time decrease. But the weekly pattern remains the same, habits are developed, and stress (and therefore learning) is applied to the areas that matter. As the season progresses, there is a slight reduction in volume, but intensity is maintained.

The same principles apply to postseason. There is no change in the weekly plan, but there is an increase in intensity and reduction in volume.

Recovery allows the intensity to be maintained into the final games, which lets us manage any possible fitness-versus-freshness issues that may arise.

THE LAW OF REINFORCEMENT
14.8.2

A victory cannot be considered as an isolated event; rather, it must be considered in the context of the results that precede and follow it. Similarly, one team practice session is not an individual entity but exists in the morphocycle and with the overall goals of the game plan in mind. Objectives and the principles needed to achieve them must be firmly established and then reinforced over and over again. As Bill Belichick has said, "There are no shortcuts to building a team each season. You build the foundation brick by brick."[106]

INCREMENTAL, GRADUAL PERFORMANCE IMPROVEMENTS REPLACE PEAKING
14.8.2.1

The aim of implementing a morphological programming morphocycle is not to peak for late-season games, when the stakes are at their highest. Yes, the team should be performing at its best at this point, but not because of periodization's false promise of peaking. Rather, when the four elements of team preparation—technical, tactical, physical, and psychological—are included in each training session and emphasized on different days to allow some systems to be stimulated while others are de-emphasized to encourage recovery, there should be consistent gradual improvement.

To ensure that players recuperate from training enough that all of their faculties are ready for game day, the coaching staff should only ever look to improve physical performance by 1 or 2 percent in each morphocycle. Otherwise, the degree of change can be too great, risking injury and increasing the chance that the players will not recover adequately before the next contest. And in fact, if there is a 1 percent increase in successive weeks, there can be a greater residual effect that sees performance increase by 3 or 4 percent. With such a philosophy in mind, every game should see a slight uptick in performance on an individual and, more importantly, a team basis. Today's sports seasons are virtually continuous, so team training must mirror this with preparation that is sustainable over the long haul.

Here's José Mourinho's take: "Weekly training sessions are solely focused on the next game. There's no plan to come good in December or May, no looking ahead. No plan to play better against the top teams."[107]

The holistic, game-centric, long-term mindset of the morphological programming approach is a stark contrast to the fragmented, training-focused, short-sighted methodology that has prevailed up until now. With previous preparation methods, every expert was responsible for an individual part of a player's preparation, and the intensity, volume, density, and collision of each training session was the prerogative of those individual coaches or consultants.

The fundamental mistake was targeting advancements and personal records during training itself rather than working toward improvements on the playing field. As such, there used to be little to no communication between each area, meaning that a player could be subjected, for example, to a high-intensity and high-collision session in the weight room, a high-volume session during practice, and a high-density workout with the speed coach.

The cumulative effect of checking the "high" box for each of the morphological programming components is not constructive but rather destructive, and over time it leads to physical, emotional, and mental burnout, injuries, and, quite probably, shorter playing careers. Such a fragmented, incoherent way of preparing the team also limits the effectiveness of strength and skill coaches, physiotherapists, psychologists, unit coaches, and the rest, as the potentially positive impact of their expertise is blunted or even negated entirely.

Not so in the morphological programming approach, in which the walls between various specialties are torn down and the head coach communicates to each and every department how much load will be placed on the team on any given day, with respect to the four coactives and the components of

the morphological programming approach. It is only by getting each person on the same page that the morphocycle will be effective and will yield continually beneficial outcomes for the duration of the season. This way of doing things is not just about how players' bodies are prepared for competition but also encompasses the way in which the staff and coaches talk to and interact with their players, as this too impacts the cognitive aspect of the morphological programming approach.

So on a day that is high volume but low intensity, coaches should avoid reprimanding, confronting, or overcriticizing the team, as the psychological element of preparation requires the same minimal intensity as the physical, tactical, and technical areas. Similarly, an owner should not be trying to resolve a contract dispute on a low-intensity day. Otherwise, the guiding principle for that day will be compromised and undermined.

To achieve such harmony, it's vital that a clear, cohesive message is composed by the head coach and sent to the entire staff, the training team, and back-office personnel. One of the keys to the six championships of the Chicago Bulls in the 1990s was the constant and open communication between head coach Phil Jackson and his talented coaching staff. In his book *Eleven Rings,* Jackson recalls, "Every morning the coaching staff and I would meet for breakfast and discuss the fine points of the practice plan, as well as the latest scouting reports. That allowed us to share information with one another and make sure we were all on the same page in terms of day-to-day strategy. Each coach had a high level of autonomy, but when we talked to the players, we spoke as one."[108]

The entire organization must be aware in advance of how the morphological programming elements will be balanced on each day of the coming morphocycle, whether it's one, two, or four weeks long. Then they must buy into the idea and agree to follow the plan to the letter.

This is not to say that there's no room for specialists to get creative in preparing the team, but such creativity must exist within the framework of the morphocycle. The way each day is set up is a conscious attempt not only to enhance players' performance but also to protect them from the excesses that have bedeviled the linear block periodization approach for so long.

OPENING
FEEDBACK CHANNELS   14.8.3

To help ensure that everyone in the organization is clear on their role in the team preparation morphocycle and what is expected of them, there should be feedback mechanisms in place and an open-door policy among the coaches and staff. This will not only reduce anxiety and combat ambiguity but also allow any confusion to be identified, communicated, and resolved before preparation begins for the next day.

It's also important that coaches have the opportunity to share their thoughts on how each day's preparation went, how well the team responded to each practice session, and what needs to be done differently. One of the reasons that agile software development has been so successful and prevalent in Silicon Valley since the 1990s is that every team member is encouraged to contribute to a continual feedback loop. It's the same in the morphocycle. If every person who interacts with players is monitoring what's going well, what's not working, and what can be improved and communicates these thoughts each day, the team will be better prepared come game day.

Such information sharing shouldn't wait for the end of the day; it should happen in real time. So if the strength coach notices that a player or the team as a whole seems lethargic during a session in the weight room, he or she can let the head coach know before the squad goes out onto the training ground. The coach can then dial back the volume or intensity so that the preparation leads to adaptation, not exhaustion.

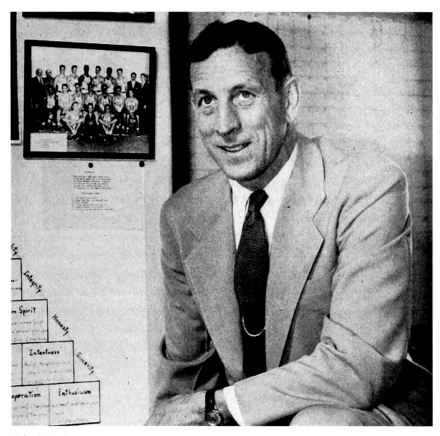

John Wooden.

Similarly, one of the hallmarks of the morphological programming approach to team preparation is that the athletes themselves have a voice. The coaching staff might believe that they've dialed in the balance between the four elements for a certain cycle, but this theory may prove false in reality. Players are the ultimate litmus test for each cycle, day, and session, and if they're allowed to share their feedback with coaches and staff members, they will not only train more effectively but also feel more involved and more committed to the organization. The overarching goal of the morphocycle method is to continually improve game-day performance, which is only possible if team preparation also evolves, adapts, and improves.

THE THREE-YEAR RULE   14.8.4

In a brilliant multipart story for the soccer magazine *The Blizzard,* Jonathan Wilson explained how José Mourinho's fortunes as manager at Chelsea took a rapid about-face, with the team going from winning the title in May 2015 to languishing in sixteenth place by December. This resulted in owner Roman Abramovich dismissing Mourinho, despite Mourinho's recent triumph. Wilson noted that Mourinho's fall realized the words of Hungarian manager Béla Guttmann, who said, "The third season is fatal."

So what went wrong for "the Chosen One" at Chelsea, and why can that third season lead to a coach's downfall no matter what success came in the first and second years? Wilson identifies several factors—including Mourinho's testy relationship with Abramovich, a questionable transfer policy, and insistence on playing the opposite style to Barcelona's tiki-taka, possession-focused strategy.[109]

These are all valid points. I'd like to add to them some commonalities I've seen among elite teams in football, soccer, rugby, basketball, Australian rules football, and other sports who experience the third-year collapse and those that maintain a standard of excellence for much longer. First is the continuity of the game plan philosophy—in other words, there's an attitude of, "This is how we play here." The San

Antonio Spurs are a great example. Any player who joins the Spurs knows that he'll be expected to buy into unselfish play predicated on ball movement. Bill Walsh started every season with the same speech on day one, outlining the team rules.

Second, the team's culture must be so solid that it's unshakeable by exterior forces, such as a bad run of form or a media scandal. Exactly what the team's values and beliefs are and how they are manifested in the way people act, speak, and carry themselves must be clear to every player, coach, and member of the back-office staff.

Third, there needs to be a consistent and cohesive message throughout the organization. No matter what the circumstances are, the way the head coach communicates the team's priorities and aims must remain constant from season to season.

Finally, any discord or difficulties need to remain in the locker room and not be leaked to the media. Sam Smith's book on Michael Jordan and the Bulls, *The Jordan Rules,* featured explosive revelations about how Jordan allegedly treated coaches and teammates. These details could only have come from people within the organization, who betrayed Jordan's trust by sharing things with Smith that they should have kept private. Players and coaches alike need to understand that what goes on within their group is not the business of the outside world, and that to maintain the values of trust and honor, they need to resolve issues within the team itself instead of airing their dirty laundry to the outside world. It can't be "us against the world" if the "us" (the team) turns on itself.

LEGISLATION WITH EDUCATION   14.8.5

The amount of time that college sports coaches can spend with their players is limited by several factors. One of these is the NCAA (or, for smaller schools, NAIA) rulebook, which stipulates when teams can start practicing with the ball, how many hours the team can spend training each day (currently four for football and other contact sports), and "countable athletically related activities" (a maximum of twenty hours per week). The days of Paul "Bear" Bryant running his players all day are long gone.[110]

Such governance and restriction mean that head coaches must be more diligent than ever about how they plan main practices and how much time they apportion to skills, unit, and strength and conditioning coaches. Every specialist wants time with the players, but the coach must be very careful to manage such expectations and prioritize education with the various experts on the staff. Balancing the morphological programming elements and four coactives should provide some guidance, as should the main game plan principles and objectives.

MANAGING IDIOCY   14.8.6

It's not just the college sports Powers That Be that limit and restrict certain elements of team dynamics and the player-coach relationship. Most major league sports have rules that govern the amount of contact coaches can have with players during the off-season, the timing of preseason practices, and other things that they'd be better off leaving alone.

As these rules can't be broken without penalties, how can a sports team better manage legislative idiocy? One way is to focus on playing the game as frequently as possible. One of the main reasons athletes get injured during the "off-season" is that when they're left to their own devices, the game fades into the rearview mirror and they develop bad practices. Outside of any bad lifestyle habits that are amplified in the off-season (see, for example, players' Instagram pics of pool parties in Vegas), the off-season also often means massive changes in training. It's typically not the load itself that gets players hurt but rather a large differential between what they do when they're with the team and what they do when they're

training by themselves or with some "guru" who doesn't understand the demands of the game or the team's preparation protocols.

If we really wanted to reduce injuries, we'd allow athletes to play the game more often, not less, with full recovery between contests. Every season the clamor for a reduced number of competitions and longer breaks seems to get louder, yet this is based on a fallacy that more competition is the root of injury. It isn't. The culprit is what goes on during breaks, when holistic, game-focused preparation goes out the window and weird and wacky self-focused physical training takes over. Before the competitive season ends, the coaching staff should educate players about what they need to be doing to maintain readiness through a daily practice in the off-season. Though not every athlete will stick to this, it might mitigate the damage that can begin the moment the final team practice is over.

> *Every action needs to be prompted by a motive. To know and to will are two operations of the human mind. Discerning, judging, deliberating are acts of the human mind.*

—Leonadro da Vinci

FIFTEEN

INDIVIDUAL EMPHASIS IN A TEAM SPORT

It's worth noting that some aspects of preparation need to be customized for the individual. Even though the morphocycle prescribes certain areas of emphasis for each day between games, every player's background, culture, genetics, and physical makeup are different. This means that if you have ten players in a training session, you will see twenty different physical and psychological responses. It's no good trying to get a median or "average" that holds true across the entire squad; this is a false premise.

For example, say you're working with three players. Player 1 gauges the intensity of the session at 70 percent, while players 2 and 3 rate the intensity at just 10 percent. That gives you an average appraisal of 30 percent intensity. But now let's say that three other players complete the same session. All three tell you that they think they were at 30 percent. So now you have the same average intensity but very different assessments among the player groups. This is why training must be somewhat individualized, even though the team may work on similar drills. Simply put, using measurement averages delivers average game-time performance.

CONCEPT OF OPTIMIZATION

15.1

The term *optimization of the player* is not intended to refer to maximizing only physical qualities. The game model and its respective principles should be subject to careful planning and dynamic preparation that emphasizes physical, technical, and psychological components but always keeps the tactical element in mind. Auxiliary training for the individual is added and manipulated based on each player's performance needs.

TAKING PLAYER PERSPECTIVE INTO ACCOUNT

15.1.1

The coaching staff must acknowledge that not every member of the squad can be treated the same way. It's a reality that players who will potentially deliver the most relative superiority on game day require a different approach than the benchwarmers who rarely play. I'm not advocating for "star treatment" per se, but it's not the right way ahead to prepare each individual for competitive play in exactly the same manner. That said, the organization must treat each and every player fairly, respectfully, and with the best possible care, and in return expect that all athletes give their best, respect team rules and policies, and adhere to core principles.

As we've already established that team preparation is not purely physical but also technical, tactical, and psychological, the coaching staff must consider the nonphysical demands of the morphocycles they design. Certain sessions require more emotional involvement, focus, and cognition than others and can leave players feeling drained even though they have not been physically overloaded. Unlike in periodization, we cannot prioritize physiology above everything else; we must take every player's emotional and mental state into account in shaping and adjusting practices between games. Essentially, the body and brain are one.

The bottom line? If athletes are being honest and say that they feel overworked, then they're being overworked, and performance in upcoming games will suffer—even if objective markers don't match perceived exertion. In such a scenario, the coaching staff should trust the squad over their monitoring measures and then sit down together as soon as possible to adjust the morphological programming loads for the next day and subsequent sessions in the current morphocycle. Giving players an active role in team preparation will also strengthen the bonds within the organization and make it clear that the players are valued as both people and athletes.

INJURY AND RECOVERY
15.1.2

Athlete feedback helps inform another beneficial application of the morphological programming approach: injury prevention and recovery. If an athlete feels like she's going to injure herself, there's a reason, and she's most likely correct. When a player voices this in a particular type of session, the coaching staff knows that they either need to hold the player out of this kind of training for the next few days or should at least limit the player's exposure to this morphological programming element.

REHAB STATUS

PHASE	EXPLANATION	DETAIL
PROTECTION	Protect from further injury	Player must protect himself from further injury and allow diagnosis
DIAGNOSIS	Complete diagnosis	Informed clarification of severity and options available
PASSIVE	Passive intervention	Establishing rom and pain-free movement
RETURN TO ACTIVITY	Player active engagement	Active establishment of rom and preparation for training
RETURN TO TRAIN	Loading introduced	Low-level isometric loading of injured tissue, while active training of the athlete. Move to eccentric, concentric, low-level oscillation, ballistic, etc.
		Loaded energy transport-absorption, slow and low-level
		Low-level concentric force generation
		Progress in the same order through medium and high loads
RETURN TO PRACTICE	Player returns to limited practice	Volume is managed/limited by increasing density
		Intensity never drops
		Slowing, reducing density increases endurance
RETURN TO COMPETE	Player competes unrestricted (volume excepted) in training	Full-contact training
RETURN TO PLAY	Player returns to unrestricted game (limited volume/density)	Player can partake in games at reduced volume
RETURN TO PERFORMANCE	Player returns to full game	Volume, intensity, contact & density are back to pre-injury levels

The morphocycle can also inform recovery. As the specific loads on each player are predetermined and every member of the organization who interacts with the team has the entire upcoming morphological programming plan, the medical staff can strategize in advance to help athletes recover better from specific stimuli. The morphological programming approach framework also provides a guide for a team dealing with player injuries.

If a coach knows that a squad member was hurt during full-contact drills, then this is a collision-related injury and the individual should avoid similar exercises until cleared by the team physio or physician. The medical staff can also treat the injury according to which type of training session it occurred in, leading to enhanced and expedited return to playing condition.

The biggest mistake made in rehabilitation, particularly in the U.S., is separating the injured player from coaches, strength training, and other forms of training—whether on purpose or unintentionally. This leaves the player not only at greater risk of reinjury but also needing a longer time frame to return to play.

The graphic below is an integrated model used for rehabilitation to speed the player back to a sustained level of performance using a holistic approach. The speed of return is critical: returning a player faster actually helps the player sustain performance and therefore improves the probability of a successful return to play. By contrast, a longer segmented approach, which is more common, decreases the chance of a successful return. The integrated model also provides an opportunity to improve the athlete's "weaknesses" in a structured way, rather than haphazardly, and therefore return the player with a new ability or more-rounded game or lifestyle, thereby exploiting the enforced reduction in playing time. Once again, note that the return to play is not physically driven but based on a complete holistic approach to the performance on the field, working backward.

HOLISTIC REHAB PROGRESSION

PHASE	PSYCHOLOGICAL	PHYSICAL	TECHNICAL	TACTICAL
PROTECTION	Support with the injury and management of context	Dietary support to reduce inflammation and support recovery process		
DIAGNOSIS	Help with the acceptance of injury and the delay process	Dietary advice and support to maintain lbm and prevent fat storage		
PASSIVE	Goal-setting education of the injury and severity, management of expectations and aims	Passive support of physical gains		
RETURN TO ACTIVITY	Education on the process, help with motivation and assist in designing an educational program (reading, learning, etc.)	Active engagement to maintain athletic qualities	Player can begin to reintroduce some technical skills	General tactical education
RETURN TO TRAIN	Helping with coach/student education Understanding of stress and stress-management skills	Improving weaknesses and beginning of rehabilitation		
RETURN TO PRACTICE	Limited support at educational practice	Beginning with isometric and eccentric work, focusing on maintaining qualities already developed and keeping player close to performance	Limited involement in practice	Specific tactical education
RETURN TO PRACTICE	Assistance with communication skills to actively and effectively communicate with coaches	As player returns to practice, manage volume and additional periods of training to compensate for fatigue		
RETURN TO COMPETE	Assistance with performance under pressure and goal management	Add volume missed in games in additional training drills	Assessment of technique (compensation & fatigue)	
RETURN TO PLAY	Management of expectations			
RETURN TO PERFORMANCE				

	SYMPATHETIC-DOMINANT ATHLETES	PARASYMPATHETIC-DOMINANT ATHLETES
OVERREACHING SYMPTOMS	Increased resting heart rate	Decreased resting heart rate
	Increased resting blood pressure	Faster return of heart rate to resting value after exercise
	Decreased maximal power output	Decreased sports performance
	Decreased sports performance	Decreased blood lactate concentrations during submax exercise
	Decreased maximal blood lactate concentrations	Decreased blood lactate concentrations during maximal exercise
	Slower recovery after exercise	Unemotional behavior
	Weight loss	May describe depressive symptoms
	Decreased appetite	Low heart-rate recovery from interval training
	Decreased desire to exercise	Increased sodium loss
	Increased irritability and depression	Increased weight loss (through dehydration) after training
	Increased incidence of injury	
	Increased incidence of infection	
	Tendency to adrenal dysfunction	

TAILORING THERAPY AND RECOVERY FOR PARASYMPATHETIC-DOMINANT AND SYMPATHETIC-DOMINANT ATHLETES   15.1.2.1

Just as every athlete has a different four-coactive profile (more on this in "The Player"), so too are players typically either parasympathetic-dominant or sympathetic-dominant. The characteristics of each type are described in "The Player" in section 7.12.1—broadly, parasympathetic-dominant players are more relaxed and may have more difficulty ramping up energy, while sympathetic-dominant players are more intense and driven and may have difficulty winding down after activity.

THE STRENGTH AND CONDITIONING MYTH   15.1.3

There is a pervasive myth in elite sports that every error that occurs during a game is caused by a physical weakness or deficiency. In response, the strength and conditioning coach is charged with making the player faster, stronger, or more explosive. The trouble is that a problem is just as often a technical, tactical, or psychological issue that has little or nothing to do with the athlete's physical qualities.

This is not to detract from strength and conditioning, but we simply cannot bring everything back to physicality if we're to truly improve game-day performance. Another problem with always putting the blame for poor execution on the athlete's body is that it ignores the profound impact that technical, tactical, and psychological coactives have on each game.

Going back to the physical dimension every time is a dangerously reductionist approach that seeks to pull out one thing, like maximum strength, develop it by itself, and then expect the athlete to go back onto the field like an enhanced Six-Million-Dollar Man who can use his cyborg powers to overwhelm opponents. In fact, as we're seeing over and over in every facet of team sports, everything is interconnected.

A CAUTIONARY TALE OF YOUTH VERSUS EXPERIENCE

15.2

I've already made some general observations about the age and experience level of the team and how this should influence playing style in the four game moments—such as a younger, less experienced squad using a high-tempo offense. However, there are no hard-and-fast rules regarding such things, and just having a team full of battle-hardened veterans is no guarantee of success, just as a young team will not necessarily perform poorly.

In some cases, the old heads in the locker room can prove to be part of a cultural problem and contribute to negative habits and mindsets that are detrimental to performance and hinder rather than help younger players. Such was the case when Bill Belichick took over the Cleveland Browns and, to some degree, during his early years in charge of the New England Patriots.

In both scenarios, Belichick discovered that some of the more-experienced players felt entitled to their starting jobs, refused to buy into the game plan, and weren't committed to working hard in practice. Belichick could not count on these players to help him change the culture and identity of the team in New England, so he began reshaping the roster through trades and the draft.[111]

In contrast, one young player on the Patriots roster stayed late into the night practicing with the receivers, hitting the weights, and studying game film.[112] As a sixth-round draft pick, Tom Brady was far from a proven entity in the NFL, but when Drew Bledsoe went down with an injury, Brady stepped up and justified his coach's faith in him. Once Bledsoe recov-

ered, the fans and media clamored for him to be reinstated as QB, but Belichick held firm and retained Brady in the starting lineup. We all know how history has vindicated this gutsy decision.

Another team where youth has trumped experience is Manchester United. Rather than going out and buying a team full of established stars like the "super teams" of today, manager Matt Busby relied on the young players developed in the team's academy to propel United to success in the 1940s, 1950s, and 1960s. Two generations later, we saw Sir Alex Ferguson follow a similar path with Ryan Giggs, David Beckham, Nicky Butt, the Neville brothers, Paul Scholes, and the rest of the now-celebrated "Class of '92." Contrary to Alan Hansen's dour prediction that "you can't win anything with kids," this youthful core led United to the Treble in 1999 and to umpteen Premier League titles, FA Cup wins, and League Cup triumphs as well.[113]

The lesson is that you have to evaluate the character of the squad and take the players on their individual merits, not just their age and experience level. Coaches must think long and hard how the available players fit with the game plan, objectives, and style rather than go on reputation or history with the club alone. They should use the four-coactive analysis model outlined in "The Player" to evaluate each athlete comprehensively and then bring in new personnel as needed to complement those players who stay.

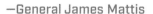

> *If I were to sum up what I've learned in 35 years of service, it's improvise, improvise, improvise.*
>
> —General James Mattis

1 Paul Kimmage, "The Big Interview: Richie McCaw," *The Sunday Times,* November 5, 2006, www.thetimes.co.uk/article/the-big-interview-richie-mccaw-ngnbxgqt9jg.

2 Leigh Sales and Julia Holman, "Richie McCaw: 'Failure Lifted My Game' Says Former All Blacks Captain," ABC News Online, October 18, 2016, www.abc.net.au/news/2016-10-18/failure-lifted-my-game-says-former-all-black-richie-mccaw/7943102.

10 CREATURES OF HABIT

3 Jeremy Dean, *Making Habits, Breaking Habits: Why We Do Things, Why We Don't, and How to Make Any Change Stick* (Boston: Da Capo Press, 2013), 14.

4 Russell G. Foster and Leon Kreitzman, "The Rhythms of Life: What Your Body Clock Means to You!," *Experimental Physiology* 99, no. 4 (April 1, 2014): 599–606.

5 Jonathan Wilson, *Inverting the Pyramid: The History of Soccer Tactics* (New York: Nation Books, 2013), 220–223.

6 Ibid.

7 David Winner, *Brilliant Orange: The Neurotic Genius of Dutch Football* (New York: Overlook Press, 2011).

8 Wilson, *Inverting the Pyramid*, 99.

9 Franz Halberg, "Quo Vadis Basic and Clinical Chronobiology: Promise for Health Maintenance," *Developmental Dynamics* 168, no. 4 (December 1983): 543–594.

10 Susan Perry and Jim Dawson, *The Secrets Our Body Clocks Reveal* (New York: Ballantine Books, 1990), 20.

11 Jeremy Campbell, *Winston Churchill's Afternoon Nap: A Wide-Awake Inquiry into the Human Nature of Time* (New York: Simon and Schuster, 1986), 75.

12 Ibid., 79.

13 Natalie Angier, "No Time for Bullies: Baboons Retool Their Culture," *New York Times*, April 13, 2004, www.nytimes.com/2004/04/13/science/no-time-for-bullies-baboons-retool-their-culture.html.

14 Mark Shwartz, "Robert Sapolsky Discusses Physiological Effects of Stress," *Stanford Report,* March 7, 2007, news.stanford.edu/news/2007/march7/sapolskysr-030707.html.

15 Ibid.

16 João Medeiros, "The Truth Behind Testosterone: Why Men Risk It All," *Wired*, January 27, 2013, www.wired.co.uk/article/why-men-risk-it-all.

17 Ibid.

18 Christian Jarrett, "Faster, Higher, Stronger!," *The Psychologist* 25 (July 2012): 504–507.

19 Ian H. Robertson, *The Winner Effect: How Power Affects Your Brain* (London: Bloomsbury, 2012), 81.

11 CREATURES OF STIMULI

20 Patrick Haggard and Benjamin W. Libet, "Conscious Intention and Brain Activity," *Journal of Consciousness Studies* 8, no. 11 (2001): 47–63.

21 Jonathan Wilson, "The Devil's Party (Part 1)," *The Blizzard,* n.d., www.theblizzard.co.uk/articles/the-devils-party/.

22 Ronald Gallimore, "What John Wooden Can Teach Us," *Education Week,* February 28, 2006, www.edweek.org/ew/articles/2006/03/01/25gallimore.h25.html.

23 David Maraniss, *When Pride Still Mattered: A Life of Vince Lombardi* (New York: Touchstone, 1999), 69.

12 THE EVOLUTION OF PREPARATION

24 Quoted in Michael E. Hyland, *Stress: All That Matters* (London: John Murray Learning, 2014), 51; Robert Sapolsky, *Why Zebras Don't Get Ulcers* (New York: Henry Holt and Company, 2004), 151–152.

25 Peter Levine, *Waking the Tiger: Healing Trauma* (Berkeley, CA: North Atlantic Books, 1997).

26 Vladimir M. Zatsiorsky and J. William Kraemer, *Science and Practice of Strength Training*, 2nd ed. (Champaign, IL: Human Kinetics, 2006), 14.

27 Dan Wathen, Thomas R. Baechle, and Roger W. Earle, "Periodization," in *Essentials of Strength Training and Conditioning*, 3rd ed., ed. Thomas R. Baechle and Roger W. Earle (Champaign, IL: Human Kinetics, 2008), 508–511.

28 Anthony Turner, "The Science and Practice of Periodization: A Brief Review," *Strength and Conditioning Journal* 33, no. 1 (February 2011): 34–46.

29 Ibid.

30 Nicholas David Bourne, "Fast Science: A History of Training Theory and Methods for Elite Runners Through 1975," PhD diss., University of Texas, Austin, 2008.

31 Tudor Bompa and Carlo Buzzichelli, *Periodization Training for Sports*, 3rd ed. (Champaign, iL: Human Kinetics, 2015), 88.

32 John M. Cissik, Allen Hedrick, and Michael Barnes, "Challenges Applying the Research on Periodization," *Strength and Conditioning Journal* 30, no. 1 (February 2008): 45–51.

33 Tudor O. Bompa, "Primer on Periodization," *Olympic Coach* 16, no. 2 (Summer 2004): 4–7.

34 Cissik, Hedrick, and Barnes, "Challenges Applying the Research on Periodization."

35 Yuri Verkhoshansky, "The End of 'Periodization' in the Training of High Performance Sport," *Leistungssport* 28, no. 5 (September 1998), translation at www.salisbury.edu/sportsperformance/Articles/THE%20END%20OF%20PERIODIZATION%20-%20VERHOSHANSKY.pdf.

36   Vladimir B. Issurin, "New Horizons for the Methodology and Physiology of Training Periodization," *Sports Medicine* 40, no. 3 (2010): 189–206.

37   Quoted in Valeriy Fomenkov, "Mourinho's 10 Commandments," (blog post), n.d., valeriyfomenkov.blogspot.com/2012/03/mourinhos-10-commandments.html.

38   Bill Walsh with Steve Jamison and Craig Walsh, *The Score Takes Care of Itself: My Philosophy of Leadership* (New York: Penguin, 2010), 206.

39   Jay R. Hoffman, "The Applied Physiology of American Football," *International Journal of Sports Physiology and Performance* 3, no. 3 (Septembr 2008): 387–392.

40   Maraniss, *When Pride Still Mattered,* 364.

41   Quoted in José Guilherme Oliveira, "Tactical Periodization: Theory and Fundamentals," slideshow presentation, n.d., www.slideshare.net/nickc/tactical-periodization-jose-guilherme-oliveira.

42   Angela Coon, "More Is Not Better" (blog post), Coach Ange's Blog, CharlieFrancis.com, February 5, 2015, www.charliefrancis.com/blogs/news/17047232-more-is-not-better.

43   Derek M. Hansen, "Eight Athlete Development Lessons I Learned from Charlie Francis," Strength Power Speed Training, January 3, 2014, www.strengthpowerspeed.com/eight-athlete-development-lessons-i-learned-from-charlie-francis/.

44   Charlie Francis, *The Charlie Francis Training System* (n.p., 2012), 1.

45   Carlos Carvalhal, Bruno Lage, and João Mário Oliveira, *Soccer: Developing a Know-How* (PrimeBooks, 2014); Israel Teoldo da Costa et al., "Tactical Principles of Football Game: Concepts and Application," *Motriz* 15, no. 3 (July/Sept. 2009): 657–668, www.nucleofutebol.ufv.br/artigos/israel principios taticos.pdf.

46   J. Garganta, "Modelação Táctica do Jogo de Futebol: Estudo da Organização da Fase Ofensiva em Equipas de Alto Rendimento," Universidade do Porto, 1997; J. Garganta, "Dissertação de Doutoramento Apresentada à Faculdade de Desporto," Universidade do Porto, 1997.

47   Oliveira, "Tactical Periodization."

48   David Gendelman, "Coaching, Portuguese Style," *Paris Review,* May 29, 2014, www.theparisreview.org/blog/2014/05/29/coaching-portuguese-style/.

49   "Football Conditioning: Interview with Dr. Mallo—Real Madrid," *PROathlete,* January 6, 2015, www.proathlete.de/2015/01/interview-dr-mallo/.

50   Marc Dos Santos, "Introduction," *F.C. Porto Academy Journal* (Leawood, KS: World Class Coaching, 2007), bilfootball.no/wp-content/uploads/2015/01/FCPortoAcademy.pdf.

51   Paul Ames, "Portugal's Army of 'Special Ones,'" *Politico,* August 7, 2015, www.politico.eu/article/portugals-army-soccer-football-coaches-sport-jose-mourinho/.

52   J. Brito, "Documento de Apoio à Disciplina de Opção II, Futebol, UTAD, Vila Real," class notes, unpublished, 2003, University of Porto.

13 FACILITATING EXPERIENCES

53   Filipe Manuel Clemente and Rúben Filipe Rocha, "Teaching and Soccer Training: An Approach Through a Tactical Perspective," *Journal of Physical Education and Sport* 13, no. 1 (2013): 14–18.

54   Clive Woodward, *Winning!* (London: Hodder & Stoughton, 2005), 135.

55   Ibid., 145.

56   David Halberstam, *The Education of a Coach* (New York: Hachette Books, 2005), 211–213.

57   John Wooden and Steve Jamison, *Wooden on Leadership* (New York: McGraw-Hill, 2005), 10.

58   Jocko Willink and Leif Babin, *Extreme Ownership: How U.S. Navy SEALs Lead and Win* (New York: St. Martin's Press, 2015), 273.

59   Richard Rapaport, "To Build a Winning Team: An Interview with Head Coach Bill Walsh," *Harvard Business Review,* January/February 1993, hbr.org/1993/01/to-build-a-winning-team-an-interview-with-head-coach-bill-walsh.

60   Katherine Thomas, "The Development of Sport Expertise: From Leeds to MVP Legend," *Quest-Illinois-National Association for Physical Education in Higher Education* 46, no.2 (May 1994): 199–210.

61   Karen E. French and Sue L. McPherson, "Development of Expertise in Sport," in *Developmental Sport and Exercise Psychology: A Lifespan Perspective,* ed. Maureen R. Weiss (Morgantown, WV: Fitness Information Technology, 2004), 417.

62   Pedro Mendonça and Tony Almeida, *Tactical Periodization: A Practical Application for the Game Model of the FC Bayern Munich of Jupp Heynckes (2011–2013)* (n.p., 2014), 4–6.

63   Xavier Tamarit, *What Is Tactical Periodization?* (Oakamoor, England: Bennion Kearny, 2015), 31.

64   Juan Luis Delgado-Bordonau and Alberto Mendez-Villanueva, "Tactical Periodization: Mourinho's Best-Kept Secret?" *Soccer Journal,* May/June 2012.

14 THE METHODOLOGY

65   Quoted in *Tactics,* U.S. Marine Corps, MCDP 1-3, July 30, 1997, www.fs.fed.us/fire/doctrine/genesis_and_evolution/source_materials/MCDP-1-3_tactics.pdf.

66   Greg Bishop, "The Case for ... Changing the Combine," *Sports Illustrated,* March 7, 2016, www.si.com/vault/2016/03/15/case-changing-combine.

67   Oliveira, "Tactical Periodization"; Inez Rovegno et al., "Teaching and Learning Invasion-Game Tactics in 4th Grade," *Journal of Teaching in Physical Education* 20, no. 4 (July 2001): 370–388.

68   Don Norman, *The Design of Everyday Things,* rev. ed. (New York: Basic Books, 2013), 11.

69   Ibid., 14.

70   Oliveira, "Tactical Periodization."

71   Charles Duhigg, *Smarter Faster Better: The Transformative Power of Real Productivity* (New York: Penguin Random House, 2016), 27–29.

72   Mark L. Latash, *Neurophysiological Basis of Movement,* 2nd ed. (Champaign, IL: Human Kinetics, 2008), 202.

73   John van der Kamp and Ian Renshaw, "Information-Movement Coupling as a Hallmark of Sport Expertise," in *Routledge Handbook of Sport Expertise,* ed. Joseph Baker and Damian Farrow (New York: Routledge, 2015), 50–63.

74   Keith Ellis, *The Magic Lamp: Goal Setting for People Who Hate Setting Goals,* rev. ed. (New York: Three Rivers Press, 1998), 194.

75   Michael Silver, "An Education in Quarterbacking: Sports' Most Difficult Position," NFL.com, September 6, 2016, www.nfl.com/news/story/0ap3000000695685/printable/an-education-in-quarterbacking-sports-most-difficult-position.

76   Robin Kirkwood Auld, "The Relationship Between Tactical Knowledge and Tactical Performance for Varying Levels of Expertise," *Master's Theses, Dissertations, Graduate Research and Major Papers Overview,* Rhode Island College, 2006, digitalcommons.ric.edu/cgi/viewcontent.cgi?article=1000&context=etd.

77   Judith L. Oslin, Stephen A. Mitchell, and Linda L. Griffin, "The Game Performance Assessment Instrument (GPAI): Development and Preliminary Validation," *Journal of Teaching in Physical Education* 17, no. 2 (January 1998): 231–243; Sue McPherson, "The Development of Sport Expertise: Mapping the Tactical Domain," *Quest* 46, no. 2 (1994): 223–240.

78   David Fleming, "No More Questions," *ESPN The Magazine,* October 4, 2016, www.espn.com/espn/feature/story/_/id/17703210/new-england-patriots-coach-bill-belichick-greatest-enigma-sports.

79   "Stephen Curry's Full NBA MVP Transcript," NBCSports.com, May 10, 2016, www.csnbayarea.com/warriors/stephen-currys-full-nba-mvp-transcript.

80   Micah Rieke, Jon Hammermeister, and Matthew Chase, "Servant Leadership in Sport: A New Paradigm for Effective Coach Behavior," *International Journal of Sports Science and Coaching* 3, no. 2 (2008): 227–239.

81   "Butler Bulldogs Mission Statement," Butler University, www.butlersports.com/information/school_bio/mission_statement.

82   Karen E. French and Jerry R. Thomas, "The Relation of Knowledge Development to Children's Basketball Performance," *Journal of Sport Psychology* 9, no. 1 (March 1987): 15–23; Janet L. Starkes, "Skill in Field Hockey: The Nature of the Cognitive Advantage," *Journal of Sport Psychology* 9, no. 2 (March

1987): 146–160; Mark Williams et al., "Cognitive Knowledge and Soccer Performance," *Perceptual and Motor Skills* 76, no. 2 (1993): 579–593; Werner F. Helsen and Janet L. Starkes, "A Multidimensional Approach to Skilled Perception and Performance in Sport," *Applied Cognitive Psychology* 13, no. 1 (February 1999): 1–27; Jean-Francis Gréhaigne, and Paul Godbout, "Tactical Knowledge in Team Sports from a Constructivist and Cognitivist Perspective," *Quest* 47, no. 4 (1995): 490–505; M. D. Hughes and M. Bartlett, "The Use of Performance Indicators in Performance Analysis," *Journal of Sports Sciences* 20, no. 10 (October 2002): 739–754.

83   Stuart James, "Brendan Rodgers: Spain Have Been a Great Model for Me Over Many Years," *The Guardian,* May 11, 2012, www.theguardian.com/football/2012/may/11/brendan-rodgers-swansea-city.

84   LeBron James, Twitter post, March 6, 2016, 8:13 p.m., twitter.com/kingjames/.

85   Gabe Mirkin, "Why Ice Delays Recovery," DrMirkin.com, October 13, 2016, www.drmirkin.com/fitness/why-ice-delays-recovery.html.

86   Jae-Sung You et al., "Dietary Fish Oil Inhibits the Early Stage of Recovery of Atrophied Soleus Muscle in Rats via Akt-p70s6k Signaling and PGF2a," *Journal of Nutritional Biochemistry* 21, no. 10 (October 2010): 929–934.

87   Rapaport, "To Build a Winning Team."

88   Garganta, Maia, and Marques, "About the Investigation of the Factors of Performance in Football."

89   José Guilherme Oliveira, "Programming and Periodization of Training in Football; Course Notes from the 4th Year," University of Porto, 2001.

90   V. Fernandes, "Implementation of the Model of Play: The Reason for Adaptability with Emotion," University of Porto, 2003.

91   Oliveira, "Tactical Periodization."

92   Delgado-Bordonau and Mendez-Villanueva, "Tactical Periodization: Mourinho's Best-Kept Secret?."

93   Raul Oliveira and Rodrigo Casarin Vicenzi, "Periodization Tactics: Structural Principles and Methodological Errors in Their Application in Football."

94   Bruno Gateiro, "The Hidden Science of Success: Mourinho in the Eyes of Science," PhD diss., University of Porto, Portugal, 2006.

95   Daniel Coyle, *The Talent Code* (New York: Bantam Dell, 2009), 91.

96   Louis Alfieri et al., "Does Discovery-Based Instruction Enhance Learning?" *Journal of Educational Psychology* 103, no. 1 (2011): 1–18.

97   Ronald Gallimore, Wade Gilbert, and Swen Nater, "Reflective Practice and Ongoing Learning: A Coach's 10-Year Journey," *Reflective Practice* 15, no. 2 (2014): 268–288.

98   Swen Nater and Ronald Gallimore, *You Haven't Taught Until They've Learned: John Wooden's Teaching Principles and Practices* (Morgantown, WV: Fitness Information Technology, 2005), 69.

99   Alexander Star, "The Way We Live Now: 5-7-00: Questions for Antonio Damasio; What Feelings Feel Like," *New York Times*, May 7, 2000, www.nytimes.com/2000/05/07/magazine/the-way-we-live-now-5-7-00-questions-for-antonio-damasio-what-feelings-feel-like.html.

100   Fomenkov, "Mourinho's 10 Commandments."

101   J. McCrone, "Como Funciona o Cérebro. Um Guia de Principiantes," *Civilização Editores,* 2012.

102   P. Haggard. and B. Libet, "Conscious Intention and Brain Activity," *Journal of Consciousness* Studies 8, no. 11 (November 2001): 47–64.

103   Donald McRae, "Pep Guardiola: 'I Would Not be Here Without Johan Cruyff. He was Unique," *The Telegraph,* October 7, 2016, www.theguardian.com/football/2016/oct/07/pep-guardiola-exclusive-interview-johan-cruyff-unique.

104   A. Delextrat and A. Martinez, "Small-Sided Game Training Improves Aerobic Capacity and Technical Skills in Basketball Players," International Journey of Sports Medicine 35, no. 5 (May 2014): 385–391.

105   Silver, "An Education in Quarterbacking."

106   James Lavin, *Management Secrets of the New England Patriots,* vol. 2 (Stamford, CT: Pointer Press, 2005), 218.

107   Fomenkov, "Mourinho's 10 Commandments."

108   Phil Jackson and Hugh Delehanty, *Eleven Rings: The Soul of Success* (New YorK: Penguin, 2013), 87.

109   Jonathan Wilson, "The Devil's Party (Part 2)," *The Blizzard,* n.d., www.theblizzard.co.uk/articles/the-devils-party-part-2/.

110   "Countable Athletically Related Activities," NCAA, n.d., www.ncaa.org/sites/default/files/20-Hour-Rule-Document.pdf.

15 INDIVIDUAL EMPHASIS IN A TEAM SPORT

111   Halberstam, *Education of a Coach,* 229, 235.

112   Ibid., 219–220.

113   "'You Can't Win Anything with Kids,'" BBC.com, August 18, 2015, www.bbc.com/sport/football/33982195.

PART FOUR

THE COACH

The athletic trainer leaves the head coach's office and walks down the long hallway. It's just after 8 p.m., and the building is dark and quiet.

A cleaner moves between doors in the silence.

Behind the head coach's hardwood desk, a fifty-something-year-old man, whose hair has been gray for as long as he can remember, looks over a list of currently injured players delivered by the head trainer. Each name has a color code. It's intuitive. Yellow means that the player is injured, at risk of missing the game in four days, and unavailable to train tomorrow. Red signifies a player who's injured and unlikely to play in the upcoming contest. Green means that a squad member is available but has not fully recovered from an injury. Players not on the list are assumed to be healthy and good to go.

There's one other color: black. That means suspended, usually for some kind of legal issue or rule infraction, such as a failed drug test.

There is only one name marked black today. A younger player. The coach sighs. It's always the ones with the most talent. He isn't sentimental, though, as he knows the heavy price for misplacing trust in someone who hasn't earned it. Sixteen years ago, when he was an assistant coach just trying to find his way in the league, he learned one of his earliest and most beneficial lessons on this subject. He was part of a back-office team that was sacked at the end of a disastrous season. The head coach of that team had put his faith in a player who

had failed multiple substance abuse tests. This individual missed key games through suspension, and as a result, the whole season went down the tubes. Like this kid, that one had come from a disadvantaged background, but the owner didn't care, and after the last game, he cut him from the roster and cleared out the entire coaching staff for good measure.

The coach refocuses his mind on the current problem. Psychologists and family members have been brought in to help, as well as a couple of veteran players willing to serve as mentors to the troubled young man. But none of them have broken through. It's the coach's responsibility to help until the player either changes his ways or blows his last chance. But for now, he has to put the issue aside. The next game is just ninety-six hours away, and it has to be his priority.

Glancing up at the whiteboard in front of him, the head coach sees the monthly calendar and the next opponent's name. He knows the intricacy of the planning that lies ahead. The list of injured players dictates some of the team's training restrictions. He is low on defensive players for some drills he'd hoped to run and needs to rethink tomorrow's session.

Of more immediate concern is one offensive player who is coming back from a hamstring injury. He will be able to train properly for the first time in three weeks, and the coach has to balance integrating him back into practice with being mindful of what that hamstring will tolerate. At thirty-two, the player is older, but while his powers of recovery aren't what they were a decade ago when he was a spry rookie, he can give much better feedback on his rehab progress than he would've then and is smart enough to manage himself in the upcoming session. This makes his comeback easier and relieves a little pressure on the coaching staff.

Looking at the trainer's sheet again, the coach sees a banged-up team. But he's lucky. One lesson he learned from his first mentor was to ensure that he has a deep roster. With all the measurables and statistics at his disposal, the one thing that cannot be quantified is availability. Who is the player who will be available week in and week out?

The coach starts to plan training and practice times for the week in a spreadsheet. Many head coaches don't do this. They prefer to delegate the scheduling to someone else, like the performance director. But the coach knows from experience that he alone sees the complete picture and fully understands what he's trying to achieve.

The rest day is the first one he puts on the schedule. The coach can then plan around it and maximize recovery from last weekend's contest while optimizing the training that precedes the next one. In doing so, he's working backward from the game. Filling in the blocks of training and team meetings, he ensures that the longest periods are equally separated from the games on both ends of the week.

Recovery is important, but so is building a tolerance for training. It's his contention that players have become softer over the past decade, but it's a delicate balance. Push them too hard and discontent can rise in the locker room—especially if the team is not winning. But if the coach is too soft, then players will expect to do less and might let complacency slip in. Both are equally risky, but losing with lack of passion would be the worst thing of all.

His days are long. When he was younger, the coach slept on the couch in his office every other night. Now that age has caught up with him, he goes home each night, but he still prides himself on getting to the team facility before anyone else. At 6 a.m., he watches two hours of film before getting breakfast and a shower at 8 a.m.

Feeling refreshed at 9 a.m., he has a block of two hours where all his non-player, non-team commitments are lined up so he can get them out of the way. This can involve anything from meeting with the team owner to doing short media interviews. Sitting down with the ownership is always a priority. Lessons from his mentors emphasized keeping the guy who writes everyone's checks closely informed so he understands the motivations for decisions and provides support. Because so much of the business is played out in the media, it's easy for a wedge to be driven between the coach and his boss. This weekly meeting stops that from happening.

The business of sports has changed a lot in recent years. Media—especially social media—has created a round-the-clock demand for current information. His personal assistant helps him manage this and keeps his interviews to a minimum. So much work goes into managing his schedule that he has thought about adding another assistant to manage the load. It's a lot for one person.

After that two-hour block, his coaching duties resume. This is his sanctuary.

Before he can get to actual game work, the coach has a meeting with the players' committee, made up of a mixture of older and younger players from most of the major position groups. This conversation offers the coach the opportunity to take the temperature of the locker room. They discuss everything from issues with player discipline to questions about the schedule.

This committee wasn't something he was keen on. It certainly wasn't his idea. But a former coordinator suggested it to him, and as it developed, the benefits became obvious. It gives the players a better understanding of the challenges the coach faces and makes them feel that they have more ownership of the team. Nothing is off-limits. Sometimes the focus is simply complaints about the food, while other times there are more serious discussions about disciplining players for DUIs or internal issues. This is where the leadership of the senior team members comes to the fore.

After that short but vital meeting, the coach meets with the offensive and defensive coordinators to talk strategy for next weekend's game. His role here is to be something of a devil's advocate, always questioning. He isn't disagreeing for the sake of it but rather to make sure he understands his coordinators' reasoning and can support their best ideas fully, while disregarding those that have no place in the game plan.

Talking with the coordinators gives the coach the information he requires to write his daily address. The two things he always needs to keep a pulse on are the players and the coaches. So every day at noon, the whole playing, coaching, and support staff meets for a ten-minute address from him. To the coach and his staff, this is the most important action of the day. It frames the message for all team activities.

Usually it's just a quick run-through of the day's schedule, but he sometimes changes his approach on the fly. If he senses that the group is tense because of a couple of recent losses, he'll portray an air of relaxation or add some humor to lighten the mood. But if the players sitting in front of him seem complacent, he'll inject a completely different attitude of caution or even anger. Over the years, he's used many tricks to set the right emotional tone and get the mindset of the players and coaches where it needs to be.

After the coach's address, the team goes back to its meetings. The coach tries to attend as often as he can, but he also sets aside time to meet with the training, conditioning, and support staffs. He makes a point of talking to everyone, from the chef to the athletic trainers to the strength coaches. The small details he picks up help add to his perspective on the team's mood and the motivation level of his staff. He can't count how many times he has bumped into someone in the hallway and, in the course of a brief conversation, heard something useful that he has put into practice to help the team improve. This exchange works both ways, giving him the chance to reinforce his vision for the team.

Doing this quick walk-through can also help the coach pick up on the real reason the star player is struggling. The player might have opened up to an assistant strength coach, explaining how his marriage is under pressure and expressing his fear that if it ends, he won't get to see his young son anymore. Such off-field issues can become big problems during a game.

After this walk-through, it's time for practice.

The fast-paced two-hour session is an escape for everyone from the trials of the business of sports. Practice is planned in great detail. The rest periods are designed to maximize intensity, and rotations and substitutions are scheduled to minimize injury risk. But everything is expected to be done at maximum effort.

The head coach watches closely. He speaks mostly to the coaches, and much of what he says is negative. He makes a point of shouting at them if something fails. Such expressions of anger are never directed at the players. To them he gives only positive feedback. This is mostly a well-rehearsed act on his part. It was something he picked up from a mentor who'd served under Bill Walsh, who made it a point never to criticize a player if a drill or scheme was wrong but instead let the coach responsible know. Praise was reserved for the players. The effect wasn't lost on the squad, and this tactic kept everyone sharp.

After practice comes a quick lunch, and then the coach joins his assistants to watch film of the practice and grade players. When this ends, he often has a dinner or function to attend for a sponsor, but occasionally he has an off night. This is when he gets to catch up on calls and respond to emails.

For now, he must finish the week's schedule.

Fighting off the encroaching tiredness, he pours one last cup of coffee, adds in the last details on the spreadsheet, and watches film of the day's practice for another hour. Finally, as the clock reaches 10:30, he turns off his computer, gets out of his chair, and heads for the parking lot.

The world of team sports today is vastly different from what is was fifty, twenty, or even ten years ago. To say that sports are big money is a large understatement. A *Washington Post* story noted that forty-eight college athletic departments in the wealthiest NCAA Division I conferences earned $2.6 billion in 2004 and spent $2.5 billion. Over the next decade, those numbers ballooned to $4.7 billion and $4.6 billion, respectively. During the first month of the 2016 summer transfer window, Premier League soccer teams shelled out $634 million on new players, which doesn't factor in the $3 million league-average annual salary for the new arrivals. NBA teams committed a cool $2 billion in player salaries in the first ten days of the 2016 NBA transfer window.[1]

Such spending doesn't happen in isolation but is a product of team revenues from a wide variety of sources. Ever-increasing college athletic department budgets are made possible by hundreds of thousands of fans cramming stadiums each weekend, millions of dollars in apparel sales, and massive TV deals—like the $2.64 billion that Fox Sports and ESPN pay for broadcasting football in the Big Ten Conference alone and an $8.8 billion extension tagged onto the existing $11 billion contract for the NCAA Tournament.[2] The NFL, supposedly a nonprofit organization, signed a $450 million deal with CBS and NBC to show games on Thursday nights over a two-year period. With all this revenue and spending come equally big expectations on coaches to win games. That's what this section is all about.

SIXTEEN

THE SIX LAWS OF WINNING

One of the most important sets of principles I've adapted from those outlined by the U.S. Army Special Operations Command are the truths that winning teams need to accept. If you had to boil down the management of any sports team to a few simple points, these are what you'd come up with.

THE LAW OF KNOWLEDGE

16.1

Know the game and know people. Every successful coach or military leader knows their game. They have a good basic understanding of what they do and what they need to do. You cannot be successful unless you possess this. The route to knowledge and perspective may be different. Some coaches have played the game; others have played very little. Some were great players; others were average or poor. But to survive in one of the most cutthroat professions there is requires a solid knowledge of the game.

Three keys to success: read, read, read.

—Vladimir Lenin

Some great managers and head coaches have confided to me that they don't have the detailed or academic knowledge of the game that others do, but these are the ones who usually have an unrivaled understanding of human instinct and nature and tend to be able to connect with people and players on a deeper level. That said, you can have all the people skills in the world, but if you don't have a fundamental knowledge and an understanding of the game, you will not be successful.

THE LAW OF HUMAN SUPERIORITY

16.2

Humans are more important than technology. As I've said elsewhere, this is a people business. For all the hype about new technology and the millions that teams spend on all the latest and supposedly greatest equipment, team sports is still at its core a people business, and it always will be. Just as at any successful organization, actual human beings are always the number-one asset, not state-of-the-art stadiums or fancy training facilities. The best possible equipment is useless unless a team has the right personnel to wield it. And because no combination of technology is perfect, you're going to have to rely on your people to pick up the slack.

It's also true that the ability of a team of talented people to work together is more important than getting computer systems to talk to each other. Teams spend a lot of money on coaching management applications, scouting software, and all the rest, but many of them invest little time or energy in their personal health and well-being. Urban Meyer, the incredibly successful Ohio State football coach, emphasized this in stark detail recently when he opened up about the stresses he has faced as a human who is a head coach. Washing down Ambien with beer is not a healthy habit for any person, least of all the person in charge of a sports program.[3]

The players must know their roles and work together in a synchronized way during a game, and it's the same for the coaches and staff in their jobs. The head coach should encourage everyone to try to better understand their colleagues' needs, objectives, and challenges and be respectful and professional in their interactions.

THE LAW OF INTENSITY AND QUALITY

16.3

Intensity and quality always trump volume and quantity. When confronting the challenges of modern warfare and international terrorism, the U.S. and British military soon recognized that just putting more boots on the ground was a dated and woefully ineffective tactic. They now rely on small, highly trained, and self-reliant groups that can be deployed anywhere at a moment's notice, putting Stanley McChrystal's "Team of Teams" approach into action.

The same is true in sports: quantity is rarely effective. It's better to have a small, tight-knit group of focused, experienced, and committed people than a massive coaching and back-office staff that doesn't fully commit to the ideals of the team and head coach. In this way, quality will always beat quantity, even at the "biggest" elite college and pro sports

organizations. You'd be surprised how many of these are run by a relatively small number of professionals who get big things done.

This quality-over-quantity philosophy extends to practice and preparation. As we saw in the principles of the four-coactive model and the morphological programming approach, there's no sense in (literally) running players into the ground. This is also true of the coaching, medical, and support staffs. According to a study conducted by John Pencavel at Stanford University, productivity starts to decline once the workweek exceeds 50 hours and, as CNBC summarized it, "falls off a cliff after 55 hours."[4] So while a head coach is right to expect hard work, forcing a culture of old-style "crack the whip" presenteeism is going to undermine productivity and alienate the staff.

THE LAW OF INDIVIDUALIZATION

16.4

Highly effective winners cannot be mass-produced in a short training cycle. An old truism in sales is that it costs ten times as much to gain a new customer as it does to keep an existing one, and when applied to personnel, the value of retention is even greater. Another reason an employee's leaving hurts a sports organization is that the knowledge that's in the employee's head when they walk out the door is lost. This doesn't apply just to coaching and specialty staff members but also to those in the operational departments who are crucial to the success of the team but are rarely acknowledged. Say the head coach's executive assistant goes to another team after many years of service. That assistant doesn't just screen calls and set up meetings but knows the ins and outs of the coach's life. For example, maybe the coach can't be disturbed between 8 and 10 a.m. because that's when she's most productive, or perhaps her husband needs to know in advance when there's a conflict with the kids' after-school activities.

It would take a replacement months to find out all these small nuances, which can't be taught during onboarding or any formal training program. This is just one example that shows how important it is to keep good people around. There are no shortcuts, and developing winners takes time. This is why it's imperative that the head coach and staff acknowledge the hard work of each individual at every level of the organization and make it a point to highlight their achievements. If you don't care for and respect good people, they'll soon find another organization that does.

THE LAW OF PREPARATION

===== 16.5

A competent coach must prepare for crises before they happen and be ready when chaos unfolds. Once problems manifest themselves, it's far too late to come up with an action plan for dealing with them. The plan must already exist and be, at a minimum, tested in practice. This is one of the reasons a weekly walk-through/talk-through the day before a game is an essential discipline. Preparing players and assistant coaches for every eventuality not only reduces their anxiety and leaves more of their functional reserve intact for the game itself, but also requires the head coach to strategize for everything that can (and probably will) go wrong, so there's a planned response for any eventuality. Expect the unexpected and prepare for it.

Once the ball is in play, emergencies will invariably occur. When the emergency is an injury, the potential replacement for the starting player must be adequately prepared in all four coactives so that they can enter the game and perform effectively. This is why having a deep bench of players who are prepared and ready to go at a moment's notice is essential if the team is to weather the injury storm that bedevils every squad at some point in the season. Similarly, the assistant coaches must be able to take over practices and games if the head coach is unable to perform his or her duties because of ill-

ness, a family emergency, or some other unexpected event. Invariably, the best-prepared teams are the ones that perform the best. To adapt a maxim from Darwin, the most successful teams are not the biggest or strongest but those that can best adapt to the stresses and challenges they face.

THE LAW OF SUPPORT

===== 16.6

Winners require outside support. When creating a tribal mentality and a team identity, it's beneficial in many ways to create an "us against the world" mentality, as this helps players commit to a higher ideal, play for each other, and be loyal to the club. However, this can go only so far, because the reality is that no player or team can win independently. Dozens of support staff contribute to the team's success. This includes those inside the organization—like the maintenance staff who keep the locker room clean, the cafeteria staff who prepare, serve, and clear away the food, and the equipment managers who make sure the kit is ready to go for each practice. It also encompasses a lot of external people who often go unnoticed, such as the bus drivers who get the team to the arena, the hotel staff who check in the team and get their rooms ready, and the airline crews who serve them in-flight drinks and meals. If all these support staff suddenly disappeared or went on strike, the team would be unable to function.

The behind-the-scenes folks who do the "little things" needed to keep a sports organization on track will put in extra effort for players and coaches who are courteous, respectful, and grateful to them. Conversely, they will not go out of their way to help those who treat them rudely and might even start underserving them when they next meet. That's why the head coach should make it clear to everyone that, whether they're at home or on the road, the team must treat others the way they want to be treated.

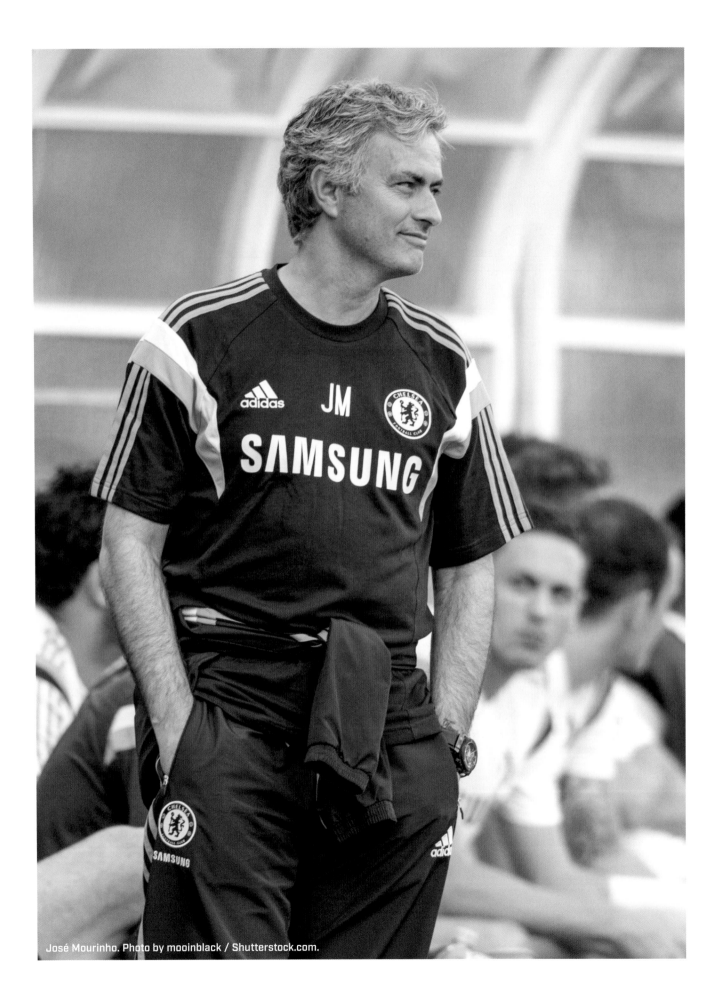

José Mourinho. Photo by mooinblack / Shutterstock.com.

SEVENTEEN

THE FOUR MACRO PRINCIPLES OF WINNING TEAMS

Over many years working with head coaches in almost every field sport and with military commanders, I've found that there are key principles that are critical to successful leadership. Combine observations of Jim Harbaugh, Eddie Jones, Alastair Clarkson, and the rest and you soon see trends in their successes and failures. Many of these coaches have what popular culture calls "growth mindsets," meaning that they believe hard work and dedication can keep progressing their abilities.

When I use the word *winning* to talk about such coaches, I'm not just referring to the on-field performance of their teams, though cultivating these traits in conjunction with the game model, four-coactive model, morphological programming approach, and player-health-centered principles will help coaches achieve that. Success is also about establishing a sustainable culture that attracts, retains, and rewards the best people. And it all starts with the head coach.

Sustainable winning is different from a one-off victory. Many coaches can build or force a team to summon all of its resources into a major effort to achieve something great in a particular event. A sustainable-winning organization is far more difficult to achieve and a far scarier proposition for the opposition.

THE MACRO PRINCIPLE OF HUMILITY

17.1

Many teams promote the idea of pride in the team jersey or shirt. While understandable, this is a misguided premise for dominant, sustainable-winning teams. They must honor the jersey, yes, but not become puffed up because they get to wear it on game day. Pride can be a dangerous value to encourage in teams because it promotes the idea of achievement and self-importance, whereas humility suggests that the honor is the players'. It is observant of the service of a team and the realization of one's place relative to everyone else in the organization.

> *It's awfully important to win with humility. It's also important to lose. I hate to lose worse than anyone, but if you never lose you won't know how to act. If you lose with humility, then you can come back.*

—Paul "Bear" Bryant

When you ask former players on great teams about their experiences on the team, they will predominantly talk positively, mention their teammates frequently, and speak of admiration they still feel for their former coaches. They might also refer indirectly to their commitment to a cause. Such a perspective shows that this player is humble and fully bought into the team concept.

Humility is at the core of every successful sports team, from the head coach down. One of the reasons humble people continue to improve is that humility discourages complacency. If you're truly humble, then you know that what you've achieved is not worth being arrogant about in a global context, so you keep striving to do better. That's not to say that you can't be satisfied with a job well done. But it's important to put titles, championships, and other achievements in the context of the club's history.

Take a coach like Bill Belichick, for example. There is no excessive celebration or taunting of opponents by his teams; there's no lapsing into overconfidence or complacency. Despite all the Super Bowl wins, Belichick is committed to a cold, ruthless, almost mechanical pursuit of success.

Humility also ensures that success is contextualized and that individuals are aware of the contributions their teammates and colleagues have made. They're not selfish or arrogant. So for a team like Red Auerbach's Boston Celtics, winning yet another NBA title was something to celebrate for a few days, but then it was back to work. And when Doc Rivers later led the Celtics to their first championship since the glory days of Larry Bird and company, he and his veteran leaders—Kevin Garnett, Paul Pierce, and Ray Allen—knew that they had to look to the legacy of Auerbach, Bill Russell, and Bird and recognize that their championship was but one of a dozen the team had claimed.

In contrast, pride has been the downfall of many great organizations. It's not one of the deadly sports sins just because it's poisonous in its own right but also because this poison quickly spreads throughout the team. Once a leader—whether that leader is a coach or a player—becomes puffed up and prideful, the focus switches from the higher ideal that the team once strived for to the individual. Rather than put the team above all, an arrogant person will look to satisfy himself and succeed for his own glory. And once this happens, the fellowship that once held the team fast starts to unravel.

When teams fail because of an absence of humility, we tend to see personalities come to the fore in a search for public acceptance and adulation. "The disease of me" takes precedence at the intended or unintended expense of other teammates and the group as a whole.

Pride breeds an outsized sense of self-entitlement and selfishness that takes the place of the sacrifice needed for sustainable organization-wide success. As spiritual leader the First Panchen Lama wrote in the fifteenth century, "The self-centered attitude is the entrance for all misery." This is why the head coach must endeavor to be anything but self-consumed and should continually demonstrate humility in all interactions with the team, the media, and fans. The coach must also make it a point to look for and snuff out pride and arrogance in the locker room before it can take root, particularly when a player is excelling and the team is winning.

Humility is also demonstrated in gratitude. It's quick and easy to say "Thank you" or "I'm grateful for that," and while it might seem like a small thing, it can have significant positive results. By expressing gratitude, head coaches can show that they know they can't go it alone and they value the help that others continually provide. Humility allows perspective on both success and failure.

Humility can be seen in subtle ways in postgame press conferences and interviews. Note the players who respond to questions with answers that give credit to their teammates, the coaches, and the organization, not themselves, even when specifically asked about their own performance. If a star player has such a humble attitude, it will percolate throughout the locker room.

The most important aspect of humility is related to self-improvement. Pride focuses players on material successes and external reinforcement of achievements. In contrast, humility allows a healthy sense of introspection that constantly keeps athletes and coaches aware of their achievements, their strengths, and their failures and weaknesses in totality. This healthy awareness is critical to continuous development and progression.

THE MICRO PRINCIPLE OF TRUST AND SERVICE · 17.1.1

Earn trust, earn trust, earn trust. Then you can worry about the rest.

—Seth Godin

When the members of a team are humble, they find it easier to trust each other simply because there is an appreciation that they are all working toward the same goals. As the Spartan culture proposed, everyone is to fight for each other, not for themselves. Plutarch asked, "Why do the Spartans punish with a fine the warrior who loses his helmet or spear but punish with death the warrior who loses his shield? Because helmet and spear are carried for the protection of the individual alone, but the shield protects every man in the line."[5] The currency of humility also kindles a spirit of serving others. One of the main jobs of the head coach as a manager of people is to empower assistants and players to be their best and reach their potential. If it's clear that the coach is continually trying to serve others, then they will reciprocate and give their best each and every day.

A team that is dedicated to service doesn't care who gets the glory when it wins and doesn't point fingers when it loses. The only thing that matters is that the athletes are playing hard for each other and putting in full effort during every moment of the game, every drill in practice, and every rep in the weight room. When all the players care about those around them, they will go out of their way to do their best and make sure everybody's needs are met.

If a team is to establish and pursue a higher ideal, its personnel also must trust each other without question, in every situation. After writing his book *War* and making its companion film, *Restrepo,* Sebastian Junger gave a TED Talk about why veterans miss being at war after they leave the military, and he described the characteristics of the brotherhood he observed when embedded with a U.S. Army unit in Afghanistan: "Brotherhood has nothing to do with how you feel about the other person. It's a mutual agreement in a group that you will put the welfare of the group, you will put the safety of everyone in the group above your own. In effect, you're saying, 'I love these other people more than I love myself.'"[6]

Such humility and service can also be driven by understanding and respecting the legacy of the club, what it means to wear the jersey, and the team's duty to the legacy they inherit. A great example of this is the sign that hangs in the Liverpool FC players' tunnel that reads, "This Is Anfield." It reminds each team member of the hallowed names that have gone before them and won multiple league and cup trophies—not to mention giving a subtle reminder to opponents that they're about to step into a hostile environment!

No team has created a greater significance for their jersey than the All Blacks, whose players refuse to honor rugby's tradition of swapping shirts after the game unless they think their opponent is worthy to receive them.[7] This gives an almost religious significance to the current squad's responsibility to honor the legacy they're inheriting.

I must follow the people. Am I not their leader?

—Benjamin Disraeli

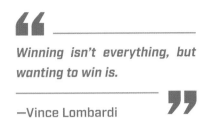

Winning isn't everything, but wanting to win is.

—Vince Lombardi

THE MACRO PRINCIPLE OF HUNGER

17.2

Ronnie Coleman, one of the greatest bodybuilders of all time, once said, "Everybody wants to be a bodybuilder, but nobody wants to lift no heavy-ass weights." In such delicate prose, Coleman summed up a clear and simple fact of life—everyone wants something big, but most people don't want to put in the effort required to obtain it. Larry Bird calls the willingness to put in that effort, drive; Jack Harbaugh calls it enthusiasm.

To be successful, you have to want something badly enough to pay the price. In the highest echelon of sport, there are many great athletes, talented coaches, and proficient specialists. They can only rise above their peers by approaching their craft with hunger and a ruthless pursuit of excellence. Great success means great self-sacrifice, self-discipline, and great self-denial, and few want to go through all that.

In recent memory, few players have poured out their emotions for hometown fans more than LeBron James, who, while succumbing to tears after leading his Cavaliers to an improbable NBA Finals comeback against the Warriors, declared, "Cleveland, this is for you." It was his hunger to win for his home city that brought James back to the team and drove him to another championship and Finals MVP award.[8]

THE MICRO PRINCIPLE OF ACCOUNTABILITY

17.2.1

We sometimes think that ambition goes hand in hand with ego or selfishness-driven arrogance. This is not the case. Every successful coach and player is highly ambitious and goal oriented. It's the job of those around them to hold them accountable for directing this drive toward the greater goals of the group rather than to selfish ends. To reach the pinnacle of achievement, each person must try to maximize his own gifts and hold everyone around him accountable for doing the same. Those who are self-motivated won't need the eyes of the head coach on them to give their best—they will just do it, even with little supervision. Every successful organization needs disciplined doers who can make decisions independently and take action.

THE MICRO PRINCIPLE OF FOCUS

17.2.2

Sports, like conflict, requires focus. In war, special operators must keep the objective in mind at all times, despite the chaos unfolding noisily around them. It's the same for a sports team, which must block out the potential distractions of media rumors, the roar of the crowd, and the weight of expectation. Each person must zero in on his or her specific role and do what it takes to execute. This encompasses seemingly routine activities, such as observation and scouting, , as well as game-day performance.

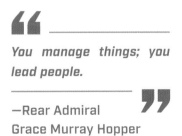

You manage things; you lead people.

—Rear Admiral
Grace Murray Hopper

THE MICRO PRINCIPLE OF HARD WORK

17.2.3

No one gets out of this world alive. There is no sense in the coaching staff, players, or back-office personnel holding back anything for later. For the team to reach its potential and achieve its goals, everybody must remain dedicated to daily hard work. This isn't just the case while chasing the first championship; it's even more true after such an achievement. It's a cliché in sports that the hardest thing is winning back-to-back titles, but if you look at the numbers, it's also a fact. Only six NBA franchises have done it (if you count the Minneapolis and Los Angeles Lakers as one franchise), and only seven NFL franchises claimed successive titles. Since Preston North End won the top-flight English soccer league in 1889 and again the next year, only ten other clubs have gone back-to-back.

One of the reasons that a team reaches the pinnacle of its sport one year and often falls short the next is that in the absence of hunger, complacency develops. In contrast, the leaders of teams that can

The reason a lot of people do not recognize opportunity is because it usually goes around wearing overalls looking like hard work.

—Anonymous

be considered dynasties don't set the goal of winning just one championship; they want to win as many as possible. After a team has been victorious, it needs to continue to practice the same habits that earned it this success in the first place if it wants to avoid the pitfalls of a one-and-done achievement. This is why one of Phil Jackson's favorite sayings is, "Before enlightenment, chop wood, carry water. After enlightenment, chop wood and carry water."[9] Hard work must be intrinsically motivated and driven by solid, repeatable habits if it's to be sustained day after day, season after season.

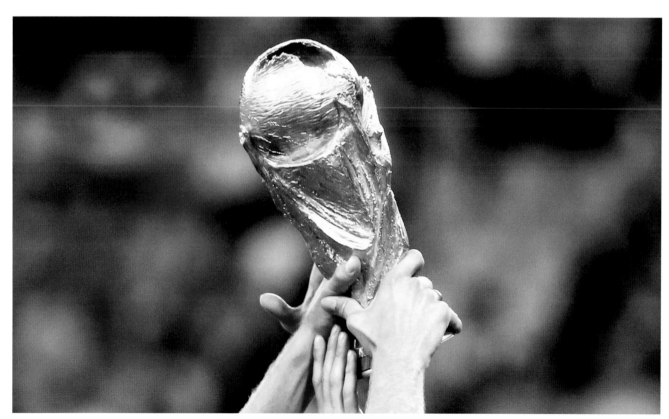

The FIFA World Cup Trophy. Photo by A.RICARDO / Shutterstock.com.

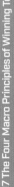

What makes a good coach? Complete dedication.

—George Halas

THE MICRO PRINCIPLE OF COMMITMENT   17.2.4

To work toward a greater goal over a number of years, each team member must display an unwavering commitment to these aims and to each other. In battle, soldiers must override the human impulse to avoid taking life, and in contact sports like rugby and football, athletes must demonstrate a similar warrior spirit. Nobody would make these kinds of sacrifices for a leader who just told them to risk everything—they have to be conditioned to follow the commanding officer or coach and strive for a higher ideal that's bigger and more important than themselves.

It's not enough for players to commit completely in their own heads. Their commitment has to be demonstrated at every game, every practice, and every team meeting. And this commitment starts with the head coach. If the players and assistants can see that their leader is all in, then they're far more likely to put everything on the line as well. You can buy star players, but you cannot buy loyalty; that comes only when there's a top-down commitment that's reinforced over and over again.

Leadership is a matter of having people look at you and gain confidence. . . . If you're in control, they're in control.

—Tom Landry

THE MACRO PRINCIPLE OF HONESTY

================== 17.3

The team must insist on brutal honesty at all levels. When a group of people are honest with each other, everyone knows exactly where they stand, what is expected, and what others think of their performance. It's the same as when you ask a good friend for advice. You don't want affirmation but rather honesty and a fresh perspective that will help you make the best possible decision.

People are often loath to criticize players and coaches who have already been very successful. This can have the knock-on effect of making such people react poorly to honest appraisal because they're not used to it and may come to think that they're above criticism. However, the best of the best want their peers to keep critiquing them, as it provides them with extra motivation to push themselves to new heights. It can also be helpful to have mentors and a small circle of close friends outside the organization whom the head coach periodically looks to for honest evaluation.

When the head coach is honest with the assistants, back-office staff, and players, it fosters trust throughout the organization. Trust helps create and sustain loyalty, dedication to one another, and adherence to a purpose that's greater than any individual goal or desire. When everyone is honest, the burden of trying to be something you're not and attempting to appear flawless is lifted. Honesty and truthfulness also help the team improve because each person can critically assess his own strengths and weaknesses.

Humility is a prerequisite for honesty because only when people are humble do they feel secure and can ask for, accept, and act on honest and constructive criticism. However, the single most important aspect of honesty is self-honesty. The ability to critically analyze one's own ability, strengths, and weaknesses is essential to creating a sustainable-winning organization. This is what separates the truly great players from the rest. Michael Jordan is not often considered outwardly humble (particularly by those opponents who endured his endless trash-talking), but his self-honesty ensured that he avoided complacency and drove himself to consistently improve his game.

> **Confrontation simply means meeting the truth head-on.**
>
> —Mike Krzyzewski

THE MICRO PRINCIPLE OF CONFLICT

17.3.1

One of the hallmarks of an honest group striving together toward a higher ideal is not peace but conflict. In teams that are continually moving forward, multiple voices speak up when they believe that something isn't right or can be improved.

The best head coaches welcome and frequently initiate conflict as they know that contradiction is a necessary part of solid decision-making. Colin Powell said, "If you have a yes-man working for you, one of you is redundant," and this is just as relevant to a sports organization as it is to Powell's military command. If people feel that they're trusted and valued, then they should have the confidence to say to the boss, "I think you're wrong, and here's why," no matter how many championships the coach has won. If coaches just go with their preconceived notions every time, they're likely to make far more mistakes, not to mention miss out on the expertise around them.

Conflict must be present to generate thoughtful insight and debate, avoid complacency, and foster innovation in all areas of performance. Safe conflict—which means that people are free to share constructive criticism and others are willing to take it on board—is not as risky as some might think among groups of coaches who are all committed to one single ideal: the success of the team.

But there is a fundamental difference between open and honest conflict that aims to further the goals of the team and dishonest conflict that someone initiates to take someone else down or pursue their own ambitions. There's no place for the latter in a winning organization, because there can be no politics or smoke-and-mirrors games.

THE MACRO PRINCIPLE OF RELENTLESSNESS

17.4

Life and sports are relentless, and the desire to win must be relentless, too. One of the hallmarks of greatness is consistency. Some people consider great teams like the New England Patriots and the San Antonio Spurs to be "boring" because they seem to win all the time. But really, this continued, sustained excellence is anything but boring—it's remarkable and should be celebrated. The same can be said of some of the greatest coaches. They don't grab headlines by courting controversy and often frustrate the media by saying the same things over and over again, but this just means that they're focused on the team and are trying to reinforce its principles in what they do and say.

When Winston Churchill took up the hobby of bricklaying and was juggling it with politics and the writing that paid his bills, he used to say that his mantra was "200 bricks and 2,000 words a day." As a result, he became a chartered bricklayer and produced forty-three books, thousands of articles, and some of the most famous speeches in history. Consistent domination is both a preparatory method and an objective.

The most successful individuals and teams are the most efficient. They devise routines to handle less-important tasks and save their energy for tackling more-significant ones. For example, Barack Obama has two styles of suits that he chooses between every morning, because he needs to save his decision-making capacity for issues that matter. Mark Zuckerburg, Steve Jobs, and Jim Harbaugh have all used the same approach: wearing the same simple uniform each day because doing so reduces decision fatigue.

Another way that a head coach can cultivate consistency is by creating a routine and habits that players come to expect and that set a baseline for the team and staff. Some of the most successful coaches in history—including Bill Walsh and Bo Schembechler—made sure that the first talk they gave at the start of each season was exactly the same as the year before. This briefing set out the expectations for what it was to be a San Francisco 49er under Walsh or a Michigan Wolverine under Schembechler. The morphocycle also helps players find comfort and consistency—they know that, for example, they'll have every Monday off, and that on the day before the next game they'll be doing a walk-through. This combination of moral and ethical routine and practical, physical habit drives the relentless pursuit of excellence that is paramount for dominant teams.

I cannot trust a man to control others who cannot control himself.

—Robert E. Lee

THE MICRO PRINCIPLE OF STEADINESS

17.4.1

In addition to putting in consistent effort, it's important for the head coach to steer the ship with a steady hand through storms and calm waters alike. This means not getting too carried away with triumph or too despondent with defeat. Perhaps Claudio Ranieri, who led Leicester City to the most unlikely title in Premier League history in the 2015–16 season, put it best when he told reporters, "There is a good quote from [poet Rudyard] Kipling, when he said, "Victory and defeat, it's the same.' It's not good or bad. You have to stay in the middle."[10] He kept his squad emotionally centered enough to finish top of the table.

Emotional consistency is key in building a sustainable organization. A great coach never panics, no matter how dire the situation appears—and if he does, he doesn't allow signs of panic to appear. This would only encourage the same state among the players and staff. Instead, the head coach needs to maintain perspective and make objective decisions driven by clear, critical thinking, even when things seem to be at their worst. This is particularly true during a losing streak and after a defeat in a multi-game series or the first match of a two-legged tie. The teams who snap such a streak and pull off comeback wins are often those whose coaches are able to maintain personal and team-wide balance during adversity. There are exceptions to the rule, however, such as if the coach wants to incite fear in players he feels are complacent and not focused enough on the challenges at hand.

No matter what the scoreboard reads at the end of the game, coaches can spin the result to ensure that the team keeps its emotional equilibrium. So in defeat, they can present positives like, "We fought hard after we conceded that second goal," and after a win they can help the players avoid complacency by finding an opportunity for improvement such as, "We did well today, but we're still not where we need to be defensively."

If you want to win, do the ordinary things better than anyone else does them day in and day out.

—Chuck Noll

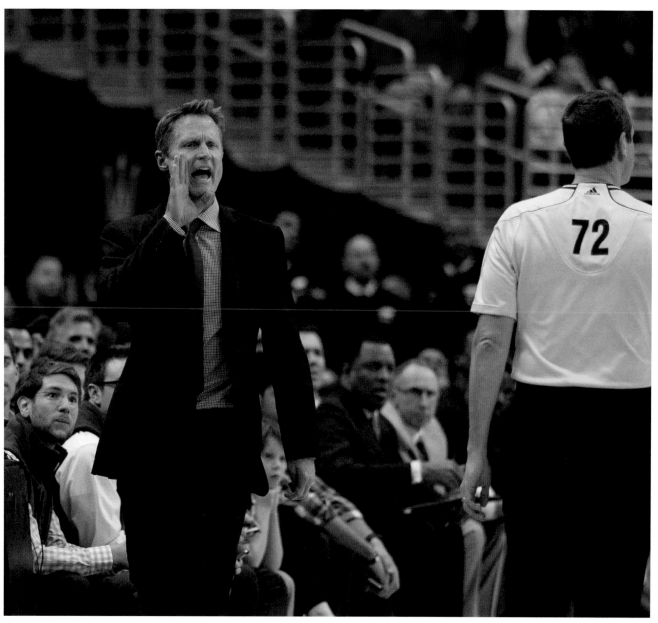

Steve Kerr, head coach of the Golden State Warriors. Photo by Keith Allison (CC BY-SA).

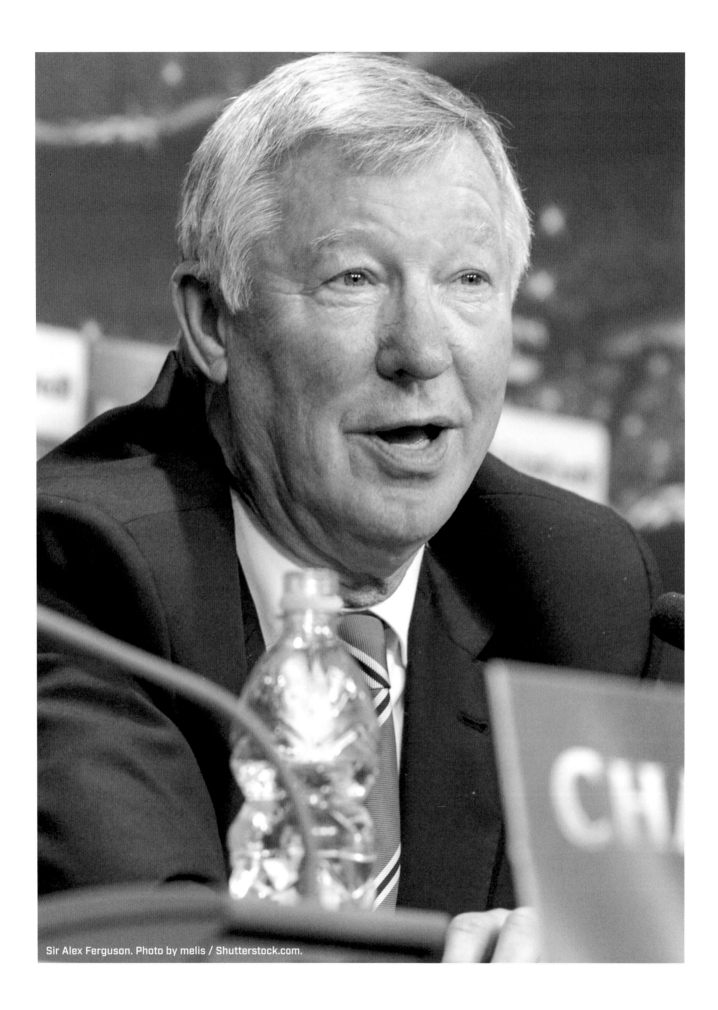

Sir Alex Ferguson. Photo by melis / Shutterstock.com.

EIGHTEEN

LEADERSHIP

There have been many great teams, but none have been successful without great leaders. Not all had great leaders at the beginning; sometimes they arose through necessity. Whether a great leader is born or made, however, there are some key traits and skillsets that are common to them all, and some rules that must be observed pitfalls that must be avoided to increase the probability of success.

KNOW THY TERRAIN

18.1

Having had the challenge and pleasure of working everywhere from Melbourne to Michigan, from Liverpool to Los Angeles, and from Cardiff to Cleveland, I've become acutely aware of the importance of understanding the role of society and culture in communicating and achieving trust and success. In "The Game," I touched on the importance of a new coach getting to know the team, city, and culture. It's vital that the head coach knows what kind of message the team's local fan base and media expects. A town that prides itself on its blue-collar, hardworking identity, like Pittsburgh or Detroit, is going to want to hear the leader of its beloved sports team talk about determination, toughness, and heart. Conversely, in a progressive city like San Francisco, fans expect their coaches to be committed to creativity and innovation. This is not to say that coaches should put on an act or try to be some-

one they're not but rather that they must be mindful and respectful of the society that their team fits within and its values.

KNOW THE BACKGROUND

18.1.1

In addition to acknowledging the surrounding society and culture that exists outside the team, coaches must make a concerted effort to understand the complex personalities that compose their staff and player roster. In the documentary *The U*, some of the University of Miami's most successful football coaches noted that a key to creating a winning organization was understanding the diverse backgrounds of the young men they'd been charged with leading. If there is one dominant leader among the players, it's crucial for the coach to create some kind of understanding with him or her, particularly if that player's background is very different from the coach's own. Gary Smith's *Sports Illustrated* story about Philadelphia 76ers coach Larry Brown ("the 60-year-old Jewish grandfather") and his star player Allen Iverson (the 25-year-old rapper) describes how this divide can be crossed:

> Larry and Allen had so much in common, if they just stopped fixating on their differences. Both were raised by single moms. Both were the smallest guys on every court they played on, all heart and hunger—Larry diving across floors so often

he now hobbled on replacement hips, Allen skidding and bouncing toward the same fate. Each so sensitive that one word or look from the other could inflict deep pain. Both, even with their 35-year difference in age, going home every day to the noise, toys and sticky hugs of small children.

Though Iverson and Brown never overcame the inherent combustibility of their relationship, they did make enough progress to forge a more productive working environment—one that ultimately led the 76ers to the Eastern Conference title and the regular season MVP award for Iverson.[11]

Another important thing for the coach to understand is the religion or predominant cultural focus of the place the team plays. So if you're going to coach football in a small Texas town, you should know that the local population likely has a strong Christian faith. But if you went somewhere like Samoa to coach rugby, you would need to recognize that the family unit comes above everything. Again, no team exists in a vacuum but must function within a society and be cognizant of its belief system.

THE POWER OF A BELIEF SYSTEM   18.1.2

One of the benefits of a belief system is that it provides context for sports. While the game is extremely important and commitment to the team's ideals must be total, it is not the only thing in life that matters, or even the most important thing. Players without such a belief system can find themselves crushed by each defeat, despondent with every injury, and adrift when their playing career ends. This brings us back to the healthy balance discussed in "The Player." For players to live healthfully, they need to maintain perspective and not prioritize sports above all else but balance it with their faith, friends, and family.

The initial purpose of organized sports was to teach young people habits—teamwork, problem-solving, a good work ethic—that they could apply to the rest of their lives. Yet this often gets lost in the multinational, multibillion-dollar business that team sports has become. The Stoic mindset can be valuable here.

Stoicism is a philosophical school of thought and perspective that was pervasive in ancient Rome and Greece. In a nutshell, Stoics believe that humans find most happiness in accepting what they're given in life, whether good or bad. When we neither succumb to desires for pleasure or suffer from fear of pain, Stoics believe, life becomes much simpler and clearer. Stoicism was founded in Athens by Zeno of Citium in the early third century BC, and his teachings were built upon by other noted philosophers, such as Seneca and Epictetus. In ancient Rome, Roman emperor Marcus Aurelius was a famous Stoic; in more modern times, decorated vice admiral James Stockdale credited Stoicism with helping him get through seven years of captivity in the Vietnam War. Ryan Holiday's book *The Obstacle Is the Way* is an excellent introduction to Stoicism and how to apply its teaching to everyday life.

Transferring this philosophy to sport can be incredibly effective. Any athlete who can endure pain and hardship without showing emotion or complaining is very difficult to defeat. The ability to look objectively at situations as they truly are, instead of getting carried away with knee-jerk reactions or emotions, helps athletes handle adversity in even the toughest of situations, as explained to great effect by Jocko Willink and Leif Babin in their book *Extreme Ownership*. A player who has a Stoic outlook doesn't run from challenges but rather embraces them, knowing that difficulties must be overcome on the way to reaching their personal goals and the team's ultimate objectives.

The sense of perspective that Stoicism encourages can also help us recognize that, while performance is important and should be pursued relentlessly, the game is still just a game. In the emotion of the game, beliefs and perspective can become unhealthily distorted. David Beckham once spoke about how he contemplated suicide after he was sent off in a World Cup game after abuse from English soccer fans. The belief system of the athlete is vital to maintaining perspective on the game and its place in life.

Another benefit of Stoicism is that it teaches coaches and athletes to focus on what's happening now and to stop dwelling on the past or worrying about the future. Stoicism also encourages people to acknowledge and disregard nonbeneficial emotions like anger and fear, which can derail preparation and dealing with the pressure of elite sports. All great boxers, for example, have tried gamesmanship and mind games to aggravate the opponent and instill anger or fear in the opponent in order to make them freeze or pause, or to make them anxious and make rash decisions. This happens in team sports, too, but often in eleven different instances on the field.

> *I do not conceive of any manifestation of culture, of science, of art, as purposes in themselves. I think the purpose of science and culture is man.*

—Fidel Castro

The Roman emperor Marcus Aurelius, who ruled from 161 to 180 AD and held the empire together in the face of attacks from the Parthians and Germanic tribes, embraced Stoicism. Unlike some of the patricians who ruled Rome and came to power because of their wealth, Aurelius was a soldier before he entered political life, so he was used to fighting and struggling to get ahead. He did not view challenges as problems, though, but rather as opportunities that prompted decisiveness and determination. Aurelius said, "The impediment to action advances action. What stands in the way becomes the way."[12] Coaches can improve their mental approach and that of their players and staff by following Aurelius's example: viewing problems as opportunities, focusing on the present, letting go of destructive emotions, and applying other basic Stoic principles to how they approach the game and the challenges of daily life.

BELIEVE

To build a dominant team, there must be a steadfast belief in the system, players, and coach. This can be developed through the clear communication of an ideal, but it cannot be faked. Some coaches can sell this belief, but others may be accused of being insincere in their methods.

In *Extreme Ownership*, their book on leadership in the Navy SEALs, Jocko Willink and Leif Babin write, "In order to convince and inspire others to follow and accomplish a mission, a leader must be a true believer in the mission. Even when others doubt and question the amount of risk, asking, 'Is it worth it?' the leader must believe in the greater cause."[13] This was true during their service as Navy SEALs and is just as vital in team sports. If the head coach believes in the team's potential and ability to reach its ultimate goal regardless of the circumstances, the assistants, players, and staff will mirror this in how they approach each training session and game.

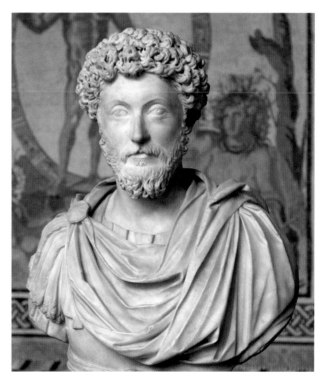

Marcus Aurelius.

SERVING TO LEAD

18.3

No matter what your role in a team, you have to both lead and serve. You represent the team in every interaction. Great leaders in extreme situations know two great rules. First, you must be able to compromise to achieve your objective, and second, you need to use your position to do whatever is necessary for your people to do what they need to do. This is genuine leadership—serving them to help them achieve what the team needs.

RULE 1: SACRIFICE

18.3.1

I've already made the point that a big part of coaching these days is knowing what to focus on and what to ignore. Another key to leadership in team sports is knowing what hills to die on and what issues to negotiate on or leave as is. Some coaches see being uncompromising and tough as a virtue, and in some situations it can be. But if head coaches are going to get everyone to work hard and sacrifice for them, they're going to have to distinguish early on between the things that merely irritate them and those that they simply cannot tolerate. Because if you fight battles on every front, you will ultimately lose. In his book *How Good Do You Want to Be?*, coach Nick Saban makes this point when he says, "You cannot possibly challenge every adverse situation or stand up to every enemy."[14]

A key to great leadership is to know what to concede on to get the desired effect from the group as a whole—and this applies to both coaches and players. In "The Player," I discussed not trying to fix elements of a player's performance if they're not broken, and a coach would do well to adopt the same attitude toward daily team operations. If something is detrimental to the players, staff, or organization, or if there's clearly a better way to do it, then fine, make the change. Yet a head coach—particularly one who's just starting out with a new team—shouldn't go shaking everything up for the sake of it or making waves because of some misguided attempt to assert authority. This will only alienate people and create disloyalty, fear, and mistrust.

> True heroism is remarkably sober, very undramatic. It is not the urge to surpass all others at whatever cost, but the urge to serve others at whatever cost.

—Arthur Ashe

RULE 2: SERVE

18.3.2

An important hallmark of leading with humility is a willingness and even a desire to serve others. This is real, practical, functional advice. When you have employed a staff and are asking them to do a job and to ensure that they do their best for you, your question should always be, "What do I need to do to help them achieve what I've asked them to do?"

So head coaches should begin each day by asking themselves two questions:

1. How I can I help those around me today?
2. What do I need to do to empower people to be their best?

In essence, the head coach is serving the staff. If the coach proceeds from this belief, the focus is already the overall good of the team and the organization, the welfare and happiness of the staff, and the health and needs of the players. If it's apparent that the head coach makes these things a priority, then everyone else will follow suit. The result is that the winning principles listed earlier—humility, hunger, trust, accountability, commitment, hard work, and consistency—go from buzzwords to things that are lived out in every interaction and every decision.

True servant leadership enriches the lives of the people the leader is responsible for, which makes them eager to come to work every day with a positive attitude and helps maintain stability by making them want to stick around, regardless of how the team is performing on the field or how much is going into their bank account every two weeks. Being a servant also helps the head coach remain grounded and humble and avoid the pitfalls of arrogance and self-centeredness that can quickly turn someone in a position of power into an insufferable tyrant. As Martin Luther King Jr. said, "Everybody can be great, because anybody can serve."

GET COMFORTABLE BEING UNCOMFORTABLE

18.4

To succeed, coaches must get used to the fact that life isn't fair, nor is it comfortable. The eloquent small book *Who Moved My Cheese?* perfectly outlines the perils of believing that comfortable is admirable. In sports, that is never the case.

Every morning in Africa, a gazelle wakes up. It knows it must outrun the fastest lion or it will be killed. Every morning in Africa, a lion wakes up. It knows it must run faster than the slowest gazelle or it will starve. It doesn't matter whether you're the lion or a gazelle—when the sun comes up, you'd better be running.

—Dan Montano

In sports, as in life, things are rarely, if ever, perfect. In fact, when we're part of a team-sports organization, we exist in a domain of chaos and instability. This has the potential to make everyone feel chaotic and unstable, not to mention unsure and fearful. That's why it's the job of the head coach to remain steady and be a source of calm and reassurance, whether there's a player in trouble, the team is fighting to stave off relegation, or the rumor mill is being particularly vicious. If the person at the top can stay comfortable when things are profoundly uncomfortable, those around him or her will draw confidence that they too can handle any crisis that arises.

RESPONSIBILITY & ACCOUNTABILITY

18.5

Pat Summitt, who has the most wins of any coach in college basketball history, rightly said, "Responsibility equals accountability equals ownership. And ownership is the most powerful weapon a team or organization can have."[15] In other words, if the staff have some skin in the game and feel like they're able to contribute their ideas and knowledge to help the team win, they'll be far more committed than if they're just taking orders. So while the strength coach will follow the morphocycle programming approach each day, just like every other specialist, it should be up to him how to apply it and which movements, exercises, and sequences the athletes are exposed to. Similarly, the physical therapist must be given responsibility for acute injury care. As Summitt said, responsibility, accountability, and ownership all go hand in hand.

THE THIN LINE BETWEEN DELEGATION AND ABDICATION

18.6

If you're the head coach of a team, it's important to realize that no matter how good you are at time management, how organized you are, and how willing to learn you are, there are simply not enough hours in the day for you to do everything. This means that you have to delegate responsibility to your staff. To show your assistants and back-office personnel that you have faith in them, you have to let them make independent decisions and apply their knowledge and expertise within their area of specialty. This fosters trust in your leadership and prevents you from becoming bogged down in minutiae that would distract you from your coaching responsibilities.

18 Leadership

Yet, as the famous rugby coach and current director of rugby at Scottish Rugby Scott Johnson once said, "There's a very thin line between delegation and abdication." As head coach, you have to know what's going on in each of the specialties that you oversee and ensure that there is open, two-way communication so that you stay informed and your staff remains accountable. Part of delegating is allowing people to experiment and make mistakes, but when these errors impact the organization and/or the players' performance, the head coach has to take responsibility and say, "I messed up." The coach who abdicates in this situation and blames staff members or players for slip-ups—particularly to the media—will turn the organization against itself and find that they have few allies when the team goes through a rough patch.

Paul "Bear" Bryant was arguably one of the toughest, most uncompromising coaches in college football history. Yet when something, anything, went wrong, he made it clear that the buck stopped with him. "Find your own picture, your own self in anything that goes bad," Bryant said. "It's awfully easy to mouth off at your staff or chew out players, but if it's bad, and you're the head coach, you're responsible. If we have an intercepted pass, I threw it. I'm the head coach. If we get a punt blocked, I caused it. A bad practice, a bad game, it's up to the head coach to assume his responsibility."[16]

THE RELENTLESS PURSUIT OF PERFECTION

18.7

For head coaches at the absolute pinnacle of their sport, nothing is ever enough. Certainly, they revel in winning trophies, and nobody would give back a Coach of the Year award, but for a select group, this satisfaction is short-lived. Soon it's back to work and business as usual. While at Stanford, where he transformed a football program with a 1–11 record into a program that finished 12–1 and number four in

the nation in 2010, Jim Harbaugh said, "I don't take vacations. I don't get sick. I don't observe major holidays. I'm a jackhammer."[17] Having worked with him at the San Francisco 49ers and again at Michigan, I can attest to this intensity and commitment, traits he also displayed as quarterback for the Bears and as head coach for the University of San Diego and Stanford.

It's a funny thing about life; if you refuse to accept anything but the best, you very often get it.

—W. Somerset Maugham

While at Manchester United, Sir Alex Ferguson wasn't just dissatisfied with a poor match performance. Poor preparation was equally unacceptable, even for just one day. "We never allowed a bad training session," Ferguson told the *Harvard Business Review*. "What you see in training manifests itself on the game field. So every training session was about quality. We didn't allow a lack of focus. It was about intensity, concentration, speed—a high level of performance. That, we hoped, made our players improve with each session."[18]

A few years ago, one of the Manchester United coaches told me a story about the morning after the team won the Premier League. They'd had a long night of celebrations and he had wisely found an alternative means of transportation for getting home, so that morning he went back to the team's training ground at Carrington to collect his car. Alex Ferguson was already at work in a meeting with the club scouts, planning for the next season. No wonder that by the time he retired in 2013, he did so as the most successful manager in Premier League history.

BURNING THE BOATS   18.7.1

Fear is a driving force in sports. As a coach, you cannot create excuses or give players a way out. Players who have doubts will take it. They'll accept the opportunity to claim a sore hamstring or tight back. This is why you sometimes need to use fear to motivate them.

When Hernán Cortés landed in Mexico in 1519, he faced a seemingly impossible task: defeating the mighty Aztecs with a tiny force of just eleven boats, sixteen horses, and six hundred men. If he had simply turned around and sailed back to Cuba, the governor there likely would have imprisoned or executed him for disobeying a direct order, which was tantamount to treason. He probably looked at his ragtag bunch and saw the fear in their eyes and sensed the doubts in their hearts. Knowing that he had zero chance of accomplishing his goal if his troops weren't all-in, he decided that the only way to ensure such commitment was to give them no alternative. So he burned their boats.

What probably seemed like a crazy act by an unstable commander turned out to be a moment of inspiration. Though the Tlaxcalans—an indigenous group in Mexico who were enemies of the Aztecs—needed a little more persuading than Cortés had hoped to join him against the Aztecs (his army had to give them a sound beating), they eventually came around. With his newly expanded force, Cortés marched to Cholula and inflicted a stunning defeat on the Aztecs. Soon enough, Montezuma's empire was no more and Mexico had been conquered, in large part due to the all-or-nothing drive of this daring leader who refused to give his men the option of turning back.[19]

This is not to say that head coaches should march into the team facilities and start setting things ablaze, but they do need to encourage a sense of adventure and show the entire organization that full-on dedication is the only way forward.

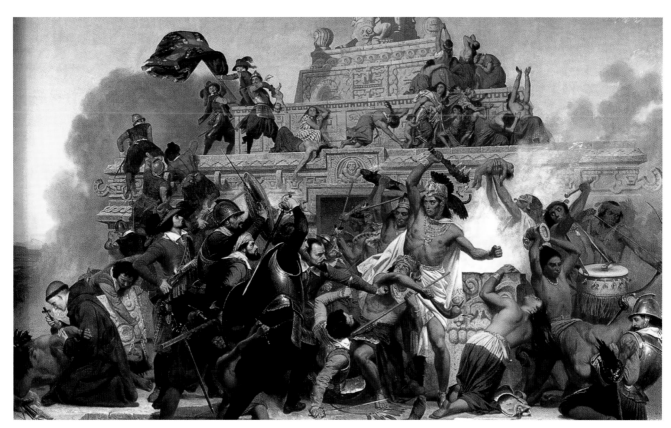

Storming of the Teocalli by Cortez and His Troops, by Emanuel Leutze.

18 Leadership

THE GIFT OF FEAR   18.7.2

In "The Player," I talked about the importance of the reptile and limbic brains and how together they act faster than the conscious mind to initiate the fight-or-flight response to danger. Fear is an important part of that response. While acting from a place of fear or even terror is incredibly demanding and so shouldn't be encouraged often, fear can occasionally be used as a powerful motivator. It's sometimes said that great teams win because they're afraid of losing, and though this is a cliché, it is a valid one. In certain circumstances, a head coach can motivate individual players or the entire team by instilling an "us versus them" fear of an opponent who threatens not only their winning record but also their basic need for security.

DEVIL'S ADVOCATE   18.7.3

Until the 1980s, every canonization proceeding in the Catholic Church was assigned an official whose job it was to take a skeptical view of the candidate and raise possible objections that would disqualify him or her from sainthood. This person was said to be taking the side of the devil in the canonization process—from which we get the term "devil's advocate." A similar concept appears in the film *World War Z*, in which Brad Pitt's character wants to know how the Israeli government anticipated the arrival of zombies. His contact tells him that after Israel ignored the intelligence that left them unprepared for the joint Egyptian-Syrian attack that started the Yom Kippur War in 1972, "we made a change. The tenth man. If nine of us look at the same information and arrive at the exact same conclusion, it is the duty of the tenth man to disagree. No matter how improbable it may seem, the tenth man has to start thinking with the assumption that the other nine are wrong." The "tenth man" concept may be fictional (though the military and intelligence communities do have something similar, as I'll discuss momentarily), but it's a valuable idea for any organization, including sports teams.

Sports teams need to combat the tendency of lower-ranking staff members to defer to the head coach and become yes-men who are afraid to disagree with a direction they think might be wrong. In fact, it helps to have someone play the role of devil's advocate in most major group decisions, even if they're not convinced that the original viewpoint is incorrect. This will at least force the head coach to explain and think more critically about the alternatives to the initial direction.

RED TEAMS   18.7.4

In the military, units can't take the risk of assuming that their position or system is secure and will be able to withstand an enemy assault. So they "red team": they employ a group whose explicit purpose is to attempt to penetrate their systems, methods, and defenses in order to identify, as an enemy would, where they're weakest. A similar practice in team sports involves the head coach inviting a peer or trusted confidant to poke holes in the game plan, strategy, and tactics. The red team outsider should come to a game inconspicuously and without the knowledge of the players or staff. It's also helpful if the outsider knows as little about the team and its personnel as possible. Then, after the game, the head coach is presented with a brutally honest assessment of what's working well and what needs improvement. The coach can then present the findings to the staff and make the necessary adjustments. This takes a lot of self-assurance and humility, but it's one of the few ways to get an objective analysis that can lead to big improvements.

EVERYONE WINS   18.7.5

When success comes, everyone wins. That has to be the mentality for coaches, players, and everybody else within an organization. Sharing credit and praising others allows individuals to enjoy the moment of victory while preserving the humility and team focus that are so essential for continued improvement. It's not just about acknowledging previous contributions but also about setting a tone of goodwill and appreciation going forward. If the star player or head coach claims too much credit, this will inflate their egos, undermine the idea of working for something bigger, and upset those who weren't thanked or praised. No victory happens in isolation and without everybody pulling together.

> *Great discoveries and improvements invariably involve the cooperation of many minds. I may be given credit for having blazed the trail, but when I look at the subsequent developments I feel the credit is due to others rather than to myself.*

—Alexander Graham Bell

THE RULE OF SUSTAINABLE LEADERSHIP

18.8

Players and personnel don't always chase the biggest paycheck when looking to find a new team—and those that do usually aren't the kind you want to recruit, anyway. For the highly motivated professional who wants to advance his or her career, the opportunity to learn from an exceptional head coach and to become part of an organization that has a reputation for excellence is often the main driving force behind the decision.

CANDOR   18.8.1

"Candor is a compliment, it implies equality; it's how true friends talk." So says Peggy Noonan, *Wall Street Journal* columnist and former assistant to President Ronald Reagan.[20] In the fast-paced, high-stress world of team sports, there is no time for ambiguity or doublespeak. What is needed is clarity and unhesitating honesty. If the head coach is candid with his or her assistants, everyone knows exactly how their

performance is measuring up to the organization's high standards and what's needed for improvement. Feedback doesn't have to be "good" or "bad" per se, just direct and BS-free.

As Noonan says, being candid is also a hallmark of friendship: it's what you expect when two people who are equals are having an open conversation with appropriate levels of disclosure. Just as in a friendship away from the team, candor runs both ways. If the head coach is going to speak candidly to the assistants, they should expect to be able to do the same in return. An assistant is often be able to offer new insight or a different perspective that the head coach has never considered. And if they feel confident that they can speak without softening their input, assistants will feel trusted and appreciated.

RECRUITING ASSISTANTS   18.8.2

An assistant coach doesn't have to be a young and eager go-getter who's on the first rung of the coaching ladder. Some of the best assistants—Tex Winter at the Chicago Bulls and Carlos Queiroz when he was at Manchester United, to name just two—are highly experienced professionals. Sometimes the head coach will bring in this type of assistant to complement their weaknesses. This approach is prevalent in football, where the defensive and offensive units and their many subunits require broad understanding and most head coaches are stronger on one side than the other.

Younger assistants can come from outside the organization or from various places within it. One of the most common routes is the one trod by former players whose on-court leadership and veteran know-how is valued by the head coach. Then there are those who take a less typical path, such as the Miami Heat's Erik Spoelstra, who earned the nickname "No Problem" for his willingness to help as the club's audio-video coordinator / concierge before serving his coaching apprenticeship under Pat Riley and Stan Van Gundy and finally becoming the team's head coach.[21]

Jack Welch's book *Winning* provides a solid blueprint for evaluating assistants, whether they're old hands, green rookies, or somewhere in between.[22] First, find candidates who have:

- *Integrity:* Will they commit to the value of honesty and work hard even when you're not watching?

- *Intelligence:* Are they dedicated to learning and able to make independent decisions without hand-holding?

- *Maturity:* Can they handle the pressure that comes with the job and maintain a balanced lifestyle?

Once you've used these criteria to narrow down the candidates, go to the next stage of Welch's evaluation, in which you should look for prospective assistants who have the "4 E's":

- *Positive energy:* Will they elevate the group with enthusiasm, a can-do attitude, and the ability to thrive in the chaos of team sports?

- *Ability to energize others:* Do they fit well with the other personalities you've assembled, and will they inspire you and the other assistants to achieve great things with a positive outlook?

- *Edge:* Will they be candid and tell you what they think? Will they be able to make difficult decisions?

- *Execute:* Can they get the job done?

Welch's final check box is for passion. When the season is dragging on and everybody is worn out physically, emotionally, and spiritually, the head coach needs to be surrounded by people who can elevate the mood and sustain joy in their work. As the head coach will work most closely with the assistants and these individuals will interact with the team and influence their attitude, having passionate assistants is a must.

WHO DO THEY LISTEN TO?   18.8.3

How an organization takes care of its own doesn't pertain only to staff members. In reality, how their families are treated is just as important, if not more so. No matter how good work relationships are, family ties are stronger, and employees listen to their significant others more than they do their colleagues or boss. Team sports can be a demanding environment that requires long and irregular hours and lots of time away. The organization needs to offset this by making each family feel valued.

This means it's a good idea to send flowers when a wife has a baby, congratulate a husband on a new job, and make kids feel special when they come to a home game. We know that a player's environment has an important influence on their emotions, habits, and performance, and the same is true of coaches, the medical team, operational personnel, and so on. If the head coach cannot attend weddings, funerals, christenings, and other important events, an assistant should go. This shows that the team truly cares about its people and is invested in their lives beyond the team. A recent example: Celtic FC manager Brendan Rodgers delayed training so that players could take their children to school on the first day back after the summer break. "It's life," Rodgers told reporters. "Your kid going to school for the very first day, you never get it back ever in your lifetime."[23]

TRAIN THEM TO LEAVE   18.8.4

There's a story told in business schools about training people to leave a company: The COO asked, "What if we invest in our people and they leave?" To which the CEO responded, "What if we don't and they stay?"

Coaches often fear that if assistants becomes too proficient, they will either leave or, if the team falters on the field, take the head coach's job. This fear and insecurity can tempt the head coach to hold back in educating and developing assistants. But such protectionism is never in anyone's best interests, and it's the opposite of what servant leadership should look like.

Head coaches have a duty to help everyone be the best they can and so must openly share their knowledge and experience with their assistants. The Commander's Intent also comes into play here. The overall aim is for the team to reach its performance potential, and the better the assistant coaches become, the closer the club will get to reaching this standard of excellence. You can't lock your assistants in the coal shed to prevent them from leaving if the right opportunity arrives, and if the head coach is truly a mentor, he should welcome his assistants' eventually moving up the ladder, even if that means going to another organization. Bill Belichick is one head coach who has exemplified such mentorship, with seven of his assistants becoming head coaches in the NFL and several more—most notably three-time national championship winner Nick Saban—finding success in charge of college football programs.[24]

WHAT YOU WANT TO BE OR WHO YOU WANT TO BE   18.8.5

When coaches are working to develop players and staff, they should encourage them to set big goals and smaller milestones that will help them get there. When talking about the future, it's easy to focus on tangible targets (like winning silverware), job-specific achievements or promotions (from bench player to starter, for instance, or from running back coach to offensive coordinator). There's nothing wrong with including such things in someone's development plan, but it's more effective to combine the "what" with the "who." When thinking about long-term advancement, helping someone become the person they want to be has more lasting appeal than giving them concrete aims that become irrelevant once they've attained them. Try asking two simple questions: "Who do you want to be in a year/three years/five years?" followed by "How can I help you get there?" This can go a long way toward proving that the head coach is invested in the future of his or her athletes and staff.

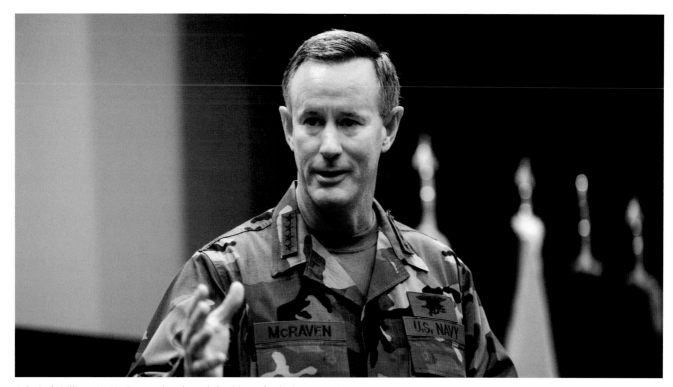

Admiral William H. McRaven developed the idea of relative superiority, which explains how a small force can overwhelm a larger one (see page 95).

18 Leadership

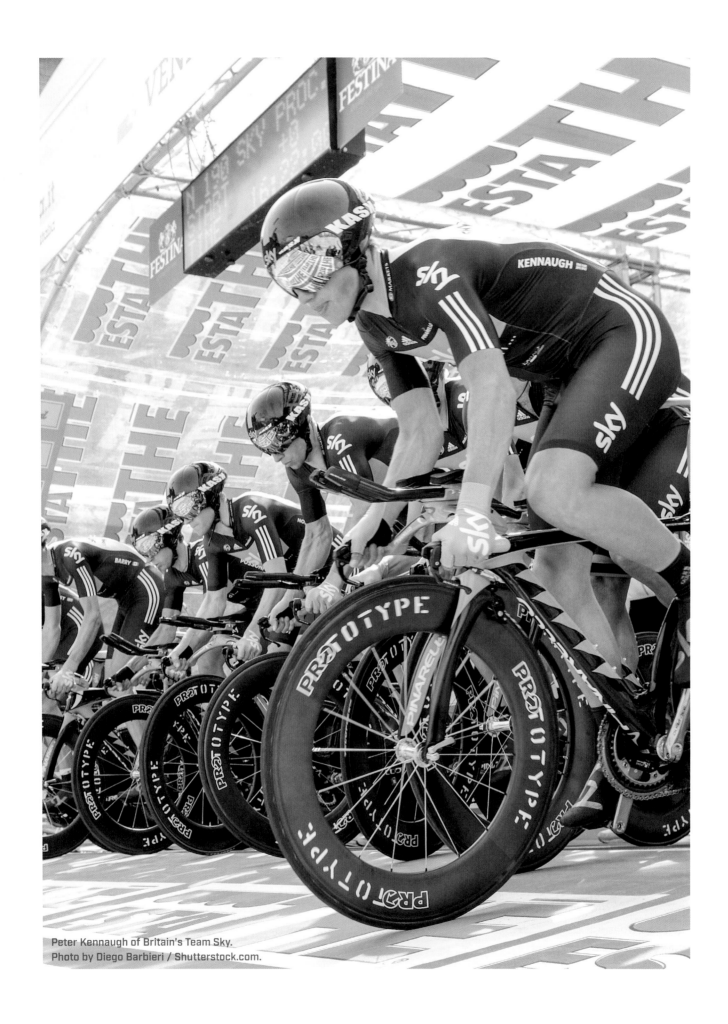

Peter Kennaugh of Britain's Team Sky.
Photo by Diego Barbieri / Shutterstock.com.

NINETEEN

PREVENTING PROBLEMS

Just as it's too late to try to create leaders once a crisis has hit, it's poor management to let problems among the squad and staff escalate to the point that they blow up the organization. The head coach must prevent such issues from taking root before the seeds are even planted. This involves getting everyone to understand the six laws of winning, continually reinforcing that the higher ideals of the group are more important than individual aims, and ensuring that there is open communication and transparency at all levels. It's also advisable to keep the back-office team as small as possible, to make it clear that responsibilities are more important than roles and titles, and to make sure everyone recognizes that the head coach is at the top of the chain of command.

SILOS, EGOS, AND INSECURITY

19.1

Ego is one of the biggest threats to the long-term health of any group, and it runs against the grain of the six principles of winning, particularly number one on that list: humility. Arrogance and insecurity often go hand in hand and together create a person with an inflated self-worth who seeks to satisfy their own needs and wants. The higher purpose of the team goes out the window.

When people are insecure and their egos are running wild, they tend to want to control everything, which leads them to form a white-knuckle grip on their area of expertise and shut others out because they're a potential threat. This hampers collaboration, slows decision-making, and creates conflict with other people and departments.

The head coach has to head off such disruptive behavior at the pass. Just as with players, the coach must ensure that every staff member feels secure and that their needs are being met. They must also reiterate that everyone has to work together, communicate openly and honestly, and be transparent. If there are one or two people who cannot change their ways and discard their own egos and ambitions in favor of the team's ideals, then it's time for them to leave the organization.

The need to prevent walls developing between staff and departments extends upward, beyond the head coach. Golden State Warriors general manager Bob Myers still keeps a 2014 quote from Gregg Popovich on his cell phone to remind himself that successful organizations must foster open communication, eliminate personal kingdoms, and set egos aside. The five-time NBA championship winner and Team USA head coach said:

> A synergy has to form between the owner, whoever his president is, whoever the GM is, whoever the coach is. There's got to be a synergy where there's a trust. There (are) no walls. There is no ter-

ritory. Everything is discussed. Everything is fair game. Criticism is welcome, and when you have that, then you have a hell of an organization. That free flow through all those people is what really makes it work. And that includes everything from draft to Os and Xs. Nothing should be left to one area—only to the president, only to the GM, only to the coach—or the culture just doesn't form.[25]

RESPONSIBILITIES, NOT ROLES

19.2

In an organization in which there are a lot of politics, one-upmanship, and personal agendas, individuals crave the status of titles and will do whatever it takes to fulfill their own selfish ambitions. This is not what a successful sports organization looks like. Rather than create fancy titles and rigid roles for narrowly focused specialists, it's wise to be more pragmatic.

Recruit staff on their ability to do tasks responsibly, not on their job titles or to fill roles. Create a small team of generalists who have a broad range of responsibilities and who are committed to success. This way, it doesn't matter what someone's title or role is, and people won't pursue status. Instead, they will work together across the numerous areas needed to coach the team, help it perform well, keep players healthy, and run the business side of the operation.

Having a small circle of trust makes management and communication easier and also enables each person to spend more time with the players. Once you start adding people and expanding this circle, each new specialist will want to interact with the athletes, and there's more risk of silos developing. This is not to say that you want to work a small team to death or spread them too thin, but neither should you go the other way and hire new staff just for the sake of it or to cater to the latest trend in performance training, sports science, or analytics. The benefits of bringing in new people have to outweigh the potential costs, not just in terms of the balance sheet but in terms of group dynamics as well.

RESPECTING THE COMMANDER'S INTENT AND COHESION

19.2.1

It's important that every member of the organization knows its overarching aims and what they're striving toward together—in other words, the Commander's Intent. A big part of this is the head coach exercising authority and people being aware that the head coach is at the top of a hierarchy. Yes, this individual should practice servant leadership, empower team members to make decisions, and respect the expertise of those around them, but they still have to lead. While a successful sports team requires hard work from multiple people, there can be only one commander, just as in the military. The staff and players must be subservient to this individual and the greater goals of the group.

Another important aspect of respecting the Commander's Intent is communicating a clear, concise, and consistent message no matter who the audience is, what stage of the season it is, or how the team is performing.

EMOTIONAL INTELLIGENCE

19.2.1.1

Due to the stressful nature of high-level sports, emotions can run high on and off the field. Head coaches can be very animated during games—picture Bobby Knight screaming at referees and players from the sidelines or Alex Ferguson allegedly throwing teacups and cleats in the locker room. Even outside of the game, the pressure to perform for staff and players alike is always present.

This means that the coaching staff, and particularly the head coach, have to not only keep their emotions in check but also be aware of how others react to criticism and praise, their hopes and fears, and how they feel when in the pressure cooker of competition. Vítor Baía believes that José Mourinho's emotional intelligence enabled him to help his Porto team keep emotions in check because he understood each person's emotional state and was able to tailor his motivational tactics accordingly.

What Sports Science Delivers (left) vs.
What Performance Science Delivers (right)

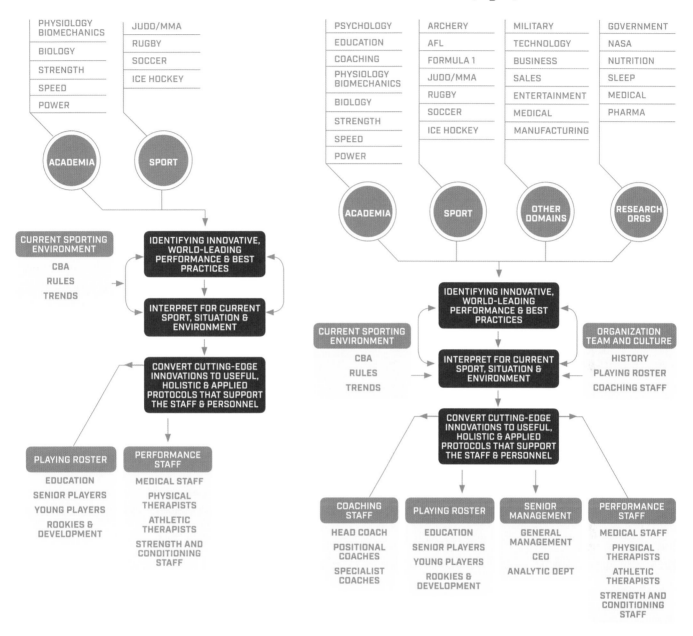

"He knew everybody so deeply that he could control our emotions in every situation," Baía said. "In my case, he would just pat me on the back and I was ready to go. However, there were players who needed motivation, who needed to be praised, and he knew which ones needed what, that's what made him so good."[26]

THE RIGHT ONE, NOT THE "BEST"

19.2.2

Many years ago, I learned a valuable lesson while working with a Tier 1 special operations commander. I used the word *best* once too often for his liking, and he abruptly explained to me that they didn't want the *best* candidate, they wanted the *right* candidate.

Why Sports Science Delivers (left) vs. Why Performance Science Delivers (right)

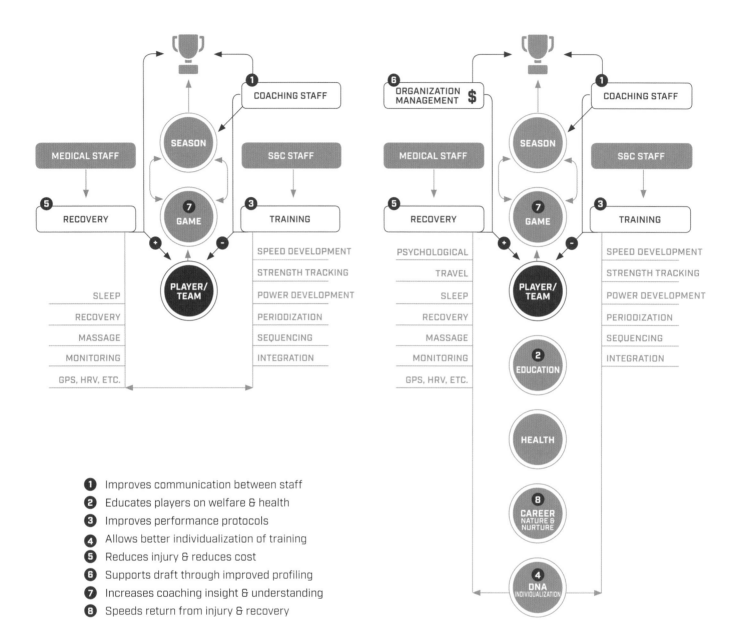

1 Improves communication between staff
2 Educates players on welfare & health
3 Improves performance protocols
4 Allows better individualization of training
5 Reduces injury & reduces cost
6 Supports draft through improved profiling
7 Increases coaching insight & understanding
8 Speeds return from injury & recovery

Within any sport, you will hear that this or that team has "the best" sports science program, "the best" strength and conditioning program, or "the best" medical team. While these programs may well be doing great new things, it's a misnomer to say that a team is the best unless the team wins.

And really, a winning team doesn't need the best of any of these specialties but rather the *right* ones. And if we are going to proclaim someone to have the best

this or that, surely it's part of the club that wins the championship at the end of the season.

Many teams can claim to have the best strength or sports science program, but if they lose, does it matter? This is one of many misguided perspectives in sports.

How Sports Science Delivers (left) vs. How Performance Science Delivers (right)

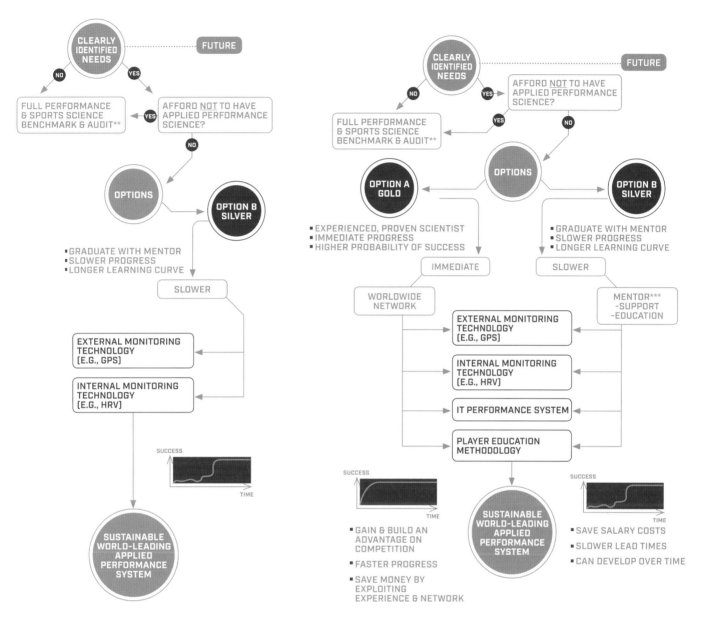

** See Performance Audit Details

*** See Elite Sport Mentoring Program

DRAFT TO YOUR STRENGTHS   19.2.2.1

In basketball, the 76ers invested in a pipe dream that former general manager Sam Hinkie referred to as "The Process." This involved purposely tanking to accumulate the "best" players through draft picks with the mistaken belief that they would all succeed in time.

Time and time again it has been proven that when the "best" players are put together, they do *not* just jell to become a great team. The right players put together in the right way and with the right coaches and support staff become the best team.

The San Francisco 49ers, under the guidance of former GM Trent Baalke, repeatedly tried to do something similar to the 76ers over a three-year period, drafting a total of nine players who were coming back from ACL injuries. These players were all initially projected as very high draft picks before their injuries, so on paper these appeared to be very smart moves. Let's look at how these picks panned out:

2013, Tank Carradine (picked 40th): Barely played during his first three seasons

2013, Marcus Lattimore (picked 131st): Retired without playing

2014, Brandon Thomas (picked 100th): Never played; recently waived by Lions

2014, Keither Reaser (picked 170th): Barely played and is hanging on to his roster spot

2014, Kaleb Ramsey (picked 242nd): Retired without playing

2014, Trey Millard (picked 245th): Traded to Kansas City; never played

2015, Deandre Smelter (picked 132nd): Waived without ever playing

2015, Rory Anderson (picked 254th): Waived without ever playing

2016, Will Redmond (picked 68th): Moved to injured list

Of course, drafting a talented player, even one who is injured, makes a lot of sense if you have a good medical team with a proven history of rehabilitating injuries. You could be selecting an individual with proven intangibles who has had one, albeit serious, injury. ACL injuries are no longer rare catastrophic accidents that we know little about. Many players return from them—look at Todd Gurley and Frank Gore. But if you have a medical team with the success rate of a blind butcher at an abattoir, then it doesn't matter who you draft, you're just wasting talented picks.

The fundamental point here is obvious: the goal is to win games, not to have the best team on paper or in theory. In reality, the team that is truly the best consists of the right people and processes, not excellence in one area at the expense of another. Recently retired lieutenant general Bennett Sacolick (who spent thirty-five years in the U.S. Army, fifteen of

them leading a Delta Force team) explained, "There was not one special thing about us [the members of his Operational Detachment Alpha, or A-team], but together as a 12-man team we did the most amazing things."[27] This is the underlying point for successful teams: they recognize that a team that works well together creates a synergy, so that 2 + 2 can lead to a score of 5 or greater, as long as no one department or individual tries to take all the credit. Such gains come back to the core value of humility.

SAFE INVESTMENT   19.2.2.2

Money and time needs to be invested first in the areas that are proven, before they're spent experimenting on the risky and unproven. The Philadelphia Eagles' sports science experiment failed after briefly flourishing and ended with players complaining about invasion of privacy, lack of compliance, and Chip Kelly's removal. The Cleveland Browns, the perennial team of pain, followed suit and spent a fortune on sports science, technology, and innovation only to fail disastrously (again). Other examples include the Port Adelaide AFL team, which has spent thousands traveling to Dubai and Oregon for warm-weather training camps, or the Welsh national rugby team, which has spent equally exorbitant sums traveling to Spala in Poland for cryotherapy, Dubai for warm-weather training, and Switzerland for altitude preparation…all ending with disappointing game results per dollar spent. In the NHL, the Buffalo Sabres invested in more than ten different sports science, training, and various back-office staff members in the 2015–16 season with no tangible results, and the season ended in the sacking of their director of player performance, among others.

Another common mistake is to misinterpret scientific principles or the systemic function of the body, as some NFL coaches have recently demonstrated with embarrassingly ill-informed public statements.[28] Look at the most successful teams, like the New England Patriots, New Zealand All Blacks, and San Antonio Spurs. All of them use simple, efficient, and cost-effective approaches to win games.

PART-TIME STAFF AND ON-CALL EXPERTS

19.2.3

Rather than creating a bloated back-office staff that includes every kind of specialist imaginable, it's often better to have a list of these experts on call. A smaller-salaried team won't be able to cover every eventuality, and you will sometimes need to bring in someone with more in-depth knowledge. For example, if a player has an emotional issue that the support staff cannot remedy, you could bring in a sports psychologist. Or if one of your athletes isn't responding to the traditional rehab methods administered by your medical team, perhaps you'll turn to a traditional Eastern medicine practitioner to help the player recover and return to competition. The counterargument is that if you have a larger staff, you're more likely to be able to cover every eventuality, so you wouldn't need the experts on call. But the problems (cost, communication, egos, and so on) that are created by carrying a larger staff are so debilitating that the large staff itself becomes an impediment to winning.

A better model is to have a small, lean core staff that should be able to handle most needs, and to bring in on-call experts for the occasional issue that requires more in-depth training and understanding.

There are, of course, very capable sports nutritionists, sports psychologists, and gurus out there who do great work, and large organizations with deep pockets may find they're helpful to have on staff. But at a smaller organization, the core coaching and medical staff can help players develop sound nutritional and lifestyle habits, for example. And the athletes themselves should also bear some responsibility, as 80 percent of nutrition is common sense and there are plenty of resources available for players to educate themselves. If a certain player is struggling with matching their nutrition to their activity and recovery needs, then you can refer them to a nutritionist. Rushing to employ experts before they are needed creates issues for staff and often ends in less buy-in from players.

ERGONOMICS OF HUMAN COMMUNICATION

19.3

When we talk about ergonomics, we're often thinking about the shapes of desk chairs or the layouts of computer keyboards. That's not what I'm talking about here. Rather, I'm referring to how the flow of staff members through team facilities either helps or hinders communication among them. In some team facilities, the medical team is in one corner, the performance specialists are in another, the coaches are on a different level, and the sports science group is in the basement, like Milton in *Office Space* (maybe a slight exaggeration). Such a dispersed layout encourages each discipline to become a fiefdom and leads to literal silos popping up throughout the organization.

If a building doesn't encourage [collaboration], you'll lose a lot of innovation and the magic that's sparked by serendipity. So we designed the building to make people get out of their offices and mingle in the central atrium with people they might not otherwise see.

—Steve Jobs

Cyberspace is just as much a consideration of ergonomics as physical space. As a culture, we're ever-ready to send a text message or IM, and such virtual "conversations" can go back and forth all day. You often see long email chains copied to multiple people that can span days, weeks, or even months. There's nothing inherently wrong with texting or IMing, but it can't take the place of face-to-face conversations. Talking with someone in person builds relationships in a way that electronic communications can't match.

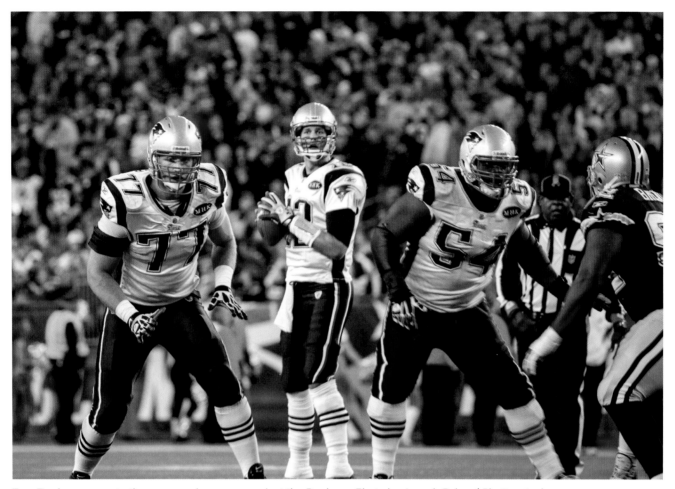

Tom Brady prepares to throw a pass in a game against the Cowboys. Photo by Joseph Sohm / Shutterstock.com.

Another pitfall of these quick-hit, stream-of-consciousness messages is that they're easily misconstrued and the recipient can perceive subtext that isn't intended. A short email rattled off before leaving for the day can seem curt or dismissive. An unanswered text message can come off as a slight, especially when the last person to text can see that the other person has read their last message. This is why it's essential in team sports to make a concerted effort to get people together and recognize that being connected by technology can lead to a profound *disconnection* in relationships.

A simple way to remedy these issues is to rethink the layout of the team facilities and create more opportunities for face-to-face conversations by removing physical walls (and hallways, levels, etc.) between individuals and departments. This doesn't mean having everyone in a single open-plan space or cube farm, as this can interfere with phone calls and meetings. Everyone can still have a designated office, but these should be close together, with no delineation between specialties. You want the strength coach to bump into the physiotherapist and the head coach to bump into the sports scientist.

Having just one place for people to get coffee, eat their lunch, and so on can yield unexpected benefits. This is why the Pixar headquarters has an atrium that houses a café, the building's only restrooms, and, of course, a theater. Steve Jobs biographer Walter Isaacson writes that Jobs wanted the building's design to be such that it "promoted encounters and unplanned collaborations."[29]

Of course, not every sports team has the resources to spend $88 million on a brand-new HQ. But it is possible to create something close to the Apple leader's vision simply by putting offices close together, removing "department X is over here, department Y is over there" divisions, and designating a single space for communal gathering. Doing so will improve problem-solving, discourage insecurity, and promote faster, more collaborative decision-making.

THE OPERATION WAS A SUCCESS ... BUT THE PATIENT DIED

19.4

Some teams invest a lot of time, effort, and money in building a sports science program and then spend even more time bragging to the media about how forward-thinking they are because of it. But if you're not winning more games, then you're just showing off and this fancy sports science department isn't delivering anything of true value. In other words, the operation was a success, but the patient died.

There's a belief in elite-level sports that sports science can fix just about anything and can create a team of super athletes who are fitter, better prepared, and more durable than any of their competitors. Not so. What effective sports science does is to bring together an understanding of how the body works and an interpretation of research that helps the coaching staff solve on-field performance issues. But just knowing that manipulating diet and sleep can increase testosterone, for example, doesn't make stronger athletes. The coaches still have to implement this knowledge in their preparation plans and the athletes still have to lift the weights. Sports science alone is never enough, and overreliance on it to produce innovation sets an unrealistic expectation for everyone.

One of the biggest trends in sports science over the past few years has been so-called injury prediction. I say "so-called" because this concept is a fine example of the emperor's new clothes: there's really nothing there. Imagine the coaching staff sitting in the boardroom with the medical and performance teams to see which players are available for the upcoming weekend's game. The physical thera-

pist and doctor agree that the star player still hasn't recovered from injury and will have to sit out at least one more game. Everyone starts mumbling and grumbling except the sports scientist, hunched over a laptop in a corner of the room, who shouts, "Yes, I predicted that." If computer modeling had done such a great job of predicting the player's injury and long layoff, surely they would have intervened and taken action before the injury occurred.

SMALL IS BIG

19.4.1

There's a common misconception that if you hire two people to do the job currently done by one person, tasks will get done faster. This is the myth that productivity is a simple calculation of division. In reality, it never works out this way, as both people will ease their feet off the gas pedal because they know that there's someone else to rely on for part of the load. Software engineer Frederick Brooks coined the phrase "mythical man-month," noting that "adding manpower to a late software project makes it later."[30]

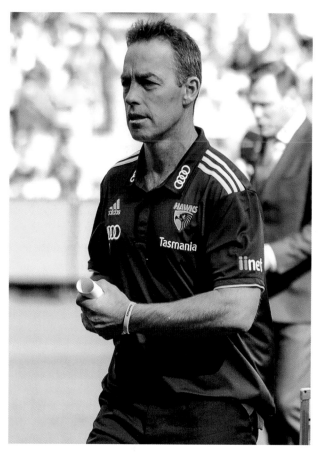

Alastair Clarkson. Photo by Flickerd (CC BY-SA).

> *Small groups of people can have a really huge impact.*

—Larry Page

In sports, bigger is rarely better when it comes to building a back-office staff. With a small group, if there needs to be water on the team bus, someone will put it there. Or if someone's out sick, one of that person's colleagues will step up and cover their responsibilities for a few days. You don't usually have to create a job or title to plug the gaps. If your organization already has a big head count, then try creating smaller teams that are independent and interdependent. This will ensure that you don't become mired in bureaucracy or the painstakingly slow decision-making that often characterizes large companies.

RELATIONSHIPS IN SMALL GROUPS   19.4.2

There's a reason that start-up companies often sell people on their culture when they're unable to compete for potential hires on salary or benefits—because when they say things like "Relationships matter here," it's typically true. In a small group, it's easier for people to get to know one another and to develop deeper connections instead of just knowing names and saying hi to a lot of colleagues, as happens at larger organizations. Think of the difference between the small back-office team and a monolithic group as the difference between talking to and regularly meeting with two or three friends you've had since high school and casually liking the posts of eight hundred Facebook "friends."

THE RESPONSIBILITY OF SMALL GROUPS   19.4.3

In a big bureaucracy, there are lots of layers and often entire classes of job titles that do nothing but assign work to other people. In a small group, everyone has

to be a producer and the structure has to be relatively flat because there's a lot to do and not much time to do it. This is why members of a small group feel a responsibility to do their jobs to the best of their ability and do whatever they can to help their colleagues do their jobs well, too. When you truly know and care about the people you work with, you're bound to be invested in their success and the achievements of the team as a whole—there's a sense of camaraderie that's difficult to replicate in a huge multilayered organization in which people barely know each other or what other people do.

THE SPEED OF SMALL   19.4.4

On the field, athletes don't have time to think before they act—execution needs to be automatic and unconscious. While the need for quick action isn't quite as urgent for coaching, medical, and support staff, they still need to move rapidly if the organization is to stay ahead of the competition. This is why, when you're putting together a small team, it needs to be composed of decisive, confident, and independent people who can think for themselves and take advantage of the speed of small. In small groups, communication is faster, autonomy is a given, and decision-making is decentralized, so there's no need to wait for permission or instructions before acting.

THE AGILITY OF SMALL   19.4.5

Soldiers must to be able to adapt standard operating procedures to the ever-changing reality of combat. The same is true of sports organizations, which need to be nimble enough to make adjustments and change tactics on the fly. When you have a large back-office

> *Man's achievements rest upon the use of symbols.... We must consider ourselves as a symbolic, semantic class of life, and those who rule the symbols, rule us.*

—Alfred Korzybski

staff, its very size creates delays. If you need to convene a meeting of ten or twelve people to make every decision or ask for the head coach's seal of approval on every detail, you're going to slow decision-making to a glacial pace, waste people's time, and reduce productivity. In contrast, small teams whose members have the authority to make independent decisions and who can collaborate with one or two other colleagues to problem-solve are better positioned to adapt to and thrive in changeable conditions.

> *I studied Italian five hours a day for many months to ensure I could communicate with the players, media and fans.*
>
> —José Mourinho

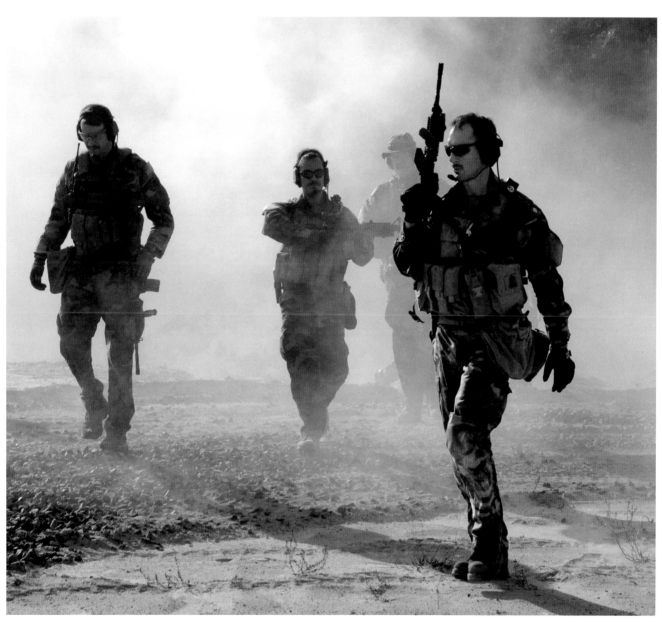

Navy SEALs conducting drills at the John C. Stennis Space Center.

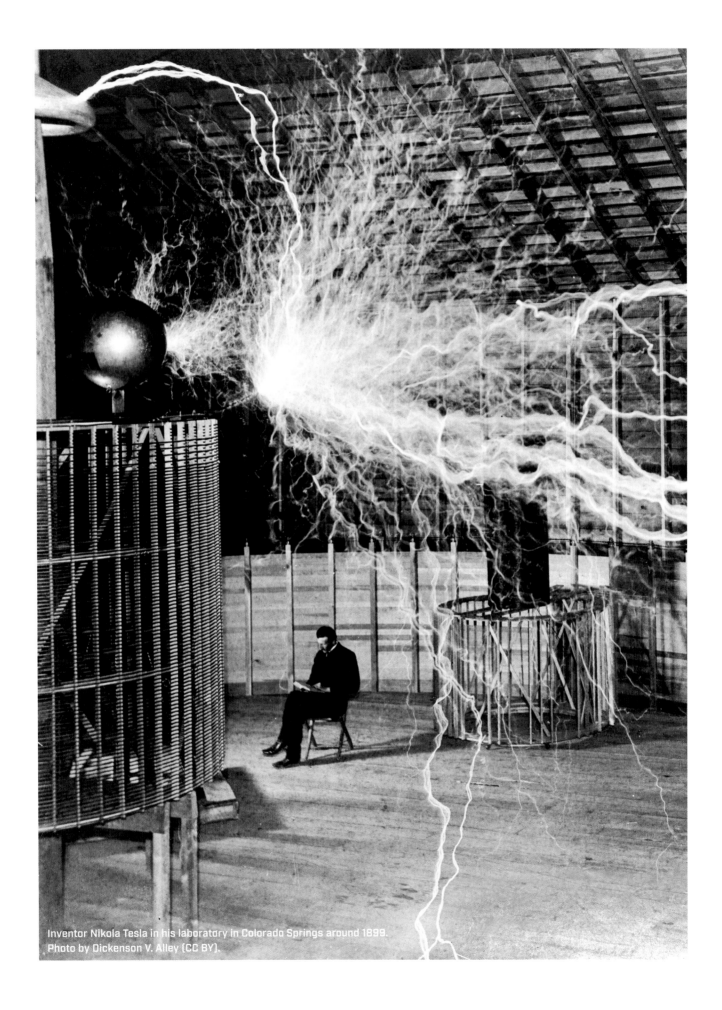

Inventor Nikola Tesla in his laboratory in Colorado Springs around 1899.
Photo by Dickenson V. Alley (CC BY).

TWENTY

INNOVATION AND THE NINE MOST-USED WORDS

The nine most-used words in coaching are, "Because this is the way it's always been done"—but that attitude often gets in the way of making real improvements. The way around this is to know what you can change and what you can't before trying to innovate. On the court, all the basketball players know that if they knock the ball past the sidelines or end lines, their team will lose possession. It's little different in an organizational setting: everybody must know where the boundaries are and what the consequences are for exceeding them. They can then start looking within the lines for opportunities to change the team's approach in small ways.

RULE BENDERS · 20.1

The media often portrays an innovator as someone who creates something new. This is occasionally the case, but many times an innovator is a person who takes something that already exists, sees its shortcomings, and improves it in a way that hasn't been done or maybe even thought of before. For example, James Dyson looked at the vacuum cleaner and saw the inefficiency of bags that lose suction, the issue with a short cord, and the trouble with ineffective accessory tools. So he fixed each of these issues to create the cyclone vacuum cleaner. He bent the rules of industrial design without breaking any.

The same should be true of creative sports organizations. They can look for the opportunities to exploit within the boundaries of the rules. Some sports-

writers complained that the Golden State Warriors' approach of launching umpteen three-pointers and playing the "death lineup" of five small, versatile players instead of the traditional two big forwards "broke basketball" or was some kind of "cheat code." Really, all the team did was look at how playing big guys slowed down the offense, the damage human Swiss Army knife Draymond Green could do in a free-flowing offense, and how Steph Curry and Klay Thompson could dismantle virtually any defense with their long-range shooting, and then tried an experiment. Teams in any sport can be just as bold and creative. There's no rule saying that you have to stick with something if it doesn't work for you.

CHEATING OR TRYING · 20.1.1

People who are willing to cheat lack the integrity and honesty needed to be positive contributors to the organization. By all means, bring in and encourage those who will go right up to the line of what's acceptable and what isn't, but make it clear that team members must never go over the line, even for a moment. There's no such thing as small-scale rule-breaking—if someone goes just an inch over the line, then they'll soon be willing to go a mile. Just as small keystone habits can have an outsize positive effect on a team's entire culture, so too can seemingly minor ethical and moral transgressions foreshadow bigger problems that are just around the corner. As we've seen in recent years in state-sponsored doping in Russia and the prevalence of performance-enhancing drugs in cycling, "win at all costs" is not a healthy or sustainable mantra in sports.

SETTLERS GET THE GOLD

20.2

If you study the development of the western United States, you quickly discover that there was a profound difference between the pioneers who went into the unknown in the late 1700s, those who traveled the Oregon and California Trails in the mid 1800s, and the settlers of the California Gold Rush era. The first two groups endured unbelievable hardship, disease, an unforgiving landscape, and conflict with Native Americans in their journey to settle the frontier. They received little material reward for their great labors, and many thousands died long before reaching their destination. It wasn't until 1848, when James W. Marshall discovered unusually shiny rocks while building a sawmill at Sutter's Creek in California, that the gold rush began and settlers started profiting from frontier land.

The same applies to team sports. It's the settlers who get the gold, not the pioneers. Coaches, players, and the media get excited about the promise of new technology, training techniques, and analysis, but the teams on the bleeding edge rarely reap the most benefits from these because they're the ones doing the trial-and-error work of figuring out how best to use innovations. It isn't until there's more data available and best practices have been created that organizations can start to profit from their own type of gold rush. This is why the head coach must dismiss his or her FOMO (fear of missing out) instinct and invest in initiatives that have been proven to improve performance.

TECHNOLOGY

20.2.1

In his landmark business book *Good to Great,* Jim Collins writes that "thoughtless reliance on technology is a liability."[31] Though the first edition was released fifteen years ago, Collins's assertion is still correct. You simply cannot spend big on technology on the assumption that there will be a return on your investment. In a reductionist approach, teams try to apply technology to improve certain isolated characteristics—usually physical ones—expecting that it will magically lead to better athletes. This is a fallacy.

Again, we have to start with the game and work backward. How will the items on a high-tech wish list positively impact elements of the team's game-time performance, and are there any problems with this area that actually need solving? Just because every other team is investing in activity trackers, sleep monitors, or other technology doesn't mean that they're gaining an advantage from doing so, and even if they are, the same gear might not work for your organization. Instead of giving in to a "me, too" mindset, first figure out what you're trying to achieve, and *then,* if necessary, find the gizmos and gadgets that fit the bill.

ANALYTICS

20.3

The analysis of data and statistics has become a major talking point in sport in recent years. In many if not most cases, it has yet to provide a distinct advantage in team sports, and it's certainly questionable in field sports.

BIG DATA

20.3.1

Big Data is one of the most overhyped and overrated buzz phrases in business and sports alike. It refers to the belief that there are hidden insights to be gained from studying and analyzing large swaths of data. For example, if a large shopping chain analyzes its sales data, it can find demographic trends for who buys at certain times or who buys certain products, and it can then tailor advertising to maximize their sales. And in true FOMO spirit, every organization thinks that they need to adopt Big Data or fall behind their competitors. As Dan Ariely, professor of psychology and behavioral economics at Duke University, puts it, "Big data is like teenage sex: everyone talks about it, nobody really knows how to do it, everyone thinks everyone else is doing it, so everyone claims they are doing it."[32]

Amid the continuing frenzy to gather as much information as possible, research group IDC predicts that spending on Big Data will balloon to $48.6 billion by 2019.[33] Elite sports teams are all in, with one report estimating that they'll spend up to $4.7 billion on analytics by 2021.[34] Part of the problem with such a huge investment is that in their eagerness to gather as much data as possible, teams are forgetting how small the sample sizes are: only 446 players compete in the NBA, 500 in the English Premier League, 700 in the Rugby World Cup, and 1,696 in the NFL. This isn't 1 percent of the population but 1 percent of 1 percent! From a scientific standpoint, trying to draw definitive conclusions about so many variables from such a tiny sample is preposterous. And if the conclusions drawn from analytics were rock solid, we'd no longer have humans coaching sports teams but would leave it to computers.

And yet sports teams continue to look at the success of Billy Beane's analytical innovations at the Oakland A's and think that they have to get on board with Big Data, immediately. But in the best-selling book that details Beane's approach, Michael Lewis's *Moneyball,* it's clear that Beane wasn't focused on just harvesting a ton of numbers for the sake of it, in keeping with a misguided "more is better" philosophy, as is often the way with Big Data. Instead, Beane's initiative was about capturing a very select set of data points that were directly applicable to on-field performance. In other words, he was focusing not on Big Data but on Agile Data.

A leader is best when people barely know he exists. When his work is done, his aim fulfilled, they will say: we did it ourselves.

—Lao Tzu

AGILE DATA   20.3.2

The biggest difference between Big Data and Agile Data, other than the fact that with Agile Data less information is collected, is that the latter seeks to solve a specific problem or answer a certain question with numbers, while the former is about gathering as much information as possible, taking the view that we'll figure out how to apply it later. I made the point earlier that you don't mess with a technical, tactical, physical, or psychological element unless it's a limiting factor on the field. We need to take a similar approach with Agile Data. Unless a data point can provide a solid answer to a predefined question and in doing so give us an edge during a game, it's a waste of everyone's time and money to crunch the numbers.

If your team is going to use a data-driven approach to tackle an issue, it's best to follow the scrum methodology that software companies—particularly fast-moving start-ups—utilize to great effect. This involves developing a new product quickly, launching it, and then improving it in response to users' experiences with frequent updates. In sports, coaches need to have something good enough that they can use now, rather than waiting months for the best possible solution. This is an organizational variation of the morphological programming approach that we apply to player preparation, in which you're constantly adapting to changing conditions and new challenges that arise.

PROBLEM-SOLVING VS. RESEARCH   20.3.3

Often when I tell people about my work with sports teams, they say, "Oh, so you must do a ton of research." This is another big misunderstanding about the role of sports scientists. Their function is not to conduct research studies at all, which would be impossible during the competitive season and whose results might not be clear or applicable for years. Rather, the sports scientist's mandate is to find information that can help solve performance problems and improve decision-making, distill their findings into layman's terms, and convey them to the coaching staff so that they can apply them to their athletes. The information has to be tightly focused, appropriate, and actionable, or else it's irrelevant. If sports scientists can't explain research findings so that they're easily understood and the coaches can't use the information to construct learning experiences that better prepare the team for competition, what's the point?

PATHWAYS OF DEVELOPMENT   20.3.4

Though the pace of sports is relentless, the desire to do everything right now can be counterproductive. This is certainly true when it comes to implementing new technology, analytics, and sports science initiatives. In a basic experiment, scientists manipulate only a single variable, so that the cause-effect relationship is obvious. We should follow a similar method in sports. It's no good introducing two, three, or four new things because if the team's performance improves, you won't know which change caused the effect or to what degree.

It's better to prioritize around the biggest problem that the team is having and deploy the product, tool, or strategy that best addresses this need. This implementation should be gradual, and education needs to be a priority so that every department understands what's being done, why, and how to make the most of it. In my experiences with professional teams in every major field and court sport, it can take up to four years for a new initiative to reach its full potential impact. However, the best ones deliver results in year one if you can get a buy-in from the coaches and players and focus on the simplest application first. It drives me crazy when people say that the first twelve months should be spent on collecting data alone. If that's the case, then your team should fire its sports scientist!

THE AGGREGATION OF MARGINAL GAINS   20.3.5

The concept of the aggregation of marginal gains involves making tiny improvements in many areas, which over time adds up to a big overall improvement. One sports organization that has used this approach is the British cycling team Team Sky. When Dave Brailsford joined the team in 2010, it had never won a Tour de France title, and its management wanted to change that. Among other initiatives, Brailsford began looking for ways to improve small things by 1 percent—including elements of bike design, sleep habits, and nutrition—believing that there would be a cumulative effect on his cyclists' performance. Rather than taking the expected five years to turn the team around, it took Brailsford just two, with Bradley Wiggins claiming the Tour de France crown in 2012. That same year, Brailsford managed the British Olympic cycling team that claimed 70 percent of the gold medals at the London Olympics.[35]

It's undeniable that Brailsford proved to be a highly effective leader and that his strategy of making marginal gains paid great dividends for Team Sky and Team GB. And yet we can't overlook the fact that where these teams started also played a big part in where they ended up. First, Team Sky already had very talented riders—most notably Wiggins and fellow Tour de France winner Chris Froome—when Brailsford implemented his marginal gains aggregation strategy, and the British Olympic cycling team had topped the sport's medal table at the 2008 Beijing Olympics, too, with eight gold, four silver, and two bronze medals.

This is not to take anything away from Brailsford or his work, because he's an exceptional coach. But teams shouldn't try to copy what he did chapter and verse without first assessing where they find themselves on the road to excellence. Many poorly performing organizations are failing to live up to expectations not because of missed marginal gains but because one or several large issues are holding them back. They'd be well advised to identify and remove a

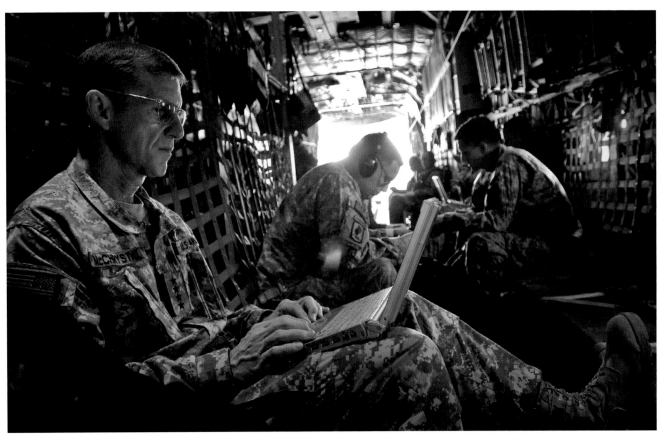

General Stanley A. McChrystal, now retired. His 2015 book *Team of Teams* shows how the best teams decentralize decision-making (see page 77).

small number of major roadblocks first, as doing so can lead to significant improvement. Then there will be a greater opportunity to take advantage of marginal gains. Before you can make marginal gains, you must have exhausted maximal gains.

UNDERSTANDING THE HUMAN-MACHINE INTERFACE

20.4

Now more than ever before, humans interact with technology regularly. This has created an interesting dynamic and raises questions about how important it is to ensure the interaction itself doesn't affect the outcomes. There can be misconceptions and false assumptions with any technology.

ARTIFICIAL INTELLIGENCE

20.4.1

Some technology devotees believe that artificial intelligence will eventually take over sports. They believe that all we need are the right models and a large enough amount of information. The flaw in this concept is that you cannot solve what you cannot understand. Is there the potential for technology to help coaches and staff make better decisions? Certainly—but only if the people working with those machines know which questions to ask and which problems need solving. At the other end of this topic is the fact that as technology becomes more sophisticated, the people who wield it need to increase their understanding in order to interpret the data. Searching for something on Google and getting twelve million results doesn't mean that you're closer to getting what you need; it just means that you have more information to sift through. This is why the human component of the human-machine interface will always be more important in sports.

WHAT ABOUT THE SINGULARITY?

20.4.2

Although futurist Ray Kurzweil believes that machines and humankind will eventually merge together and become indistinguishable—the singularity in action—it won't happen in sports in our lifetime on the level he predicts. Even the most expensive supercomputer can apply its processing power only if it's given the right instructions, providing the problem is understood first. A random generator program doesn't even really churn out a completely random sequence of numbers, because it needed a programmer to set the parameters. Kurzweil's line of thinking might be good fodder for science fiction writers, but in the real world of sports it is largely irrelevant.

One of the reasons that computers will never replace decision-making staff in the sports world, such as trainers, strength coaches, or sports coaches, is that we have such limited understanding about so many elements of the human body. Though our grasp of certain areas, like anatomy, is fairly solid, in so many others—neuroenterology, neurobiology, and genetics, for example—entire disciplines are still in their infancy. This lack of comprehension and the many knowledge gaps that might never be filled prevent us from creating accurate models for computers to use. Then there's the largely unquantifiable realm of emotion, mindset, and motivation, none of which can be reduced to lines of code or fit within convenient buckets.

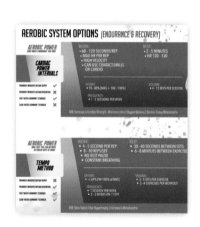

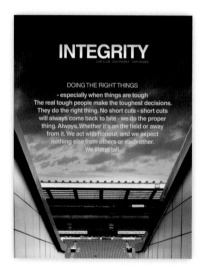

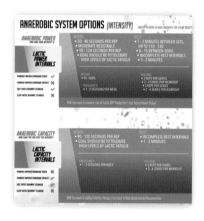

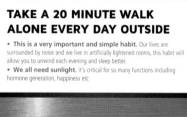

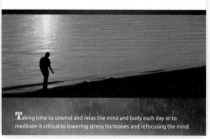

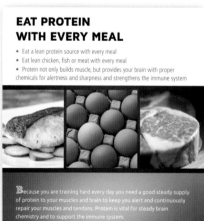

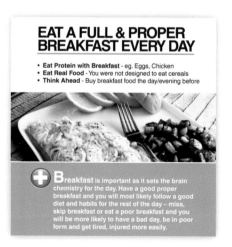

A small example of imagery used to create culture and educate.

IMPLEMENTATION

20.5

When it comes to making sports science actionable, coaches don't want to get into the nitty-gritty or sit through a seventy-eight-slide PowerPoint deck that the presenters think makes them sound smart. They typically want answers to just three simple questions: what is this rehab program or this strength program, why should we do it, and how will we do it?

As shown in the figure on page 396, there are three main applied performance pathways that can be implemented:

1. Mentored interim model: The implementation of a sports science model is often most successful with a mentor who has walked the path before. The professional growth of the sports scientist in the team environment is important to consider. Often, when an organization simply hires the "best" sports scientists, it ends up not having the desired effect because these people have to adjust to working at a slower speed and doing more mundane tasks than they have been used to. An apprentice-and-mentor model, however, in which more senior scientists train and mentor younger ones, can help avoid that pitfall. It also saves the organization money.

2. Sports science model: The traditional sports science models that teams have implemented until now have been very modular in their approach. This does "check the box": technically, the teams and players have sports-science services. However, this is not a very integrated system and is limited in its potential for growth.

3. Performance science model: A proper performance science model is much more comprehensive than a traditional one, specifically focused on improving performance and results, not on sports science for its own sake. It identifies problems and challenges and sources the best solutions using a combination of qualitative and quantitative approaches. A performance science model recognizes that only approaches that will positively affect the scoreboard should be applied.

The more complex the program is, the longer it will take to implement. However, the payoff for a more sophisticated model can be significantly greater. The team needs to consider its internal resources; the time investment needed up front, in the mid term, and in the long term; and how long the organization is willing to wait to see the program reach its ultimate potential. Another factor is how fast a competing team is typically able to deploy a similar model. (See the figures on page 396.)

"WHAT IS THIS PROGRAM?"

20.5.1

One of the most important skills a sports scientist can possess is the ability to take complex, research-driven concepts and put them into simple terms that the coaching staff can comprehend and convey to the players. If you can't explain the "what" inside a minute, then you need to simplify the plan and rethink how you frame it.

"WHY SHOULD WE DO IT?"

20.5.2

The head coach has an almost unlimited to-do list that includes items in just about every area of the organization. Anything new is going to cause some level of disruption, so the payoff needs to exceed the cost. If a sports science initiative solves a problem, creates an opportunity for improved game performance, and can be implemented with minimum upheaval, the coach is more likely to buy into it.

Lead me, follow me, or get out of my way.

—General George Patton

WORLD-LEADING APPLIED PERFORMANCE PATHWAY

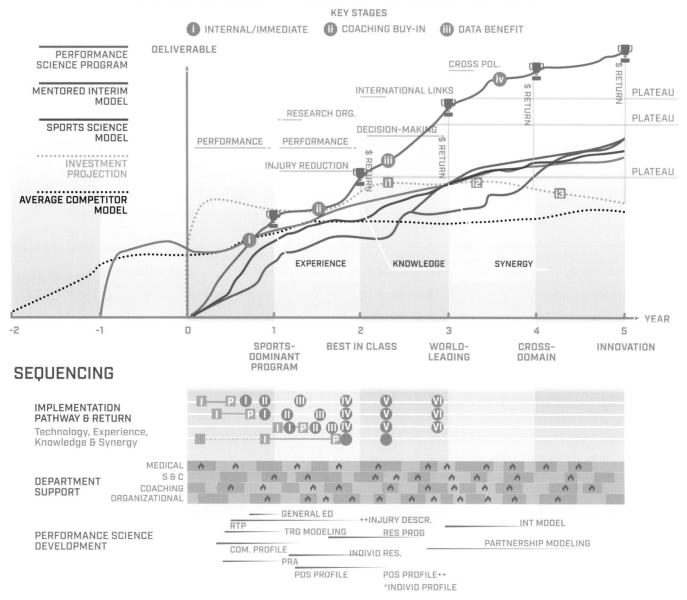

"HOW WILL WE GET A RETURN FROM IT?"   20.5.3

Sports scientists need to be innovative within reason and not out in the Wild West on their own. As we covered in "The Settlers Get the Gold," it's easier to figure out the "how" part of implementing a new technology or approach if it's in its second or third iteration, so you're not an early adopter who's going to spend a lot of time figuring things out through trial and error. When the head coach asks, "How will we get a return from it?" she's not going to want a rambling, unsure response but a definitive answer.

Ⓘ IMMEDIATE FEEDBACK
Ⓘ COMPARISON & CONTEXT
Ⓘ INTEGRATION
Ⓘ STATISTICAL ANALYSIS
Ⓥ DATA RG ANALYSIS

> *The best executive is the one who has sense enough to pick good men to do what he wants done, and self-restraint enough to keep from meddling with them while they do it.*
>
> —Theodore Roosevelt

TWENTY-ONE

GROUP PSYCHOLOGY

In this section, we're going to explore how individuals behave in group settings, how the team should and should not communicate with the outside world (media, fans, etc.), and how such messaging can positively or negatively affect the team's mindset. We'll also discuss the importance of creating a common identity and sense of family within the organization, some new ways to think about leadership in a team context, and the significance of body language and other nonverbal cues in impacting the mood in the locker room. In addition, I'll share how the best teams in the world create a distinctive brand and identity and ensure current players understand their role in continuing the team's legacy. We'll also examine how different belief systems manifest themselves in the team setting, how Maslow's hierarchy of needs comes into play, and the vital importance of values in creating and sustaining a winning culture.

EXTERNAL AND INTERNAL MESSAGES

21.1

In today's sports-obsessed culture, every word a head coach says is captured and broadcast and can have a positive or negative impact on the team. Sometimes there's a need to look at internal messaging a little differently from external messaging, but they should still be unified and clear. For example, if your organization has an innovative sports science facility, like the Milan Lab at AC Milan, you'll want to tell the players that they have the best facilities in the world, because they need to feel like they're well prepared and taken care of. You'd give a similar message to the media, but for a different purpose—to make opposing coaches and players fear that your preparation is superior to theirs. The delivery might vary slightly to suit each purpose, but you're essentially saying the same thing to different audiences. The myth that your team is the best (whether the myth is true or not) remains unchanged.

In "The Player," I explained why a clear, coherent, and cohesive message has to be communicated to the players about the game plan, Commander's Intent, and objectives for each game moment. The same must be true of the messages communi-

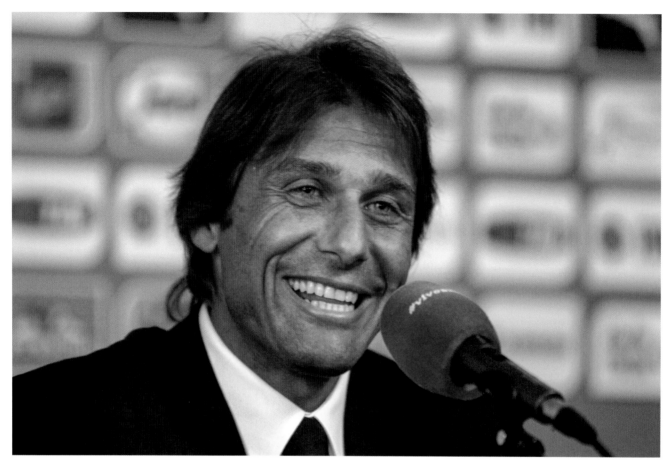

Antonio Conte. Photo by Marco Iacobucci EPP / Shutterstock.com.

cated inside the organization and to the outside world. One of the reasons that certain managers are accused of giving boring interviews is that they know the importance of reinforcing the same points over and over. So if the team's priority on offense is to move the ball quickly and unselfishly, the manager might say either that the team did this well or that "we need to improve our ball movement before the next game." The latter variation would not only reinforce the principle of ball movement to any player who's watching but also prepare them to work on it in the upcoming morphocycle.

In addition, media-savvy coaches recognize that while they might not want to watch themselves talking on TV, their players and staff often do. If the coach says something that undermines the team's mission or values, it's going to sow doubt in people's minds. This is why it's better for a coach to say almost the same thing in every pregame and postgame interview than to lapse into a stream of consciousness and deliver headline-grabbing sound bites that are off message and can do more harm inside the organization than outside it.

Finally, a press conference or interview is another opportunity to reinforce the principles of winning teams. For example, the head coach can show humility by giving credit to the players after a win and by taking responsibility for a loss without blaming the squad. This enhances the feeling of trust between players and coaches. England rugby coach Eddie Jones is a master in this area. Will Greenwood, who earned fifty-five caps for the England team, wrote that Jones "has protected all his players by making sure that all of the media spotlight is on him. He has consistently got the narrative exactly where he wanted it. Rod Kafer, the former Wallaby, reckons there has not been one negative article or comment about an English player. He's a media black belt. Mischievous, charming, always putting pressure back on the opposition."[36]

PHYSIOLOGY OF PSYCHOLOGY

Empowering your team to make decisions, take ownership of their area of expertise, and take risks is another way to make them happy. According to a Gallup poll, 24 percent of workers feel "actively disengaged" in their jobs—in other words, they don't like where they work and have checked out. A further 63 percent reported being "not engaged" in what they do.[37] This means almost nine out of ten people either dislike or hate their job! This cannot be the case at a winning organization.

BE PASSIONATE

It's all too easy to point fingers at players for not listening or appearing bored, but their level of engagement starts with the head coach's demeanor (although banning cell phones from team meetings might not be a bad idea). As Bill Walsh writes in *The Score Takes Care of Itself,* "Your enthusiasm becomes their enthusiasm; your lukewarm presentation becomes their lukewarm interest in what you're offering.... When the audience is bored, it's not their fault."[38]

Passion starts with thankfulness. If coaches are grateful to be doing what they enjoy every day, then this sentiment will show. If the leader is positive and energetic, this is contagious and impacts everyone else.

WATCH YOUR POSTURE

There's a reason that members of the military are expected to carry themselves with an upright posture instead of slouching. It not only means that they're in a position of physical readiness but also conveys strength, confidence, and control of the environment. An excerpt from a 1946 U.S. Army training manual lists another important reason for soldiers to maintain an organized bearing: "It is an accepted psychological fact that good posture is associated with good morale—a man with a good posture feels better and is more positive."[39] Indeed, research shows that maintaining good posture makes people feel more confident and reduces the number of negative thoughts. So there's a real connection between how we stand and move and our brain chemistry.[40]

The posture of a head coach can be just as influential as that of a four-star general. This is particularly apparent in the locker room before a game, at halftime, and after the final whistle has blown. How coaches carry themselves can either reinforce a positive message or undermine it. If they hang their heads when the team is losing, it will be difficult to inspire a comeback. Similarly, if the head coach comes in and slumps in the corner after the team loses, the game can't be framed as anything other than a crushing defeat. As we've seen from neurologist Robert Sapolsky, every tribe looks to its alpha members to set the tone for behavior and attitude. So coaches need to ensure that their body language is united with their verbal message.

SMILE

Facial expressions are another important element of nonverbal communication that head coaches can use to impact their own mood and that of the players and staff. The simple act of smiling prompts our brain to release stress-fighting neuropeptides, serotonin, endorphins, and dopamine.[41] And the benefits of smiling don't stop with the individual. A Swedish study showed that participants who were shown pictures of people grinning were more likely to mirror this with their own smiles than to display any other facial expression.[42]

USE POSITIVE LANGUAGE

Clearly, body language is very important when it comes to creating and sustaining excellence. But coaches also need to back this up with what they say. Positive reinforcement, publicly recognizing outstanding contributions, and offering encouragement (especially in difficult circumstances) can all help people feel special. When researching their book *How Full Is Your Bucket,* Tom Rath and Donald Clifton found that when leaders made a habit of praising their staff, it increased productivity and engagement with colleagues, improved loyalty, and led people to stay in their jobs longer.[43]

CULT AND BELIEF

21.3

One of the biggest surprise stories in modern team sports was Kevin Durant's decision to leave the Oklahoma City Thunder and join the team that the Thunder had pushed to seven games in the 2015–16 NBA playoffs, the Golden State Warriors. During the introductory press conference with his new team, Durant shared that a big factor in his decision was the family-like relationship among the Warriors players who pitched the trade to him: "To see them together, they were almost holding hands…it was all about family." The Warriors' Andre Iguodala told him, "It will be the most fun you've had in your life." Durant decided that despite his strong community ties in Oklahoma City and the success he'd had there—winning the league MVP award and guiding the team to the NBA Finals—the chance to be part of the Warriors' close-knit group was too great to pass up.[44] The same is true when it comes to coaches and staff. An organization with a stellar reputation hardly needs to recruit because the kind of talented, self-motivated winners they want to bring in already have the team on their radar.

ADVENTURE AND FUN

21.3.1

Explorers like Ernest Shackleton and Edmund Hillary didn't cross frozen wilderness or climb the world's highest peaks to get their names in newspaper headlines. Rather, it was their sense of adventure that motivated them to try expeditions that nobody had successfully completed before. If a sports team is going to keep improving, pushing forward, and striving for greatness, the game can't become a grind. There needs to be a sense of fun and enjoyment in the journey itself. This is not to say that there won't be times when, as for those famous explorers, things go wrong, conditions get tough, and people think about turning back. But it's the relentless pursuit of a goal—the sports equivalent of summiting a mountain peak or reaching a pole—and the adventure along the way that will keep everyone going.

COMMITMENT TO IDEALS

21.3.2

When he said, "Once a Raider, always a Raider," Oakland Raiders coach and owner Al Davis wasn't expressing wishful thinking or hollow sentiment but rather an ideal that resonated among former players and staff. Even those who didn't play for the team for very long echo Davis's line. "Being a former Raider, it's always in you," said Bucky Brooks, who suited up for the Raiders for just half a season. "It never changes. Silver and Black 'til I die."[45] Eddie DeBartolo is still held in almost a religious regard by players of the San Francisco 49ers. His caring nature, fun personality, loyalty, and generosity are still spoken of by those who played decades before.

The key takeaway is that a successful sports organization has to have higher ideals and get personnel to commit to them, whether that's players on the field, coaches on the sideline, or staff at the ticket counter—not to mention, of course, fans in the stands.

LEGACY

21.3.3

At SEAL Qualification Training graduation, newly minted Navy SEALs are presented with a knife that bears the name of a former SEAL and where he was killed in action on the blade.[46] The knife presentation is this elite special operation group's way of conveying the weight and importance of legacy throughout the generations. While a sports team might not have a ritual that carries similar significance, they can do certain things in a way that emphasizes the lessons that can be learned from previous players and coaches.

Certain shirt numbers are also strongly tied with legacies. LeBron James and, late in his career, David Beckham adopted the number 23 jersey in honor of the most legendary number 23 of them all, Michael Jordan. Beckham also wore the hallowed number 7 shirt at Manchester United, which club legends George Best, Eric Cantona, and Bryan Robson had previously worn and which Cristiano Ronaldo would later inherit.

One of the most important things about legacy is that it takes the focus off the individual and places it on history and heritage. It also encourages players and staff to try to live up to the accomplishments of those who have gone before them and to look to the past for inspiration.

Leaders aren't born, they are made. And they are made just like anything else, through hard work. And that's the price we'll have to pay to achieve that goal, or any goal.

—Vince Lombardi

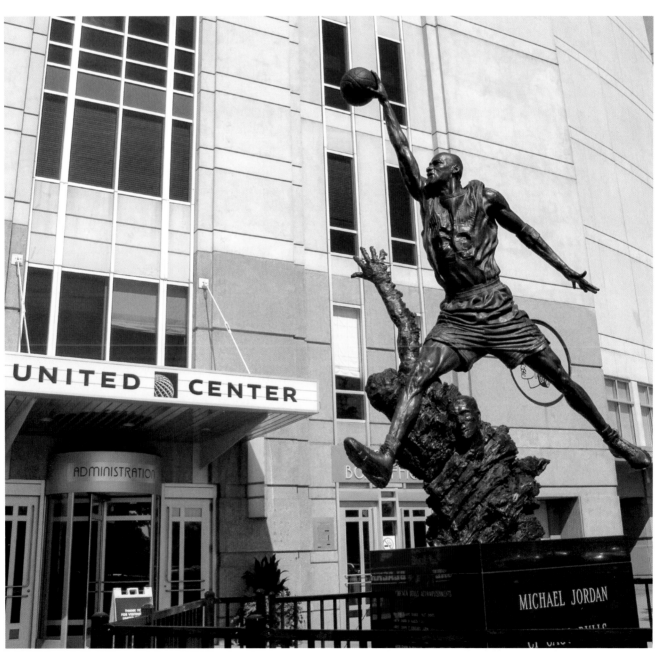

The statue of Michael Jordan outside the United Center sports arena in Chicago. Photo by Zarah Vila / Shutterstock.com.

THE SUCCESS BRAND

========= 21.4

Why do sports-related brands like Nike and Gatorade pay top athletes so much money to represent them? Part of it is name recognition and getting their gear shown on TV. But the main reason is that they want people to associate them with these individuals' success. Ad campaigns that resonate with the public are typically aspirational and/or motivational—"Be Like Mike" or "Just Do It"—but a tagline or cool graphic alone won't sell more drinks or shoes. You need to add a champion like Michael Jordan, LeBron James, or Serena Williams to the mix to connect aspiration and motivation to success.

Sports organizations can learn a lot from this approach. Some teams play up the storied history of their stadiums—like the Boston Red Sox's Fenway Park, Liverpool's Anfield, and England Rugby's Twickenham. Doing so ties in to the concept that I introduced in "The Gift of Fear" (page 372): opposing teams coming to these grounds are meant to be fearful and intimidated. Other teams gain an advantage in the transfer/free-agent market by selling a proven track record and the allure of playing for a legendary coach. The chance to become part of an organization with a longstanding reputation for excellence can trump more lucrative offers from other clubs, particularly for veterans looking to win late in their careers—the San Antonio Spurs, Manchester United, and the New England Patriots all excel in this area. If your team can create a brand built around success, then players, staff, and fans will come.

THE PSYCHOLOGY OF TRIBE

========= 21.5

I covered this topic from the standpoint of evolutionary biology in "The Player," but the psychology of tribe also impacts the coach and the organization, in different ways. The first is that all tribes look for natural leaders within their ranks. It could be a head coach who is physically imposing and dominant, like Mike Ditka, or a strict disciplinarian, like Bear Bryant. Or perhaps the identity of the team is best reflected by a more methodical and studious leader, like Steve Kerr, or someone who can switch between being hard-driving in practice and being gregarious when talking to the press, like Jürgen Klopp. No matter what a coach's demeanor and style is, players and staff will look to them for guidance.

It's also possible, of course, for players to set the tone. Think of Ray Lewis's pregame antics or the collective intimidation factor that the All Blacks' haka (based on a traditional Maori war dance) creates. The very act of a player putting on her shirt before a game can be likened to a superhero donning a cape. The fans themselves get in on the act by wearing their team's jersey with almost equal pride, painting their faces like they're trying to audition for a remake of *Braveheart,* and even getting team-focused tattoos. The head coach needs to understand what the primary traits of the team's tribe are and respect these traits as they apply their own approach.

A HIGHER PURPOSE

================================== 21.6

It's a basic human desire to want to belong to a group that has shared beliefs—it's a major reason for membership in religious organizations, for example. Some individual athletes have vocally shared that they are motivated by serving a higher power, perhaps most notably Muhammad Ali. While team members who share a faith can bond through this affiliation, the team itself can provide a similar affinity for those who have no religious or spiritual beliefs. This is not to say that team spirit should or does take the place of faith in a higher power, but rather that full dedication to a greater purpose can meet the need for belonging and change the self-centered focus that can be so destructive within an organization.

GROUP BELIEF SYSTEMS

================================== 21.7

Having worked closely with special operations groups in the U.S. and the U.K., I've seen firsthand that their basic training programs are not designed to break people. Yes, they are supposed to be physically demanding, but this is merely one small part of the picture. Those few who make it through Hell Week for the SAS, the Marines, or the Navy SEALs create an unbreakable bond forged by suffering together. All those who complete this rite of passage join an exclusive club whose members recognize the sacrifice it took to become truly elite and to have earned the insignia on their uniforms. Such special operations groups live by a code and a set of beliefs that inform everything they do, and they are conditioned to act as one on the battlefield.

A successful sports organization needs to establish and protect a similar culture and ensure that every person in the club buys into it. People need to know that "this is the way we do things here" and that the way the team practices, plays, and carries itself reflects unique principles that are on display for all to see. This can be reinforced by rituals, pregame and postgame routines, and ceremonies for players and staff.

> To have long-term success as a coach or in any position of leadership, you have to be obsessed in some way.
>
> —Pat Riley

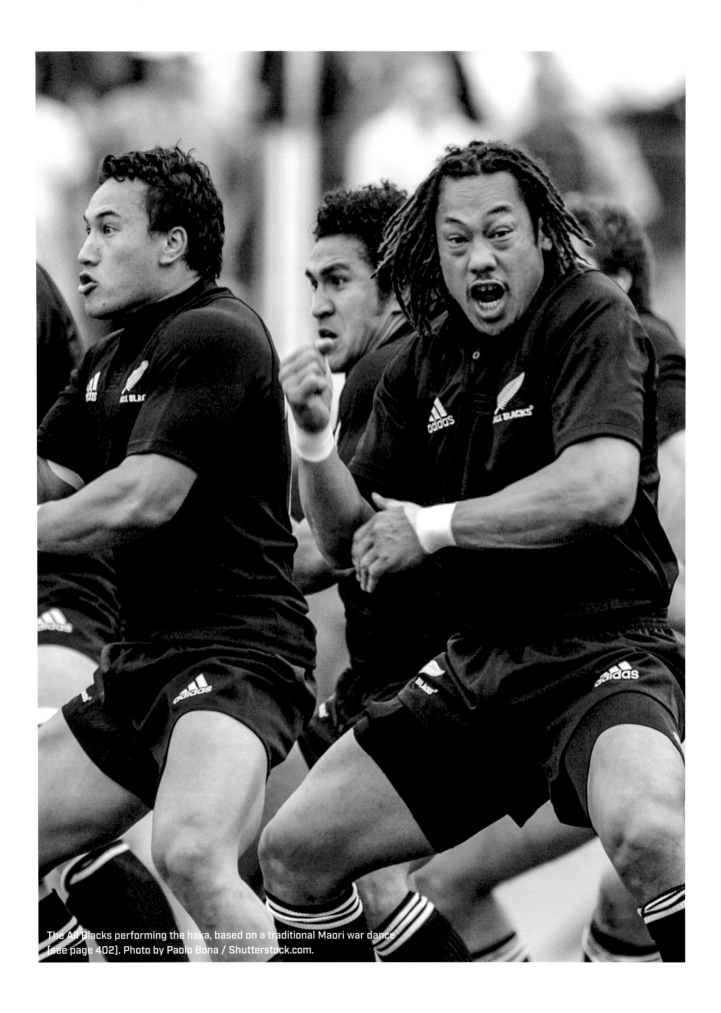

The All Blacks performing the haka, based on a traditional Maori war dance (see page 402). Photo by Paolo Bona / Shutterstock.com.

TWENTY-TWO

THE CULTURE MODEL

One of the most misused words in both sport and business is *culture*—as much as it's thrown around, it's not understood by many. Culture is undoubtedly important and critical to success and affects all aspects of performance, but how to develop it has not been well understood.

HIERARCHY OF NEEDS

22.1

One of the fundamental purposes of military training is to get recruits to override their instinct to meet their own personal needs. For a combat unit to simply survive the mission, let alone execute its orders, its members must put the good of their comrades above their own safety. This is why you hear stories of soldiers throwing themselves on grenades—their desire to protect their brothers has overcome their need for self-preservation. In a sports setting, teammates might not die for one another, but they do need to be willing to sacrifice their own selfish needs and wants for the good of the team.

THE BELIEF PRINCIPLE

22.2

One key way that a culture—or team—defines and distinguishes itself is through a set of ideas that are held in common. Shared beliefs can drive the thoughts and actions of an organization's members in the same direction, toward the Commander's Intent and the mission objectives. Beliefs also provide a moral compass that guides everyone to make the best decisions with good intentions.

THE VALUE PRINCIPLE   22.2.1

The beliefs of a team inform and help determine its values and the way its personnel view their jobs and the world. The side blocks that hold John Wooden's Pyramid of Success in place are values that any organization would do well to cultivate, including honesty, sincerity, patience, and reliability. If these guide every individual interaction, decision, and action, then group success is almost inevitable. Following are the four main ways values can be affected:

- *Moralizing:* "Do as I say"—giving verbal instruction, such as, "You must treat each other with respect." Moralizing can get quick results among those who welcome structure and respect authority, but it usually fails to win over those who like to think for themselves.

- *Modeling:* "Do as I do"—leading by example. This style takes longer to show results but can be more effective in the long run than moralizing.

- *Experimenting:* "You figure it out"—laissez-faire leadership, in which several concepts are introduced and then people are left to go their own way. Exploratory learners gravitate to this style.

- *Clarifying:* "We're going to meet to talk about our values." This approach reiterates what the leaders believe and what the organization stands for. Clarifying can be combined with the previous three styles to great effect. Unlike with moralizing, here the group together explores and investigates what the values of the team mean to each person.

Some values that you might want your organization to emphasize, using one or more of these methods, include:

integrity

leadership

discipline

courage

respect

innovation

loyalty

teamwork

humility

fortitude

honor

commitment

service

excellence

legacy

professionalism

Of course, you don't want to create an exhaustive list like this and expect people to remember it; instead, pick three to five core values that you feel embody your organization's beliefs and reiterate them through modeling and clarifying throughout the season. On this topic of keystone values, Winston Churchill said (paraphrasing Samuel Johnson), "Courage is rightly esteemed the first of human qualities because, as has been said, it is the quality which guarantees all others."

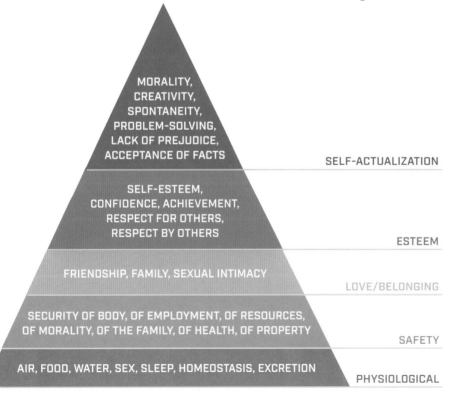

HOLISTIC PLAYER WELLNESS MODEL

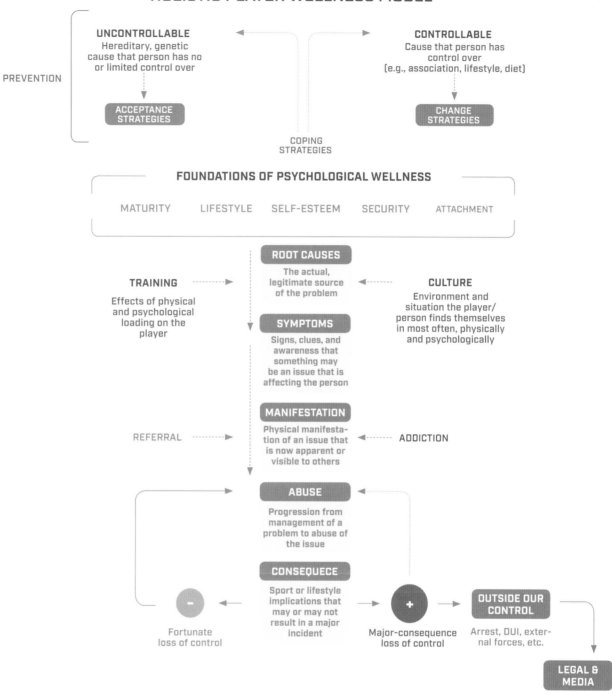

THE ATTITUDE PRINCIPLE

22.2.2

If beliefs help determine values, then values influence and inform attitude. For example, going back to Wooden's pyramid, the belief that caring for others is important elevates the value of humility, which fosters an attitude of cooperation and helpfulness. Attitude is the spirit in which members of the organization perform their tasks and interact with each other every day.

THE BEHAVIOR MICRO PRINCIPLE

22.2.3

When you visit a team, you'll usually form an opinion about its culture based on two things. First is the behavior and actions of the people you meet and how they treat you. Behavior is the combination of beliefs, values, and attitude put into action. There are four main techniques that leaders use to mold the behavior of those they work with:

- *Demand it:* "I'm in charge, and this is how we do things." This authoritarian technique is effective with rule followers and those who respect or even crave discipline. It's not so effective with creative personality types.

- *Ceremony:* "These are the special things we do here." Ceremonies can be a useful way to create togetherness and reinforce an "it's us against the world" mentality, which can lead to improved effort.

- *Conditional:* "If you do this, then you'll be rewarded." This is an effective motivational approach for those who are extrinsically motivated, like salespeople who enjoy the challenge of chasing a quarterly bonus. However, intrinsically motivated individuals won't need or respond well to this kind of incentive-based method.

- *Teach:* "This is why we should behave like this, and these are the benefits." This final tactic appeals to those who continually seek to learn more and are never satisfied with their most recent achievements.

THE ARTIFACTS MICRO PRINCIPLE   22.2.4

The second thing that impacts how you perceive an organization's culture is the artifacts you encounter. These are tangible and visual things, like the appearance of the team facilities, the uniforms of the players and staff, and the cleanliness of the locker rooms.

This area is often overlooked by teams and organizations, yet it has an important impact on a person's perception of culture. Most of us know exactly what it means to walk into a restaurant or hotel and get a sense of the type of place it is, a feeling of what is

essentially its culture. That sense comes from a combination of the attitude and behavior of the staff and the artifacts (the building and the items in it). Think of a time when you were eating at a restaurant where staff are rude or abrupt, perhaps not even to you but to other customers. What kind of culture did that suggest? Or what about eating somewhere where the cutlery and chairs were untidy and dirty? Again, your understanding of the culture can be influenced by moments and experiences like these.

THE APPLE EXPERIENCE

22.3

Do you own an iPhone? Or a MacBook? If so, do you remember its packaging? The light, easy-to-remove plastic film over the white box, how the top part slipped easily off over the bottom box and exposed the beautifully crafted device in front of you. Remember how you opened it and with one touch of the power button the product started right away?

Everyone who has an Apple product notices the same things, and not by accident. This experience of getting a new device was carefully designed and planned by Steve Jobs. He focused on what the customer feels, knowing that we value experiences above anything else.

How many pages were in the user manual for the iPhone? Correct, none. There is no user manual. This is because Jobs also focused on creating intuitive products that ultimately allow people to use them fast, effectively, and efficiently. He focused on the user's experience.

This approach is critical in creating an optimal environment for players and staff, which directs them toward optimal performance. Good sports teams, coaches, and organizations look at everything from the perspective of the "player experience," just as Apple thought carefully about the totality of how users feel when looking at, buying, unboxing, and using their products. Simple details about team facilities, such as paint color, temperature, lighting, signage, as well as more complex details, such as the ergonomics, personnel, and layout of the buildings, all affect culture, player experience, and performance.

Cell phones, texting, and email all existed before Steve Jobs and Jony Ive created the iPhone, but they had never been combined in a slick package that looked good, was easy to use, and was far more reliable than the old flip phones. The iPhone also had a built-in iPod and made it easy to browse the internet on your phone. But beyond all the cool and useful features, what Jobs, Ive, and company wanted to provide was a unique and special experience for the consumer.

That's why they thought about every detail—from the box to the instant start-up to the lack of the clunky instruction manual. What was left out was just as important as what was included. Every product and accessory, and even the Apple stores, were now color-coordinated. The thread running through all of these details was simplicity. "It's Apple's devotion to Simplicity that forms an unbreakable connection with its customers," writes Ken Segall in *Insanely Simple: The Obsession That Drives Apple's Success.* "Simplicity not only enables Apple to revolutionize—it enables Apple to revolutionize repeatedly. As the world changes, as technology changes, as the company itself adapts to change, the religion of Simplicity is the one constant."[47]

The sports organization that wants to innovate can draw a couple of lessons from Apple. The first is that it's important to look at how things have always been done with a critical eye and find flaws in this approach that can be fixed. The second is that leaders should make things as easy and straightforward as possible for personnel. It's not just Apple's customers who benefit from simplicity and the clarity that comes with it but also their employees. Segall elaborates: "When you work at Apple, you know exactly where you stand, what the goals are and how quickly you need to perform."[48] This means that people in

your organization won't get bogged down in extraneous details and trying to figure out what they should be doing. Instead, they're given a clear mission and are empowered to figure out innovative ways to help the team meet its objectives.

A TALE OF TWO EXPERIENCES 22.3.1

A couple of years ago I visited two of the top Premier League soccer clubs, located in the same city. Yet despite being geographically close, it was obvious from the get-go that their cultures were a world apart.

At the first club, the security guard was in a uniform, but it wasn't new or well cared for. He was slouching and smoking as my taxi pulled up to the gate. Though he wasn't rude to me, he had no record of my visit and asked me what I wanted. I explained that I had been invited by the sports science team, and he let me through. Though I spent an enjoyable day at the club, this unprofessional encounter set a bad tone.

My reception at the second club was a completely different and altogether more pleasant experience. The security guard was wearing what looked like a new uniform, and while he wasn't as rigid as a soldier patrolling in front of Buckingham Palace, he carried himself with an upright posture. As soon as my car got to the gate he greeted me kindly and then checked a list. "They should be all ready for you, Mr. Connolly," he said as he waved me through. This opening encounter was reflected in every interaction I had that day—everyone was professional, genial, and welcoming. Their demeanor was a reflection of the club's storied history.

WHAT THEY DO WHEN YOU'RE NOT AROUND 22.3.2

As head coach, you cannot be everywhere at once, and you have far too many responsibilities to be looking over your staff's shoulders—just like any leader. So you need to hire people of high character whom you can trust to do the right thing at all

> *The true test of a man's character is what he does when no one is watching.*
>
> —John Wooden

times, whether you're present or not. If someone has the kind of character that moves the organization forward, they will represent you, themselves, and the team well at all times, be self-motivated, and always give their best. They will care for colleagues, players, and their families, treat visitors and support staff respectfully, and constantly try to improve. In contrast, if someone slacks off, is disrespectful and uncaring to others, and can't perform unless there's someone behind them cracking the whip, they're going to be a drain on the organization's performance and need to be removed.

HOW YOU WANT YOUR STAFF TO TREAT PEOPLE   22.3.2.1

When interviewing candidates for a coaching or staff position, most organizations look for glowing reports from the big names at the applicants' former teams—the head coach, the GM, and so on. But while these recommendations can be valid, everyone goes out of their way to impress their bosses. A better way to find out how potential hires treat people is to talk to the interns who worked for them, in addition to their supervisors. If what you hear from an intern is consistent with positive statements from the GM or head coach, then this is the type of person you want working for you. If, however, someone gets a glowing review from their former boss but a poor one from somebody who worked for them, then you should be wary.

EVOLUTION, NOT REVOLUTION

22.4

When you fail to expect change, you set yourself up to fail to adapt to it when it arrives. And in sports as in life, change is inevitable. A head coach who wants to create change should do so gradually and in stages. As with players' on-field performance, it's best to leave alone things that aren't holding the organization back. Things that simply must be altered should be prioritized and changed one at a time. Stakeholders, from players to staff to management, should be told what's being changed, why, and how the new way will be better. It should be clear that the new direction is not a referendum on the performance of the people involved in the old way of doing things; instead, it's an opportunity to improve. Asking these individuals how they would further enhance the new plan will help them feel invested in the changes. Clarity, transparency, and realistic expectations will help prevent anxiety, misunderstanding, and miscommunication about changes.

AIMING FOR A TARGET YOU CAN'T SEE   22.4.1

Leaders often have a crystal-clear vision of where they would like their organization to be in a year, five years, or ten years. In truth, though, they cannot know exactly what this will be. Due to the randomness of life, the chaos of sports, and the unique mix of characters and personalities within any team, it's impossible to plan out each small step and control everything. Things don't necessarily happen in a linear and sequential way. Leaders have to submit to letting the destination reveal itself and empower people to help guide the club day-to-day.

CHOOSING BATTLES   22.4.2

Don't change things for the sake of doing so or because of a mistaken belief that your way is the best way to do everything. No matter how competent and experienced you are, you have to accept that experts typically know their discipline better than you do, and in team sports there isn't time to start from scratch. Instead, choose initiatives that will yield the highest return with the lowest cost, so that the differential is the greatest for those few things you decide to alter.

If you're going to remove something, you must have a plan for what's going to replace it. Finding a bottleneck or inefficiency and eliminating it is just one half of the problem. So before you announce that the organization will no longer do X, you'd better have a clear vision of why and how you're going to start doing Y.

RECOGNIZING STRENGTHS   22.5

The most effective leaders don't hire people who will just affirm their decisions or look at the world exactly as they do. That would be the equivalent of creating twenty clones of a head coach and put them to work at every sports team—a recipe for disaster. No, the best leaders build their teams with people who complement their strengths, fill the gaps created by their weaknesses, and are able to execute in their area without oversight.

If you're new to a team, don't let gossip dictate how you view certain people. Find out the truth for yourself. Similarly, if in the first few days on the job it's abundantly clear that a coach or staff member is bad at something, don't let that color your perception of them. It doesn't mean that they're bad at everything, just that you've identified a growth opportunity. Everyone has at least one strength and unique way to contribute, and it's the leader's job to find this

and emphasize it, while minimizing weaknesses. If that sounds an awful lot like what we try to do with even our best players using the four-coactive profile, that's because it uses the same principle of maximizing dominant qualities and improving limiting factors.

THE BOOK OF REVELATION   22.6

There are a couple of different ways to approach changing a dysfunctional culture. When Stuart Lancaster took over the England rugby team, he quickly decided what needed to be fixed and set about fixing it. He later gave presentations about how he changed the culture of England rugby in just ten days. One of the key things Lancaster did was to oversee a $100 million revamp of Twickenham Stadium, where artifacts representing a new culture that emphasized the team's legacy were prominently placed in the locker room. "When we got in there we could show the players the history wall, the debut board and also behind each player's changing spot were the names of those who had played in their position before," Lancaster told the *Daily Telegraph*. "So you get across the point that you are not just playing for your friends and family but also those who have played previously in your position."[49]

When Eddie Jones became England's head rugby coach, he took a different tack, waiting for the culture to reveal itself before deciding which keystone values and habits needed to be rewired. He also looked for small potential changes to the way the team prepared and played. A lot of Jones's changes were not to facilities or team preparation but were rather based on the core identity of the team. After coaching Japan to a World Cup upset of South Africa, Jones told *The Rugby Site* that "culture is based on values. With the Japan team we have three key values. These are how players cooperate with each other, compete with each other and as the head coach, how do I get the best out of each individual."[50]

When he took the England job, Jones combined this values-centric approach with a renewed focus on playing to the traditional strengths of the national side, which Will Greenwood wrote are "set piece power, great defense, world class goal kicking." Jones also made a concerted effort to bring his players closer together, according to Mako Vunipola. "There has been a lot more emphasis on team bonding, which showed on the pitch where we were willing to go out and fight for each other."[51]

This is not to say that Jones's approach is better or worse, just that there are alternatives to a "come in, take charge, shake things up" mindset.

CULTURE

Environment and situation the player/person finds themselves in most often, physically and psychologically

Visual: Banners, posters, quotes

Presentation: Dress, symbols, color

Environment: Building & support itself

ARTIFACTS

Tangible, overt or verbally identifiable elements in an organization

BEHAVIORS

The outcome of attitude, the action

Forced: Demanded behavior, useful & useless

Ceremony: Facilitated behavior

Taught: Mentoring, lectures, etc.

ATTITUDE

Learned predisposed response to a person, place, or experience

VALUES

Values are dominant and lack flexibility

BELIEFS

An idea that the person/organization holds as fundamentally true. It may be true or false.

Moralizing (DO as I SAY): Instruction

Modeling (DO as I DO): Following example

Experimenting: Life experience

Clarification: Discussion and explanation

TWENTY-THREE

THE ROSTER

The team that takes the field is only the "tip of the spear." The management of the whole roster of players and staff is critical to the success of the few who play at any moment.

THE SECOND-BEST TEAM

23.1

While Jim Harbaugh was head football coach at Stanford, Bill Walsh was athletic director, and Walsh passed on one of his last and most valuable lessons before he passed away in July 2007. Walsh told Harbaugh that almost anyone can pick out the superstars, but the most underrated coaching skill is finding the reserves who can be the second-best team in the league. You never know when a starting player will be lost to illness, injury, or a trade or transfer, and you often don't have enough time to bring in a replacement from the draft or another club. So it's vital that every single one of your reserves knows the system, understands the Commander's Intent, and is physically and mentally ready to perform when called upon.

Second- or third-choice players must also push the starters hard in practice and help the coaching staff create an environment in which no player's job is safe and competition is constant. This will encourage even the superstars to continue putting in their best effort and will help ensure that the learning experiences the head coach sets up will be high quality.

FINDING THEM

23.1.1

To put together the second-best team, you need to look for players of high moral character who are dedicated to excellence. They must be a good fit for your training system and the club beliefs, values, and attitudes, which inform how players perform, behave, and treat others. Those who will most likely not be starters from the get-go also need to understand what their role on the team will be. For older veterans, this may mean contributing their leadership and experience; for younger players, this may mean learning and growing in their abilities.

Finding players who can thrive in pressure moments is also key. Remember that it was shots from John Paxson and Steve Kerr that won the final games in the Chicago Bull's 1993 and 1997 title runs, not Michael Jordan or Scottie Pippen. In the huddle before he hit that shot, Kerr told Jordan that if Stockton left him to double-team Jordan, "I'll be ready." Not only did Kerr prove himself to be up to the task, but Jordan—the ultimate closer—trusted him enough to make the pass.[52]

MAINTAINING AMBITION

When asked what continues to motivate him despite all of his individual accolades and team trophies, Lionel Messi explained, "You cannot allow your desire to be a winner to be diminished by achieving success." If all great players shared in this sentiment, coaches' jobs would be a lot easier! As not every player thinks like Messi, it's important that the head coach helps continually fuel his or her players' ambition. This starts with understanding what resonates with each player. Bob Bowman has said that he was able to keep Michael Phelps going after he'd already won so many Olympic golds and set so many world records because he understood how to tap into Phelps's unparalleled drive: "When it's me and Michael in the pool, I have to know the things that motivate him, that don't motivate him."[53]

For some athletes who've already achieved a lot, their historical standing can be the key motivator. Going into the Olympics, in which he would fulfill his aim of becoming the first man to win the one hundred and two hundred meters and the 4x100-meter relay, Usain Bolt was asked what his goal was. "I am trying to become a legend," the Jamaican replied.[54] For players on the other end of the scale, who haven't yet reached the pinnacle of the sport, gaining that first division title or championship can be the aim.

It's important that whatever goals coaches set for their players, they stay within the context of team success and the shared targets of the group. Otherwise you can have a lineup of talented yet self-focused individuals who are only chasing stats, records, and their own glory.

THE PLAYER DEVELOPMENT PATHWAY

23.2

Though statistics are not the be-all and end-all that some sports scientists try to portray them as, it can be useful to collect data on the typical career trajectory for players at any level of a team sport. These can be used to create lines of best fit that enable the coaches to evaluate the roster based on a player's age, the level they've already attained, and where their performance level is likely to be in the seasons to come.

When thinking about a player's age, it's important to recognize that there's a difference between athletes' chronological age and their playing age. A young player may have already moved up through a very good club's youth system and perhaps even played for international junior teams (rugby and soccer) or proven herself in a competitive high school environment (like New York for basketball or Texas for football) and then for an elite college program. In this case, chronological age would be a lot younger than their playing age.

Conversely, an older player's age might suggest experience, but he may have only played a few minutes on teams that weren't very good, and perhaps he wasn't challenged at a junior level before he scraped into the pro ranks. This player's chronological age would be greater than his playing age. The point is that we shouldn't just say "She's too young" or "He's too old" when assessing the prospects of any athlete.

YOU BUY WHAT YOU SELL

23.2.1

When a team buys a player or acquires him through trade or the draft, the rationale has to extend beyond what the athlete can do for the team in the first year or two to what his contribution will probably be in years three and four and beyond. A further consideration is that in today's fickle transfer market, the rate at which players change teams is faster than ever. This means that when thinking about the mid- to long-term plan, the team must consider what it will lose if a player leaves and how well the replacements it has on hand will fill this hole.

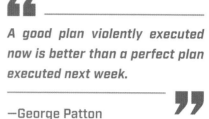

A good plan violently executed now is better than a perfect plan executed next week.

—George Patton

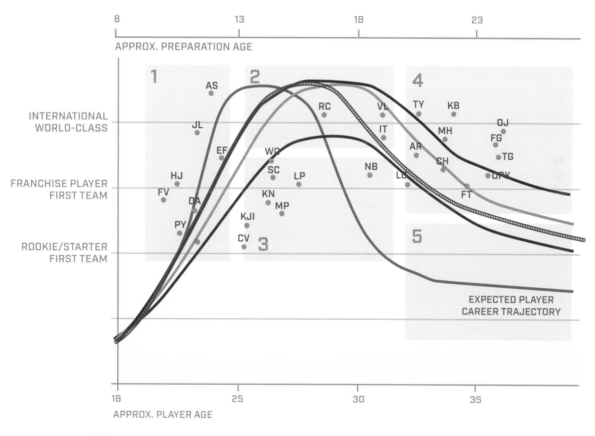

ROSTER DISTRIBUTION & PLAYER CAREER TRAJECTORY

1 INCOMING ROOKIES, ACADEMY & DRAFTEES

2 GAME WINNERS (ELITE KEY TEAM PLAYERS)

3 BACKUP AND RESERVE TEAM PLAYERS (MOST DIFFICULT TO CORRECTLY IDENTIFY)

4 EXPERIENCED, SEASONED PROFESSIONAL

5 TRANSITIONING TO COACHING

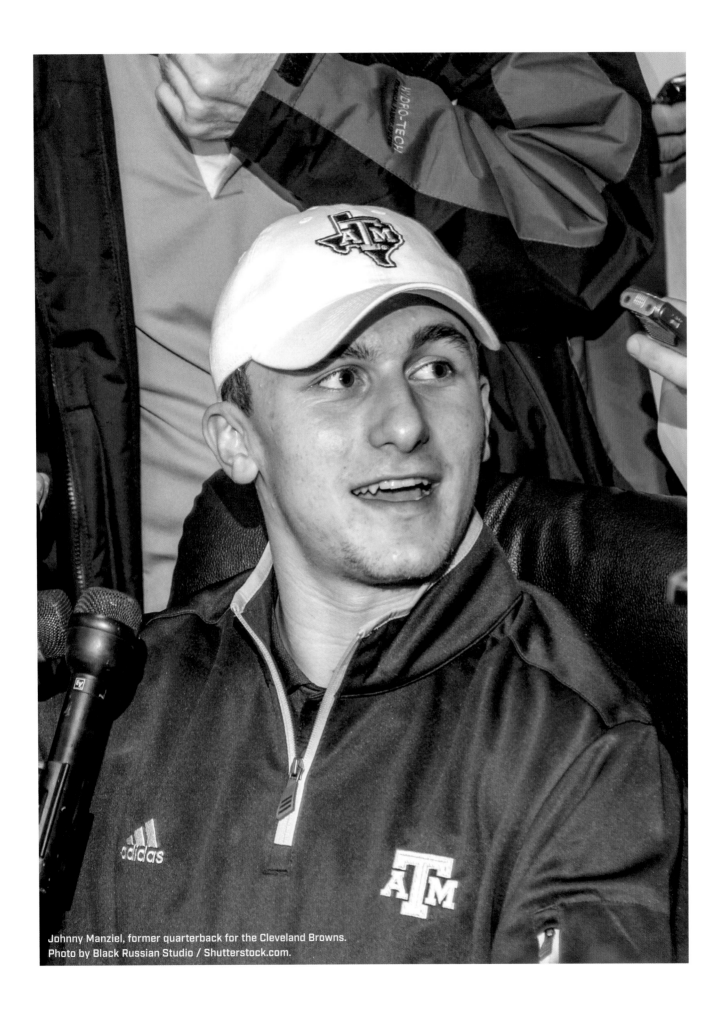

Johnny Manziel, former quarterback for the Cleveland Browns.
Photo by Black Russian Studio / Shutterstock.com.

TWENTY-FOUR

MODERN SOCIAL CHALLENGES

In my experience in modern professional sport, the majority of issues that we see on the field have nothing to do with playing. They are usually caused by stressors off the field. They can be anything from relationships to substance abuse issues to financial or contract concerns. This is truer the higher up the professional ladder you go.

ADDICTIONS AND ABUSES

24.1

The pressure of modern team sports are difficult for players (and often coaches) to deal with. Some turn to alcohol and drugs to take the edge off and help them unwind and deal with the realities of being in a media fishbowl. Players might believe that the use of such substances is under their control, but all too often, it ends up morphing into addiction and controlling them. There are all too many instances of athletes who careers have been cut short by substance abuse, including Paul Gascoigne in soccer and Lawrence Taylor in football. Then there are those tragic cases, like that of basketball phenom Len Bias, whose lives are claimed by their addiction.

SUBSTANCE ABUSE

24.1.1

If a player is caught driving under the influence of alcohol or drugs, there's only a very small chance that it's a one-off incident, as the odds of being pulled over by the police for any reason are extremely low. According to the Bureau of Justice Statistics, just 12 percent of U.S. drivers were involved in a traffic stop in 2011.[55] A DUI or similar charge—or failing a drug test for a banned performance enhancer—most likely indicates that a player has been abusing this particular substance (and possibly others) for quite a while. When the red flag of abuse becomes apparent, the team must act quickly to determine what the issue is and how it can help the player break the cycle of abuse before it becomes a life-dominating addiction.

In *The Power of Habit*, Charles Duhigg writes that to change a habit, it must be replaced by another, one that has a defined cue and reward. He also states, "For a habit to stay changed, people must believe change is possible. And most often, that belief only emerges with the help of a group."[56] While Duhigg is a firm believer in the benefits of group therapy, the network of a troubled player's coaches, teammates, and organization can also provide much-needed support.

If players can admit to themselves and those who are trying to help them that they have an issue, if they want to change their abuse pattern, and if they believe they can still control their actions, then the team can employ a change strategy, working with a third-party consultant if necessary. But if the player slides into an addiction in which the behavior pattern becomes uncontrollable and the player cannot acknowledge or express the desire to change, then an acceptance strategy must be adopted first. This means that the player must accept that there is an issue before they can start to solve the issue. The athlete also needs to accept that they cannot manage or overcome their issue without help.

FOUNDATIONS OF PSYCHOLOGICAL WELLNESS AND RESILIENCY

COPING STRATEGIES

FOUNDATIONS

MATURITY

Sophistication, streetwise intelligence, education, problem-solving

LIFESTYLE

Living situation, community, environment, living skills

SELF-ESTEEM

Alcohol and substance addiction issues. self-esteem, confidence, self-respect

SECURITY

Financial state or concern, finances, dependents, safety-security

ATTACHMENT

Emotional support, tribe, people outside of work, love, friendship, support

ADDICTION 24.1.2

Addiction occurs when a player's sustained bad habits create a behavioral reliance on alcohol or drugs, and often a psychological and physiological dependence as well. Once a player is in the grip of addiction, it is much more difficult to help them to recognize their problem and begin to deal with it.[57] When someone is addicted to a substance, physical changes occur in the brain that affect judgment and decision-making, and the user craves the rush of dopamine and other neurotransmitters that the substance provides.[58] The trouble is that as the body builds up tolerance, it needs higher and more frequent doses to produce the same feelings.

CAUSES 24.1.3

When it comes to helping players overcome dependencies, abuses, and addictions, it's not good enough to just try to eliminate or manage the symptoms. What's really needed is to delve deeper into the player's life and past to find the underlying causes. Sometimes these are environmental, such as if the athlete is in a living situation or friendships that encourage drug or alcohol abuse. In the case of performance-enhancing drugs (PEDs), it can be a coach, personal physician, or off-season training group that is the bad influence.

Athletes can also get caught in cycles of abuse that they find hard to break. For example, a player might come from a family in which one or both parents were alcoholics or drug addicts. Or maybe it's a society or cultural cycle, such as if the individual grew up in an area where substance use was rampant or even the accepted norm. Perhaps the athlete is dealing with psychological issues rooted in abuse or neglect. Regardless, the coaching staff has an obligation to get their players the help they need, rather than just discarding them when a negative behavior pattern manifests itself in actions that are destructive to the individual and detrimental to the team.

John Lucas, a former NBA player who became one of the league's all-time assists leaders after overcoming his own substance abuse issues, says that his rehabilitation program helps current basketball and football players only when they're finally honest with him and themselves about the root of their issues: "People let me into their closet," Lucas told ESPN.com. "I get to go into the bedroom instead of sitting in the living room and listening to all that artificial stuff. I need to know what I'm dealing with."[59] Just as honesty is one of the core principles of a winning organization, it can also be key for individual players who've lost their way to transform their lives.

THE ETHICS OF AN ORGANIZATION

24.2

Vince Lombardi once said, "Morally, the life of the organization must be of exemplary nature. This is one phase where the organization must not have criticism." If a culture is to be healthy all the way through, it has to have a solid moral and ethical core. You might bite into an apple that looks fine on the outside and discover that the core is rotten and the whole fruit tastes awful. It's the same with an organization. If there is a rotten middle, outside appearances count for very little. Eventually moral and ethical decay will spread until the entire thing is rancid.

MORALS AND ETHICS   24.2.1

Every culture has a combination of laws, norms, and mores that have to be observed most of the time by most of the people if the society is to thrive. This isn't just true on a broader societal level but also within groups that make up that society, such as the government and corporations. As humans, we behave better when there are boundaries and clear definitions of what is acceptable and unacceptable behavior. There also needs to be reinforcement of these lines. This is why "threaten and repeat" parenting is ineffective—if you don't follow through after saying you're going to put your child in a time-out, there's ambiguity and no cause-effect relationship between behavior and consequences.

The same holds true in a sports environment. Players and staff alike need to know what the mor-

als and ethics of the team are, what is acceptable and unacceptable, and what the consequences are for stepping over boundary lines. Though researchers have found that athletes often have lower moral reasoning scores than nonathletes, they also found that when coaches and senior players act as positive role models and the team environment encourages ethically sound decision-making, players follow this lead.[60]

THE COACH-PLAYER RELATIONSHIP   24.2.2

A GM or athletic director's main aim for their head coach often seems to be getting the best possible performances out of the athletes during the game. But every coach has a moral and ethical duty that goes beyond just winning on the field. They also have to help those in their charge—players, assistants, and support staff—win at life. UCLA legend John Wooden stated that while he could be tough on players, he always tried to show that his "concern for their interests and welfare" superseded his concern for their contributions on the court.[61]

Though coaches must demonstrate that they care for players and have their best interests at heart, they should not try to be peers. As Benjamin Franklin put it, "Love thy neighbor, but don't pull down your hedge." For a sports organization to avoid dysfunction, there has to be a clear barrier between coaches and athletes. This is not to say that head coaches shouldn't have an open-door policy or make themselves available to hear player concerns, but just as a general in the army must maintain absolute authority, so too must a coach make it clear who is in charge. Alex Ferguson told the *Harvard Business Review* that this principle was key to his longevity and unprecedented record at Manchester United: "You have to achieve a position of comprehensive control. Players must recognize that as the manager, you have the status to control events.... Before I came to United, I told myself I wasn't going to allow anyone to be stronger than I was. Your personality has to be bigger than theirs. That is vital."[62]

NICE GUYS DON'T WIN. GOOD GUYS DO. 24.2.3

Let's be frank here, the only thing that matters is winning, and occasionally in doing so you cannot be nice. However, you must bring in a lot of fundamentally good people to build a sustainable-winning team. I'm not talking about competence here but character. You cannot be rude or untrustworthy, as word travels fast in the small, tight-knit elite sports community. But being "good" is not the same as being "nice." Nice guys win nothing. You cannot allow yourself to be walked over by those who try to bully you.

It's important to make the distinction between a team's morals and ethics of a team and its demeanor. You can have players who channel Marshawn Lynch's "beast mode" aggression on the field and are similarly intense off the field. Don't mistake this for being mean or unprincipled—these players can be morally and ethically solid individuals who need anything but a nice guy demeanor to get the job done. The same can also be true of coaches. Many of the greats have reputations for being hard taskmasters or difficult with the media, yet their records and how beloved they are by their players tell the true story.

THE PLAYER DEVELOPMENT MODEL

24.3

There are five factors that impact the development of players as people and determine their long-term development: maturity, lifestyle, self-esteem, security, and attachment. When these are applied across the entire team, they heavily impact the organization's culture. In my experience in professional sports, players who are strong and capable in these areas have a greater chance of success.

THE MATURITY PRINCIPLE 24.3.1

We often make the mistake of thinking that age and maturity are one and the same. Not so. Young players can be mature beyond their years, while older athletes might still be very immature. In sports, we should think of maturity as the ability to make good decisions, handle pressure, and take on responsibility.

Mature players are those who can isolate the key issues in front of them and prioritize decisions. They have amassed enough experience to know that tough decisions are often needed. The ability to prioritize comes with time, but the faster they learn, the better. Experienced scouts know that players who have had most decisions made for them by parents tend to make the most maturity mistakes.

THE LIFESTYLE PRINCIPLE 24.3.2

Players who can demonstrate self-discipline and self-control off the field bring the same qualities to practice and game day. Maturity is an ineluctable aspect of lifestyle: as players mature, they become better able to create a balanced, well-rounded life away from the team, which in turn gives them the poise needed to grow as a student of the game and a teammate.

Physically and psychologically healthy athletes are most often those who remain injury-free and have longer careers. Manchester United's Alex Ferguson famously encouraged his players to marry young, as he knew a wife would slow the partying lifestyle many players fell into. There's no doubt that lifestyle is a major factor in keeping players away from undesirable company.

THE SELF-ESTEEM PRINCIPLE

Young players who act recklessly and selfishly often do so because they lack self-esteem. Developing an accurate sense of self-worth and sense of how they fit within the team is a crucial step if athletes are to have a long career. The coaching staff can help players increase their self-esteem, as can veteran players who act as mentors.

Spirituality is closely linked to self-esteem. Faith and religious beliefs provide players with an understanding of where their sports achievements and challenges fit in the bigger scheme of things. Players who have this spiritual framework tend to have a good perspective on life and its challenges and a good measure of self-esteem. Those who lack such a framework tend to search for external compliments and recognition, rather than find confidence within themselves.

THE SECURITY PRINCIPLE

The most basic of human desires is security, whether in relationships, finances, or career. When security is threatened, all other issues fade into the background. Of course, the nature of the perceived threat depends on what the coach or athlete sees as most important to them. For example, a person who is driven by purely financial ambition will view any threats to job security and, therefore, monetary security as very serious. But for others, the gravest threat could be one that targets ego, prestige, or even location. Usually, though, security is most important.

The more experience individuals get in such things as navigating contract negotiations, working with the coaching staff, and developing relationships with teammates, the more secure they're likely to feel. It is important that their material needs are met, of course, but beyond this, feeling like they're valued contributors to the organization's success is also important. In contrast, those who are insecure and believe their needs aren't being met will feel threatened, which can lead to their becoming either confrontational or withdrawn, both of which will adversely affect how they train, play, and act towards coaches and other players.

THE ATTACHMENT PRINCIPLE

No one is an island—all people have a basic human desire to be loved and appreciated. Relationships, on every level, are important. If players have strong attachments to their coaches and teammates, they're going to be fully committed and will give total effort every day. Tight bonds with others in their personal lives will also create stability and help reduce stress and anxiety. If players are also connected to their community, such as their religious denomination or charities that they give their time to, they will find it easier to maintain an even keel throughout the topsy-turvy sports season.

COACHING IN THE AGE OF SOCIAL MEDIA

Today's coaches have unparalleled budgets, technologies, and facilities that their predecessors could never have even dreamed of. On the flip side, they also face challenges that even the likes of Bear Bryant, John Wooden, and Bill Shankly would have struggled to overcome. One of the biggest is the constant chatter of the blogosphere and social media, not to mention cable sports channels and networks intent on churning out sensationalist stories (which Denzel Washington rightly called "opi-news"—or the intersection of opinion and news—in a 2017 BBC interview) around the clock.

Some old-school coaches have tried to bury their heads in the sand, and I completely understand this instinct. They want to focus on the matter at hand—preparing the team to be its best on game day—and don't want to get distracted by the constant demand for their take on everything from a recent winning

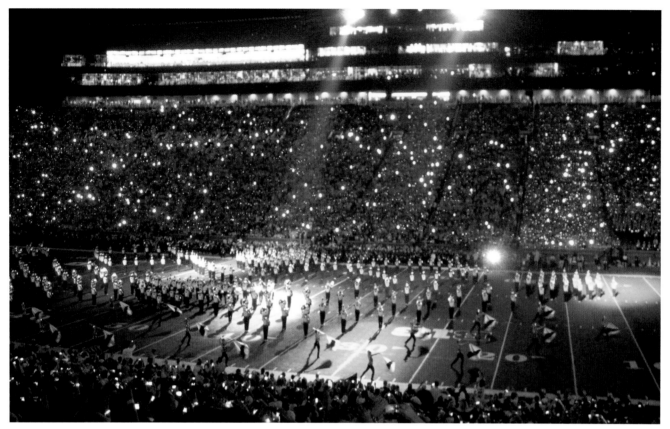

The Michigan Marching Band performing during halftime at a Notre Dame vs. Michigan football game. Sports as a product is entertainment first and foremost. Photo by Michael Barera (CC BY-SA).

streak to players' personal dramas to political issues. But this is very difficult to do nowadays, even for the likes of Gregg Popovich, the famously taciturn San Antonio Spurs head coach, who likes to give monosyllabic answers to sideline reporters' questions during games. In Popovich's case, he does a good job of portraying and even amplifying his true personality and making it clear that he just wants to get on with the business of coaching. But other coaches take it too far, attempting to stonewall reporters and thus alienating the press corps. On the other hand, you have those coaches who love the attention and try to make media appearances all about them instead of the team, or who undermine morale by using the media to call out players for subpar performances rather than taking responsibility as a true leader should. So if staying stony and silent isn't practical and grandstanding is obnoxious, what's a coach to do? That's what we're going to cover in this section.

THE MOST ADVANCED SPORT IN THE WORLD 24.4.1

The never-ending hype machine of media means that sports teams, players, and coaches are living in a continual glare of attention that burns brightly far longer than the floodlights at any game. It's not just a 24/7 news cycle but a second-by-second running commentary on every facet of sports imaginable. Everything a player does, says, and wears is broadcast around the globe in real time and scrutinized to a subatomic level. A Google search for "Lionel Messi's haircut" returns 632,000 results. There are multiple TV shows dedicated to the shopping and bickering of players' wives and girlfriends.

But while players' homes and once-private lives have become reality TV fodder, there's a vast disconnect between what is said about sports teams and actual reality. The rumors, gossip, and speculation that form the foundation of the sports media–industrial complex exist to perpetuate this multibillion-dollar business. Don't be misled into thinking that most of what you read or watch bears any relation to what goes on day-to-day at an elite level sports team, because it doesn't.

The reality is that sports as a product is entertainment first and foremost. I have often said that the most advanced sport in the world is WWE wrestling. It is pure entertainment. This is the direction that most professional sports are heading in. They are entertainment entities first, sports teams second. The NFL has become a very similar to WWE, with heroes, villains, and storylines—many of them not related to the game or performance. Roger Goodell and Vince McMahon have much in common when you think about it! Whether you turn on ESPN for an hour or a twelve-hour period, the majority of the discussion is on stories that don't surround the actual game. Much less time is spent on what happens on the field than you'd think. Storylines range from failed drug tests, to transfer and trade crises, to athlete protests, to just about every other non-game topic imaginable. Larry Bird once said, "The game should be enough." Unfortunately, in our media-saturated society, it doesn't seem to be enough for many people, or for the networks feeding them content.

MEDIA INFLUENCE   24.4.2

Sports media touts its ability to provide scoops, inside information, and you-saw-it-here-first exclusives. Yet despite the flood of information, the public knows as little about the inner workings of its favorite sports teams as ever. No one outside the organization can really know what goes on inside its walls, no matter what those "unnamed sources" tell sports reporters. But what reporters write and say reaches a vast audience across multiple platforms, which makes it very difficult for coaches and players to insulate themselves and focus on what should be the main task at hand: winning. This invasion of the entertainment business has an incredibly wide-reaching influence.

Even if coaches and players don't read newspapers or magazines, cut the cable cord, and shun social media, their friends and family members will invariably share what's being said about them and their team. That's why it's important to always remem-

ber that such reports are mostly inaccurate, and even when there's some truth in them, outsiders can't understand the intricacies of what's going on in the locker room. As you can now appreciate, a significant result of this phenomenon is that coaches must ensure their players listen to the storyline they want them to hear, not the storyline the media is reporting.

During the 2016 Rio Olympics, USA head basketball coach Mike Krzyzewski relayed a story from when he served under Chuck Daly as an assistant on the 1992 Olympic Dream Team, considered the greatest basketball team ever assembled. As eager college coaches, Krzyzewski and fellow assistant P.J. Carlesimo had notebooks and pens out to write down what Daly said during the first team meeting. Daly told them to put the writing materials away. "I want you to do one thing really well: You have to learn to ignore. For you college guys, everything is important. In our world, not everything is important, but the things that are important need to have complete focus. So don't get caught up in all this minutiae."[63]

Chuck Daly said to ignore what's not important and better understand what is so they can focus on it. I can't guarantee Dream Team–like performance, but the principles named here will equip coaches at any level to build an organization that strives for excellence, gets the best from its players and staff, and is a place where people want to come and give their best every day.

MESSAGE MANAGEMENT   24.4.3

One of the most dangerous lines you'll hear a sports reporter say is, "According to a source close to the team…" Sometimes such a source is a figment of the reporter's imagination, created to lend credence to a rumor. But in other cases, a player, assistant coach, or staff member has either deliberately leaked something to the media or inadvertently let something slip. It's the job of the head coach to establish a clear information management policy. Only the head coach should address the media on issues concerning the team, unless someone else in the organization is given express permission to talk to the media, on a case-by-case basis. What's discussed in team meetings and practices and in the locker room before and after games has to remain confidential. If a problem of any kind arises, everyone needs to understand that it will be dealt with within the confines of the team and that others outside this tight circle cannot be trusted with even a tidbit of information. Everyone has to act as a gatekeeper to preserve the trust and integrity of the organization.

Airplanes are not designed by science but by art, in spite of some pretense and humbug to the contrary.... There is a big gap between scientific research and the engineering product which has to be bridged by the art of the engineer.

—John D. North

There are some coaches who stonewall reporters or remain tight-lipped around them to preserve secrecy and avoid saying something the internet might make them regret. Some others—particularly those new to the job—seem to be a bit intimidated by all the attention. But many others are finding that traditional media outlets and social media provide opportunities to frame their club's narrative, influence public opinion, and even pressure referees into more favorable treatment of their players. Postgame interviews can also be used to direct attention away from bad performances without pointing the finger at players. José Mourinho is a master of this strategy, as was his Manchester United predecessor, Alex Ferguson. In the NBA, Phil Jackson would blast referees for not protecting Michael Jordan and Scottie Pippen after a defeat, and then, as if by magic, his stars would get more calls and win the next game.

Media-savvy athletes and their sponsors can also use media to elevate their reputation and market-

ability. Today's sports stars have millions of followers on Instagram, Twitter, and the rest, and tech-obsessed fans hang on their every word (or photo). David Beckham was one of the first players to understand how to reach a global audience and to understand that players' style—what they're wearing, their latest hairstyle—is every bit as important to the modern fan as what they do on the pitch.

IGNORING CRITICISM AND ADULATION   24.4.4

Players of all ages and experience levels—but especially those at the elite end who are going to be in the spotlight for fifteen to twenty years—need to accept that they cannot control the media. So they need to ignore what is written about them, whether that's good or bad. When negative stories about players pop up, they're often exaggerated, sensationalist, or both. Despite the claims of some magazines and TV shows that they can take the casual fan inside athletes' private lives, the opposite is true. Only players, their families, their coaches, and their teammates can truly know the truth. Everything else is just speculation devised to generate more clicks and social media engagement. The media likes to play judge and jury, and it's easy for fans get sucked into the trap of making assumptions about athletes without truly knowing them.

At the opposite end of the spectrum is athlete adulation. When players are performing well and being successful, they're bound to generate positive headlines and stories that can at times almost deify them. But in many cases these puff pieces exist merely to create a contrast with the negative press that often follows. Players should be encouraged to avoid reading positive stories about themselves because it just softens them up, so the negative pieces end up hurting on a more profound level. And as spouses and significant others can get even more emotionally caught up in media coverage than the athletes, they'd also do well to steer clear of the sports and celebrity rumor mill.

It is better to lead from behind and to put others in front, especially when you celebrate victory when nice things occur. You take the front line when there is danger. Then people will appreciate your leadership.

—Nelson Mandela

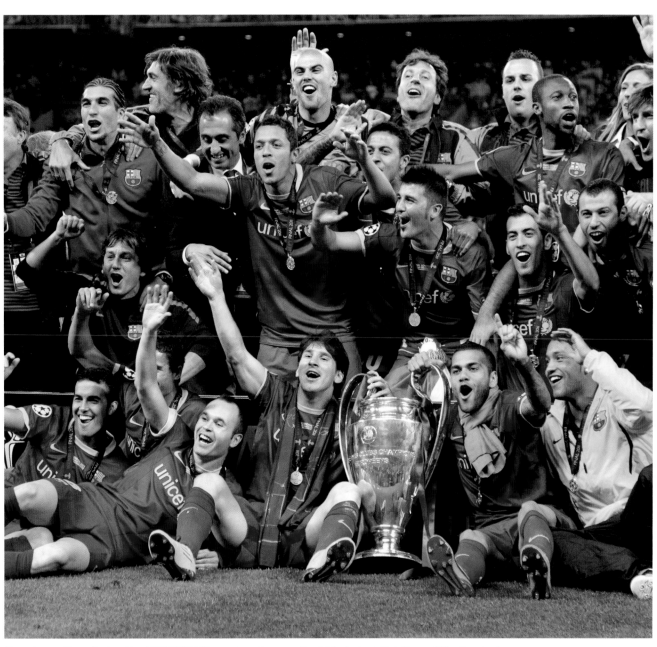

Barcelona after winning the 2011 UEFA Champions League final. Photo by Mitch Gunn / Shutterstock.com.

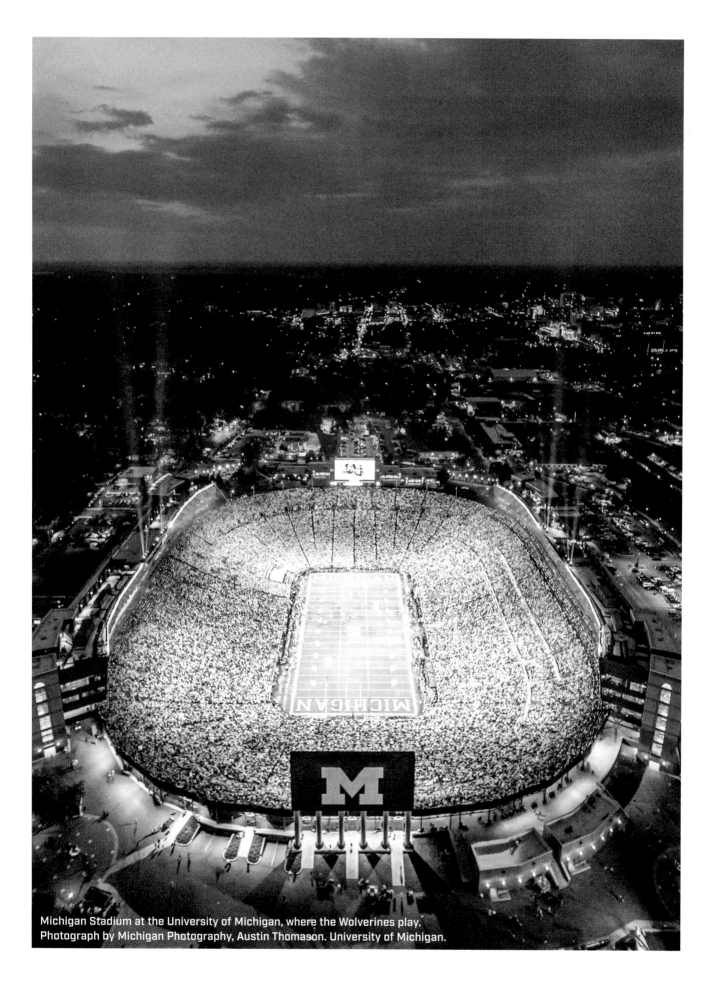

Michigan Stadium at the University of Michigan, where the Wolverines play.
Photograph by Michigan Photography, Austin Thomason. University of Michigan.

TWENTY-FIVE

YOU WIN WITH PEOPLE

It can be easy for athletes to allow their sports career to become the be-all and end-all of their existence. Their performance becomes the only thing that defines their identity and determines their self-worth and perceived value to others, and suddenly what happens during the game is all that matters. The trouble is that if players then get injured, they're more psychologically and emotionally devastated than they should be, and they struggle to fill the void of competition when their playing days are over. They can also become selfish and egotistical, and develop a win-at-all-costs mentality that can lead to the use of performance-enhancing drugs and other rule-breaking.

It's the job of the coaching staff to make sure this doesn't happen and to put sports in context. Should their sport be very important to an athlete? Certainly, but it shouldn't be the *only* thing in their life. Family, friends, community, the team—all of these should also be priorities. The great coach Woody Hayes titled his book *You Win with People,* and that sums up the key point: this is a people business. It's healthy for players to have hobbies that don't relate to the sport itself. To achieve longevity and maintain health, it's necessary to first find balance, and, particularly for younger players, the coaching staff can play an important role in teaching life lessons and ensuring that athletes don't elevate themselves to the status of a deity.

WHAT'S THE MESSAGE?

25.1

A while ago I read about a current-events assignment that a schoolteacher gave her students. She had them read a news article about classes being canceled after a meteorite fell near the school and then asked each student to write a story about it for the school newspaper. She'd pick the one that best conveyed the central message and it would be published in the next edition.

Well, kids being kids, the teacher got some very creative and imaginative stories back. Some students claimed that aliens were involved, while others focused on how big the crater was and painted a very vivid picture of the damage it had done. The more analytical of the bunch wrote about the science of meteors, how fast they fly through space, and how fast they're going when they hit the ground. But only one child, who turned out to have the winning entry, centered his story on the real news: school was canceled.

This lesson applies to how coaches address the players in the locker room. What's the real story that they want to get across? They need to think about what they're going to say from their point of view but also from the audience's perspective. What are the players going to focus on, and how do they need to structure what they say so the main message comes across?

IT'S THE ECONOMY, STUPID   25.1.1

When Bill Clinton was campaigning against incumbent George H. W. Bush in the 1992 presidential election, his campaign team was struggling to find a definitive central phrase to anchor the push to the White House. Clinton and his staff walked into the war room one morning to find that strategist James Carville had placed a simple yet declarative four-word statement on the whiteboard for all to see: "It's the economy, stupid."[64] Carville's purpose was not only to focus the campaign strategy but also to remind Clinton and his staffers what the American people really cared about: how much money was in their pocket, what it would allow them to buy, and how much the government would take in taxes.

Similarly, players on any team want to know what the coaches and staff members are going to do for them. If a new initiative is introduced during preparation, they want to know how it's going to make them better during the game and why it's better than the old way. The head coach must keep such things in mind when communicating with players and assistants, and should incorporate clear and concise "It's the economy, stupid," thinking into their decision-making. If it can help win a presidential election, this approach can certainly help win sports games.

WHAT DISNEY CAN TEACH US   25.1.2

Walt Disney once said, "Animation can explain whatever the mind of man can conceive." Disney recognized that using cartoons allowed him to convey themes and ideas without having to say anything about them directly. The best cartoon characters aren't one-dimensional but rather multilayered representations of certain traits or characteristics. It took Victor Hugo hundreds of pages to convey the loneliness and isolation of his *Hunchback of Notre Dame,* but this was evident the first time the character appeared on screen in Disney's film version. The story's powerful message—that we shouldn't judge people by their appearance—was also vividly imagined by Disney's illustrators.

There may be few budding cartoonists or animators in the coaching ranks, but coaches can follow Disney's lead in using graphics, metaphors, and visual themes to share important ideas with their players. These don't even have to be original. If the defense needs to step up its intensity, what better picture is there than the whirling Tasmanian Devil? Or if the offense needs to move more quickly, showing a thirty-second clip of Roadrunner evading Wile E. Coyote should get the message across.

STORYTELLING, PARABLES, AND FABLES   25.1.3

In the Bible's New Testament, Jesus didn't explain every little detail of his teachings. Instead, he used parables to convey meaning through imagery, allegory, and narrative. The same is true of fables and fairy tales like "Hansel and Gretel," "The Tortoise and the Hare," and "The Ant and the Grasshopper." These stories teach us valuable lessons without bashing us over the head with heavy-handed moralizing. Talented film directors also embed layers of symbolism into their movies, as designer Mike Hill showed to great effect in his twenty-eight-minute presentation on "Spielberg's Subtext" in *Jurassic Park* at the 2016 THU Conference.[65]

Coaches would do well to follow this example when attempting to talk to their players about beliefs, values, attitude, and behavior. Most players don't want to listen to long sermons on such things, but they will pay close attention to a succinct, meaning-rich story that captures their imagination.

NURSERY RHYME AND MEMORY   25.1.4

"Rock-a-bye baby on the treetop, when the wind blows the cradle will rock…" There's a reason that we can recall this and many other nursery rhymes years after our parents last sang them to us. The rhyming and rhythm create an indelible imprint on our minds from the first line onward, and the simplicity of a nursery rhyme makes it even catchier. Then there's the impact of repetition, which ingrains our favorite rhymes in our long-term memory. We see the same concept in action in the chants sports fans sing in the stands every weekend.

Now, if you start singing "Rock-a-Bye Baby" to a locker room full of rugby or football players, you might get some very weird looks, to say the least. That's not what I'm suggesting. Rather, you and your staff can come up with your own simple rhymes that convey the goals, principles, or values of your team, and which the players can use to center their group identity by repeating them during pregame and postgame rituals. For example: "We're all in, we all win." Repeating such a simple line might seem literally elementary, but it can become a powerful ritual, unique to your group, that encourages everyone to rally around a common theme. In the TV show *Friday Night Lights*, the high school football team repeated a chant before every game: "Clear eyes, full hearts, can't lose." This is a great example of how a chant can convey the principles and values of a team: here, the "clear eyes" of good judgment and decision-making, the "full hearts" of commitment and camaraderie, and the "can't lose" of determination and perseverance.

DRIVER OR MECHANIC   25.1.4.1

A mechanic in a Formula 1 pit crew needs to know how virtually every part of a car works and interacts with other parts, as well as understand common problems and how to fix them quickly. But to squeeze every potential mile per hour out of the vehicle, a race car driver doesn't need the same level of comprehension. The coach-player dynamic is similar. The athlete just needs to know what to do. If they're told the why or how behind everything, they'll start overthinking, to the detriment of their decision-making and execution in practice and competition. This is why coaches must make things as simple as possible for their players, so that players can maintain as much of their functional reserve as possible and not be overloaded with information. In the words of coach Red Auerbach, who led the Boston Celtics to nine NBA titles, "It's not what you say as much as what they absorb."

WHY COCA-COLA NEEDS PEPSI

Some people might think that a company would want to be the only one in its field, so that it could have a total monopoly. But in reality, organizations need targets to aim at, and often these are provided by the performance of their closest competitors. Coke needs Pepsi. Nike needs Adidas. Southwest needs American Airlines. Apple needs Microsoft. Competition breeds excellence, fosters a spirit of togetherness, and prevents complacency from setting in. It's the same in the world of team sports. The Springboks need the Wallabies. Arsenal needs Tottenham. The Cavaliers need the Warriors. The Patriots need the Colts. It's these intense rivalries (and in European sports, particularly fiercely contested derbies that pit local antagonists against each other) that push teams onward, no matter how much they've achieved in the past or how well they're doing in any particular season.

GIVE IT A NAME   25.1.4.2

Any initiative that the coaching staff wants to implement needs a name if it's to resonate with the players and stick in their minds. For example, when I was with Munster, we implemented a program to help older players extend their careers. It would've been useless to waffle on about longevity for half an hour, so instead we introduced it to Ronan O'Gara and the other senior veterans as "the Maldini Project" (named after former Italy captain Paolo Maldini, who played for AC Milan until he was forty-one). It's the same with any plan or strategy—you've got to give it a name to make it memorable.

ONE-LINERS   25.1.4.3

Catchphrases can stick in our minds for years. Think of some of the best ad campaigns, like "Stay thirsty, my friends," from Dos Equis's "Most Interesting Man in the World," or Budweiser's "Whassup?" Super Bowl commercial. The impact of catchphrases even spawned an entire subgenre of comedy in the U.K., with skits in programs such as *Harry Enfield and Chums* and *The Fast Show* anchored by their characters' catchphrases.

One-liners, catchphrases, and acronyms can also be used to great effect to communicate in the locker room. I have often used catchphrases to teach: for instance, I use "Glo, Slo, Flo" to outline three phases of player recovery. Each phase had three or four modalities, which I identified with the Superman's "S" symbol—a familiar image, and one the athletes identified with. So in the "Glo" stage, we had:

- Shake: Get protein and carbs in to kick-start muscle repair

- Shiver: Use the ice bath to reset the central nervous system

- Skins: Put on compression gear to stimulate the circulatory system

So by using the Superman theme and a three-word rhyme, I was able to distill some complex sports science into language that was easily understood and remembered. That way, the players didn't need multiple lectures or a thick handout to remind them what

to do. Coaches used to complain they would give the players forty-minute lectures from which they'd remember nothing, but I found that after a ten-minute presentation, almost all the players could recall the key takeaways. Many former 49ers have told me they still remember the Superman S's and "Glo, Slo, Flo."

RIDING CHAOS
25.2

For a sports team to continually progress, it must learn lessons from its own prior experiences and also apply best practices from other successful teams. This involves not only correcting mistakes that led to things going wrong but also reinforcing the habit and behaviors that led to success. There are few, if any, scenarios that a sports team can find itself in that another club hasn't been in before and thrived. Trying to stay at the top of the league table or fighting relegation, fighting injuries or making the most of a full squad, breaking a losing streak or keeping a winning streak going—there are plenty of case studies for all of these situations, and more, that coaches can learn from and apply to their own team.

CONTROL THE CONTROLLABLES   25.2.1

As we saw when exploring the frictions of the game in "The Game," every sports game presents unexpected circumstances and is subject to some degree of chaos and chance—that is, uncontrollables. To help players maintain the functional reserve they need to react to and deal with these, the head coach needs to identify what the controllables are—those things that are predictable and can be kept in check. The walk-through/talk-through the day before every game is one setting in which the coaches can delineate between controllables and uncontrollables. Defining "if this, then that" protocols can help reduce player anxiety, as can taking a page from the military's book and establishing standard operating procedures for every controllable—from travel to pregame warm-ups to postgame nutrition and

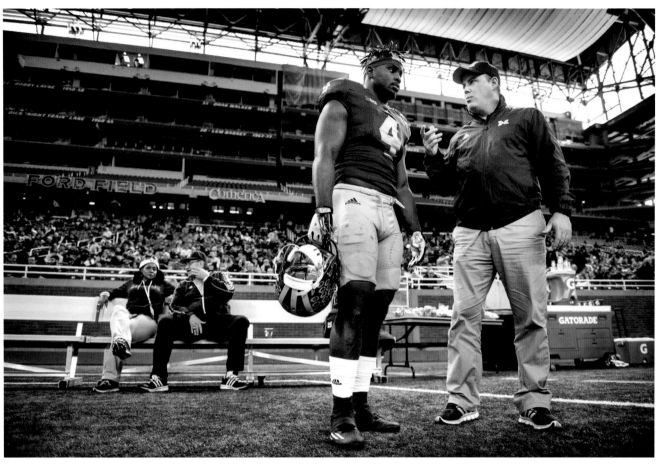

The author with former Michigan running back De'Veon Smith, now with the Miami Dolphins. Photo by David Turnley

recovery. When players know what they can control and how to do so, they feel more comfortable, are less stressed out, and can focus their full energy and effort on playing the game.

AGILITY   25.2.2

As much as we would like things to be perfect, in team sports they rarely, if ever, are. Whether it's an injury right before the game, adverse weather conditions, new training gear getting lost during shipping, or hundreds of other potential problems, chaos happens. It's the teams that accept this and are agile enough to adapt at a moment's notice that thrive no matter what the circumstances. One way to improve this agility is for everyone to be willing to pitch in as needed, even if it's outside the typical expectations for their job. This willingness to help will be compounded if everyone is committed to helping their colleagues and wants to see them and the entire group do its best at all times.

IT'S MURPHY'S WORLD   25.2.3

Murphy's Law states that anything that can go wrong, will. Even the best planning and preparation cannot account for every possible eventuality, and difficulties invariably arise during every game, preparation morphocycle, and day-to-day team management. The key thing to remember is that nothing has to be perfect for the team and the organization to succeed: they just need to be the right thing at the right time. Having such a mindset will prevent people from making excuses and putting failure down to just bad luck. You don't want to always think the worst, that someone made a mistake; instead, acknowledge that things outside your control will go wrong and all you can do is your best in any given situation. It's those teams whose personnel get caught up in whining and complaining that fail to respond adequately when Murphy's Law comes into play, which has negative consequences for everyone.

KNOWING PEOPLE

25.3

In sports it's easy to get caught up in stats, fixated on trophies and accolades, and obsessed with the latest and supposedly greatest technology. But when you boil it down, sports is a people business. You don't need to prioritize just the health of your players but also the well-being of your coaching and back-office staff. Glittering stadiums, new gear, and fancy facilities do not win sports games: a dedicated, committed team of happy, healthy people does.

LESSONS FROM A PICKUP ARTIST

25.3.1

We can learn a couple of valuable lessons from how romances blossom or wither. In his book *The Game: Penetrating the Secret Society of Pickup Artists,* Neil Strauss reveals how important posture is in dating. "Strangers size each other up in seconds," he writes. "A hundred tiny details, from dress to body language, combine to create a first impression."[66]

Players, assistant coaches, executives, and reporters are just as quick to assess a head coach when he or she enters the room, walks onto the practice field, or enters a press conference. How the coach sits or, preferably, stands goes a long way to setting the tone. Their positioning can either enhance or undermine what they say.

LISTENING TO WORDS

25.3.2

Two people can hear the same message or have the same interaction and interpret it in very different ways due to their past experiences, emotional state, and many other individual variables. In the 1970s, John Grinder and Richard Bandler introduced neurolinguistic programming (NLP) as a way of looking at communication that goes far beyond what is said. This system looks at how language, the brain, and the body interact with the environment to create different perceptions of reality.[67] From a sports stand-

point, we can apply the basic NLP principle of subjective communication to how coaches talk to their players. It can be valuable to find out whether each athlete is analytical or creative, as this will determine how they see the world around them and, as a result, what kind of communication they respond to most readily.

For example, when I was at the 49ers, the coaching staff realized that Vernon Davis was very artistic and so needed to view football in a creative, expressive way. Some of the other players had minds more like engineers or mathematicians and responded better to very clear, precise instructions. While the message the head coach delivers to their team needs to be cohesive and consistent, varying the delivery can make what's being said hit home more effectively.

"MY GREATEST FEAR": MISINTERPRETING ACTIONS

25.3.3

If we don't understand someone's motivations and fears, it can be very easy to misinterpret what they say and how they act. Nowhere is this truer than in team sports, where many seemingly inexplicable events are driven by fear. This is why the head coach must try to understand the collective fears of the team and the individual apprehensions and anxieties of each player. If a rugby player misses a crucial drop goal, it might not be because he's mentally weak or lacks power but because his attempt was marred by the memory of a previous miss that cost the team a win. If the coach knows and understands this, then he can recognize that this player needs to feel some success under gamelike kicking conditions in practice in order to feel comfortable when the next drop goal opportunity presents itself. This is a far better approach than dropping the athlete to the bench or sending him to the weight room to work on his leg strength.

HOW WE TREAT OTHERS

25.4

Head coaches can talk all they want about how their staff and players should treat others inside and outside the organization, but if they set a bad example and treat people poorly, it undermines the sentiment. Everyone sees how the coach relates to athletes and assistants in practice, back-office staff in meetings, and fans, family members, and members of the media before and after games. These interactions set the tone for how everyone else behaves, too. If the head coach wants to create an atmosphere of trust and consistency, then she must be careful to act and speak appropriately in each and every situation. Remember, someone is always watching.

THE IMPORTANCE OF EXAMPLE

25.4.1

When his sons Jim and John were young, Jack Harbaugh took them on a recruiting trip to a high school game in Cedar Rapids, Iowa. The guest of honor was legendary sprinter Jesse Owens, who illuminated the falsehood of Hitler's "master race" belief as he won four gold medals at the 1936 Berlin Olympics. The boys came back to their father raving about how nice Owens was and how he patiently signed autographs for what seemed like hours. In turn, Owens complimented Harbaugh for raising two polite, respectful young men. This is why today, as head coaches of the University of Michigan and the Baltimore Ravens, Jim and John are patient with fans and all too eager to sign one autograph after another, just like their boyhood hero. Players can be similarly impacted by a coach who sets a good example in how they treat people every day.

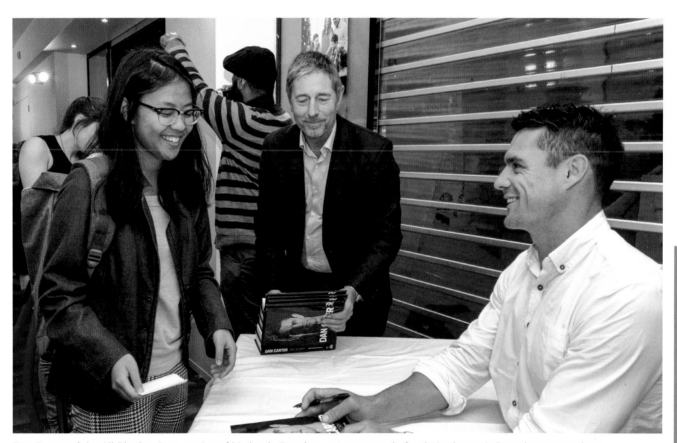

Dan Carter of the All Blacks signs copies of his book. Coaches set an example for their players in how they treat others.
Photo by ChameleonsEye / Shutterstock.com.

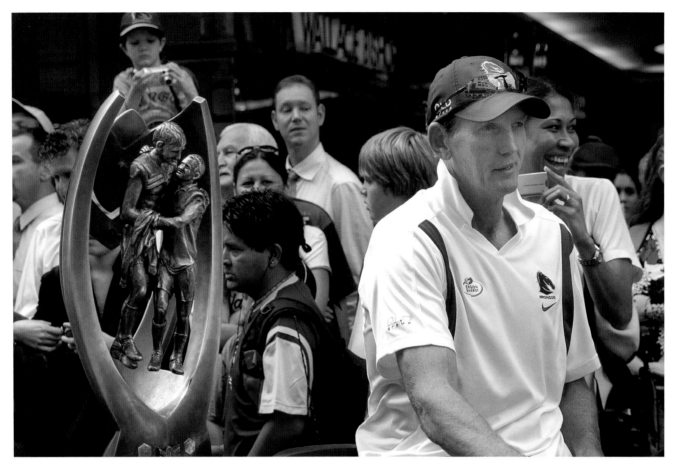

Wayne Bennett, coach of the Brisbane Broncos. His players say he's like a father to him, and he was once named Father of the Year in Australia. Photo by John (CC BY-SA).

BELIEVE THE
BEST OF PEOPLE

25.5

Australian Rugby League coach Wayne Bennett is one of the biggest believers in players' ability to change their character for the good of the team. Shane Webcke, one of Bennett's players who helped the Brisbane Broncos win several of their six league titles, said that his coach's philosophy is, "If you make someone a better person, every aspect of their life improves, including their football." Despite cultivating a prickly image when talking to reporters, Bennett was once named Father of the Year in Australia, and former players like Allan Langer have said he deserves the title because "he is like a father to all the players."[68]

If you believe the best of people, they will sometimes let you down. But the lesson of Wayne Bennett is that you have to give players and staff the benefit of the doubt and, like a doting dad, never give up on a young person whose well-being is in your hands until there's no other alternative. This is especially important when you're just starting a new coaching role with a group you don't really know yet. Avoid the temptation to judge people on first impressions or by reputation; rather, make an effort to discover what they're good at and how you can help them become even better.

1   Will Hobson and Steven Rich, "Playing in the Red," *Washington Post,* November 23, 2015, www.washingtonpost.com/sf/sports/wp/2015/11/23/running-up-the-bills/; "Transfer Window: Premier League Clubs Spend £475m in First Month," BBC.com, August 2, 2016, www.bbc.com/sport/football/36952866; Joe Bernstein, "Wayne Rooney Will Earn Around £73 million on His Current Manchester United Deal While Five Manchester City Players Are Among the 10 Best Paid in the Premier League," *Daily Mail,* September 9, 2015, www.dailymail.co.uk/sport/football/article-3227651/Wayne-Rooney-earn-73million-current-Manchester-United-deal-five-Manchester-City-players-10-best-paid-Premier-League.html; Tony Nitti, "The Real Winner of NBA Free Agency? California," *Forbes,* July 5, 2016, www.forbes.com/sites/anthonynitti/2016/07/05/the-real-winner-of-nba-free-agency-california/#3d4a64935ecc.

2   Rodger Sherman, "The NCAA's New March Madness TV Deal Will Make Them a Billion Dollars a Year," *SB Nation,* April 12, 2016, www.sbnation.com/college-basketball/2016/4/12/11415764/ncaa-tournament-tv-broadcast-rights-money-payout-cbs-turner; Ben Baby, "Report: Big Ten Signs Lucrative TV Deal to Push Revenue Totals Past SEC, Big 12," *Dallas News,* June 20, 2016, sportsday.dallasnews.com/college-sports/collegesports/2016/06/20/report-big-ten-signs-lucrative-tv-deal-ahead-push-revenue-totals-past-sec-big-12; Tony Evans, "Premier League's New TV Deal Will Make It More Competitive Than Ever," ESPN.com, November 23, 2015, www.espnfc.us/english-premier-league/23/blog/post/2724541/premier-league-new-tv-deal-will-usher-in-bold-era.

16 THE SIX LAWS OF WINNING

3   Brandon Sneed, "I'm Not the Lone Wolf," *Bleacher Report,* September 13, 2016, thelab.bleacherreport.com/i-m-not-the-lone-wolf/.

4   Bob Sullivan, "Memo to Work Martyrs: Long Hours Make You Less Productive," CNBC.com, January 26, 2015, www.cnbc.com/2015/01/26/working-more-than-50-hours-makes-you-less-productive.html.

17 THE FOUR MACRO PRINCIPLES OF WINNING TEAMS

5   Quoted in Steven Pressfield, *The Warrior Ethos* (New York: Black Irish Entertainment, 2011), 42.

6   Sebastian Junger, "Why Veterans Miss War," TED Talk, May 2014, www.ted.com/talks/sebastian_junger_why_veterans_miss_war/transcript?language=en.

7   David Walsh, "No Half Measures," *The Sunday Times,* December 12, 2010, www.thetimes.co.uk/article/no-half-measures-lc3tmq732sd.

8   Teddy Mitrosilis, "Emotional LeBron James Pays Tribute to Cleveland: 'This Is for You!'" FoxSports.com, June 19, 2016, www.foxsports.com/nba/story/cleveland-cavaliers-nba-title-lebron-james-honors-city-postgame-interview-061916.

9   Phil Jackson and Hugh Delehanty, *Eleven Rings: The Soul of Success* (New York: Penguin, 2013), 173.

10 "Claudio Ranieri's Best Quotes," *Red Bulletin,* n.d., www.redbulletin.com/int/en/sports/claudio-ranieris-greatest-quotes.

18 LEADERSHIP

11 Gary Smith, "How Allen Iverson and Larry Brown Learned to Live Together," *Sports Illustrated,* May 15, 2015, www.si.com/nba/2015/05/15/allen-iverson-mvp-larry-brown-2001-philadelphia-76ers-vault.

12 Quoted in Greg Bishop, "How a Book on Stoicism Became Wildly Popular at Every Level of the NFL," *Sports Illustrated,* December 8, 2015, www.si.com/nfl/2015/12/08/ryan-holiday-nfl-stoicism-book-pete-carroll-bill-belichick.

13 Jocko Willink and Leif Babin, *Extreme Ownership: How U.S. Navy SEALs Lead and Win* (New York: St. Martin's Press, 2015), 76.

14 Nick Saban, *How Good Do You Want to Be?: A Champion's Tips on How to Lead and Succeed at Work and in Life* (New York: Ballantine, 2007), 133.

15 Stephen Stowell and Stephanie Mead, *The Art of Strategic Leadership: How Leaders at All Levels Prepare Themselves, Their Teams, and Organizations for the Future* (Hoboken, NJ: John Wiley and Sons, 2016), 58.

16 Creed King and Heidi King, *Don't Play for the Tie: Bear Bryant on Life* (Nashville, TN: Rutledge Hill Press, 2006), 91.

17 Chelena Goldman, "Jim Harbaugh and His Golden Quotes," *SF Bay,* September 3, 2012, sfbay.ca/2012/09/03/jim-harbaugh-and-his-golden-quotes/.

18 Anita Elberse, "Ferguson's Formula," *Harvard Business Review,* October 2013, hbr.org/2013/10/fergusons-formula.

19 "Cortés Burns His Boats," Cortés, From Explore to Conquer, *Conquistadors,* PBS.com, www.pbs.org/conquistadors/cortes/cortes_d00.html.

20 Peggy Noonan, *What I Saw at the Revolution: A Political Life in the Reagan Era,* 20th anniversary ed. (New York: Random House, 2003), 218.

21 Kevin Arnovitz, "The Mystery Guest Has Arrived," ESPN.com, June 1, 2011, www.espn.com/nba/truehoop/miamiheat/columns/story?page=Spoelstra-110601.

22 Jack Welch, *Winning: The Ultimate Business How-To Book* (New York: HarperBusiness, 2005), 83-87.

23 Craig Swan, "Brendan Rodgers Makes Sure Celtic Players Put Family First as He Prepares Hoops for Champions League Battle," *Daily Record,* August 17, 2016, www.dailyrecord.co.uk/sport/football/football-news/brendan-rodgers-makes-sure-celtic-8645034.

24 Erik Frenz, "Bill Belichick's Coaching Tree Has Branches Both Lush and Barren," Boston.com, January 3, 2015, www.boston.com/sports/extra-points/2015/01/03/bill_belichicks_coaching_tree_has_branches_both_fu.

19 PREVENTING PROBLEMS

25 Scott Davis, "Warriors GM Keeps a Striking Quote from Gregg Popovich in His Cellphone About How to Build the Perfect Franchise," *Business Insider,* December 11, 2015, www.businessinsider.com/warriors-gm-bob-myers-inspired-by-gregg-popovich-quote-2015-12.

26 Jonathan Wilson, "The Devil's Party (Part 1)," *The Blizzard,* n.d., www.theblizzard.co.uk/articles/the-devils-party/.

27 Drew Brooks, "The Man Who Commanded Delta Force, and a New Breed of War," *Fayetteville (NC) Observer,* July 9, 2016, www.fayobserver.com/55d2dd63-7dea-5563-896c-4a8dc1fcd5d6.html.

28 Joe Lemire, "Chip Kelly's HGH Science Is Bad, Say Scientists," *Vocativ,* September 16, 2016, www.vocativ.com/359807/chip-kellys-hgh-science-is-bad-say-scientists.

29 Walter Isaacson, *Steve Jobs* (New York: Simon and Schuster, 2011): 431.

30 Frederick P. Brooks Jr., *The Mythical Man-Month: Essays on Software Engineering* (Boston: Addison-Wesley, 1975).

20 INNOVATION AND THE NINE MOST-USED WORDS

31 Jim Collins, *Good to Great: Why Some Companies Make the Leap…and Others Don't* (New York: HarperCollins, 2001), 159.

32 Dan Ariely, Facebook post, January 6, 2013, www.facebook.com/dan.ariely/posts/904383595868.

33 Thor Olavsrud, "IDC Says Big Data Spending to Hit $48.6 Billion in 2019," *CIO,* November 11, 2015, www.cio.com/article/3004512/big-data/idc-predicts-big-data-spending-to-reach-48-6-billion-in-2019.html.

34 "Sports Analytics Market Worth $4.7 Billion by 2021" (press release), ReportsnReports, *MarketWatch,* June 25, 2015, www.marketwatch.com/story/sports-analytics-market-worth-47-billion-by-2021-2015-06-25-142032056.

35 James Clear, "This Coach Improved Every Tiny Thing by 1 Percent and Here's What Happened" (blog post), jamesclear.com, n.d., jamesclear.com/marginal-gains.

21 GROUP PSYCHOLOGY

36 Will Greenwood, "How Eddie Jones Has Transformed England," *The Telegraph,* June 27, 2016, www.telegraph.co.uk/rugby-union/2016/06/27/how-eddie-jones-has-transformed-england/.

37 Susan Adams, "Unhappy Employees Outnumber Happy Ones by Two to One Worldwide," Forbes.com, October 10, 2013, www.forbes.com/sites/susanadams/2013/10/10/unhappy-employees-outnumber-happy-ones-by-two-to-one-worldwide/#193603e5362a.

38 Bill Walsh with Steve Jamison and Craig Walsh, *The Score Takes Care of Itself: My Philosophy of Leadership* (New York: Penguin, 2010), 124.

39 Quoted in Brett McKay and Kate McKay, "WWII Workout Week: Posture Training," *The Art of Manliness,* January 17, 2015, www.artofmanliness.com/2015/01/17/wwii-workout-week-posture-training/.

40 Vivian Giang, "The Surprising and Powerful Links Between Posture and Mood," *Fast Company,* January 30, 2015, www.fastcompany.com/3041688/the-surprising-and-powerful-links-between-posture-and-mood.

41 Sarah Stevenson, "There's Magic In Your Smile," PsychologyToday.com, June 25, 2012, www.psychologytoday.com/blog/cutting-edge-leadership/201206/there-s-magic-in-your-smile.

42 M. Sonnby–Borgström, "Automatic Mimicry Reactions as Related to Differences in Emotional Empathy," *Scandinavian Journal of Psychology* 43, no. 5 (December 2002): 433–443.

43 Tom Rath and Donald O. Clifton, "The Power of Praise and Recognition," *Gallup,* July 8, 2004, www.gallup.com/businessjournal/12157/power-praise-recognition.aspx.

44 "Warriors Dream Comes True; Durant Signed to a Contract," *CBS SF Bay Area,* July 7, 2016, sanfrancisco.cbslocal.com/2016/07/07/kevin-durant-inks-deal-with-warriors/.

45 Rui Thomas, "Once a Raider, Always a Raider: No Exceptions," *Golden Gate Sports,* June 27, 2013, goldengatesports.com/2013/06/27/once-a-raider-always-a-raider-no-exceptions/.

46 "An Insignia and a Knife," *Navy Dads,* June 30, 2011, www.navydads.com/forum/topics/an-insignia-and-a-knife.

22 THE CULTURE MODEL

47   Ken Segall, *Insanely Simple: The Obsession That Drives Apple's Success* [New York: Penguin, 2012], 3.

48   Ibid., 14.

49   Steve James, "Revealed: How Stuart Lancaster Transformed England from National Laughing Stock into World Cup Hopefuls," *The Telegraph,* November 1, 2014, www.telegraph.co.uk/sport/rugbyunion/international/england/11196506/Revealed-How-Stuart-Lancaster-transformed-England-from-national-laughing-stock-into-World-Cup-hopefuls.html.

50   "Eddie Jones—Creating Team Culture," *The Rugby Site,* n.d., www.therugbysite.com/blog/leadership-management/coming-soon-eddie-jones-creating-team-culture.

51   Greenwood, "How Eddie Jones Has Transformed England"; Rory Keane, "Eddie Jones Changed the Environment at England When He Arrived … We Had More Fun and a Few Beers, Says Mako Vunipola," *MailOnline,* March 30, 2016, www.dailymail.co.uk/sport/rugbyunion/article-3516066/Eddie-Jones-changed-environment-England-arrived-fun-beers-says-Mako-Vunipola.html.

23 THE ROSTER

52   Bruce Jenkins, "Steve Kerr Was Leader Enough to Stand Up to Jordan in 1995," *SF Gate,* May 17, 2014, www.sfgate.com/sports/jenkins/article/Steve-Kerr-was-leader-enough-to-stand-up-to-5486547.php.

53   Jeremy Hobson, "Michael Phelps' Coach on How to Set Goals—And Achieve Them," *Here & Now,* WBUR.org, May 19, 2016, www.wbur.org/hereandnow/2016/05/19/phelps-coach-book.

54   Jeff Miller, "Usain Bolt Brings Showmanship to Olympics in a Flash," *Orange County Register,* August 14, 2016, www.ocregister.com/2016/08/14/miller-usain-bolt-brings-showmanship-to-olympics-in-a-flash/.

24 MODERN SOCIAL CHALLENGES

55   "Traffic Stops," Bureau of Justice Statistics, www.bjs.gov/index.cfm?ty=tp&tid=702.

56   Charles Duhigg, *The Power of Habit: Why We Do What We Do in Life and Business* [New York: Random House, 2012], 92.

57   Jennifer Kunst, "Why Addictions Are So Hard to Break," PsychologyToday.com, August 15, 2012, www.psychologytoday.com/blog/headshrinkers-guide-the-galaxy/201208/why-addictions-are-so-hard-break.

58   "Drugs, Brains, and Behavior: The Science of Addiction," National Institute of Drug Abuse, July 2014, www.drugabuse.gov/publications/drugs-brains-behavior-science-addiction/preface.

59   Jason King, "Lucas Offers the Gift of a Lifetime," ESPN.com, December 18, 2012, www.espn.com/mens-college-basketball/story/_/id/8757777/john-lucas-offers-gift-lifetime-college-basketball.

60   Sharon K. Stoll and Jennifer M. Beller, "Do Sports Build Character?," in *Sports in School: The Future of an Institution,* ed. John R. Gerdy [New York: Teachers College Press, 2000], 18–31; Angela Lumpkin, Sharon Kay Stoll, and Jennifer M. Beller, *Sport Ethics: Applications for Fair Play,* 3rd ed. [New York: McGraw-Hill Education, 2002].

61   Quoted by David Brunner, "Creating a Culture of Values That Will Promote Sustained Excellence in Competitive Football," PhD diss., University of Idaho, 2009.

62   Elberse, "Ferguson's Formula."

63   "Coach K: I Learned to 'Ignore' from Chuck Daly" [video], ESPN.com, August 11, 2016, www.espn.com/video/clip?id=17249858.

25 YOU WIN WITH PEOPLE

64   Robert J. Samuelson, "It's Still the Economy, Stupid," *Washington Post,* February 3, 2016, www.washingtonpost.com/opinions/its-still-the-economy-stupid/2016/02/03/b47fc5b8-caa0-11e5-ae11-57b6aeab993f_story.html.

65   Mike Hill, "Spielberg's Subtext" [video], MikeHill.Design, May 9, 2016, www.mikehill.design/spielberg-subtext.

66   Neil Strauss, *The Game: Penetrating the Secret Society of Pickup Artists* [New York: ReganBooks, 2005], 64.

67   Robert Dilts, "What Is NLP?," NLP University, n.d., www.nlpu.com/NewDesign/NLPU_WhatIsNLP.html.

68   Wayne Smith, "Wayne Bennett—Maker of Men," *The Australian,* February 25, 2012, www.theaustralian.com.au/sport/wayne-bennett-maker-of-men/news-story/3cb044b98b3f1cca7b33dd90a97cc786.

THE 12 TAKEAWAYS

I'm not vain enough to believe that everything I've written is so scintillating that you'll recall every word, or that every law, rule, or principle will apply to you. So if you were to remember only a few key things from this entire book, these are the points I'd like you to take away:

1. The game itself is the only true test of player and team performance, and it's also a measuring stick for the game plan. So center everything on the game, then work backward from it when planning preparation.

2. An athlete is a person first and a player second. The coaching staff has a duty to help each member of the squad maintain optimal health, which not only underpins players' continued development and sustainable team excellence but also allows them to live long, productive lives.

3. It's a mistake to look at the game only through a physical lens. The technical, tactical, and psychological coactives are just as important. Again, the game is where we assess how dominant qualities and limiting factors in each area manifest themselves and should inform what a player needs to work on during preparation sessions for future contests.

4. Periodization is dead. A far better way to plan team training is to use a performance model that focuses on tactical, technical, physical, and psychological qualities simultaneously. These are balanced with volume, intensity, density, and contact/collision in a morphological programming approach that introduces sufficient stimuli to prompt adaptation yet ensures that every player is fresh for the next game.

5. Coaches should not instruct or dictate but rather facilitate rich learning experiences in which players can discover how to find the best possible outcomes. Repeating such guided discovery opportunities will reinforce positive habits and give players the freedom to problem-solve during games.

6. The game plan must be simple, clear, and cohesive. In addition to the Commander's Intent—win!—each player should be given a maximum of three directives for each game.

7. Tactics vary from game to game based on the preferences and strengths of the opponent, but principles and strategy remain the same. Successful execution depends on your team's ability to execute faster and better in each subsequent game so that the opposition can't stop you—even if they know what you're planning to do.

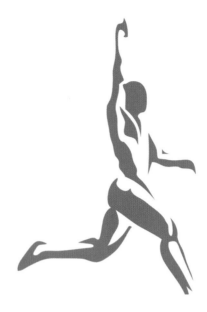

8. The biggest challenge for an athlete is managing and adapting to stress, which can be physical, psychological, cognitive, and/or spiritual. The head coach's job is to ensure that the cumulative load of preparation and games is never too great. Such load balancing will reduce the risk of injury and burnout.

9. Winning is extremely important, but it's not confined to the game. A sustainably successful organization practices top-to-bottom excellence daily and is committed to a set of shared values and beliefs that inform every action.

10. You cannot build a truly dominant team without first hiring an excellent head coach. Leadership is the key factor in the success of every organization. Such leaders don't need to surround themselves with the "best" people; rather, they seek out the *right* people, who can come together to create a culture of excellence.

11. With big budgets often come large back-office teams. But even at an elite organization, it's better to maintain a small, tight-knit group of people who are fully committed to each other and communicate well.

12. Fancy facilities, endless statistical reports, and the latest technology will *not* deliver more wins. Quantitative analysis is useless without qualitative assessment using the four-coactive model, while new technologies must be applied purposefully and one at a time to measure their effectiveness. Facilities just need to be good enough, not perfect.

GLOSSARY

Aerobic: The aerobic part of the energy substrate system provides sustainable output using oxygen.

Alactic: The alactic part of the energy substrate system can generate huge amounts of power using ATP (adenosine triphosphate).

Allostasis: The process that achieves homeostasis over time by recruiting various systems and mechanisms to respond to stimuli, take the necessary steps to produce adaptation, and then return to a "normal" baseline.

Anaerobic: The anaerobic part of the energy substrate system provides short bursts of energy without using oxygen.

Chaoplexity: A term that brings together the theory of complexity and chaos theory. A key principle of chaoplexity is that complex dynamic patterns are underpinned by an unexpected simplicity.

Chaos theory: A model for understanding nonlinear, unpredictable systems, such as the weather, the stock market, and team-sports games.

Coactive: One of the four interrelated, complementary elements of player performance present in every event in games and during team preparation: tactical, technical, psychological, and physical.

Coherence: In sports, the idea that all principles and methods must complement one another and not conflict.

Cohesion: The working together of all players on the field toward a common goal, aligned with the game plan.

Collision/contact: The amount of vibrational force the athletes absorb. All sports have some amount of collision/contact, but it's more pronounced in contact sports such as rugby and football.

Commander's Intent: The overarching aim of any team: to win.

Concentric: Muscle shortening.

Density: How many breaks there are within a training session or game.

Eccentric: Muscle lengthening.

Epigenetics: Biological changes that occur in gene function as a result of exposure to a certain environment.

Fitness-fatigue model: A theory of sports training that holds that the key to designing any training program is to maximize the fitness benefit while giving the body enough time to overcome resulting fatigue so that fitness isn't diminished.

Fog of the game: The confusion that occurs in the middle of a game when there are multiple players acting at the same time, creating an enormous amount of information in a very short amount of time. The fog of the game often makes it difficult for players to remember exactly what happened afterward.

Fractal: A figure in which a close-up detail resembles the figure as a whole.

Frictions of the game: Events resulting from the random, chaotic nature of team sports and military conflict.

Functional reserve: The remaining capacity of an organism or organ to fulfill its physiological activity; in a sports context, stress and the energy needed to manage stress and fatigue drain functional reserve.

Game model: A team's overall system of play, based on the team's philosophy of its sport.

Game moment: One of the four primary ways that any moment in a game can be described from the perspective of the players: offensive, defensive, transition-to-offense, or transition-to-defense.

Game plan: The plan that guides players' decisions and actions during a game.

General adaptation syndrome: Austrian endocrinologist Hans Selye's theory of the body's neurobiological response to stress, which consists of three stages: alarm, resistance, and exhaustion.

Homeostasis: The sustainable status quo of the human body.

Intensity: How rigorous and demanding a training session or game is.

Morphocycle: The structure and format of a preparation cycle between two games.

Morphological programming: A preparation approach that calls for the morphocycle to be balanced among learning experiences that stress volume, intensity, density, and collision/contact.

OODA Loop: The decision-making cycle described by American fighter pilot John Boyd. It consists of four steps: observe, orient, decide, act. Also known as the "observation-action cycle."

Periodization: The training model developed by Russian sports scientist Leonid Matveyev that focuses on introducing timed doses of physical stimulation to produce a desired effect, such as increased strength, power, speed, or endurance. Periodization uses sequential programming that varies the intensity, density, and volume of certain types of training in order to allow an athlete to peak at a certain time.

Matveyev and other Russian and Eastern European periodization pioneers initially designed their systems with individual athletes and Olympic medals in mind.

Physical coactive: A player's physical traits. There are three main components of physical execution: biomechanics, bioenergetics, and biodynamics.

Plyometrics: Exercises that rapidly stretch and contract muscles.

Programming: A training approach specifically for team sports that is based on the immediate status of the athlete, with consideration to the overall plan for the next game. Compared to periodization, it's much more flexible and responsive and can determine strategies of action much faster. Programming involves not only exploiting adaptation principles but also taking into account how individual athletes respond psychophysiologically to the cumulative effects of training.

Psychological coactive: A player's ability to mentally and emotionally manage the elements of play and competition. This dimension includes three micro coactives: spiritual, emotional, and cognitive.

Reductionism: The principle of Western science that divides a subject into the largest possible number of sections and focuses on each individually. In sports, it refers to preparing athletes by focusing on individual elements rather than the player as a whole.

Schwerpunkt: A German term meaning "organizational focus" and originally a German military idea that helped direct military strategy toward singular aims without preventing ground troops from taking the initiative. In sports, it refers to players and groups of players acting in sequence and harmony with each other toward a common tactical goal.

Small-sided games / scrimmage: Learning experiences with less than the full complement of players that echo real-world game scenarios.

Tactical coactive: A player's ability to employ tactical decision-making during play. Tactical competencies include ball circulation, player movement, positioning, and the sequencing of all three.

Tactical periodization: A training approach designed for team sports that first established the four game moments and the elements of the four-coactive model.

Technical coactive: A player's ability to employ sport-related skills, such as passing, throwing, kicking, etc.

Tempo: A team's ability to change pace and alter the speed of ball and player movement; it's not speed itself but rather the gearing that enables a team to choose and move between different speeds.

Tiki-taka: A style of play in soccer in which the only thing that seems to move when a team has possession is the ball.

Vertical integration: Originally a business term referring to the process whereby a company combines two or more stages of production, in sports this refers to the training method developed by sprint coach Charlie Francis that sequences high-intensity and low-intensity sessions to allow athletes to recover more quickly.

Volume: The amount of work done in a training session or game.

DETAILED CONTENTS

PART 3: THE PREPARATION

PART 4: THE COACH

INDEX